W9-BEH-126

Health Psychology

AN INTRODUCTION TO BEHAVIOR AND HEALTH

FOURTH EDITION

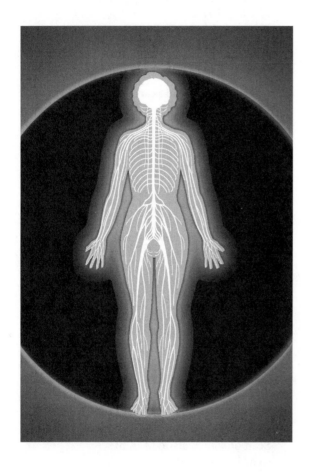

Linda Brannon

McNeese State University

Jess Feist

McNeese State University

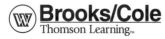
Brooks/Cole
Thomson Learning™

Australia • Canada • Denmark • Japan • Mexico • New Zealand • Philippines
Puerto Rico • Singapore • South Africa • Spain • United Kingdom • United States

Psychology Editor: Marianne Taflinger
Assistant Editor: Jennifer Wilkinson
Editorial Assistants: Rachael Bruckman, Suzanne Wood
Marketing Manager: Jenna Opp
Print Buyer: Karen Hunt
Permissions Editor: Susan Walters
Production: Matrix Productions Inc.

Text and Cover Designer: Lisa Mirski Devenish
Copyeditor: Bonnie Allen
Illustrators: John & Judy Waller, ColorType
Cover Image: John & Judy Waller
Compositor: ColorType/San Diego
Printer: R.R. Donnelley & Sons, Crawfordsville
Signing Representative: Ragu Raghaven

COPYRIGHT © 2000 by Wadsworth,
a division of Thomson Learning

Brooks/Cole Counseling is an imprint of
Wadsworth

All rights reserved. No part of this work
covered by the copyright hereon may be
reproduced or used in any form or by
any means—graphic, electronic, or
mechanical, including photocopying,
recording, taping, or information storage
and retrieval systems—without the written
permission of the publisher.

Printed in the United States of America

1 2 3 4 5 6 03 02 01 00 99

For permission to use material from this
text, contact us by
   web: www.thomsonrights.com
   fax: 1-800-730-2215
   phone: 1-800-730-2214

Wadsworth/Thomson Learning
10 Davis Drive
Belmont, CA 94002-3098
USA
www.wadsworth.com

International Headquarters
Thomson Learning
290 Harbor Drive, 2nd Floor
Stamford, CT 06902-7477
USA

UK/Europe/Middle East
Thomson Learning
Berkshire House
168-173 High Holborn
London WC1V 7AA
United Kingdom

Asia
Thomson Learning
60 Albert Street #15-01
Albert Complex
Singapore 189969

Canada
Nelson/Thomson Learning
1120 Birchmount Road
Scarborough, Ontario M1K 5G4
Canada

Library of Congress Cataloging-in-Publication Data

Brannon, Linda, (date t/k)
  Health psychology/Linda Brannon, Jess Feist—4th ed.
     p. cm.
  Includes bibliographical references and index.
  ISBN 0-534-36850-6
    1. Medicine and psychology, 2. Sick—Psychology. 3. Health behavior. I. Feist, Jess. II. Title.
  R726.5.B72 1999
  616'.001'9—dc21   99-25890

 This book is printed on acid-free recycled paper.

BRIEF CONTENTS

CONTENTS

Part 2 Stress, Pain, and Coping

Part 3 Behavior and Chronic Disease

Part 4 Behavioral Health

Part 5 Looking Toward the Future

PREFACE

As we enter the 21st century, we can look back on the last 100 years as a time of unprecedented change. A person whose life spans the entire 20th century would have seen greater changes in agriculture, manufacturing, transportation, and communication than a person born at any other time in human history. Concurrent with these vast developments has been a major shift in the areas of disease and health.

At the beginning of the 20th century, most serious diseases were caused by contact with viruses and bacteria. People had little individual responsibility for preventing diseases because these microorganisms were nearly impossible to avoid. Today, most serious diseases and disorders occur as the result of individual behaviors—or failures to behave. As health and disease become more closely linked to behavior, psychology—the science of behavior—became involved in many health-related issues. This involvement led to the birth and development of *health psychology,* the scientific study of behaviors that relate to health enhancement, disease prevention, safety, and rehabilitation.

At about the same time, two other disciplines began to emerge—behavioral medicine and behavioral health. *Behavioral medicine,* an interdisciplinary field oriented toward treatment, has grown rapidly as a result of the recognition that behavior is an important and controllable contributor to illness. *Behavioral health* includes the wide variety of research and interventions that explore ways to keep healthy people from becoming sick.

The field of health psychology has continued to grow and progress since the publication of the first three editions of *Health Psychology: An Introduction to Behavior and Health.* The first edition of the book, for example, contained a rationale for the existence of a textbook for health psychology at the undergraduate level, but now no such rationale is necessary: Undergraduate health psychology courses have appeared at many universities, colleges, and community colleges. The field is no longer fighting for acceptance as a teaching area in undergraduate curricula.

Our purpose in writing a fourth edition of *Health Psychology: An Introduction to Behavior and Health* was to reflect changes in the field of health psychology, to update the material in the book by including more of the crucial research on behavior and health, and to give students a balanced view of health psychology—one that includes both behavioral medicine and behavioral health.

The Fourth Edition

We have organized the fourth edition of *Health Psychology: An Introduction to Behavior and Health* into five parts. Part 1, which includes the first four chapters, lays a solid foundation for understanding subsequent chapters; Part 2 deals with stress, pain, and coping; Part 3 discusses heart disease, cancer, and other chronic diseases; Part 4 includes chapters on safety, tobacco, alcohol, diet, and physical activity; and Part 5 looks toward future challenges in health psychology.

More specifically, Chapter 1 introduces the field of health psychology and stresses the need for psychology's involvement in health. Chapter 2 compares research methodology in psychology and epidemiology, a comparison that allows students to appreciate and understand the research presented in later chapters. Chapter 3 presents information on seeking health care and includes a critique of several theories that attempt to explain why people seek health care. In addition, this chapter includes a review of factors involved in seeking medical care and being hospitalized. Chapter 4 reviews participants' compliance with medical advice, presenting not only research evidence but also theories that are relevant to adherence.

After these foundation chapters, students are ready for Part 2, which includes topics within behavioral medicine and begins with two chapters on stress. Chapter 5 covers the theories, sources, and measurement of stress. Chapter 6 examines the relationship between stress and disease. Chapter 7 discusses the topic of pain, including the physiology of the somatosensory system, pain syndromes, theories, and measurement. Because of the similarities in their techniques, stress management and pain management both appear in Chapter 8 along with an extensive evaluation of the effectiveness of each technique.

Part 3 deals with chronic disease, beginning with cardiovascular disease in Chapter 9. This chapter identifies factors involved in cardiovascular disease and updates the extensive research on this topic. Chapter 10 reviews behavioral factors in cancer and notes a recent downturn in cancer deaths in the United States. Chapter 11 focuses on problems of living with chronic disease, problems experienced both by the person with the disease and by family members. These diseases include cardiovascular disease, cancer, diabetes, HIV/AIDS, and Alzheimer's disease.

Chapters 12 through 16 comprise Part 4 and examine the health consequences of unsafe behaviors, smoking, drinking and drug use, eating and weight control, and exercising. All these chapters contain updated information about these health-related behaviors.

Part 5 consists of Chapter 17, which offers predictions about the role of health psychology in the future with respect to health goals for the United States during the first 20 years of the 21st century.

New Features

Readers of earlier editions of *Health Psychology: An Introduction to Behavior and Health* will notice a new look to the present edition. We have added several features to the fourth edition—features that stimulate critical thinking and facilitate learning. These new features include chapter-opening questions, a "Check Your Health Risks" box, and a "Becoming Healthier" box. The purpose of these additions is to actively engage readers in the process of acquiring health-related information to enhance their personal well-being.

Questions and Answers

Each chapter begins with a series of *Questions* designed to organize the chapter, preview the material, and enhance active learning. As each chapter unfolds, answers to these questions are revealed through a discussion of relevant research findings. At the end of each major topic, an *In Summary* statement offers a succinct summary of that topic. Then, at the end of the chapter, *Answers* to the chapter-opening questions appear. This *preview, read, and review* method facilitates learning and improves recall.

Check Your Health Risks

Near the beginning of most chapters is a "Check Your Health Risks" box that personalizes material in that chapter. This box consists of several health-related behaviors or attitudes that readers should check before looking at the rest of the chapter. After checking the items that apply to them and then becoming familiar with the chapter's material, readers can ascertain their current level of risks for injury, disease, or disability.

Becoming Healthier

Embedded in most chapters is a "Becoming Healthier" box with advice on how to acquire a healthier lifestyle. Although some of this advice may not seem to agree with some people's existing notion of a healthy lifestyle, all of it is based on the most current available research data. We believe that if you follow these guidelines, you will increase your chances of a long and healthy life.

Online Suggested Readings

Another new feature to this edition is the inclusion of suggested readings that are available from **InfoTrac® College Edition.** At least one such suggested reading appears at the end of each chapter along with three or four other suggested readings. These readings have been carefully chosen for their recency, their readability, and their importance to the chapter subject. They will direct students to further study.

The online suggested readings are available as a bonus to students who purchase *Health Psychology: An Introduction to Behavior and Health,* fourth edition, published by Wadsworth Publishing Company. Each of these online suggested readings, available from InfoTrac College Edition, is marked with a special symbol. This service is an easy way for students to successfully negotiate the Internet. To access the full text of the article, enter http://www.infotrac-college.com/ wadsworth as the address. The screen that appears will have a box to enter a password that adopters and students receive. Once you enter a valid password, you can find not only the marked article, but also the full text for thousands of other publications from over 600 popular and technical publications. In addition, InfoTrac College Edition offers full search capabilities through topic or keyword searches and a linking function that allows users to find related publications. This innovative service can introduce students to the Internet or allow experienced users to hone their search skills.

Other New Features

In addition to these four innovations, the fourth edition of *Health Psychology* contains several other new features that we believe make it an even stronger book than its three predecessors. First, we have added nearly 500 recent references, updating existing topics and adding new ones. Second, we have presented the chapters in a somewhat different order, adding chapters on seeking health care and adherence to the introductory chapter and the research chapter and creating a unified foundation for *Health Psychology*. This reorganization provides a firm basis for understanding the subsequent chapters on stress, pain, and coping, as well as for understanding the remaining chapters that deal with chronic disease and behavioral health.

Third, we have added a new chapter on preventing injuries (Chapter 12). The prevention of both unintentional and intentional injuries is rapidly becoming a crucial topic in health psychology. Although injury prevention receives little or no attention in many textbooks on health psychology, we believe that it is an important issue for health psychologists. Unintentional injuries (previously known as accidents) are the fourth leading cause of death in the United States and the leading cause of death for young people. Intentional injuries (homicide and suicide) are each ranked among the top 13 causes of death in the United States and are the second and third leading cause of death for young people age 15 to 24. Fourth, we have updated all tables and figures to reflect the constantly changing patterns of death and disease. For example, Table 15.4 shows the relationship between obesity and disease or death. In addition to updating nearly all the tables, we have added three new ones, and we have added 12 new figures. For example, Figure 16.2 records some of the physical and psychological benefits of exercise, and Figure 17.5 compares health care expenditures in Canada, Germany, Great Britain, and the United States.

Familiar Features

Readers of earlier editions of *Health Psychology: An Introduction to Behavior and Health* will recognize several familiar features in the fourth edition. First, we continue to take a biopsychosocial approach to health psychology, examining issues and data from a biological, psychological, and social viewpoint. Second, we continue to recognize and emphasize issues of gender and ethnic factors whenever appropriate. Third, we retain our emphasis on theories and models that may both explain and predict health-related behaviors.

Fourth, we have kept the popular "Would You Believe . . .?" boxes, retaining some of the previous ones and adding new ones. These boxes, which appear in nearly every chapter, all begin with the question "Would You Believe . . . ?" and then highlight a particularly intriguing finding in health psychology. These boxes are designed to explode some preconceived notions and to challenge students to take an objective look at issues that previously they may have seen from a nonscientific viewpoint.

Writing Style

While including much new content in this book, we have streamlined most of the material by introducing a more concise writing style, removing outdated information, and eliminating redundant references. Although the fourth edition of *Health Psychology: An Introduction to Behavior and Health* frequently explores complex issues and difficult topics, we use clear, concise, and comprehensible language as well as an informal writing style. The book is designed for upper-division undergraduate students and should be easily understood by those with a minimal background in psychology and biology. Health psychology courses typically draw students from a variety of college majors, necessitating the inclusion of some elementary material that may be repetitive to some students. For other students, this material will fill in the background they need to comprehend the material unique to health psychology.

Technical terms appear in **boldface type**, and a definition usually appears at that point in the text. These terms also appear in the glossary at the end of each chapter.

Instructional Aids

Besides chapter glossaries, we have supplied several other features to help both students and instructors. These include annotated suggested readings, case studies, and frequent summaries within each chapter.

Case Studies

We begin every chapter except the final one with a case study. Some of these case studies are new to the fourth edition, and others have appeared in the previous editions; all illustrate the topics for each chapter. The cases are never perfect examples, and we have often been asked why we included specific features or behavior in a certain case. The case studies fail to be perfect examples because they are about real people. We have never invented any specific characteristics for these people but have chosen real cases we believe will help students relate the chapter's scientific information to real people. Each case matches research findings only imperfectly, but we hope this imperfection will illustrate to students that real people do not fit the statistical profiles in every way.

We would like to thank the people who shared their stories with us so that we could write these case studies. We have changed some details of their lives to protect their privacy, but we have preserved those details of their cases that relate to their health and behavior.

Within Chapter Summaries

Rather than waiting until the end of each chapter to present a lengthy chapter summary, we have placed shorter summaries at key points within each chapter. In general, these summaries correspond to each major topic in a chapter. We believe these shorter, more frequent summaries will keep readers on track and promote a greater understanding of the chapter's content.

Study Guide

We have authored the study guide for the fourth edition of *Health Psychology: An Introduction to Behavior and Health* because we feel that a study guide written by the textbook's authors provides students with a more accurate and meaningful account of the contents of the text. Like the textbook, the study guide is divided into 17 chapters. Each chapter of the study guide begins with a challenge to students to "Fill in the Rest of the Story," a feature that should facilitate learning through active participation. In addition, the study guide contains a variety of *test questions* and a "Let's Get Personal" feature that allows students to integrate health information into their personal lives. We believe these features will help students organize their study methods and will also enhance their chances of achieving their best scores on class quizzes.

Instructor's Manual

This edition of *Health Psychology: An Introduction to Behavior and Health* is accompanied by a comprehensive instructor's manual. Each chapter begins with a lecture outline designed to assist instructors in preparing lecture material from the text. Many instructors will be able to lecture strictly from these notes; others will be able to use the lecture outline as a framework for organizing their own lecture notes.

A test bank of nearly 1,200 multiple-choice test items makes up a large section of each chapter of the instructor's manual. Some of these items are factual, some are conceptual, and others ask students to apply what they have learned. These test items were written by the authors and will reduce the instructor's work in preparing tests. Each item, of course, is marked with the correct answer.

Essay questions are included for each chapter, along with an outline answer of the critical points that should appear in answers to these questions.

Also included for each chapter are suggested activities. These activities vary widely—from video recommendations to student research to classroom debates. We have tried to include more activities than any instructor can feasibly assign during a semester so as to give instructors a choice of activities.

The growing availability of electronic resources prompted us to include a Surf the Net activity. In this section, we suggest online activities, including websites that are relevant to each chapter. This activity supplements Wadsworth's InfoTrac College Edition, expanding the electronic resources students may use to explore health-related topics.

Acknowledgments

Many people have contributed to the completion of this book, and we wish to express our gratitude. First, we thank Patrick Moreno, who has acted as adviser, librarian, reviewer, and proofreader. His untiring efforts to make the book better have made the book better.

Next we acknowledge the considerable assistance of all the staff at the McNeese library, whose help has been essential for the completion of this project. Joanne Durand, Leslye Quinn, and Brantley Cagle have been especially helpful—each has exhibited outstanding skill and constant good humor in acquiring material for our use. We also thank Imogene Park, Medical Librarian at St. Patrick Hospital in Lake Charles, Louisiana, for her help.

In addition, we would like to thank the people at Wadsworth for their assistance. Marianne Taflinger supervised this edition, and we are grateful for her interest and assistance. We are also indebted to a number of reviewers who read all or parts of the manuscript for this and earlier editions. We are grateful for the valuable comments of the following reviewers:

Richard Contrada, Rutgers, The State University of New Jersey

Michael Felts, East Carolina University

Arthur Gonchar, University of La Verne

David Hines, Ball State University

Kristi Lane, Winona State University

Richard Lazarus, University of California, Berkeley

Ralph Paffenbarger, Jr., Stanford School of Medicine

David Mostofsky, Boston University

Paul B. Paulus, University of Texas, Arlington

Raymond Zurawski, St. Norbert College

Authors typically thank their spouses for being understanding, supportive, and sacrificing. We thank our spouses, Barry Humphus and Mary Jo Feist, because they were understanding, supportive, and sacrificing. But they have given much more than the traditional emotional support. Both have made contributions that have helped to shape the book. In addition to his creative contributions to the book, Barry provided generous, patient, live-in, expert computer consultation that proved essential in the preparation of the manuscript, and Mary Jo has made suggestions on style and content.

CHAPTER 1

Introducing Health Psychology

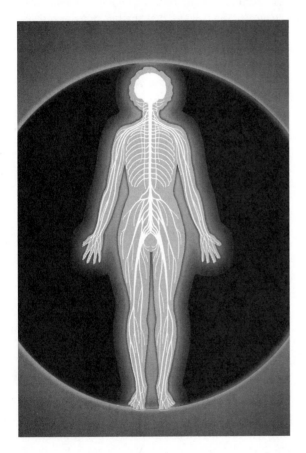

QUESTIONS

This chapter focuses on two basic questions:

1. How have views of health changed?

2. What is psychology's involvement in health?

DWAYNE AND ROBYN: TWO ATTITUDES TOWARD HEALTH

Dwayne, a 21-year-old college junior, seldom thinks about his health—either his present or his future health. In fact, Dwayne seems to believe that he is invincible. He sees his present lack of illness as a sign of good health and assumes that he will always be free of disease and disability.

Perhaps Dwayne should be more concerned, because many of his present habits may have some effect on his future health. Probably his most damaging health practice is his diet, which consists mostly of fast-food hamburgers, with an occasional fried fish sandwich for variety. However, variety is a very low priority for Dwayne, who eats three meals a day, six days a week at the same fast-food restaurant. For breakfast he almost always eats a biscuit, scrambled eggs, sausage, and a soft drink (because he doesn't like coffee). Lunch invariably consists of french fries, a hamburger, and another soft drink. Dwayne's evening meal is usually a repeat of lunch, except that occasionally he will have a fried fish sandwich in place of the hamburger. In addition to these meals, he eats lots of sweets between meals; he is especially fond of ice cream, candy bars, and doughnuts.

Dwayne's diet is not his only health risk. He seldom exercises, never uses his car seatbelts, and has few close friends. Also, he tends to believe that his future health is beyond his personal control. He believes that heart disease, cancer, and accidents are matters of genetics, chance, or fate rather than his behavior. Thus, he has thought little about ways of enhancing his future health or decreasing his chances of developing disease or avoiding premature death. When he gets sick, he adopts a passive attitude toward his own treatment, hoping that the over-the-counter medication he takes will help him feel better.

On the other hand, Dwayne does some things right. He does not smoke cigarettes or drink alcohol, and he reports very little stress in his life. When he filled out the popular Social Readjustment Rating Scale (Holmes & Rahe, 1967; see Chapter 5 for a discussion of this scale), he reported only one stressful life event—Christmas. Although Dwayne does not smoke, his reasons for refraining have nothing to do with health. When he smoked a cigarette as a young adolescent, he became sick and lost any motivation to try again. He avoids alcohol for religious reasons and not because he thinks it is harmful to his health.

Robyn is also a 21-year-old college junior, but her attitude toward health is quite different from Dwayne's. She believes that she has primary responsibility for her own health, and she has adopted a lifestyle that she believes will keep her healthy. Like Dwayne, she does not smoke. She tried to take a puff from a cigarette when she was in the fourth grade but, after coughing for a while, she decided that smoking wasn't for her. She never tried again. Her father is a smoker, but several years ago she and her mother convinced him not to smoke in their house. Robyn is acutely aware of the potential dangers of passive smoking, and when possible, she avoids all enclosed places where people are allowed to smoke. She has confidence that she will never smoke, and she believes that smoking contributes to both heart disease and cancer. Unlike Dwayne, Robyn drinks in moderation. Her parents are also moderate drinkers, and Robyn has lived all her life with a variety of alcoholic beverages in her home. She feels confident that her drinking will not escalate and has no fear of becoming a problem drinker.

Robyn's diet is quite different from Dwayne's. She seldom eats eggs, whole milk products, beef, or pork; she concentrates on eating lots of fruits and vegetables. She occasionally allows herself a dessert, such as a small piece of cake, pie, or pudding. In selecting her meals, she chooses food that is low in fat, calories, sodium, and cholesterol. Her grandfather died of heart disease at 63, and Robyn is convinced that his smoking and high-fat, high-cholesterol diet hastened his death.

Robyn has also begun a regular exercise routine. She is currently enrolled in an aerobic dancing class that meets three times a week. On three of the other days she walks briskly for 30 minutes a day. When not enrolled in an aerobics class, she walks six days a week. She seldom allows weather, class work, job, or social engagements to interfere with exercising.

Unlike Dwayne, who thinks that disease is caused by agents beyond his control, Robyn believes that disease results from a combination of biological, psychological, and social causes and that a person has considerable control over those psychological and social forces. This book examines these psychological and social factors as they apply to health and disease.

The Changing Field of Health

At the beginning of the 20th century, most people in the United States had views of disease and health similar to Dwayne's. People's diseases were largely the result of contact with impure drinking water, contaminated foods, or sick people. Once they were ill, people were expected to seek medical care to be cured, but medicine had few cures to offer. The duration of most diseases—such as typhoid fever, pneumonia, and diphtheria—was relatively short; a person either died or got well in a matter of weeks. People felt very limited responsibility for contracting a disease because they believed it was impossible to avoid contagious disease. At that time, Dwayne's view of disease would have been with the majority. But as we enter the 21st century, such a view is becoming obsolete.

During the 20th century, health in the United States changed in several important ways. First, the leading causes of death have changed from infectious diseases to those that relate to unhealthy behavior and lifestyle. Second, the escalating cost of medical care has spotlighted the importance of educating people about how health-related practices can lower their risk of becoming ill. Third, a new definition of health has emerged, so that health is now seen as the presence of positive well-being, not merely the absence of disease. Fourth, some people in the health care field have advocated a broader perspective of health and disease, questioning the usefulness of the traditional biomedical model.

Patterns of Disease and Death

Today the major health problems in the United States no longer come from infectious diseases but from **chronic diseases** that develop, persist, or

---

 ### CHECK YOUR HEALTH RISKS

Check the items that apply to you.

☐ 1. I believe that if I feel well, I must be healthy.

☑ 2. My weight is not within the range that the charts say it should be.

☑ 3. I smoke cigarettes.

☐ 4. My drinking would not qualify as moderate—I either do not drink, or I drink too much to be considered a moderate drinker.

☐ 5. I rarely get 7 or 8 hours of sleep.

☑ 6. I do not follow a regular exercise program.

☐ 7. I believe that most diseases have a genetic basis.

☐ 8. I believe that modern medicine will find cures for most diseases before I am old enough to be affected by these diseases.

☐ 9. As long as I am not overweight, I believe that my diet will not affect my health.

☐ 10. I can wait until I am older to adopt a healthier lifestyle.

Each of these items represents a behavior or attitude that increases the risk for illness or premature death. As you read this book, you will learn how these (and other) behaviors and attitudes relate to health.

Table 1.1   The 10 leading causes of death in the United States, 1900 and 1997 (rates per 100,000 population)

1900	Rate	1997	Rate
1. Cardiovascular diseases (heart disease, stroke)	345	1. Cardiovascular diseases (heart disease, stroke)	331
2. Influenza and pneumonia	202	2. Cancer	201
3. Tuberculosis	194	3. Chronic obstructive pulmonary diseases	41
4. Gastritis, duodenitis, enteritis, and colitis	143	4. Accidents (unintentional injuries)	34
5. Accidents (unintentional injuries)	72	5. Influenza and pneumonia	33
6. Cancer	64	6. Diabetes	23
7. Diphtheria	40	7. Suicide	11
8. Typhoid fever	31	8. Kidney disease	10
9. Measles	13	9. Chronic liver diseases and cirrhosis	9.3
10. Chronic liver diseases and cirrhosis		10. Septicemia (blood infection)	8.4
		Alzheimer's disease	8.4

Source: Figures for 1900 from *Historical Statistics of the United States: Colonial Times to 1970,* Pt. 1, by U.S. Bureau of the Census, 1975, Washington, DC: U.S. Government Printing Office. Figures for 1997 from *National Vital Statistics Report,* vol. 47, No. 4 (p. 7), by S. J. Ventura, R. N. Anderson, J. A. Martin, and B. L. Smith, 1998. Births and Deaths: Preliminary Data for 1997.

recur over a long period of time. Chronic disorders include heart disease, cancer, chronic obstructive pulmonary disease, and stroke—the four major causes of death in the United States. These diseases are not new, of course, but the proportion of people who die of them has changed dramatically since 1900. Table 1.1 reveals important differences in the leading causes of death in the United States as recorded in 1900 and 1997. Although cardiovascular diseases (including both heart disease and stroke) head both lists, there are few other similarities. In 1900 the majority of deaths were from diseases that were rooted in public or community health problems, such as influenza, pneumonia, tuberculosis, diphtheria, and typhoid fever. Throughout the last half of the 20th century, most deaths were attributable to diseases associated with individual behavior and lifestyle. Cardiovascular disease (including stroke), cancer, chronic obstructive pulmonary disease (including emphysema and chronic bronchitis),

unintentional injuries, diabetes, suicide, and cirrhosis of the liver have been linked to cigarette smoking, alcohol abuse, unwise eating, stress, and sedentary lifestyle. In addition, some current cases of infectious and parasitic diseases are linked to human immunodeficiency virus (HIV) infection, which is largely the result of unsafe behaviors.

According to one estimate (McGinnis & Foege, 1993), about half the deaths in the United States in 1990—more than one million deaths—had preventable causes. In this calculation, tobacco accounted for about 400,000 deaths, or 19% of all deaths. In addition, diet and physical inactivity were responsible for about 300,000 deaths (14%), and alcohol, firearms, sexual behaviors, motor vehicles, and illicit drug use killed about 200,000 more (9%). These figures highlight the importance of behavior and lifestyle as significant contributors to mortality.

However, ranking causes of death for the entire population may be misleading with regard to

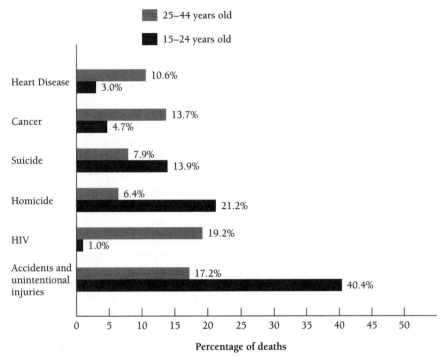

Figure 1.1 **Leading causes of death among adults, 15 to 24 versus 24 to 44, United States, 1995.** *Source:* Data from "Report of Final Mortality Statistics, 1995," by R. N. Anderson, K. D. Kochanek, & S. L. Murphy, 1997, *Monthly Vital Statistics Report, 45*(11), supp. 2, Table 7.

specific age and ethnic groups. The chronic diseases that are the leading causes of death for the population as a whole are more likely to affect middle-aged and older people. Young people between 15 and 24 years old die from accidents or unintentional injuries more often than from any other cause. In 1995, unintentional injuries were responsible for about 40% of the deaths in this age group, homicide about 21%, and suicide nearly 14% (Anderson, Kochanek, & Murphy, 1997). As Figure 1.1 reveals, other causes of death account for much smaller percentages than unintentional injuries, homicide, and suicide.

For adults 25 to 44 years old, the picture is somewhat different. Beginning in 1993, HIV infection surpassed unintentional injuries as the primary killer of people in this age range. As Figure 1.1 shows, HIV remains the leading cause of death for

people 25 to 44, followed by unintentional injuries, cancer, heart disease, suicide, and homicide (Anderson et al., 1997).

Ethnic background is also a factor in life expectancy and cause of death. If African Americans and European Americans in the United States were considered to be different nations, European America would rank 12th in the world in mortality rate, whereas African America would rank 33rd (Dwyer, 1995). The same dramatic relationship does not occur for Hispanic Americans, who are similar to other European Americans in mortality (Liao et al., 1998). The underlying reason for the discrepancy between African Americans and European Americans is not clear. Social class differences seem to be more important than ethnic differences in predicting health risks (Pappas, 1994), but social class is a complex construct that includes income level, education, and occupation, and each of these components relates to life expectancy.

Poverty is unquestionably a factor in disease rates and decreased life expectancy. Separating ethnic background from poverty is difficult in the United States, because disproportionate numbers of African Americans, Hispanic Americans, and Native Americans are poor. About 12% of European Americans are poor, but about one-third of African Americans live below the poverty line (Gorman, 1991), and these economic differences have an impact on health and health care. One study (Fisher, 1995) found that ethnic minority Americans were less likely than European Americans to have insurance coverage, which is an important factor in access to medical care. Access to medical care is not the only factor that makes poverty a health risk: Poverty is also associated with poorer health habits (Gibbons, 1991). Because of this association, poverty puts poor people at increased risks for disease as well as presenting difficulties in accessing medical care.

The health risks associated with poverty begin before birth. With no prenatal care, poor women are more likely to deliver low-birth-weight infants, who are more likely to die than infants with normal birth weight (Gorman, 1991). Cutbacks in federal immunization programs during the 1980s resulted in an increasing percentage of poor children without protection against measles and other childhood diseases. Children and adolescents living in urban poverty are vulnerable to neighborhood violence. They are also less likely than wealthier children and adolescents to receive regular health care. Poor adults also have limited access to regular health care, with local hospital emergency rooms providing the only accessible care for many low-income individuals. These conditions present health risks to the poor.

Income level is strongly related to health, not only at poverty level but at higher income levels as well (Kent, 1997). Within any income group, such as the middle class, those at higher levels have better health and lower mortality than those

at lower levels, but the reasons for this relationship remain unclear. One possibility is the relation of income to educational level, which, in turn, is related to occupation, social class, and ethnicity (Navarro, 1990; Rogers, 1992). In addition, education level is also related to behaviors that increase health risks such as smoking, eating a high-fat diet, and maintaining a sedentary lifestyle; that is, the higher the educational level, the less likely people are to engage in unhealthy behaviors (Lantz et al., 1998). Thus, the possibilities for influence are numerous, and the mechanisms that underlie the relationship of health to income, ethnicity, educational level, and social class remains to be clarified.

During the 20th century, life expectancy rose dramatically in the United States and other industrialized nations. In 1900, life expectancy was 47.3 years (USBC, 1975), whereas today it is around 76 years (United States Department of Health and Human Services [USDHHS], 1998a). In other words, infants born today can, on average, expect to live more than a generation longer than their great-great-grandparents born at the beginning of the 20th century.

What factors have accounted for the nearly 30-year increase in life expectancy during the 20th century? A more health-conscious lifestyle is a factor, but the control of many infectious diseases and the reduction of infant mortality rates have been more important. Widespread vaccination, safer drinking water and milk supplies, and more efficient disposal of sewage have helped contain infectious diseases. In addition, improved nutrition has increased people's resistance to infection, and antibiotics have provided a cure for many infectious diseases. Improved medical care, such as surgical technology, improved paramedic teams, and better intensive care units, also have made some contribution to longevity.

Although these advances have helped extend lives, the lowering of infant mortality has contributed even more to average increased life expectancy. When infants die before their first birthday, these deaths lower the population's average

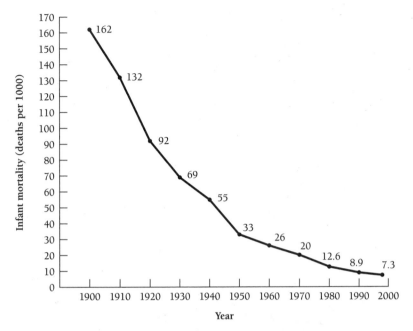

Figure 1.2 **Decline in infant mortality in the United States, 1900 to 1996. (rates per 1,000).** *Source:* Data from *Health, United States, 1998* (p. 93), by U.S. Department of Health and Human Services, 1998, Washington, DC: U.S. Government Printing Office and from *Historical Statistics of the United States: Colonial Times to 1970* (p. 60) by U.S. Bureau of the Census, 1975, Washington, DC: U.S. Government Printing Office.

life expectancy much more than the deaths of middle-aged or older people. Thus, decreasing deaths at a young age can have a substantial statistical impact. As Figure 1.2 shows, a dramatic decline in infant death rates occurred between 1900 and 1996. Death rates for all ages have declined as well, but not as rapidly as for infants. Indeed, life expectancy at age 65 has increased little, indicating that lifestyle changes, public health measures, and improvements in medical care have not had as great an impact on life expectancy for older people.

Escalating Cost of Medical Care

The second major change within the field of health has been the escalating cost of medical care. These costs have some relationship to increased life expectancy: As people live to middle and old age, they tend to develop chronic diseases, which require extended (and often expensive) medical treatment. Medical costs, however, are increasing at a much faster rate than inflation, and year to year they represent a larger and larger proportion of the gross domestic product. Figure 1.3 shows that from 1975 to 1995, the total yearly cost of health care increased from $582 to $3,633 per person, a jump of more than 600% and a much faster annual increase than that reported for the years 1960 to 1975. By 1996, Americans were spending more than $1,030 billion a year on health care. This figure represented 13.6% of the gross domestic product, nearly triple the percentage in 1960 (USDHHS, 1998a).

Although medical treatment during the 20th century has yielded nearly miraculous cures for some individuals, the mounting monetary costs of medical miracles militate against the traditional

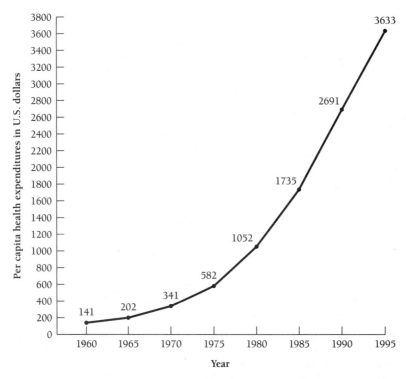

Figure 1.3   **Per capita health expenditures, United States, 1960 to 1995.**
Source: Data from *Health, United States, 1998* (p. 342) by U.S. Department of Health and
Human Services, 1998, Washington, DC: U.S. Government Printing Office.

philosophy of health, which emphasizes diagnosis, treatment, and cure. Expensive medical procedures such as heart surgery, hemodialysis, and
high-technology imaging techniques contribute
substantially to the rising cost of health care
in the United States, even though they are used
with only a relatively small proportion of the
population.

Curbing mounting medical costs requires a
greater emphasis on the early detection of disease
and on changes to a healthier lifestyle and to behaviors that help prevent disease. For example,
early detection of high blood pressure, high serum
cholesterol, and other precursors of heart disease
allows these conditions to be controlled, thereby
decreasing the risk of serious disease or death.
Screening people for risk is preferable to remedial

treatment because chronic diseases are quite difficult to cure and living with chronic disease decreases quality of life. Even more preferable to
treating diseases or screening for risks is maintaining health through a healthy lifestyle. Staying
healthy is typically easier and less costly than getting well. Thus, prevention of disease through a
healthy lifestyle, early detection of symptoms,
and reduction of health risks have all become part
of the changing philosophy within the health
care field.

What Is Health?

What does it mean to be healthy? Is health an absence of disease, or is it the presence of some positive condition? How do people know they are

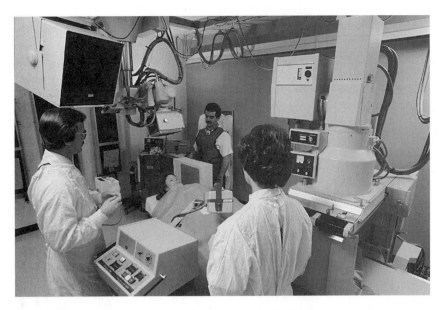

Technology in medicine is one reason for escalating medical costs.

healthy? Is health a single condition, or is it multidimensional?

According to George Stone (1987), definitions of health fall into two categories: those that portray health as an ideal state and those that portray health as movement in a positive direction. The first definition implies that any disease or injury is a deviation from good health and that the ideal state can be restored by removing the disease or disability. With this limited definition of health, a blind concert violinist would not be healthy, despite his or her accomplishments, productivity, and contribution to society. The second definition avoids this problem by considering health as a direction on a continuum. This definition implies that movement toward greater health is better than movement in the opposite direction. But because health is multidimensional, all aspects of living—biological, psychological, and social—must be considered. By this definition, a scientist who disregards personal safety or physical health to search for a cure for contagious disease would be moving away from biological health but toward social and perhaps psychological health.

One part of good health, in Stone's view, is improved biological functioning, such as normal blood pressure, superior cardiac output, a high level of respiratory volume, and the ability to withstand stress, infection, and physical injury. Stone proposed that the psychological manifestation of health is a subjective feeling of well-being. Social manifestations of health include the capacity for high levels of social productivity and low demands on the health care system.

Is health merely the absence of disease, or are some additional elements necessary for health? Does health result from the removal of a negative state, or must some positive state be attained? As Table 1.2 summarizes, people in various cultures during different times have held varying views of health. In 1946, the United Nations established the World Health Organization (WHO) and wrote into the preamble of its constitution a modern, Western definition: "Health is a state of complete physical, mental and social well-being, and not merely the absence of disease or infirmity." This definition clearly affirms that health is a positive state.

Table 1.2   Definitions of health held by various cultures

Culture	Time period	Health is
Prehistoric	10,000 B.C.E.	endangered by spirits that enter the body from outside
Babylonians and Assyrians	1800–700 B.C.E.	endangered by the gods, who send disease as a punishment
Ancient Hebrews	1000–300 B.C.E.	a gift from God, but disease is a punishment from God
Ancient Greeks	500 B.C.E.	a wholistic unity of body and spirit
Ancient China	1100–200 B.C.E.	a balance of the forces of nature
Galen in Ancient Rome	130 C.E.–200 C.E.	the absence of pathogens, such as bad air or body fluids, that cause disease
Early Christians	300 C.E.–600 C.E.	not as important as disease, which is a sign that one is chosen by God
Descartes in France	1596–1650	a condition of the mechanical body, which is separate from the mind
Vichow in Germany	late 1800s	endangered by microscopic organisms that invade cells, producing disease
Freud in Vienna	late 1800s	influenced by emotions and the mind
World Health Organization	1946	"a state of complete physical, mental and social well-being"

To Dwayne, health is an absence of disease. Because he does not feel sick most of the time, he believes that he is healthy, even though his lifestyle includes few behaviors that move him toward greater health. In contrast, Robyn sees health as a positive condition, not merely freedom from disease. As a consequence, she works hard to achieve an enhanced sense of total well-being. Her reasons for eating a healthy diet, exercising, not smoking, and drinking alcohol moderately have little to do with avoiding disease. She engages in healthy behaviors not to guard against disease but to achieve a positive state of health. And her lifestyle is paying off. She is able to study for long hours without becoming bored or lethargic; she enjoys being with other people but also likes solitude; she is able to exercise for 30 minutes a day without undue fatigue; and she very seldom suffers from headaches, depression, or general malaise. In short, she approaches the level of complete health described by the World Health Organization.

Dwayne and Robyn personify the two separate definitions of health. To Dwayne, health is a condition of not being sick, whereas Robyn regards health as a positive state of physical, mental, and social well-being that can be achieved through healthy behavior and lifestyle.

Changing Models of Health

Throughout the 20th century, the biomedical model has allowed medicine to conquer or control many of the diseases that once ravaged humanity. The notion that diseases are caused by a specific **pathogen**, a disease-causing organism, spurred the development of synthetic drugs and medical technology, which in turn engendered the belief that many diseases could be cured. However, the belief that a disease is traceable to a specific agent places more focus on disease than on health. In addition, this biomedical model defines health exclusively in terms of the absence of disease.

Although the biomedical model of disease has been the predominant view in medicine, an alternative model advocates a holistic approach to medicine—that is, one that considers social, psychological, physiological, and even spiritual aspects of a person's health. During the last quarter of the 20th century, more physicians, many psychologists, and some sociologists have even begun to question the usefulness of the biomedical model. Although they concede that the model has stimulated much progress in disease treatment, they question its limited definition of health and its usefulness in dealing with the current patterns of disease and death.

Currently, people in the health care field are debating which model researchers and practitioners should use. Some have become dissatisfied with the traditional biomedical model and have challenged its adequacy. Dissatisfaction, however, is not sufficient grounds to prompt a change. An alternative model must be available, and this alternative must have the power of the old model plus the ability to solve problems that the old model failed to solve. The alternative model is the *biopsychosocial model,* which incorporates not only biological but also psychological and social factors. In this model, health is once again seen as a positive condition. Advocates of the biopsychosocial model believe it has both these advantages.

The biopsychosocial model of disease incorporates not only physical factors but also psychological and social factors:

> To provide a basis for understanding the determinants of disease and arriving at rational treatments and patterns of health care, a medical model must also take into account the patient, the social context in which he lives and the complementary system devised by society to deal with the disruptive effects of illness, that is, the physician role and the health care system. This requires a biopsychosocial model. (Engel, 1977, p. 132)

Although the biomedical model has been the dominant view of medicine in the 20th century, before 1900 most physicians held a view of disease that emphasized the patient more than the symptoms. Joseph Matarazzo (1994), a pioneer in the development of health psychology, argued that before the widespread use of drugs, a compassionate, empathic bedside manner was about all that a physician had to offer patients. He also contended that the relatively recent explosion of scientific knowledge in such areas as biology, physiology, chemistry, and microbiology has produced several generations of physicians who know little about that type of bedside manner.

Nevertheless, some research has suggested that today's physicians may also conceptualize disease in ways that include psychological and social factors. Medical students distinguish between physiologically based diseases and those that appear to have heavy psychological involvement (Schmelkin, Wachtel, Schneiderman, & Hecht, 1988). This analysis demonstrates that even those who should be most indoctrinated in the biomedical approach still tend to include psychological factors in their thinking, a finding that supports the biopsychosocial model.

Other research also supports a biopsychosocial view of health. Only 28% of adolescents (Millstein & Irwin, 1987) defined health as an absence of disease. Instead, these adolescents tended to include both physical and psychosocial factors, such as the ability to perform certain activities and the presence of positive emotional states. Thus, the young people in this study defined both health and disease in multidimensional terms and saw health and lack of disease as being related but not identical. Not being sick was part of their definition of health, but it was not the whole picture. These studies indicate that both physicians and young people view health as a complex of biological, social, and psychological factors; that is, their concepts of health are consistent with the biopsychosocial model.

In Summary

Four major trends have changed the field of health care in the past century. One trend is the changing pattern of disease and death in the United States and other industrialized nations. Chronic diseases have replaced infectious diseases as the leading causes of death and disability. These chronic diseases include heart disease, stroke, cancer, emphysema, and adult-onset diabetes, all of which have causes that include individual behavior.

The increase in chronic disease has contributed to a second trend: the escalating cost of medical care. Costs for medical care have risen dramatically in the past 25 years and show few signs of stabilizing. These costs are due to a growing elderly population and innovative but expensive medical technology as well as to inflation.

A third trend is the changing definition of health. Many people continue to view health as the absence of disease, but a growing number of health care professionals and the public view health as a state of positive well-being. To accept this definition of health is to reconsider the biomedical model that has dominated health.

The emergence of the biopsychosocial model of health is the fourth trend that has changed the health care field. Rather than defining disease as the simple presence of pathogens, the biopsychosocial model emphasizes positive health and sees disease, particularly chronic disease, as resulting from the interaction of biological, psychological, and social conditions.

Psychology's Involvement in Health

Although chronic diseases have many causes, no one seriously disputes the evidence that individual behavior and lifestyle are strongly implicated in their development. Because most chronic diseases stem at least partly from individual behavior, psychology—the science of behavior—has become involved in health care.

A large part of psychology's involvement in health care is a commitment to keeping people healthy rather than waiting to treat them after they become ill. Psychology shares this role with medicine and other health care disciplines, but unlike medicine (which tends to study specific diseases), psychology contributes certain broad principles of behavior that cut across specific diseases and specific issues of health. Among psychology's contributions to health care are techniques for changing behaviors that have been implicated in chronic diseases. In addition to changing unhealthy behaviors, psychologists have also used their skills to relieve pain and reduce stress, improve compliance with medical advice, and help patients and family members live with chronic illnesses.

Psychology in Medical Settings

Psychology has been concerned with people's physical health almost from the beginning of the 20th century. In 1911 the American Psychological Association (APA) convened a panel to discuss the role of psychology in medical education (Rodin & Stone, 1987). Psychologists of the time agreed that medical students would profit from instruction in psychology and recommended psychology as part of premedical training or the medical school curriculum. As reasonable as this proposal now seems, most medical schools failed to pursue the recommendation. The APA again broached the topic in 1928 and once more in 1950, but medical schools implemented few changes during this time. According to a 1913 survey of medical schools, only 27% of those with academic affiliations collaborated with psychology departments (Franz, 1913).

During the 1940s, medical training typically incorporated the study of psychological factors as they relate to disease, but this training was usually conducted by physicians and was limited to the medical specialty of psychiatry. Before 1950, only a handful of psychologists were employed in medical schools (Matarazzo, 1994), and the duties of most of those were limited largely to teaching. A few of these clinical psychologists provided psychological services, such as testing and psychotherapy for patients with emotional problems, but few were involved in research. Also, psychologists seldom collaborated with medical specialists other than psychiatrists. That relationship be-

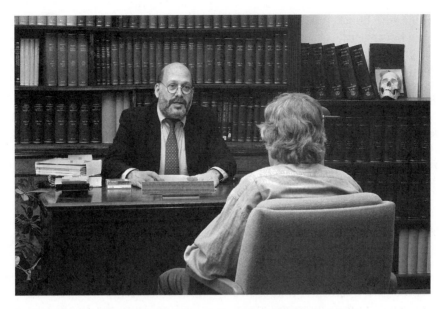

By the 1990s psychologists had become staff members of many hospitals.

tween psychology and psychiatry can be summarized by saying, "Behavioral science and psychiatry was a good marriage . . . until the behavioral scientists were sought out by other medical departments such as family medicine, pediatrics, internal medicine, and preventive medicine for clinical and research collaboration" (Pattishall, 1989, p. 45). As psychology became more widespread in medical training and as the research base increased to give behavioral science academic credibility, psychology's role in medicine began to expand.

Behavioral science became part of the curriculum in most medical schools in the 1960s, when many new medical schools were established and new curricula for these schools were developed. Matarazzo (1994) estimated that the number of psychologists who held academic appointments on medical school faculties nearly tripled from 1969 to 1993. By 1993, 3,500 psychologists were employed in medical settings, a number greater than the total membership of Division 38 (Health Psychology) of the American Psychological Association. By the 1990s, physicians no longer thought of health psychologists as merely statistical con-

sultants, test administrators, or therapists with skills largely limited to psychosomatic illness. Psychologists, along with neuropsychologists and rehabilitation psychologists, had become accepted members of most major hospital staffs (Sweet, Rozensky, & Tovian, 1991).

Psychosomatic Medicine

Psychosomatic medicine concerns the emotional and psychological components of physical diseases and the psychological and somatic (or physical) factors that interact to produce disease. The notion that psychological and emotional factors can contribute to physical ailments is older than history (Kaplan, 1985). Prehistoric humans saw disease as spiritual as well as physical, and many cultures in ancient history included psychological and social factors in their views of disease. The more modern concept of psychosomatic medicine received some impetus from Sigmund Freud, who emphasized the importance of unconscious psychological factors in the development of physical symptoms. But Freud's methods relied on clinical experience and intuitive hunches that were largely unverified by laboratory research.

The research base for psychosomatic medicine began with Walter Cannon's observation in 1932 that physiological changes accompany emotion (Kimball, 1981). Cannon's research demonstrated that emotion could cause physiological changes that might be related to the development of physical disease; that is, emotion can cause changes, which in turn, can cause disease. From this finding, Helen Flanders Dunbar (1943) developed the notion that habitual responses, which people exhibit as part of their personalities, are related to specific diseases. In other words, Dunbar hypothesized a relationship between personality and disease.

Franz Alexander (1950), a one-time follower of Freud, saw psychosomatic disorders as resting on a link between personal conflicts and specific diseases. During Alexander's time, such diseases as peptic ulcer, rheumatoid arthritis, hypertension, asthma, hyperthyroidism, neurodermatitis, and ulcerative colitis were thought to be psychosomatic. Alexander believed that certain people were more vulnerable than others to the effects of stress on their organ systems and that when organ vulnerability and stress coincided, these susceptible people would develop the disease to which they were vulnerable.

Although stress and its effects on physiology and the development of disease has remained a prominent subject of psychosomatic medicine, by the 1970s the emphasis had shifted away from specific diseases, and the term *psychosomatic* was no longer applied to diseases but to an approach to the study and treatment of disease. Physicians supporting this newer psychosomatic approach believe that illness is complex and that the single-factor pathogen approach would not be successful (Kimball, 1981). These physicians were the first in modern medicine to accept a biopsychosocial model for disease and to call for an expansion of the prevailing biomedical model.

Psychosomatic medicine can be seen as a reformist movement within medicine (McHugh & Vallis, 1986), but it has not lived up to its objectives of emphasizing the psychological and social components of somatic disease. Psychosomatic medicine remains in the domain of psychiatry, a branch of medicine, and the collaborative goals of the psychosomatic movement have not been attained; that is, the psychological and physiological aspects of disease have not yet been totally integrated. Instead, the objectives of the psychosomatic movement have been subsumed under the subject of *behavioral medicine*.

Behavioral Medicine

Although some psychologists have worked in medical settings since the beginning of the 20th century, only during the past 25 years has the medical establishment begun to recognize their contributions. Until the 1970s the role of psychologists in medicine was mostly restricted to medical education, psychological testing, psychosomatic medicine, and psychotherapy. Psychologists rarely participated in the psychological aspects of medical treatment, and their expertise was generally thought to be limited to mental health problems. Although psychologists considered their discipline the science of behavior, their skills were rarely called on to help people stop smoking, eat a healthy diet, exercise wisely, reduce stress, or control pain.

A growing awareness of the link between behavior and disease and psychology's development of effective techniques to change problem behaviors led to an increased role for psychology in health care. A 1977 conference at Yale University led to the definition of a new field, **behavioral medicine**, defined as "the interdisciplinary field concerned with the development and integration of behavioral and biomedical science knowledge and techniques relevant to health and illness and the application of this knowledge and these techniques to prevention, diagnosis, treatment and rehabilitation" (Schwartz & Weiss, 1978, p. 250).

This definition indicates that behavioral medicine is designed to integrate medicine and the various behavioral sciences, especially psychology (Pomerleau, 1982). The goals of behavioral medicine are similar to those in other areas of health care: improved prevention, diagnosis, treatment, and rehabilitation. Behavioral medicine, then, attempts to use psychology and the behavioral sciences in conjunction with medicine to promote health and treat disease. Chapters 3 through 11 cover topics in behavioral medicine.

Behavioral Health

A new discipline called **behavioral health** began to emerge at about the same time behavioral medicine was establishing its identity. Behavioral health emphasizes the enhancement of health and the prevention of disease in healthy people rather than the diagnosis and treatment of disorders in sick people. Furthermore, it is an "interdisciplinary subspecialty within behavioral medicine specifically concerned with the maintenance of health and the prevention of illness and dysfunction in currently healthy persons" (Matarazzo, 1980, p. 807). Behavioral health includes such concerns as injury prevention, cigarette smoking, alcohol use, diet, and exercise, topics discussed in Chapters 12 through 16.

The focus of behavioral health is on individual responsibility for health and wellness rather than on physician-based diagnosis, treatment, or rehabilitation (Matarazzo, 1984, 1994). All those behaviors and lifestyles that maintain or enhance health fall within the purview of behavioral health. Although people are generally accepting more responsibility for their health, the formal discipline of behavioral health has not emerged as a rival to the fields of behavioral medicine or health psychology (Matarazzo, 1994).

Health Psychology

Related to both behavioral medicine and behavioral health is a discipline within the field of psychology called **health psychology**, the branch of psychology that concerns individual behaviors and lifestyles affecting a person's physical health. Health psychology includes psychology's contributions to the enhancement of health, the prevention and treatment of disease, the identification of health risk factors, the improvement of the health care system, and the shaping of public opinion with regard to health. More specifically, it involves the application of psychological principles to such physical health areas as lowering high blood pressure, controlling cholesterol, managing stress, alleviating pain, stopping smoking, and moderating other risky behaviors, as well as encouraging regular exercise, medical and dental checkups, and safer behaviors. In addition, health psychology helps identify conditions that affect health, diagnose and treat certain chronic diseases, and modify the behavioral factors involved in physiological and psychological rehabilitation. As such, health psychology contributes to and overlaps with both behavioral medicine and behavioral health (see Figure 1.4).

The Development of Health Psychology   As an identifiable area, health psychology received its first important impetus in 1973, when the Board of Scientific Affairs of the American Psychological Association (APA) appointed a task force to study the potential for psychology's role in health research. Three years later, this task force (APA, 1976) reported that few psychologists were involved in health research and that research conducted by psychologists in the area of health was not often reported in the psychology journals. However, the report envisioned a future in which health psychology might help to enhance health and prevent disease. The task force stated that

> there is probably no specialty field within psychology that cannot contribute to the discovery of behavioral variables crucial to a full understanding of susceptibility to physical illness, adaptation to such illness, and prophylactically motivated behaviors. (American Psychological Association, 1976, p. 272)

This directive led to the establishment of the Section of Health Research within APA's Division

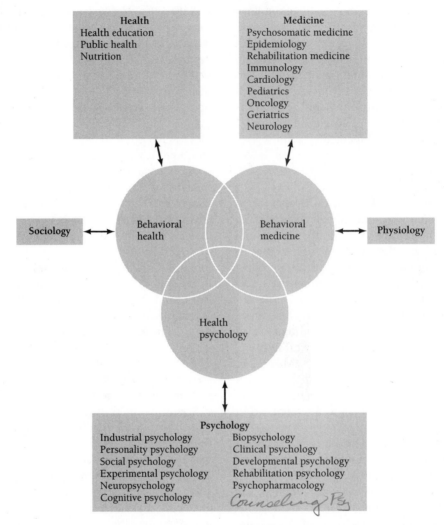

Figure 1.4   Relationship of health psychology to other health-related fields.

of Psychologists in the Public Service. In 1978, the American Psychological Association established Division 38, Health Psychology, as "a scientific, educational, and professional organization for psychologists interested in (or working in) areas at one or another of the interfaces of medicine and psychology" (Matarazzo, 1994, p. 31). Four years later, in 1982, the journal *Health Psychology* began publication as the official journal of Division 38.

Health Psychology's Position within Psychology

Health psychology is presently a well-established division within the American Psychological Association and is well recognized by the American Psychological Society—the two primary professional psychology organizations in the United States. Indeed, health psychologists are first and foremost psychologists, with the same basic training as any other psychologists. This training core was determined by the landmark Boulder Conference of 1949, which established psychology as both a scientific discipline and a practicing profession. From that time, every doctoral program within a department of psychology has offered nearly the same core of generic course work for psychologists. Along with the core courses required of all psychologists, health psychologists take courses in such fields as biostatistics, epidemiology, physiology, biochemistry, and cardiology. Like other psychologists, health psychologists rely on and contribute to the basic core of psychological research and then apply this knowledge to a particular field of specialization. In other words, health psychologists are psychologists first and specialists in health second. According to Matarazzo (1987b), "psychology" is the *noun* that identifies the subject matter; and "health" is the *adjective* that describes the client, problem, or setting to which psychology is applied. Like other fields of psychology, health psychology applies the principles of generic psychology to a particular area. Health psychology does not exist as a profession separate from generic psychology; rather, "health psychology is today nothing more than the application of the accumulated knowledge from the science and profession of generic psychology to the area of health" (p. 55).

Health psychology is now beginning to emerge as a clearly unique profession. It has (1) founded its own national and international associations; (2) established a number of its own journals in addition to *Health Psychology;* and (3) received acknowledgment from professionals in other fields of psychology that its subject matter, methods, and applications are different from theirs (Matarazzo (1987b). Moreover, health psychology has (4) begun to set up postdoctoral training specific to health psychology and distinct from other fields of psychology; (5) received recognition from the American Board of Professional Psychology; and (6) been recognized by the new American Psychological Association Commission on the Recognition of Specialties and Proficiencies in Professional Psychology (Belar, 1997). In addition, health psychology is becoming recognized within medical schools, schools of public health, universities, and hospitals.

In Summary

Psychology's involvement in health dates back to the beginning of the 20th century, but few psychologists were involved in medicine until recently. The psychosomatic medicine movement sought to bring psychological factors into the understanding of disease, but that view never moved beyond psychiatry. By the 1970s, psychologists had begun to develop research and treatment aimed at health promotion and chronic disease; this research and treatment led to the founding of two new fields, behavioral medicine and behavioral health.

Behavioral medicine is concerned with applying the knowledge and techniques of behavioral research to physical health, including prevention, diagnosis, treatment, and rehabilitation. Behavioral health is concerned with health maintenance and disease prevention in people who are healthy. Psychology and psychologists have been important in both these fields, but health psychology is the specialty within psychology that is concerned with issues of physical health. Health psychology strives to enhance health, prevent and treat disease, identify risk factors, improve the health care system, and shape public opinion regarding health issues.

Answers

This chapter addressed two basic questions:

1. **How have views of health changed?**

   Views of health are changing, both among health care professionals and among the general public. Several trends have prompted these changes, including (1) the changing pattern of disease and death in the United States from infectious diseases to chronic diseases; (2) increasing medical costs that represent a progressively larger percentage of gross domestic product for the United States; (3) growing acceptance of a view of health that includes not only the absence of disease but also the presence of positive well-being; and (4) an emerging new biopsychosocial model of health, which departs from the traditional biomedical model by including not only biochemical abnormalities but also psychological, and social conditions.

2. **What is psychology's involvement in health?** Psychology has been involved in health almost from the beginning of the 20th century. During those early years, however, only a few psychologists worked in medical settings and most were considered adjuncts rather than full partners with physicians. Psychosomatic medicine emphasized psychological explanations of somatic diseases and increased the need for psychologists in the health field. By the 1960s and early 1970s, psychology and other behavioral sciences were beginning to play a role in the prevention and treatment of chronic diseases and in the promotion of positive health, giving rise to two new fields: behavioral medicine and behavioral health.

Behavioral medicine is an interdisciplinary field concerned with applying the knowledge and techniques of behavioral science to the maintenance of physical health and to prevention, diagnosis, treatment, and rehabilitation. *Behavioral health* is a subspecialty within behavioral medicine concerned with health maintenance and disease prevention in currently healthy individuals. Although both behavioral medicine and behavioral health are related to psychology, both are disciplines outside the field of psychology. In 1978, the American Psychological Association established Division 38, *Health Psychology,* a specialty within psychology that contributes to both behavioral medicine and behavioral health and uses the science of psychology to enhance health, prevent and treat disease, identify risk factors, improve the health care system, and shape public opinion with regard to health.

Glossary

behavioral health   A discipline concerned with preventing illness and enhancing health in currently healthy people.

behavioral medicine   An interdisciplinary field concerned with developing and integrating behavioral and biomedical sciences.

chronic diseases   Illnesses that develop or persist over a long period of time.

health psychology   A field of psychology that contributes to both behavioral medicine and behavioral health; the scientific study of behaviors that relate to health enhancement, disease prevention, and rehabilitation.

pathogen   Any disease-causing organism.

Suggested Readings

 Bhopal, R. (1998). Spectre of racism in health and health care: Lessons from history and the United States. British Medical Journal, 316, 1970–1973.

Raj Bhopal analyzes the complexities of ethnic differences in health, including the economic and other factors that make a simple analysis of this area impossible. Available through InfoTrac College Edition by Wadsworth Publishing Company.

Matarazzo, J. D. (1994). Health and behavior: The coming together of science and practice in psychology and medicine after a century of benign neglect. *Journal of Clinical Psychology in Medical Settings, 1,* 7–39.

Matarazzo covers many of the same issues discussed in this chapter; in addition, he briefly discusses some examples of misbehaviors, such as smoking, overeating, and living a hostile lifestyle.

Stone, G. C. (1982). Health Psychology: A new journal for a new field. *Health Psychology, 1,* 1–6.

This editorial appeared in the first issue of Health Psychology and helped to define the field by outlining the types of articles considered appropriate for publication.

CHAPTER 2

Conducting Health Research

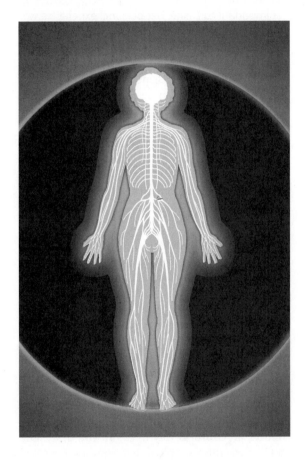

QUESTIONS

This chapter focuses on five basic questions:

1. How has psychology contributed to health?

2. How has epidemiology contributed to health?

3. How can scientists determine if a behavior causes disease or death?

4. What is the role of theory in scientific research?

5. What is the role of measurement in scientific research?

DIANE: PERSONAL DECISION OR PERSONAL BIAS?

Diane, a 22-year-old college senior, wanted to quit smoking but didn't know how to stop. Her roommate, who was enrolled in a health psychology class, told Diane that smoking was one of the topics included in the course and advised Diane to talk to the professor. When Diane visited the health psychology professor, she asked her to recommend a therapist to hypnotize her so she could quit smoking.

The professor asked Diane why she wanted to use hypnosis rather than some other smoking cessation program, and Diane replied that she had enrolled in a group class in hypnosis 2 years earlier and had quit smoking for almost a year. The professor explained that hypnosis has a number of uses and can be effective for some problems but that hypnosis is not very useful in helping people quit smoking. Diane believed that if hypnosis had been successful for her once, it would be successful a second time. She did not see her resumption of smoking as a failure of the hypnotherapy; instead, she blamed herself and the stresses in her life for her return to smoking.

Diane was adamant that hypnosis was the technique she wanted, despite the professor's contention that research had not shown hypnosis to be an effective treatment for smoking. Research evidence was not important to Diane; her personal experience was more important than results from scientific studies. She was convinced that hypnosis would work for her, even if it did not work for other people.

Like many people, Diane was relying more on personal experience than on research evidence. She believed that her own observations were more valid (especially for her) than research conducted on large groups of people. She did not see that her own biases were interfering with her judgment of the value of hypnosis—that is, Diane had trouble accepting the value of scientific research on a personal level.

Scientific Foundations of Health Psychology

Interestingly, Diane believed that scientific research had proved that smoking was dangerous to health. Although she was aware of much of the data linking cigarette smoking to heart disease and cancer, she chose to ignore the research suggesting that hypnosis was not an effective means of quitting smoking, believing instead unfounded claims that hypnosis was a simple and painless way to stop smoking. Much unfounded information on health-related behaviors comes from individuals and organizations trying to sell a product. Fortunately, scientists have discovered a vast body of health-related information that is relatively objective and free from self-serving claims. This information has been produced by researchers trained in the behavioral and biomedical sciences who typically are associated with universities and research hospitals. Because these men and women use the methods of science in their work, evidence usually accumulates gradually over an extended period of time. Dramatic breakthroughs are rare.

When scientists are familiar with one another's work, use controlled methods, keep personal biases from contaminating results, make claims cautiously, and are able to replicate their studies, evidence is more likely to be evolutionary than revolutionary. Claims to the contrary are most often motivated by financial or other personal interests. News reports must get readers' attention, so the headlines and news coverage are often misleading. (See the Would You Believe . . . ? box.) And, of course, commercial advertisements that champion their product as a revolutionary new cure for insomnia, an effortless way to eat all you desire and still lose weight, a simple way to stop smoking, or a food that protects you against cancer or heart disease either are not using, or are distorting, scientific evidence when they make their claims.

Like many people, Diane was concerned about her health. She not only wanted to quit smoking, but she tried to exercise regularly, watch her diet, and avoid too much stress. But how do people such as Diane know that these health practices will indeed contribute to better health? What is the source of health information? Who conducts

CHECK YOUR HEALTH RISKS

Check the items that are consistent with your beliefs.

☐ 1. Personal testimonials are a good way to decide about treatment effectiveness.

☐ 2. Newspaper reports of scientific research give an accurate picture of the importance of the research.

☐ 3. The personal information from case studies usually provides more valid data than information from longitudinal studies.

☐ 4. Placebo effects apply only to suggestible people and are not an important factor in the treatment of most people.

☐ 5. Placebo effects can influence psychological but not physical disorders.

☐ 6. Different research methods are not important in determining the validity of research because all scientific methods yield equally valuable results.

☐ 7. The number of participants in a research study is not important to the validity of the study.

☐ 8. Studies with nonhuman subjects can be just as important as those with human participants in determining important health information.

☐ 9. Experimental rather than observational research is required to learn about patterns of disease.

☐ 10. Valuable research is done by people outside the scientific community, but scientists try to discount the importance of such research.

☐ 11. Scientific breakthroughs happen every day.

☐ 12. Each new report of health research seems to contradict previous findings, so there is no way to use this information to make good personal decisions about health.

Each of these items represents a naive or unrealistic view of research that can make you an uninformed consumer of health research. Count your check marks to see if you have any naive or unscientific views about health-related research. Information in this chapter will help you become more accurate in your evaluation of and expectations for health research.

---

the basic research that suggests which behaviors are healthy and which are harmful?

Much health-related information comes from studies conducted by behavioral and biomedical scientists using a variety of research methods. The choice of methods depends in large part on what questions the scientists are trying to answer. Questions regarding heart disease, for example, may require many different research methods in order for scientists to reach a comprehensive understanding of this disease. This chapter looks at the way scientists work, emphasizing the behavioral and biomedical sciences—that is, psychology and epidemiology. These two disciplines share some

methods for investigating health-related behaviors, but each has made its own contributions to scientific methodology.

Contributions of Psychology

As the scientific study of behavior, psychology has made many important contributions to the understanding of those behaviors and lifestyles that relate to health and illness. As reported in Chap-ter 1, most of the leading causes of death in the United States are chronic diseases that result in large part from individual behavior and lifestyle.

WOULD YOU BELIEVE...?

Media Messages May Be Misleading

Would you believe that reading the daily newspaper can be hazardous to your understanding of health? Some research exists that news print media significantly misrepresent most of the leading risks and nearly every major cause of death in the United States. Karen Frost, Erica Frank, and Edward Maibach (1997) measured the amount of space devoted to the nine leading risks for death in the United States as well as the 11 leading causes of death by the most popular (1) weekly news magazine (*Time*), (2) women's interest magazine (*Family Circle*), (3) general interest monthly magazine (*Reader's Digest*), and (4) daily newspaper (*USA Today*).

The analysis revealed some interesting results. News reports of four of the risks for death—diet, alcohol, firearms, and sexual behavior—were reasonably close to their actual risks in terms of percentage of space devoted to them. However, three risks were greatly overreported and one dangerously underreported. People getting their health-related news solely from these four sources would be led to believe that (1) illicit drug use is more than 17 times as deadly as it actually is, (2) motor vehicle crashes are nearly 13 times as frequent as law enforcement records indicate, (3) toxic agents are nearly 11 times more lethal than they really are, and (4) microbial agents are almost 3 times the risk that they actually are. Interestingly, the one risk that was dangerously underreported was tobacco use. Although use of tobacco products accounts for 19% of deaths in the United States, only about 4% of the space in these news reports was devoted to tobacco.

As for the 11 leading causes of death, only suicide was reported in proportion to its frequency. Others were either grossly overreported or significantly underreported. For example, although cardiovascular disease kills nearly twice as many people in the United States than cancer, it receives far less news coverage. However, two other causes of death are even more overrepresented—unintentional injuries and homicide. Unintentional injuries received more than one-fourth of all the space devoted to mortality but account for only about 4% of deaths; and homicide—the 11th leading cause of death during the target year—received almost as much publicity as cardiovascular disease, the leading cause.

In their conclusions, Frost et al. rightly pointed out that most of the overreporting involved health risks or causes of death that are largely beyond an individual's personal control, such as toxic agents and microbial agents; or they are the result of dangerous acts of others, such as illicit use of drugs, motor vehicle crashes, unintentional injuries, and HIV infection.

Studies of risk perception indicate that threats that are perceived to be externally imposed loom larger than self-imposed threats. Thus, not only do the news media emphasize relatively rarer causes of and risk factors for death, but those causes emphasized are those that are instinctively overestimated. (p. 844)

Many of these chronic illnesses can be prevented by changing people's learned response patterns.

Psychology has made several important contributions to health and medicine. First, it has provided a variety of techniques for changing behaviors that have been implicated in chronic disease. Second, psychology is committed to keeping people healthy rather than waiting to treat them after they become ill. Third, psychology has a long history of developing reliable and valid measuring instruments for assessing factors related to health and illness. Fourth, psychologists have constructed and used theoretical models to explain and predict behaviors associated with health and illness. Fifth, psychology has contributed a solid foundation of scientific methods for studying such behaviors. We discuss the first four of these contributions throughout this book, but now we look at research methods used in psychology.

Research Methods in Psychology

When scientists wish to learn as much as possible about a single individual, they usually employ a *case study;* when they are interested in what factors predict or are related to either disease or healthy functioning, they use *correlational studies;* when they want to compare people across different ages or ethnic groups, they rely on *cross-sectional studies;* when they desire information on stability or instability of health status over a period of time, they use *longitudinal studies;* and when they wish to compare one group of participants with another, they can use either *experimental designs* or *ex post facto designs.* Case studies, correlational studies, cross-sectional studies, longitudinal investigations, experimental studies, and ex post facto designs, then, are all methods from the discipline of psychology that have application in the field of health.

Case Studies   Although most psychological investigations employ many participants, studies using only one person have a legitimate role in science. **Case studies** provide an in-depth analysis of only one individual and are one type of single-subject design.

In a case study, a researcher extensively studies one subject, usually because that person presents a particularly interesting or unusual case. The advantage of the case study is that it ordinarily provides a more complete analysis of an individual than can be obtained by investigations of large numbers of participants. The principal disadvantage is that it magnifies sampling errors. One purpose of any scientific investigation is to allow generalization to other participants or even to an entire population. Although all studies on population samples suffer from problems of generalization, case studies are an extreme example, permitting even fewer inferences about people in general than studies with multiple participants.

Many areas of health psychology can be studied from a variety of angles, and in our discussion of psychology and epidemiology studies we examine myriad ways of looking at cardiovascular disease (CVD), the leading cause of death in the United States and in all other industrial nations (World Health Organization, 1998). For example, the case study method can be used to learn about cardiovascular disease. One such study was described by Joel Gore and John Fallon (1994) who presented the case study of a 25-year-old man with congestive heart failure and a recent diagnosis of diabetes. The vast number of measures gathered from this single case yielded information that is not ordinarily available in studies with many participants. From the description given by Gore and Fallon, we know that this man was an only child, living at home with both parents, and working in a clerical job when he developed an irregular heart beat and a severe upper respiratory tract infection. After a week of bed rest, the infection subsided, but continual heart palpitations led him to seek the care of a **cardiologist**—that is, a medical doctor who specialized in heart disease. Gore and Fallon described the man as weak, fatigued, and having symptoms of diabetes. Their description also included dozens of other pieces of information on such heart-related measures as blood glucose concentration, **electrocardiogram (ECG)** signals, cholesterol levels, pulse, blood pressure, jugular vein pressure, and white-cell count. One year after treatment for both heart disease and liver ailment, the patient had no symptoms of heart disease, was working full time, and had become engaged to be married. Such detailed reports allow health psychologists and physicians to learn about heart disease in a relatively young patient and to see how this disease may, in some cases, be related to diabetes.

Correlational Studies   **Correlational studies** yield information about the degree of relationship between two variables, such as personality factors and heart disease. Correlational studies *describe* this relationship and are, therefore, a type of **descriptive**

research design. Although scientists cannot determine causal relationships through a single descriptive study, the degree of relationship is valuable information that can be used as an exploratory tool before designing an experimental study. On the other hand, information about the degree of relationship may be exactly what a researcher wants to know, and thus a correlational study may be the preferred method of investigation.

To assess the degree of relationship between two variables, the researcher measures each variable in a group of participants and then computes a correlation coefficient. Many types of correlation coefficients exist, but the one most commonly used in psychology is the *Pearson product-moment correlation coefficient*. This **correlation coefficient** is described by a formula, and the correlation is computed by applying the formula to the data that the researcher has gathered. The computation yields a number that varies between −1.00 and +1.00. Correlations that are closer to 1.00 (either positive or negative) indicate stronger relationships than do correlations that are closer to 0.00. Small correlations—those less than 0.10— can be *statistically significant* if they are based on a very large number of scores. However, such small correlations, though not random, offer the researcher very little ability to predict scores on one variable from knowledge of scores on the other variable.

Positive correlations occur when the two variables increase or decrease together. Negative correlations occur when one of the variables increases as the other decreases. For example, a researcher might wish to study the relationship between psychological factors, such as stress, and a variety of factors known to relate to heart disease. This was one of the purposes of a study by Jack Hollis and his associates (Hollis, Connett, Stevens, & Greenlick, 1990). To learn whether stressful life events are correlated with other risks for coronary heart disease, Hollis et al. gathered information from nearly 13,000 men with multiple risks for heart disease and correlated stressful experiences with such coronary risks as age, education, income, di-

astolic blood pressure, serum cholesterol level, and cigarette smoking. (A **risk factor** is any characteristic or condition that occurs with greater frequency in people with a disease than in people free from that disease.) All resulting correlations, though statistically significant, were quite small. Negative correlations ranged from −0.03 for diastolic blood pressure to −0.10 for age; positive correlations ranged from 0.03 for education to 0.10 for number of cigarettes smoked per day. In other words, this study found that stressful life events were somewhat positively related to such coronary risk factors as cigarette smoking and somewhat negatively associated with other risks, such as age.

Compared with the case study, correlational studies are rather impersonal, but they offer much more information concerning the factors that are associated with or predict a particular risk factor, disorder, or other event.

Cross-Sectional and Longitudinal Studies   **Cross-sectional studies** are those conducted during only one point in time, whereas **longitudinal studies** follow participants over an extended period. In a cross-sectional design, the investigator studies a representative sample of people from at least two different age groups or developmental periods or from two different ethnic groups to determine the possible effects of age or ethnicity on a particular variable.

For example, researchers may want to know whether total cholesterol levels are related to heart disease in people of different age ranges. Although high cholesterol levels are associated with high incidence of heart disease among younger people, one study (Kronmal, Cain, Ye, & Omenn, 1993) discovered that cholesterol was *not* positively related to heart disease among people over the age of 50. This finding, however, cannot suggest that older people somehow outgrow their need to maintain moderate cholesterol levels. Because people 70 or 80 years old were born at an earlier time than 40- to 50-year-old participants and thus had different experiences that might relate to heart disease, we cannot conclude that younger people with high cholesterol levels can avoid heart problems if they can only survive into their 70s or 80s. Older people with high cholesterol may have simply outlived their age-mates with high cholesterol because they were blessed with better genes for coronary health.

Longitudinal studies can yield more useful results than cross-sectional studies because they assess the same people over time. However, longitudinal studies have one obvious drawback: They take time. In addition, longitudinal studies are usually more costly than cross-sectional studies, and they frequently require a large team of researchers.

Although cross-sectional studies have the advantage of speed, they have a disadvantage as well. Whereas longitudinal studies compare individuals to themselves, cross-sectional studies compare two separate groups of individuals. Cross-sectional studies can show differences, but they cannot yield information about changes in peo-ple over a period of time. For example, a cross-sectional study may find that a group of 20- to 30-year-olds have lower cholesterol levels than a group of 50- to 60-year-olds, but such information does not demonstrate that cholesterol levels go up as people become older. Only a longitudinal study, looking at the same people over a long period of time, can show that cholesterol increases with age. Thus, longitudinal studies allow researchers to assess developmental trends and draw conclusions concerning the course of a particular condition. The choice between a longitudinal method and a cross-sectional method depends partly on which questions the researcher is asking and partly on the amount of time and resources available.

Cross-sectional and longitudinal studies can be combined, allowing researchers to examine differences among people at different ages and then to follow them over time to measure developmental differences. Such a design was conducted by Liisa Keltikangas-Järvinen and Katri Räikkönen (1990a, 1990b). These investigators selected a large group of healthy adolescents and young adults, ages 12, 15, and 18, and assessed their coronary risk factors three times over a 6-year period. The cross-sectional phase of the study allowed the researchers to compare coronary risk factors among three different age groups, whereas the longitudinal aspect of the study permitted an examination of risk factor changes. Keltikangas-Järvinen and Räikkönen found that participants with high risk factors—that is, those with high blood pressure, high cholesterol, and a high body-mass index—were more likely than those with low risk factors to be aggressive-competitive but less likely to be closely involved with other people. They also found that male and female participants were quite similar in risk factors, a finding that suggests that early risk factors do not explain the later higher death rates from heart disease experienced by men.

Experimental Designs   Case studies, correlational studies, cross-sectional designs, and longitudinal studies all have important uses in psychology, but none of them is able to determine causality. Sometimes psychologists want information on the ability of one variable to cause or influence another. Such information requires an experimental design. Experimental designs are valuable because they generally yield information about cause-and-effect relationships that no other method can reveal.

In an experimental study, the experimenter begins with a sample of participants, divides them randomly into two or more groups, administers the condition of interest to one group, and administers a different condition to the other group or groups. The group receiving the condition of particular interest is called the *experimental group;* the participants receiving the comparison condition make up the *control group.* Often the experimental condition consists of administering a treatment whereas the control condition consists of withholding that treatment, but other combinations of treatment and control conditions are possible.

In an experimental design, the participants in the experimental group must receive treatment identical to that of participants in the control group except for one factor. The only difference between the two groups must be that they differ in their exposure to the **independent variable.** The experimental group receives one level of the independent variable, and the control group receives a different level. The independent variable is systematically manipulated to observe its influence on behavior—that is, on the **dependent variable.** If manipulation of the independent variable causes a change in the dependent variable, which can be evaluated by contrasting the experimental and control groups, the independent variable has a cause-and-effect relationship with the dependent variable.

For example, psychologists may be interested in the effects of a health-related behavior (such as eating a low-fat diet) on a disease (such as heart disease). In this example, the experimental group would be placed on a low-fat diet and the control group would eat a regular diet (see Figure 2.1). If the two groups are equal in all other important respects—such as baseline levels of diastolic and systolic blood pressure, age, gender, weight, and other cardiovascular risk factors—and if the two groups differed only in diet during the course of the experiment, then any posttest differences between the two groups in cardiovascular disease could be attributed to differences in diet. Such an experimental design allows the investigator to speak of causation or at least of probable causes of a particular disorder.

Experimental designs with health outcomes are problematic for ethical reasons. Participants who might be put in the control group could not be prevented, for example, from eating a low-fat diet, and neither could those in the experimental group be compelled to eat such a diet. Two experimental studies illustrate how this problem can be avoided. In one experiment, Dieter Kramsch and his associates (Kramsch, Aspen, Abramowitz, Kreimendahl, & Hood, 1981) used nonhuman subjects to investigate the effects of a high-fat diet on serum cholesterol levels, **atherosclerosis** (narrowing of the arteries), and sudden death from heart failure. These researchers randomly divided 27 monkeys into three groups. All animals were

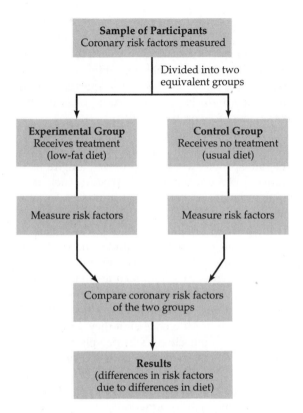

Figure 2.1 **Example of the experimental method.**

fed a very high-fat diet, but those in the two control groups were permitted little exercise whereas those in the experimental group were forced to run on a treadmill for 1 hour, three times a week. After 3½ years, monkeys in the exercise group had the same total cholesterol levels as the sedentary monkeys, but they had higher levels of "good" cholesterol, lower levels of "bad" cholesterol, and less atherosclerosis. In addition, the only monkeys that died suddenly were the sedentary ones. This study demonstrated that exercise can protect against coronary risk factors in monkeys; it could also suggest similar results for humans, if one is willing to generalize from monkeys to humans.

Another experimental study, the Multiple Risk Factor Intervention Trial (MRFIT), used humans as participants, but researchers did not force some people to eat a high-fat diet or prevent others from doing so. The study was a large-scale investigation of men between 35 and 57 years of age at the start of the study (Caggiula et al., 1981; Dolecek et al., 1986). At the beginning of this study, all the men were at risk for heart disease by virtue of being cigarette smokers with elevated blood pressure and high serum cholesterol levels. The participants were randomly assigned to either an intervention group or a control group. The intervention was not a low-fat diet; rather, it consisted of a program of counseling and advice about the benefits of a low-fat diet. Men in the control group were referred to their physicians for "usual care." Although participants in both groups reduced their daily intake of dietary cholesterol to some extent, those in the experimental group changed their diets and lowered their serum cholesterol levels much more than did men in the control group.

Achieving equivalence between the two groups is often a challenging problem in experimental studies. If one group receives a special type of intervention, then that group differs in two ways from the control group that does not receive the intervention: (1) the presence of the intervention and (2) the knowledge that they are in a group getting special attention. This knowledge may lead to people developing expectancies about the treatment that interfere with assessment of the treatment's effectiveness. To balance this expectancy researchers often give some form of a placebo to the control group, so that these people will have the same expectations as people in the experimental group. A **placebo** is an inactive substance or condition that has the appearance of the independent variable and which may cause participants in an experimental study to improve or change behavior as a result of their belief in the placebo's efficacy.

For researchers, however, the placebo effect makes the evaluation of treatment difficult. Placebos have been found to cure a remarkable range of disorders, including insomnia, headache, fever, the common cold, and warts. Placebos have also caused side effects, just as drugs do. They have been shown to produce dependence, and their re-

moval may prompt withdrawal symptoms. The adverse effects of a placebo have been called the **nocebo effect** (Turner, Deyo, Loeser, Von Korff, & Fordyce, 1994). Thus, the effects of placebos are complex and physiologically real.

Ex Post Facto Designs   Although a well-designed experiment can yield information about causal relationships, not all variables of interest in psychology can be manipulated. If the independent variable is not (or cannot be) manipulated, the study does not meet the requirements of the experimental method. When researchers are prevented by either ethical or practical restrictions from manipulating variables in a systematic manner, they sometimes rely on *ex post facto designs*.

Ex post facto designs, which are one of several types of quasi-experimental studies, resemble experiments in some ways but differ in others. Both types of studies involve contrasting groups to determine differences, but ex post facto designs do not involve the manipulation of independent variables. Instead, researchers choose a variable of interest and select participants who differ on this variable, called a **subject variable.** By placing participants in groups according to different values of the subject variable, researchers can contrast these groups according to responses in a dependent variable. The most common reasons for this research strategy are practical and ethical limitations on the manipulations that an experimenter can perform.

Ex post facto designs are very common in health psychology because researchers are interested in investigating variables they cannot manipulate. For example, researchers interested in investigating the effect of a high-fat diet on the development of atherosclerosis have used nonhuman animal subjects rather than humans. An alternative approach would be to select a group of participants who already eat a high-fat diet and also select a comparison group of those who eat a diet lower in fat. However, the comparison group in an ex post facto design is not an equivalent control group because these participants were not equivalent to those in the experimental group at the beginning of the study. Thus, any differences in the two groups in level of atherosclerosis cannot be attributed to diet, and one cannot draw any conclusions concerning cause and effect.

An example of an ex post facto design is the Nurses' Health Study (Fuchs et al., 1995) which looked at the effects of different levels of alcohol consumption on death from heart disease. The investigators began with a large group of healthy women, ages 34 to 59, and divided them into nondrinkers, light drinkers, moderate drinkers, and heavy drinkers. After 12 years, women in both the light drinking and the moderate drinking groups had lower death rates from cardiovascular disease than women who were either nondrinkers or heavy drinkers.

In this study, the classification of women into nondrinkers, light drinkers, moderate drinkers, and heavy drinkers was ex post facto; that is, the participants were divided into groups according to criteria that the researchers selected rather than manipulated. The researchers then looked at death rates 12 years later and found a U-shaped relationship between level of alcohol consumption and cardiovascular death rate, meaning that nondrinkers and heavy drinkers had the highest death rates while light and moderate drinkers fared best.

Ex post facto designs allow comparisons between or among groups, but they do not permit researchers to determine that one variable *causes* changes in another variable. In the study on alcohol consumption, for example, the researchers could not conclude that light to moderate consumption caused the difference in death rates from cardiovascular disease, but the study does provide information about one risk factor for CVD.

In Summary

We have seen that health psychology has benefited from several psychology research methods, including case studies, correlational studies, cross-sectional and longitudinal studies, experimental designs, and ex post facto studies. The case study is an intensive investigation of one person. Correlational studies indicate the degree of association between two variables, but they can never prove causation. Cross-sectional studies investigate a group of people at one point in time. Longitudinal studies, which follow the participants over an extended period of time, are generally more likely to yield useful results. However, they are more time-consuming and expensive than cross-sectional studies. With experimental designs, researchers manipulate the independent variable so that any resulting differences between experimental and control groups can be attributed to their differential exposure to the independent variable. Experimental studies typically include a placebo given to people in a control group so that they will have the same expectations as people in the experimental group. Ex post facto studies are similar to experimental designs in that researchers compare two or more groups and then record group differences in the dependent variable.

Contributions of Epidemiology

In addition to contributions from psychology methods, the field of health psychology has profited from the research of epidemiologists. **Epidemiology** is a branch of medicine that investigates factors contributing to increased health or the occurrence of a disease in a particular population (Beaglehole, Bonita, & Kjellström, 1993). Epidemiology literally means the study of (*logos*) what is among (*epi*) the people (*demos*).

Epidemiology is among the oldest branches of medicine, having its origins in ancient Greece and Babylon when observers first began to compare people who had a particular disease or characteristic to those who did not (Lilienfeld & Lilienfeld, 1980). However, epidemiology did not evolve as a science until the 19th century, when infectious diseases such as cholera, smallpox, and typhoid fever threatened the lives of millions of people. Many of these infectious diseases were controlled or conquered largely through the work of the epi-

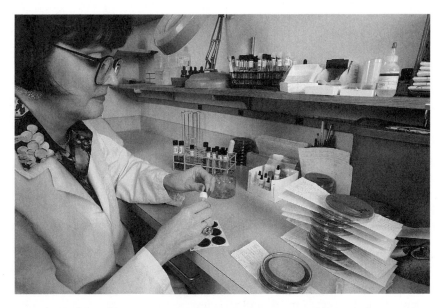

One purpose of epidemiological research is to determine the origins of a disease.

demiologists who gradually and laboriously identified their causes. With the increase in chronic diseases during the 20th century, epidemiologists continued to make fundamental contributions to health by identifying those behaviors and lifestyles that were related to heart disease, cancer, and other chronic diseases. For example, epidemiology studies were the first to detect a relationship between the behavior of smoking and the disease of lung cancer.

Two important concepts in epidemiology are prevalence and incidence. **Prevalence** refers to the proportion of the population that has a particular disease at a specific time; **incidence** measures the frequency of *new cases* of the disease during a specified period (Ahlbom & Norell, 1990). With both prevalence and incidence, the number of people in the *population at risk* is divided into either the number of people with the disease (prevalence) or the number of new cases in a particular time frame (incidence). The prevalence of a disease may be quite different from the incidence of that disease. For example, the prevalence of hyper-

tension is much greater than the incidence because people can live for years after a diagnosis. In a given community, the annual *incidence* of hypertension might be .025, meaning that for every 1,000 people in that community, 25 people per year will receive a diagnosis of high blood pressure. But because hypertension is a chronic illness, the *prevalence* in that community will be far more than 25 per 1,000. On the other hand, for a disease such as influenza with a relatively short duration (due either to the patient's rapid recovery or quick mortality) the incidence per year will exceed the prevalence at any specific time during that year.

Epidemiology studies have at least three basic purposes (Lilienfeld & Lilienfeld, 1980). The first is to determine the etiology or origins of a specific disease. For example, epidemiologists have looked at the prevalence of AIDS in certain populations and discovered possible causes of the disease. When researchers first noted an increased prevalence of AIDS within the male homosexual communities and within a population of intravenous

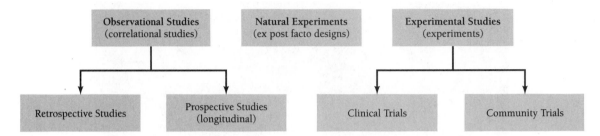

Figure 2.2   Research methods in epidemiology with their psychology counterparts in parentheses.

drug users, they hypothesized that the disease may somehow be transmitted through body fluids. Clinical tests have subsequently supported this hypothesis.

A second purpose is to determine whether hypotheses developed from other studies are consistent with epidemiological data. For example, physicians might notice that heart attack is more common in women who are overweight. Could obesity be related to heart disease in women? Only a large-scale epidemiological study could answer this question, and indeed, epidemiology studies have found such an association (Willett et al., 1995).

Also, epidemiological studies can be used to test more specific hypotheses regarding possible causes of a disease. For example, it has been noted that Seventh-Day Adventists have lower rates of CVD than the population in general. Could this lower rate be due to their vegetarian diet? Could it be their low rate of smoking? Do Seventh-Day Adventists have other behavioral differences from the general population that could lower their rate for CVD? Again, epidemiological studies can test these hypotheses by comparing Seventh-Day Adventists with others on several possible factors that might logically relate to CVD.

A third purpose of epidemiological studies is to provide a basis for developing and evaluating various preventive procedures. Treatment programs developed to control CVD need to be tested to determine how well they work to prevent the development or progression of CVD. Testing that

involves a large group of people would be necessary to demonstrate the overall rate of effectiveness.

Research Methods in Epidemiology

To achieve these purposes of epidemiological studies, researchers can use three broad methods: observational studies, "natural" experiments, and experimental epidemiology. Each method has its own requirements and yields specific information. Although epidemiologists use some of the same methods and procedures employed by psychologists, their terminology is not always the same. Figure 2.2 lists the broad areas of epidemiological study and shows their approximate counterparts in the field of psychology.

Observational Methods   Epidemiologists use observational methods to look at and analyze the occurrence of a specific disease in a given population. These methods do not show causes of the disease, but researchers can draw inferences about possible factors that relate to the disease. Observational methods are similar to correlational studies in psychology; both show an association between two or more conditions, but neither can be used to demonstrate causation.

Epidemiology studies have been used to identify psychosocial factors in cardiovascular disease. One such factor is the Type A behavior pattern, which has received extensive interest from both epidemiologists and psychologists. An epidemiology study led by Ray Rosenman—one of the originators of the Type A concept—found that men with the Type A behavior pattern were more than twice as likely as other men to experience coronary heart disease (Rosenman et al., 1975). Although this investigation did not use correlation coefficients, it suggested a correlation or association between Type A behavior and death from heart disease. In addition to being observational, this is an example of a prospective study.

Prospective studies begin with a population of disease-free participants and follow them over a period of time to determine whether a given condition, such as cigarette smoking or high blood pressure, is related to a later condition, such as cardiovascular disease or death. Prospective observational studies are identical to longitudinal studies in psychology: Both provide continuing information about a group of participants. **Retrospective studies** use the opposite approach; they begin with a group of people already suffering from a particular disease and then look backward for characteristics or conditions that marked them as being different from people who do not have that disease. For example, epidemiologist Carlos Mendes de Leon (1992) began with two groups of hospitalized patients; one consisted of men with heart disease, the other of men with diseases of the musculoskeletal system. Mendes de Leon found that one component of Type A behavior (the expression of anger) was related to coronary heart disease but not to musculoskeletal diseases. Retrospective studies such as this one are also referred to as **case-control studies** because cases (people affected by a disease) are compared with controls (people not affected). In general, prospective investigations provide more specific data than do retrospective studies, but prospective studies are expensive and time-consuming.

To compare retrospective studies to prospective designs, consider again the relationship between Type A behavior and heart disease. In the prospective study by Rosenman et al. (1975), the researchers measured Type A behavior of a large **cohort** (a group of participants starting an experience together) and then tracked the health of

these participants to learn whether men with Type A behaviors would differ from other men in their incidence of heart disease. The retrospective study by Mendes de Leon, in contrast, began with a group of heart disease patients and looked back at earlier records to determine whether their levels of anger expression differed from those of a matched group of controls. Both studies can show an association between a condition (such as Type A behaviors) and a subsequent disease (such as heart disease). The prospective study does so by looking forward whereas the retrospective study looks back in time.

Natural Experiments   A second area of epidemiological study is the natural experiment, in which the researcher can only select the independent variable, not manipulate it. Natural experiments are similar to the ex post facto designs used in psychology and involve the study of natural conditions that approximate a controlled experiment.

When two similar groups of people naturally divide themselves into those exposed to a pathogen and those not exposed, natural experiments are possible. The Nurses' Health Study (Fuchs et al., 1995) described earlier as an ex post facto design also fits the description of a natural experiment. In this study, women who had preexisting rates of alcohol consumption were divided into four groups—nondrinkers, light drinkers, moderate drinkers, and heavy drinkers—and then compared for death rates from cardiovascular disease. Because these groups are alike in other important conditions, the researchers were able to conduct a natural experiment by merely selecting levels of alcohol consumption as the variable of interest and using CVD death rates as one dependent variable. Ethical considerations would have prevented them from creating the four levels of alcohol consumption; that is, manipulating the independent variable.

Experimental Investigations   The third type of epidemiological study, the experimental investigation, is essentially identical to experiments in psychology. With this method the researcher ma-nipulates the independent variables rather than merely selecting them. Researchers match or ran-domly assign participants to an experimental or control group so that two (or more) groups are equated on all pertinent factors except the values of the independent variable. Although prospective studies are typically observational, some are ex-perimental. The feature that makes a prospective study experimental is the selection of equal groups at the beginning of the investigation, the manipu-lation of an independent variable or variables, and long-term follow-up of the participants.

In studying the effects of a high-fat diet on car-diovascular disease, an experimental group would receive a diet high in fat content while a matched group would eat a lower fat diet. If the two groups are equal in other respects, then differences be-tween the two in rates of CVD might be attributed to the high-fat diet. Obviously, this study would present a major ethical problem with human partic-ipants. People are not always willing to be subjected, merely for scientific reasons, to such a potentially unhealthy behavior as eating a high-fat diet. True, many people already eat high-fat diets, but a valid experiment would need to begin with participants who were not currently doing so. People who vol-unteer for such an experiment must be willing to be placed in either the experimental group or the control group; that is, they must agree either to eat a high-fat diet or to continue with their usual low-fat diet.

On the other hand, if people were allowed to choose to be placed in either the experimental group or the control group, then **self-selection** would be a problem. People who are willing to eat a high-fat diet are different from those who are not. This difference invalidates any experimental study that does not control for self-selection, and findings from such a study do not prove a cause-and-effect relationship.

Because of their scope and problematic ethical considerations, experimental prospective studies are quite rare. One such study, however, is the Multiple Risk Factor Intervention Trial (MRFIT),

discussed as an example of a psychology experi-ment (Multiple Risk Factor Intervention Trial Re-search Group, 1977). The MRFIT study minimized the problem of self-selection because all the men had multiple risks for heart disease at the start of the study and all were free of any visible evidence of heart disease. Participants were randomly placed into two groups: those who received a spe-cial intervention and those who received usual health care. The intervention (experimental) group received three types of treatment: (1) advice on sodium restriction, (2) counseling on giving up cigarette smoking, and (3) dietary advice to reduce cholesterol levels. Both the treatment group and the control group were invited to return yearly for a medical history, physical examination, and labo-ratory work.

A 7-year follow-up showed a decline in heart disease risk factors for both groups (MRFIT Re-search Group, 1982). Mortality rates from coronary heart disease were 17.9 per 1,000 for men in the in-tervention group and 19.3 per 1,000 for men in the control (usual health care) group, a difference that was not statistically significant. During the next 3 years, the intervention group reported somewhat fewer deaths from coronary heart dis-ease (MRFIT Research Group, 1990), a finding that suggested potential value in a program designed to change the behavior of men at risk for coronary heart disease.

Aside from prospective studies, there are two categories of experimental methods in epidemiol-ogy: clinical trials and community trials (Lilien-feld & Lilienfeld, 1980). *Clinical trials* test the effects of the independent variable on individuals, where-as *community trials* (also called field studies) test the effects of the independent variable on a group of individuals. An example of a clinical trial would be an experiment designed to test the efficacy of a drug designed to lower cholesterol. In such an experiment, participants with high serum choles-terol are randomly assigned to either an experi-mental group that receives the active drug, such as lovastatin, or a control group that receives a pla-cebo pill (Lovastatin Study Group III, 1988). Dif-

ferences between the two groups in subsequent total cholesterol levels could be attributed to the differences in treatment—that is, the independent
variable. Such an experiment would require a
double-blind design in which neither the participants nor the people who administer the pills
would know which pills contained the active ingredient and which were placebos. All drugs approved by the U.S. Food and Drug Administration
(FDA) must first undergo extensive clinical trials
of this nature.

In a field study, researchers compare one community to another. For example, people in one
city might receive extensive information on the
benefits of reducing cholesterol and high blood
pressure, whereas those in a city with similar characteristics would not be exposed to this information campaign. One such study is the Stanford
Five-City Project (Winkleby, Flora, & Kraemer,
1994). In this investigation, people in two experimental cities received increased educational messages from newspapers, television, radio, and
other sources on the value of controlling coronary
risk factors. People in the three control cities received no extra messages. After 6 years, people in
the experimental cities had reduced their blood
pressure and cholesterol somewhat more than
people in the three control cities.

Two Examples
of Epidemiological Research

Epidemiology provides useful techniques for taking a first look at a health-related problem. Two
examples of these techniques are the pioneering
work of John Snow in London and the ongoing
Alameda County Study in California.

The Pioneering Work of John Snow   A dramatic
example of how epidemiologists function is the
work of John Snow, the brilliant English epidemiologist and anesthetist and one of the founding
members of the London Epidemiological Society
(Lilienfeld & Lilienfeld, 1980; Winkelstein, 1995).
During the 1848 outbreak of cholera in London,

Snow made careful observations of the distribution of cholera deaths in the southern section of
the city. At that time, two different companies supplied the residents of south London with drinking
water. The water mains of the two companies were
interwoven so that residences on the same side of
the street received their water from two separate
sources. One water company pumped its water
from a polluted area of the Thames River; the
other had recently relocated its pumps to a less
polluted area. Snow noted which houses received
water from each company and calculated that the
cholera death rate was more than five times
higher in homes receiving their water from the
Thames than in homes receiving water from the
other south London company. He then compared
both sets of death rates with those from the rest of
London. Snow observed that the pattern of
cholera deaths closely paralleled the distribution
of polluted water. In 1855, without yet understanding the specific organism responsible for
cholera, Snow published a report in which he suggested the existence of a cholera "poison" and expressed his views of how the disease started and
how it spread. He also devised an ingenious plan
of intervention: He simply turned off the source of
polluted water. Not until 30 years later did Robert
Koch isolate the cholera bacterium, thus establishing the essential validity of Snow's views.

Snow had identified a risk factor for a deadly
disease; he had not discovered a specific cause.
During the last half of the 20th century, epidemiological work has shifted from tracking infectious
diseases to discovering factors associated with positive health or with chronic illnesses, but the procedures are quite like Snow's. Identifying these
factors does not prove causation, but it is a necessary first step leading to the control or eradication
of a particular disease.

The Ongoing Alameda County Study   A more
recent example of the way epidemiologists work is
the Alameda County Study, an ongoing prospective community study designed to identify health
practices that may protect against death and disease.

We have seen that epidemiologists identify risk factors by studying large populations over some period of time and by sifting out behavioral, demographic, or inherent elements that show a relationship to subsequent disease or death. Dozens of large-scale community studies have been reported during the past 2 or 3 decades. Unlike community trials (which are experimental and compare one community with another), community studies are observational and look at a single community. Examples of community studies include the Alameda County Study (Berkman & Breslow, 1983), the Framingham Heart Study (Dawber, 1980), the Honolulu Heart Program (Yano, Rhoads, Kagan & Tillotson, 1978), the North Karelia Project in Finland (Puska & Mustaniemi, 1975), the Seven Countries Study (Keys, 1980), and the Tecumseh Community Health Study (Higgins, Kjelsberg, & Metzner, 1967). Some of these studies appear in later chapters. For now, a review of a single project, the Alameda County Study, should reveal the flavor of community studies and the ways in which they have contributed to our knowledge of the influence of behavior and lifestyle in either promoting or endangering health.

The Alameda County Study began as an attempt to identify the health practices and social variables that relate to mortality from all causes. In 1965, epidemiologist Lester Breslow and his colleagues from the Human Population Laboratory of the California State Department of Public Health began a survey of a sample of all the households in Alameda County (Oakland), California. After determining the number of adults living at these addresses, the researchers sent detailed questionnaires to each resident 20 years of age or older. Usable returns were eventually received from nearly 7,000 people. Among other questions, these participants answered questions about seven basic health practices: (1) getting 7 or 8 hours of sleep daily, (2) eating breakfast almost every day, (3) rarely eating between meals, (4) drinking alcohol in moderation or not at all, (5) not smoking cigarettes, (6) exercising regularly, and (7) maintaining weight near the prescribed ideal.

At the time of the original survey in 1965, only cigarette smoking had been implicated as a health risk. Evidence that any of the other six practices predicted health or mortality was quite tenuous. Because several of these practices require some amount of good health, it was necessary to investigate the possibility that original health status might confound subsequent death rates. To control for these possible confounding effects, the Alameda County investigators asked residents about their disabilities, acute and chronic illnesses, physical symptoms, and current levels of energy.

A follow-up 5½ years later (Belloc, 1973) revealed that Alameda County residents who practiced six or seven of the basic health-related behaviors were far less likely to have died than those who practiced zero to three. This decreased mortality risk was independent of their 1965 health status, thus suggesting that healthy behaviors lead to lower rates of death. Surprisingly, these seven health practices turned out to be better predictors of mortality than level of income.

In 1974, a major follow-up of living participants took place. At that time a new sample was also surveyed to determine whether the community in general had adopted a new lifestyle between 1965 and 1974. The 9-year follow-up determined the relationship between mortality and the seven health practices, considered individually as well as in combination (Berkman & Breslow, 1983; Wingard, Berkman, & Brand, 1982). Five of the health practices predicted mortality rates independently of participants' use of preventive health services and their physical health in 1965. Cigarette smoking, lack of physical activity, and alcohol consumption were strongly related to mortality, whereas obesity and too much or too little sleep were only weakly associated with increased death rates. As it turned out, skipping breakfast and snacking between meals were not significantly related to mortality.

Men who practiced zero to two health-related behaviors were nearly three times more likely to have died than were those who engaged in four to five of the behaviors. For women, the effect was even more dramatic: When compared to women who practiced four or five of these behaviors, those who engaged in zero to two were over three times more likely to have died. Moreover, the number of close social relationships also predicted mortality: People with few social contacts were two and a half times more likely to have died than were those with many such contacts (Berkman & Syme, 1979).

If some health practices are inversely related to *mortality,* then a second question would be how these same factors relate to *morbidity* or disease. A condition that predicts death need not also predict disease. Many disabilities, chronic illnesses, and illness symptoms do not inevitably lead to death. Therefore, it is important to know whether basic health practices and social contacts predict later physical health. Stated another way: Do health practices merely contribute to survival time, or do they also raise an individual's general level of health?

To answer this question, researchers (Camacho & Wiley, 1983; Wiley & Camacho, 1980) studied a subset of the original sample of Alameda County participants. In addition to the five health practices that related to mortality, this investigation included a Social Network Index that combined marital status, contacts with friends and relatives, and membership in church and other organizations. Each of the five health behaviors as well as the Social Network Index were related to changes in health. More specifically, (1) both former smokers and nonsmokers had better health than smokers; (2) moderate drinkers were healthier than either heavy drinkers or abstainers; (3) people who slept 7 or 8 hours per night did better than those who got either more or less sleep; (4) both men and women who engaged in high levels of physical activity were healthier than their more sedentary counterparts; (5) normal weight people achieved higher health status than either overweight participants (30% or more above desirable weight) or underweight individuals (10% or more below desirable weight); and (6) people who scored high on the Social Network Index were healthier than those who received a low rating. Interestingly, the

Social Network Index showed that marriage did not have equal effects on the health of men and women. With both men and women, individuals who were formerly married—separated, divorced, or widowed—had greater negative changes in health, but women who had never been married were much healthier than were men who had never married. Never-married men had slightly negative health scores compared to married men, but never-married women had considerably higher health scores than either married or formerly married women. Marriage, it seems, agrees with men, but the single life is apparently healthier for women.

Evaluation of Research Methods

Like other scientists, psychologists and epidemiologists use controlled observations, try to be objective and cautious in drawing conclusions, and conduct studies that they or others can replicate. Nevertheless, all psychological and epidemiological studies have weaknesses, and those pertaining to health psychology are not exceptions. A major limitation to most studies in this field is that they simply indicate an association between a behavior and a subsequent outcome. Much research shows a relationship between a single independent variable (such as the Type A behavior pattern) and later morbidity (such as heart disease). But by looking at a single illness outcome from a variety of perspectives and by using multiple research methods, scientists learn much valuable information about that disease. We have seen that both psychology and epidemiology have examined cardiovascular disease from different angles and with a variety of methods. Such an approach has led to an increasingly better understanding of the behavioral factors in cardiovascular disease.

Nevertheless, little research exists showing how various psychological and behavioral factors interact with each other to influence the onset, progression, and severity of certain illnesses. In addition, researchers typically rely on limited assessment measures. Ideally, health psychologists

BECOMING AN INFORMED READER OF HEALTH-RELATED RESEARCH

How can you judge the worth of the abundance of health-related information you read or hear? Several questions serve as criteria for evaluating such information.

1. Is the information based solely on testimonials of "satisfied" consumers, with financial gain an obvious motive?

2. Is the information based on studies conducted by trained scientists who are affiliated with universities, research hospitals, or governmental agencies? Useful information does not typically spring from secret sources.

3. Is the information generally consistent with previous research? Dramatic breakthroughs and isolated evidence are rare in science.

4. Have the research findings been replicated by other researchers? Valid evidence should emerge from different laboratories.

5. Is the information based on studies using many participants? Information from small studies is usually less reliable than that which comes from large-scale studies.

6. Conversely, is the information based on huge studies or **meta-analyses** involving hundreds of thousands of people? With very large sam-

ples, even tiny differences can be statistically significant and can thus appear important even though they have little ability to predict health outcomes for a single individual.

7. Is the information based on correlational or experimental studies? Correlational studies cannot prove causation.

8. If the information comes from an experimental study, did the researchers control for the placebo effect?

9. Have the researchers reached conclusions that are consistent with their data?

10. Are the participants representative of some identified population?

11. Did the researchers use reliable and valid measures of the independent and dependent variables?

12. If the design is experimental, did the experimenters assure that the control and experimental groups were alike on everything except the independent variable?

13. If the design is prospective or retrospective, did the researchers adequately control for smoking, diet, exercise, and other possible confounding variables?

and epidemiologists should use a variety of instruments, including self-reports and physiological indices, as well as measures that are both clinically and theoretically relevant. Such research is difficult, expensive, and time-consuming, but it is essential for a complete understanding of how behavioral and psychological factors influence illness and health.

In addition, useful health-related research must take into consideration the placebo effect. Because health psychologists use behavioral interventions and because the patients they work with often receive drug or other medical treatment, the placebo

effect is an ever-present factor in psychological research and practice. Researchers in the health care fields, including health psychology, must assess the effectiveness of therapy cautiously, because expectancy is a factor in both medical and behavioral therapies. Without careful research design, the effectiveness of therapies can be overestimated. It is interesting that psychological placebos have been found to be about as effective as medical placebos (Blanchard & Andrasik, 1982). Both types of placebos have been shown to provide about a 35% rate of improvement for a wide variety of conditions (Evans, 1985). This means

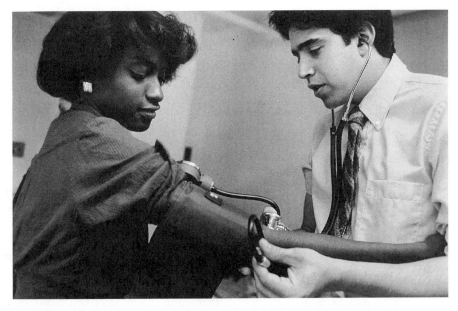

Blood pressure is a risk factor for cardiovascular disease, indicating that people with high blood pressure are at elevated risk but not that high blood pressure causes cardiovascular disease.

that in most experimental studies, the reported level of effectiveness of the intervention is actually a combination of the specific effects of the treatment plus a possible placebo effect of about one-third. Results of experimental research must be evaluated in the light of this strong expectancy effect.

In Summary

In order to investigate those factors that contribute either to health or to the frequency and distribution of a disease, epidemiologists use scientific methods that are quite similar to those used by psychologists. Among these methods are observational studies, natural experiments, and experimental studies. Observational studies, which are similar to correlational studies, can be either retrospective or prospective. (Retrospective studies begin with a group of people already suffering from a disease and then look for characteristics of these people that are different from those of people who do not have that disease, whereas prospective studies are longitudinal designs that follow the forward

development of a group of people). Natural experiments, which are similar to ex post facto studies, are used when the independent variable cannot be manipulated. Experimental designs, which are similar to experimental designs in psychology, include clinical trials and community trials.

Epidemiologists frequently use the concepts of risk factor, prevalence, and incidence. A risk factor is any condition that occurs with greater frequency in people with a disease than it does in people free from that disease. Prevalence refers to the proportion of the population that has a particular disease at a specific time, whereas incidence measures the frequency of new cases of the disease during a specified period of time.

Determining Causation

We have seen that both prospective and retrospective studies can identify risk factors in a disease, but they do not demonstrate causation. Obesity, hypertension, high total cholesterol, and cigarette smoking, for example, are all demonstrated risk factors for cardiovascular disease. People with one or more of these risks are more likely than people with none of these risks to develop CVD. However, some people with no known risks will develop cardiovascular disease and some people with multiple risks may never have CVD. This section looks at the risk factor approach as a means of suggesting causation and then examines evidence that cigarette smoking *causes* disease.

The Risk Factor Approach

The risk factor approach was popularized by the Framingham Heart Study (Dawber, 1980; Voelker, 1998), a large-scale epidemiology investigation that began in 1948 and included more than 5,000 men and women in the town of Framingham, Massachusetts. From its early years and continuing to the present, this study has allowed researchers to identify such risk factors for cardiovascular disease (CVD) as serum cholesterol, gender, high blood pressure, cigarette smoking, obesity, and the Type A behavior pattern. These risk factors do not necessarily cause cardiovascular disease, but they are related to it in some way. Obesity, for example, may not be a direct cause of heart disease, but it is generally associated with hypertension, which is strongly associated with cardiovascular disease. Because obesity is related to a known risk factor, it too is a relative risk factor for CVD.

Relative risk must be distinguished from absolute risk. **Relative risk** (RR) refers to the ratio of the incidence or prevalence of a disease in an exposed group to the incidence or prevalence of that disease in the unexposed group. The relative risk of the unexposed group is always 1.00, so that a RR of 1.50 indicates that the exposed group is 50% more likely to develop the disease in question than the unexposed group. A relative risk of 0.70 means that the rate of disease in the exposed group is only 70% of the rate in the unexposed group. **Absolute risk** refers to the person's chances of developing a disease or disorder independent of any risk that other people may have for that dis-

ease or disorder. For example, cigarette smokers have a relative risk of about 9.0 for dying of lung cancer (Lubin, Blot, et al., 1984), meaning that they are nine times as likely to die of lung cancer than nonsmokers. However, a smoker's absolute risk of dying of lung cancer in any one year is only about 0.001, or about 1 in 1,000, a very low absolute risk. A further illustration is seen in comparing the risk that cigarette smokers have of dying from cardiovascular disease with their risk of dying from lung cancer. Smokers have a relative risk of only about 2.0 for dying from cardiovascular disease (Centers for Disease Control and Prevention, 1993) but about 9.0 for dying from lung cancer. Nevertheless, because far more people in the United States die from cardiovascular disease than from lung cancer, smokers have a higher *absolute risk* of dying from CVD than they have of dying from lung cancer. More specifically, about 180,000 smokers die each year from CVD but only about 120,000 die from lung cancer (U.S. Department of Health and Human Services [USDHHS], 1995). When a disease is very rare, a person may have an extremely high relative risk for that disease but only a small absolute risk.

Although risk factors do not derive from experimental studies, they can determine the *probability* that a person will develop a particular disease. Not all cigarette smokers will develop heart disease, but if you smoke, you are about twice as likely to die of cardiovascular disease than if you do not smoke (CCD, 1993). Clearly, smoking cigarettes places one at risk for developing CVD. In a similar fashion, high cholesterol levels, high blood pressure, obesity, and stress are all risk factors for cardiovascular disease, but there is no *experimental* evidence that any of these conditions *cause* coronary heart disease or stroke.

Cigarettes and Disease: Is There a Causal Relationship?

In 1994, representatives from all the major tobacco companies came before the United States Congress House Subcommittee on Health to defend charges that cigarette smoking causes a variety of health problems, including heart disease and lung cancer. The crux of their argument was that no scientific study has ever proven that cigarette smoking causes heart disease or lung cancer in humans. Technically, their contention was correct, because only experimental studies can absolutely demonstrate causation, and no such experimental study has ever been or ever will be conducted on humans.

During the past 50 years, however, researchers have used nonexperimental studies to establish a link between cigarette smoking and several diseases, especially cardiovascular disease and lung cancer. Accumulated findings from these studies present an example of how nonexperimental studies can turn that link into a causal relationship. In other words, experimental studies are not required before scientists can infer a causal link between the independent variable (smoking) and the dependent variables (heart disease and lung cancer). Epidemiologists (Beaglehole, Bonita, & Kjellström, 1993; Susser, 1991) infer a causal relationship if certain conditions are met. Does sufficient evidence exist to infer a cause-and-effect relationship between cigarette smoking and heart disease and lung cancer?

The first criterion is that a *dose-response relationship* must exist between a possible cause and changes in the prevalence or incidence of a disease. A **dose-response relationship** is a direct, consistent association between an independent variable, such as a behavior, and a dependent variable, such as a disease. In other words, the higher the dose, the higher the death rate. A body of research evidence (Doll & Hill, 1956; USDHHS, 1990) has demonstrated a dose-response relationship between both the number of cigarettes smoked per day and the number of years one has smoked and the subsequent incidence of heart disease and lung cancer.

Second, the prevalence or incidence of *a disease should decline with the removal of the possible cause.* Research (Ben-Shlomo, Smith, Shipley, & Marmot, 1994; Kawachi et al., 1993; USDHHS,

1990) has consistently demonstrated that quitting cigarette smoking lowers one's risk of cardiovascular disease and greatly decreases one's risk of lung cancer. Moreover, quitting adds years to one's life (Fielding, 1985). People who continue to smoke continue to have increased risks of these diseases.

Third, the *cause must precede the disease.* Cigarette smoking almost always precedes incidence of disease. (We have little evidence that people tend to begin cigarette smoking as a means of coping with heart disease or lung cancer.)

Fourth, *a cause-and-effect relationship between the condition and the disease must be plausible;* that is, it must be consistent with other data and it must make sense from a biological viewpoint. Although scientists may not completely understand the exact mechanisms responsible for the effect of cigarette smoking on the cardiovascular system and the lungs, such a physiological connection is plausible. It is not necessary that the underlying connection between a behavior and a disease be known, only that it be a possibility.

Fifth, *research findings must be consistent.* For nearly 50 years, evidence from ex post facto and correlational studies, as well as from various epidemiological studies, has demonstrated a strong and consistent relationship between cigarette smoking and disease. As early as 1950, British researchers Richard Doll and A. B. Hill noted a straight linear relationship between average number of cigarettes smoked per day and death rates from lung cancer. Although a positive correlation such as this is not sufficient to demonstrate causation, hundreds of additional correlational and ex post facto studies since that time have yielded overwhelming evidence to suggest that cigarette smoking causes disease.

Sixth, the *strength of the association between the condition and the disease must be relatively high.* Again, research has revealed that cigarette smokers have about a two-fold risk for cardiovascular disease (CDC, 1993) and are nine times more likely than nonsmokers to die of lung cancer (Lubin, Blot, et al., 1984). Because other studies have found comparable relative risk figures, epidemiologists accept cigarette smoking as a causal agent for both CVD and lung cancer.

The final criterion for inferring causality is the *existence of appropriately designed studies*. Although no experimental designs with human participants have been reported on the relationship between cigarettes and disease, a sufficient number of well-designed observational studies have consistently revealed a close association between cigarette smoking and both cardiovascular disease and lung cancer.

Because each of these seven criteria are clearly met by a preponderance of evidence, epidemiologists are able to discount the argument of tobacco company representatives that cigarette smoking has not been proven to cause disease. When evidence is as overwhelming as it is in this case, scientists infer a causal link between cigarette smoking and a variety of diseases, including heart disease and lung cancer. Criteria for determining causation are summarized in Table 2.1.

In Summary

A risk factor is any characteristic or condition that occurs with greater frequency in people with a disease than it does in people free from that disease. Although the risk factor approach alone cannot determine causation, epidemiologists use several criteria for determining a cause-and-effect relationship between a condition and a disease: (1) A dose-response relationship must exist between the condition and the disease; (2) the removal of the condition must reduce the prevalence or incidence of the disease; (3) the condition must precede the disease; (4) the causal relationship between the condition and the disease must be physiologically plausible; (5) research data must consistently reveal a relationship between the condition and the disease; (6) the strength of the relationship between the condition and the disease must be relatively high; and (7) the relationship between the condition and the disease must be based on well-designed studies. When all seven of these criteria are met, scientists can infer a cause-

Table 2.1 Criteria for determining causation between a condition and a disease

1. A dose-response relationship exists between the condition and the disease.
2. Removal of the condition reduces the prevalence or incidence of the disease.
3. The condition precedes the disease.
4. A cause-and-effect relationship between the condition and the disease is physiologically plausible.
5. Relevant research data consistently reveals a relationship between the condition and the disease.
6. The strength of the relationship between the condition and the disease is relatively high.
7. Studies revealing a relationship between the condition and the disease are well-designed.

and-effect relationship between an independent variable (such as smoking) and a dependent variable (such as heart disease or lung cancer).

Research Tools

Psychologists frequently rely on two important tools to conduct research: theoretical models and psychometric instruments. Many, but not all, psychology studies are driven by a theoretical model and are attempts to test hypotheses suggested by that model. Also, many psychology studies rely on measuring devices to assess behaviors, physiological functions, attitudes, abilities, personality traits, and other independent and dependent variables. This section provides a brief discussion of these two tools.

The Role of Theory in Research

As the scientific study of human behavior, psychology shares with other disciplines the use of scientific methods to investigate natural phenomena. The work of science is not restricted to research methodology; it also involves constructing theoretical models to serve as vehicles for making sense of research findings. Health psychologists have developed a number of models and theories to explain health-related behaviors and conditions, such as stress, pain, smoking, alcohol abuse, and unhealthy eating habits. To the uninitiated, theories may seem impractical and superfluous, but scientists regard them as practical tools that give both direction and meaning to their research.

Scientific **theory** has been defined as "a set of related assumptions from which, by logical deductive reasoning, testable hypotheses can be drawn" (Feist & Feist, 1998, p. 4). Theories have an interactive relationship with scientifically derived observations. A theory gives meaning to observations, and observations in turn fit into and alter the theory erected to explain these observations. Theories, then, are dynamic and become more powerful as they expand to explain more and more relevant observations.

Near the beginning of this cycle, when the theoretical framework is still rudimentary and not yet sufficiently comprehensive to explain a large number of observations, the term **model** is more appropriate than theory. In practice, however, *theory* and *model* are sometimes used interchangeably.

The role of theory in health psychology is basically the same as it is in any other scientific discipline. First, a useful theory should generate research—both descriptive research and hypothesis testing. The goal of descriptive research is to expand the existing theory. This type of research deals with measurement, labeling, and categorization of observations. A useful theory of psychosocial factors in heart disease, for example, should generate a multitude of investigations that describe the psychological and social factors of people who have been diagnosed with heart disease. On the other hand, hypothesis testing is not specifically carried out to expand the theory but rather to contribute valid data to the body of scientific knowledge. Again, a useful theory of psychosocial factors in heart disease should stimulate the formulation of a number of hypotheses that, when tested, produce a greater understanding of the psychological and social conditions that relate to heart disease. Results of such studies would either support or fail

to support the existing theory; they ordinarily do not enlarge or alter it.

Second, a useful theory should organize and explain the observations derived from research and make them intelligible. Unless research data are organized into some meaningful framework, scientists have no clear direction to follow in their pursuit of further knowledge. A useful theory of the psychosocial factors in heart disease, for example, should integrate what is currently known about such factors and allow researchers to frame discerning questions that stimulate further research.

Third, a useful theory should serve as a guide to action, permitting the practitioner to predict behavior and to implement strategies to change behavior. A practitioner concerned with helping others change health-related behaviors is greatly aided by a theory of behavior change. For instance, a cognitive therapist will follow a cognitive theory of learning to make decisions about how to help clients and will thus focus on changing the thought processes that affect clients' behaviors. Similarly, psychologists with other theoretical orientations rely on their theories to supply them with solutions to the many questions they confront in their practice.

Theories, then, are useful and necessary tools for the development of any scientific discipline. They generate research that leads to more knowledge, organize and explain observations, and help the practitioner (both the researcher and the clinician) handle a variety of daily problems, such as predicting behavior and helping people change unhealthy practices. Later chapters discuss several theoretical models that are frequently used in health psychology.

The Role of Psychometrics in Research

From the work of Sir Francis Galton (1879, 1883) during the 19th century until the present time, psychology has had a close relationship with the measurement of human abilities and behaviors. Indeed, one of psychology's most important contributions to behavioral medicine and behavioral health is its sophistication in assessment techniques. Nearly every important issue in health psychology demands the measurement of the phenomenon being investigated. Psychologists have reacted to this demand by constructing a number of instruments to assess such behaviors and conditions as stress, pain, the Type A behavior pattern, eating habits, and personal hardiness.

For these or any other measuring instruments to be useful, they must be both *reliable* (consistent) and *valid* (accurate). The problems of establishing reliability and validity are critical to the development of any measurement scale.

Establishing Reliability   The **reliability** of a measuring instrument is the extent to which it yields consistent results. In health psychology, reliability is most frequently determined by comparing scores on two or more administrations of the same instrument (*test-retest reliability*) or by comparing ratings obtained from two or more judges observing the same phenomenon (*interrater reliability*).

Reliability is most frequently expressed in terms of either correlation coefficients or percentages. The correlation coefficient, which expresses the degree of correspondence between two sets of scores, is the same statistic used in correlational studies. High reliability coefficients (such as .80 to .90) indicate that participants have obtained nearly the same scores on two administrations of a test. Percentages can be used to express the degree of agreement between the independent ratings of observers. If that agreement between two or more raters is high (such as 85% to 95%), then the instrument is capable of eliciting nearly the same ratings from two or more interviewers.

Establishing reliability for the numerous assessment instruments used in health psychology is obviously a formidable task, but it is an essential first step in developing useful measuring devices.

Establishing Validity   A second step in constructing assessment scales is to establish their validity. Measuring scales may be reliable and yet lack validity, or accuracy. **Validity** is the extent to which an instrument measures what it is designed to measure.

Psychologists determine the validity of a measuring instrument by comparing scores from that instrument with some independent or outside criterion—that is, a standard that has been assessed independently of the instrument being validated. In health psychology, that criterion is often some future event, such as a diagnosis of heart disease. An instrument capable of predicting who will receive such a diagnosis and who will remain disease free is said to have *predictive validity.* For example, life events scales (see Chapter 5) have been used to measure stress and to predict future mortality or morbidity. For such a scale to demonstrate predictive validity, it must be administered to participants who are currently free of disease. If people who score high on the scale eventually have higher rates of death or disease than participants with low scores, then the scale can be said to have predictive validity; that is, it differentiates between participants who will remain disease free and those who will die or become ill.

In Summary

The work of scientists is aided by two important tools—useful theories and accurate measurement. Useful theories (1) generate research, (2) predict and explain research data, and (3) help the practitioner solve a variety of problems. Accurate psychometric instruments are both reliable and valid. *Reliability* is the extent to which an assessment device measures consistently, and *validity* is the extent to which an assessment instrument measures what it is supposed to measure.

Answers

This chapter addressed five basic questions:

1. **How has psychology contributed to health?**

   Psychology has made several contributions to health: (1) a long tradition of techniques to change behavior; (2) an emphasis on health rather than disease; (3) the development of reliable and valid measuring instruments; and (4) the construction of useful theoretical models to explain health-related research.

This chapter was concerned mostly with a fifth contribution, namely, the various research methods used in psychology. These include (1) case studies, (2) correlational studies, (3) cross-sectional studies and longitudinal studies, (4) experimental designs, and (5) ex post facto designs. Each of these makes its own unique contribution to the understanding of behavior and health. The *case study* is an intensive investigation of one person. *Correlational studies* indicate the degree of association or correlation between two variables, but by themselves, they cannot be used to determine a cause-and-effect relationship. *Cross-sectional studies* investigate a group of people at one point in time whereas *longitudinal studies* follow the participants over an extended period. In general, longitudinal studies are more likely to yield useful and specific results, but they are more time-consuming and expensive than cross-sectional studies. With *experimental designs,* researchers manipulate the independent variable so that any resulting differences between experimental and control groups can be attributed to their differential exposures to the independent variable. Experimental studies typically include a placebo given to people in a control group so that they will have the same expectations as people in the experimental group. *Ex post facto designs* are similar to experimental designs in that researchers compare two or more groups and then record group differences in the dependent variable. However, in the ex post facto study, the experimenter merely selects a subject variable on which two groups have naturally divided themselves rather than creating differences through manipulation.

2. **How has epidemiology contributed to health?**

Modern epidemiology began making significant contributions to health during the 19th century, when it helped conquer such infectious diseases as cholera, smallpox, and typhoid fever. During the 20th century, epidemiology continued to provide basic research that uncovered risk factors for heart disease, cancer, and other lethal diseases.

Many of the research methods used in epidemiology are quite similar to those used in psychology. Epidemiology uses at least three basic kinds of research methodology: (1) observational studies, (2) natural experiments, and (3) experimental studies. *Observational studies,* which parallel the correlation studies used in psychology, are of two types: retrospective and prospective. *Retrospective studies* begin with a group of people already suffering from a disease and then look for characteristics of these people that are different from those of people who do not have that disease; *prospective studies* are longitudinal designs that follow the forward development of a population or sample. *Natural experiments,* which are similar to ex post facto studies, involve selection rather than manipulation of the independent variable. Epidemiology also makes use of *experimental designs,* the two most common of which are *clinical trials* and *community trials.* Occasionally, experimental epidemiological studies are also longitudinal, and these demonstrate cause-and-effect relationships.

Epidemiology has also contributed the concepts of risk factor, prevalence and incidence. A *risk factor* is any characteristic or condition that occurs with greater frequency in people with a disease than it does in people free from that disease. *Prevalence* is the proportion of the population that has a particular disease at a specific time; *incidence* measures the frequency of new cases of the disease during a specified time.

3. **How can scientists determine if a behavior causes disease or death?**

Seven criteria are used for determining a cause-and-effect relationship between a condition and a disease: (1) A dose-response relationship must exist between the condition and the disease;

(2) the removal of the condition must reduce the prevalence or incidence of the disease; (3) the condition must precede the disease; (4) the causal relationship between the condition and the disease must be physiologically plausible; (5) research data must consistently reveal a relationship between the condition and the disease; (6) the strength of the relationship between the condition and the disease must be relatively high; and (7) the relationship between the condition and the disease must be based on well-designed studies.

4. **What is the role of theory in scientific research?**

   Theories are important tools used by scientists to (1) generate research, (2) predict and explain research data, and (3) help the practitioner solve a variety of problems.

5. **What is the role of measurement in scientific research?**

   Psychometric instruments, to be useful, must be both reliable and valid. *Reliability* is the extent to which an assessment device measures consistently, and *validity* is the extent to which an assessment instrument measures what it is supposed to measure.

Glossary

absolute risk A person's chances to developing a disease or disorder independent of any risk that other people may have for that disease or disorder.

atherosclerosis The formation of plaque within the arteries.

cardiologist A medical doctor who specializes in the diagnosis and treatment of heart disease.

case-control study A retrospective epidemiological study in which people affected by a given disease (cases) are compared to others not affected (controls).

case study A type of single-subject design in which one individual is studied in depth.

cohort A group of subjects starting an experience at the same time.

correlation coefficient Any positive or negative relationship between two variables. Correlational evidence cannot prove causation, but only that two variables vary together.

correlational studies Studies designed to yield information concerning the degree of relationship between two variables.

cross-sectional study A type of research design in which subjects of different ages are studied at one point in time.

dependent variable A variable within an experimental setting whose value is hypothesized to change as a consequence of changes in the independent variable.

descriptive research A type of research that describes the relationship between variables, rather than determining causation.

dose-response relationship A direct, consistent relationship between an independent variable, such as a behavior, and a dependent variable, such as an illness. For example, the greater the number of cigarettes one smokes, the greater the likelihood of lung cancer.

double blind An experimental design in which neither the subjects nor those who dispense the treatment condition have knowledge of who receives the treatment and who receives the placebo.

electrocardiogram (ECG) A measure of electrical signals of the heart.

epidemiology A branch of medicine that investigates the various factors that contribute to either positive health or to the frequency and distribution of a disease or disorder.

ex post facto designs Scientific studies in which the values of the independent variable are not manipulated, but selected by the experimenter *after* the groups have naturally divided themselves.

incidence A measure of the frequency of new cases of a disease or disorder during a specified period of time.

independent variable A variable that is manipulated by the experimenter in order to assess its possible effect on behavior; that is, on the dependent variable.

longitudinal studies Research designs in which one group of subjects is studied over a period of time.

meta-analysis A statistical technique for combining results of several studies when these studies have similar definitions of variables.

model A set of related principles or hypotheses constructed to explain significant relationships among concepts or observations.

nocebo effect   Adverse effect of a placebo.

placebo   An inactive substance or condition that has the appearance of the independent variable and that may cause subjects in an experiment to improve or change behavior due to their belief in the placebo's efficacy; a treatment that is effective because of a patient's belief in the treatment.

prevalence   The proportion of a population that has a disease or disorder at a specific point in time.

prospective studies   Longitudinal studies that begin with a disease-free group of subjects and follow the occurrence of disease in that population or sample.

reliability   The extent to which a test or other measuring instrument yields consistent results.

relative risk   The risk a person has for a particular disease compared with the risk of other people who do not have that person's condition or lifestyle.

retrospective studies   Longitudinal studies that look back at the history of a population or sample.

risk factor   A characteristic or condition that occurs with greater frequency in people with a disease than it does in people free from that disease.

self-selection   A condition of an experimental investigation in which subjects are allowed, in some manner, to determine their own placement in either the experimental or the control group.

subject variable   A variable chosen (rather than manipulated) by a researcher to provide levels of comparison for groups of subjects.

theory   A set of related assumptions from which testable hypotheses can be drawn.

validity   Accuracy; the extent to which a test or other measuring instrument measures what it is supposed to measure.

Suggested Readings

Beaglehole, R., Bonita, R., & Kjellström, T. (1993). *Basic epidemiology.* Geneva, Switzerland: World Health Organization.

An introduction to basic epidemiological methods, including types of studies, definitions, and an insightful discussion of the necessary and sufficient conditions for establishing causes of a disease.

Brown, W. A. (1997). The best medicine? *Psychology Today, 30*(5), 56–60, 80, 82.

This review of placebo effects includes the benefits of placebos in curing a variety of disorders and advice concerning boosting the positive effects of placebos. Available through InfoTrac College Edition by Wadsworth Publishing Company.

Morgan, W. P. (1997). Methodological considerations. In W. P. Morgan (Ed.), *Physical activity and mental health* (pp. 3–32). Washington, DC: Taylor & Francis.

In this chapter, William Morgan offers an insightful review of the methodological problems involved in discovering evidence for a link between physical activity and psychological health, but his recommendations can be extended to the association between any health-related behavior and its consequence.

Susser, M. (1991). What is a cause and how do we know one? A grammar for pragmatic epidemiology. *American Journal of Epidemiology, 133,* 635–648.

Since the 1950s, epidemiologists have developed ways of showing causality in nonexperimental designs, and in this practical article, Susser presents criteria for making these causal inferences.

CHAPTER 3

Seeking Health Care

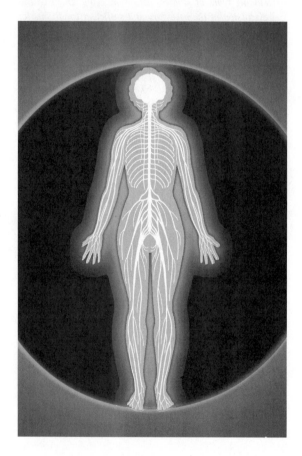

QUESTIONS

This chapter focuses on four basic questions:

1. Why do people adopt health-related behaviors?

2. What factors are related to seeking medical attention?

3. What is involved in the experience of hospitalization?

4. How can people prepare for stressful medical procedures?

JEFF: WHEN TO SEEK MEDICAL ATTENTION

While playing a game of half-court basketball, Jeff jabbed his right hand on the backboard and felt an immediate pain. However, he continued playing, as minor injuries were merely "part of the game." For the rest of the day, his hand continued to hurt, and he had difficulty writing, eating, or using the hand for other tasks. The next day, Jeff's hand was somewhat discolored and quite swollen. To reduce the swelling, he wrapped an ice pack around the hand for 20 to 30 minutes two or three times that day. Still, Jeff continued with his daily activities as well as he could, believing that the swelling would soon disappear. On the third day, however, his hand was no better, so he decided to seek advice. But the advice he sought was not from a physician or other health practitioner; rather, it was from two colleagues at his law office, neither of whom had any medical training. Both colleagues advised Jeff to have his hand X-rayed to learn whether it was broken. Still Jeff hesitated. He did not want to miss work, and he knew that being X-rayed and seeing a doctor would be time-consuming.

When he finally decided that an X ray was warranted, Jeff went to a local imaging center that specialized in X rays. The person at the imaging center informed Jeff that his hand could not be X-rayed there unless he was referred by a physician. Indeed, she seemed shocked that anyone would come to the imaging center without a physician's referral. So Jeff called his internist and asked her to order an X ray, which she did. The internist also referred him to an orthopedic specialist, whom he saw the next day. Results of the X ray revealed a broken metacarpal—that is, the part of the hand between the wrist and the fingers. Jeff's hand was put into a cast, and 6 weeks passed before he played any more basketball or used his right hand for nearly anything else.

Why was Jeff reluctant to seek medical care? Why was the pain he experienced not sufficient to prompt him go to the doctor? Why did he ask the opinion of people with no medical training before getting advice from a trained professional?

Adopting Health-Related Behaviors

Most people in the world value health and want to avoid disease and disability. Nevertheless, many people do not behave in ways that maximize health and minimize disease and disability. Why do some people, such as Jeff, seem to behave unwisely on issues of personal health? Why do others seek medical treatment when they are not ill? What explains people's reluctance to believe that their own risky behaviors are safe and their willingness to believe that those same behaviors place other people in jeopardy? No final answers to these questions are possible at this point, but psychologists have formulated several theories or models in the attempt to predict and make sense of behaviors related to health. This chapter looks briefly at some of these theories as they relate to health-seeking behavior, whereas Chapter 4 examines theory-driven research about people's adherence to medical advice.

Theories of Health-Protective Behaviors

In Chapter 2, we said that useful theories (1) generate research, (2) organize and explain observations, and (3) guide the practitioner in predicting behavior. Health psychologists frequently use theoretical models to meet each of these criteria. These models include the health belief model, which originally grew out of the work of Geoffrey Hochbaum (1958) and his colleagues at the Public Health Service; the theory of reasoned action by Martin Fishbein and Icek Ajzen (Ajzen & Fishbein, 1980; Fishbein & Ajzen, 1975); the concept of planned behavior, which Ajzen developed as an alternative to the theory of reasoned action (Ajzen, 1985, 1991): the self-regulation theory of Albert Bandura (1977, 1986); the precaution adoption process model of Neil Weinstein (Weinstein, 1988), and the transtheoretical model of James Prochaska and his colleagues (Prochaska, DiClemente, & Norcross, 1992).

CHECK YOUR HEALTH RISKS

Check the items that apply to you.

☐ 1. If I feel well, I believe that I am healthy.

☐ 2. I know that it is important to have regular medical and dental checkups, but somehow I don't manage to do so.

☐ 3. The last time I sought medical care was in a hospital emergency room.

☐ 4. Only severe symptoms of disease are worth worrying about.

☐ 5. If I had a disease that would be a lot of trouble to manage, I would rather not know about it until I was really sick.

☐ 6. I try not to allow being sick to slow me down.

☐ 7. I feel reluctant to ask questions of my physician, even when I don't understand the explanation or instructions.

☐ 8. I think it's better to follow medical advice than to ask questions and cause problems, especially in the hospital.

☐ 9. When facing a stressful medical experience, I think the best strategy is to try not to think about it and hope that it will be over soon.

☐ 10. I would rather not have a lot of information about my medical condition because I can't do anything anyway.

☐ 11. In order not to frighten children faced with a difficult medical procedure, it is best to tell them that they won't be hurt, even if they will.

Each of these items represents an attitude or behavior that may present a risk or lead you to less effective health care. As you read this chapter, you will see the advantages of adopting other attitudes or behaviors to make more effective use of the health care system.

Each of these items represents a naive or unrealistic view of research that can make you an uninformed consumer of health research. Count your check marks to see if you have any naive or unscientific views about health-related research. Information in this chapter will help you become more accurate in your evaluation of and expectations for health research.

The Health Belief Model   Since the early work of Geoffrey Hochbaum (1958), several versions of the *health belief model* (HBM) have been devised. The one that has attracted the most attention and generated the most research is that of Marshall Becker and Irwin Rosenstock (Becker, 1979; Becker & Rosenstock, 1984; Rosenstock, 1990; Strecher, Champion, & Rosenstock, 1997).

Like all health belief models, the one developed by Becker and Rosenstock assumes that beliefs are important contributors to health-seeking behavior. This model includes four beliefs or perceptions that should combine to predict health-related behaviors, such as Jeff's eventual decision to seek the aid of an orthopedic physician when he broke his hand: (1) perceived *susceptibility* to disease or disability, (2) perceived *severity* of the disease or disability, (3) perceived *benefits* of health-enhancing behaviors, and (4) perceived *barriers* to health-enhancing behaviors. After first hurting his hand, Jeff did not believe that his injury was serious or that he was vulnerable to disability. Thus, he saw little benefit in going to a doctor, an action that would have been costly in terms of money and time. After two of his colleagues expressed their belief that his injury might be serious and after two days of eating, driving, writing, and dressing with his left hand, Jeff changed his beliefs and subsequently sought medical attention.

The health belief model corresponds with common sense, but does it predict health-related behavior? Research on the utility of the health belief model has been extensive, but the results have been inconsistent, partially because researchers have not always used reliable and valid measures of its various components (Strecher, Champion, & Rosenstock, 1997).

If the health belief model is useful, then interventions to change beliefs should be effective. Beginning with this assumption, Victoria Champion (1994) used the HBM to inform women with no family history of breast cancer about the benefits of **mammography.** Women who received an intervention aimed at enhancing their knowledge and changing their beliefs were nearly four times more likely to seek mammography testing than an equivalent group of women in a control group. However, a prospective study (Hyman, Baker, Ephraim, Moadel, & Philip, 1994) indicated that perceived susceptibility to breast cancer did not predict a woman's mammography use, although both perceived benefits and perceived barriers did. Moreover, ethnicity was a better predictor than either benefits or barriers, with African American women being more likely to use mammography than European Americans. Although the health belief model has some utility in predicting mammography services, some research (Aiken, West, Woodward, & Reno, 1994) has found that having a regular place to go for health care and having a physician who recommended a mammogram were better predictors than the combined factors of the health belief model. Incidentally, none of these studies included the factor of perceived severity as a predictor of mammography use because they assumed that nearly all women view breast cancer as a severe disease.

The health belief model, of course, has been used to predict health-related behaviors other than mammography use. Some studies have found the HBM to predict safe sex behaviors (Abraham & Sheeran, 1994; Zimmerman & Olson, 1994). How-ever, studies that showed the strongest predictive value of the HBM generally used an expanded version of the model, including cues to action, self-efficacy, intentions to behave, and perceived social norms. For this reason, some researchers have begun to combine aspects of the health belief model with concepts from other models, including the theory of reasoned action.

The Theory of Reasoned Action   The *theory of reasoned action* (Ajzen & Fishbein, 1980; Fishbein & Ajzen, 1975) assumes that people are quite reasonable and make systematic use of information when deciding how to behave. Moreover, they "consider the implications of their actions before they decide to engage or not engage in a given behavior" (Ajzen, 1985, p. 5). In addition, the theory of reasoned action assumes that behavior is directed toward a goal or outcome and that people freely choose those actions that they believe will move them in the direction of that goal. They can also choose not to act, if they believe that such an action would move them away from their goal, as when Jeff decided not to seek immediate medical attention because he believed that a cast on his hand would hamper his regular work routine.

The immediate determinant of behavior is the *intention* to act or not to act. Intentions, in turn, are shaped by two factors. The first is a personal evaluation of the behavior—that is, one's *attitude toward the behavior.* The second is one's perception of the social pressure to perform or not perform the action—that is, one's *subjective norm.* One's attitude toward the behavior is determined by beliefs that the behavior will lead to positively or negatively valued outcomes. One's subjective norm is shaped by one's perception of the evaluation that a particular individual (or group of individuals) places on that behavior and one's *motivation* to comply with the norms set by that individual (or group of individuals). In predicting behavior, the theory of reasoned action also considers the relative weight of personal attitudes measured against subjective norms (see Figure 3.1).

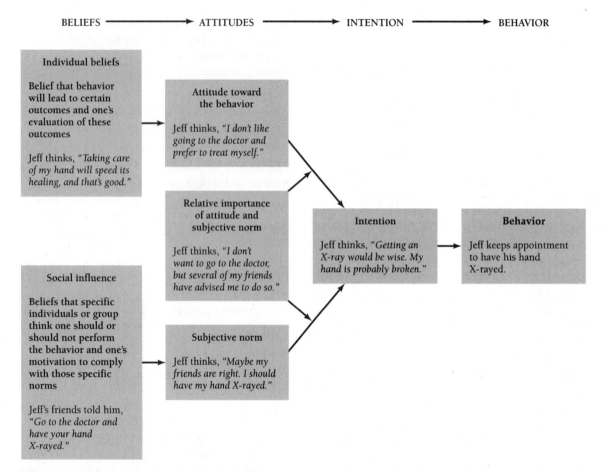

Figure 3.1   Theory of reasoned action applied to health-seeking behavior.   *Source:* Adapted from *Understanding Attitudes and Predicting Social Behavior* (p. 8), by I. Ajzen and M. Fishbein, 1980, Englewood Cliffs, NJ: Prentice-Hall. Copyright © 1980 by Prentice-Hall, Inc. Reprinted by permission.

In predicting whether Jeff, with a painful, discolored, and swollen hand, will seek medical attention, the theory of reasoned action relies on several pieces of information. First, does he believe that going to the doctor's office is related to his goal of a healthy hand? Second, how strong is his belief that other people expect him to seek medical attention balanced against his need to comply with others' expectations? The answer to the first question reveals Jeff's attitude toward seeking medical assistance, and the answer to the

second question suggests the level of social pressure on him to seek assistance. These two answers reflect his attitude toward seeking medical care and his subjective norm about seeking care. Because Jeff's attitudes and his subjective norms were initially in conflict, his early intention was somewhat mixed, making prediction of his behavior difficult. Nevertheless, the theory of reasoned action has the potential to make valid predictions when investigators accurately measure both the strength of a person's attitude toward a behavior and the person's need to conform to social norms.

Does the theory of reasoned action predict health-seeking behavior? In general, researchers have found the theory to be useful for predicting certain health-related behaviors, including use of mammograms, breast self-examination, and attendance at health-information classes. In the study on mammography (Montano, Thompson, Taylor, & Mahloch, 1997), low-income women were questioned regarding their attitude, subjective norms, intentions, and previous use of mammography. All basic components of the model were significantly related to intention to get a mammogram, and intention predicted use of mammography. In the study of breast self-examination, intention to perform breast self-examination (Lierman, Kasprzyk, & Benoliel, 1991), a modified version of the theory of reasoned action was a strong predictor of who would perform breast self-examination and who would not. Research (Michie, Marteau, & Kidd, 1992), has also found that pregnant women's intention to attend health-information classes after delivery was a good predictor of attendance, but other factors also contributed, including social norms and the attitude of the baby's father.

In each of these studies, intention to perform was a strong predictor of behavior. However, past performance may be an even more powerful predictor of future performance. One study that compared the usefulness of the theory of reasoned action, the theory of planned behavior, and an extension of the theory of reasoned action that included past behavior (O'Callaghan, Chant, Callan, & Baglioni, 1997) found that the extended theory of reasoned action offered the best prediction of alcohol use among young adults. Intention to drink was a strong predictor of who would drink and who would not, but past drinking experience and perception of what peers thought they should do (subjective norms) both predicted intention.

Although these studies did not directly compare the usefulness of the theory of reasoned action with the health belief model, the results indicate that the theory of reasoned action is at least as adequate as the health belief model in explaining and predicting health-seeking behaviors. A key element in the theory of reasoned action seems to be the intention to perform a behavior.

The Theory of Planned Behavior Ajzen has extended the theory of reasoned action to include the concept of perceived behavioral control, an extension he calls the *theory of planned behavior*. The primary difference between the theory of reasoned action and the theory of planned behavior is the latter's inclusion of the *perception of how much control* people have over their behavior (Ajzen, 1985, 1988, 1991). The more resources and opportunities people believe they have, the stronger are their beliefs that they can control their behavior. Figure 3.2 shows that predictions of behavior can be made from knowledge of (1) people's attitude toward the behavior, (2) their subjective norm, and (3) their perceived behavioral control. All three components interact to shape people's intentions to behave. In addition, perceived behavioral control may have a direct influence on people's behavior (Ajzen, 1991). Perceived behavioral control is the ease or difficulty one has in achieving desired behavioral outcomes; it reflects both past behaviors and perceived ability to overcome obstacles. Perceived behavioral control operates both directly and indirectly to influence behavior. The direct path is the actual control a person has over performing the behavior. This direct path may occur when people perform behaviors almost automatically, such as brushing their teeth. In addition, perceived personal control operates indirectly to shape behavior by influencing people's intention to behave. The theory assumes that people who believe they can easily perform a behavior are more likely to *intend* to perform that behavior than people who believe they have little control over performing that behavior.

The theory of planned behavior has not yet produced the quantity of health-related research

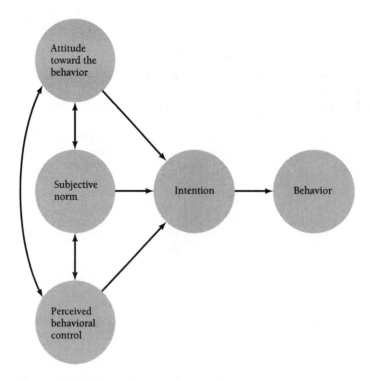

Figure 3.2   Theory of planned behavior.   *Source:*   From "The theory of planned behavior," by I. Ajzen, 1991, *Organizational Behavior and Human Decision Processes,* 50, p. 182. Reprinted by permission of Academic Press.

that the health belief model has generated, but a few studies have provided some confirmation of the theory. For example, two recent studies (Hill, Boudreau, Amyot, Dery, & Godin, 1997; Maher, & Rickwood, 1997) found that the theory of planned behavior predicts adolescent smoking, and another study (Norman & Conner, 1993) found the model to be useful in predicting attendance in a health check program. In this last study, intention and perceived behavior control were strong and independent predictors of attendance. A fourth study (McCaul, Sandgren, O'Neill, & Hinsz, 1993) reported that the model's concepts of attitude toward the behavior, subjective norms, and perceived control each predicted undergraduate students' health-related behaviors such as breast

self-examination, testicular self-examination, and dental flossing.

Self-Regulation Theory   Like the theory of reasoned action and the theory of planned behavior, Albert Bandura's social cognitive *self-regulation theory* is a general theory of behavior and not limited to predicting health-seeking behaviors. Bandura's theory of self-regulation stresses the interaction of behavior, environment, and person factors, especially cognition. Bandura (1986) referred to this interactive triadic model as **reciprocal determinism.** An important component of the person variable is self-efficacy.

Self-efficacy refers to "people's beliefs about their capabilities to exercise control over events that affect their lives" (Bandura, 1989, p. 1175). Self-efficacy is a specific rather than a global concept; that is, it refers to people's beliefs that they can perform those behaviors that will produce desired outcomes in any *particular* situation. Bandura (1986) suggested that self-efficacy can be acquired, enhanced, or decreased through one of four sources: (1) performance, or enacting a behavior; (2) vicarious experience, or seeing another person with similar skills perform a behavior; (3) verbal persuasion, or listening to the encouraging words of a trusted person; and (4) physiological arousal states such as anxiety, which ordinarily decrease feelings of self-efficacy. Bandura believes that the combination of self-efficacy and specific goals is an important predictor of behavior.

Although self-efficacy has attracted a great deal of research attention, it is but one aspect of Bandura's self-regulation theory. Bandura (1986) contended that our behavior is motivated and regulated by the continual exercise of self-influence, including (1) monitoring the determinants and the effects of our behavior, (2) judging our behavior in terms of personal standards and environmental circumstances, and (3) responding positively or negatively to our behavior depending on how it measures up to our personal standards.

Research on self-regulation and self-efficacy theories generally shows a positive relationship between levels of self-efficacy and health-seeking behaviors. For example, participants in the Stanford Five-City Project who had most difficulty changing behaviors related to cardiovascular disease also had low self-efficacy concerning their ability to make such changes (Winkleby, Flora, & Kraemer, 1994). Another study, (Borrelli & Mermelstein, 1994) examined the role of self-efficacy and goal setting among participants in a smoking cessation program and found that self-efficacy, or the confidence in being able to quit smoking and maintain abstinence, accurately predicted who would reach their subgoals and who would attain abstinence. A more recent study (Conn, 1998) looked at the ability of self-efficacy to predict exercise, stress management, and eating behavior

among older women and found that self-efficacy was a stronger predictor than outcome expectations for each of these three behaviors.

Despite some success of self-efficacy theory to predict health-seeking behaviors, research concerning its added advantage over the theories of reasoned action and planned behavior has produced inconsistent results. For example, McCaul et al. (1993) found the theory of planned behavior to be a better predictor of breast self-examination than a self-efficacy model. However, Tedesco, Keffer, Davis, and Christersson (1993) found that self-efficacy added significantly to the theory of reasoned action in predicting self-reports of brushing and flossing of people suffering from dental disease.

The Precaution Adoption Process Model Neil Weinstein (Weinstein, Rothman, & Sutton, 1998) has criticized the health belief model, the theory of reasoned action, the theory of planned behavior, and self-regulation theory for ignoring people's transition from one stage to another in their readiness to adopt health related behaviors. Arguing that these theories merely identify variables that might influence each individual's actions, he combines them in a single equation that might predict that person's likelihood of enacting a particular behavior. The *precaution adoption process model* (Weinstein, 1988) assumes that when people begin new and relatively complex behaviors aimed at protecting themselves from harm, they go through several stages of belief about their personal susceptibility. No single equation can predict behavior in all stages. Weinstein holds that stage theories, such as his precaution adoption process model and Prochaska's transtheoretical model, are superior to theories that fail to consider a person's transition from one stage to another. People do not move inevitably through the stages, and they may even move backward, as when a person who previously had considered stopping smoking abandons that consideration.

Weinstein's precaution adoption process model holds that people move through seven stages in

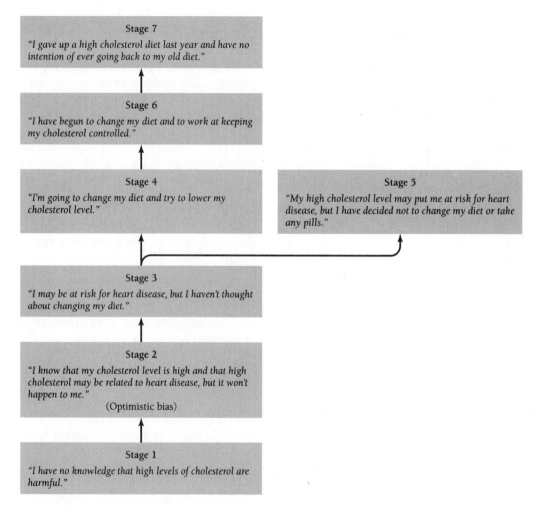

Figure 3.3   Weinstein's seven stages of the precaution adoption process model.

their readiness to adopt a health-related behavior (see Figure 3.3). In Stage 1, people have not heard of the hazard and thus are unaware of any personal risk. In Stage 2, they are aware of the hazard and believe that others are at risk, but they hold an **optimistic bias** regarding their own level of risk. Stage 3 people acknowledge their personal susceptibility and accept the notion that precaution would be personally effective, but they have not yet decided to take action. In Stage 4, people decide to take action, whereas in the parallel Stage 5, people decide

that action is unnecessary. In Stage 6, people have already taken the precautions aimed at reducing risks. Stage 7 involves maintaining the precaution, if needed. Maintenance would be unnecessary in the case of a lifetime vaccination, but it is essential for smoking cessation or dietary changes. Before people take action, they must first perceive that the relative benefits of the precaution outweigh its costs. The variables that influence action fluctuate, so that people who do not act at one point in time may do so at another time.

Although Weinstein's notion of optimistic bias has generated substantial research, his more global concept of the precaution adoption process model has attracted less attention from researchers. One study (Blalock et al., 1996) of 35- to 45-year-old women reported that this model was useful in predicting calcium consumption and weight-bearing exercise, two behaviors recommended to reduce the risk of osteoporosis. These researchers found that: (1) the women's stages of change paralleled their knowledge of and attitude toward osteoporosis; (2) Weinstein's stages of change were related to the women's perceived benefits of exercise and calcium consumption as well as to the inconvenience of these two behaviors; (3) women at the different stages differed in their requests for information on osteoporosis, with those at the higher stages wanting to know more about the illness; and (4) contrary to expectations, women who had given up exercise and extra calcium consumption did not have the *least* favorable attitudes toward those two behaviors. The authors of this study concluded that these findings offered considerable support for the precaution adoption process model.

An earlier test of the precaution adoption process model (Boney McCoy et al., 1992) looked at the relationship between smoking status and perceptions of smoking risk. As expected, smokers in a cessation clinic reported the highest perceived risk for smoking and the greatest perceived benefit of not smoking whereas current smokers reported the lowest perceived risk and the least benefit of quitting. Also, current smokers in this study showed an optimistic bias. When asked to estimate their own risks and the risks of the "typical smoker" for developing coronary heart disease, emphysema, and lung cancer, most current smokers who were not trying to quit saw that smoking was dangerous, but they retained an optimistic bias that harm would not come to them. Thus, these smokers had not advanced to Stage 3 of Weinstein's model. However, Stage 5 smokers—those in the cessation clinic—saw their risks as very high and had already made a decision to

quit. Former smokers—those who had actually quit—perceived that smoking was a health hazard. This study supported Weinstein's contentions that people adopt a precaution only after they perceive personal susceptibility, see that the hazard is detrimental to them, evaluate the precaution as personally effective, and appraise the benefits of the precautions over the risk of taking them.

The Transtheoretical Model   Another stage theory that attempts to explain and predict changes in health-seeking behavior is the *transtheoretical model* developed by James Prochaska and his colleagues (Prochaska, DiClemente, & Norcross, 1992). This model assumes that people progress through five stages in making changes in behavior: precontemplation, contemplation, preparation, action, and maintenance.

People in the precontemplation stage have no intention of changing their behavior and may fail to see that they have a problem. The contemplation stage involves awareness of the problem and thoughts about changing behavior within the next 6 months, but people in this stage have not yet made an effort to change. The preparation stage includes both thoughts and action, and people in this stage make specific plans about change. The modification of behavior comes in the action stage, when people make overt changes in their behavior. During the maintenance stage, people try to sustain the changes they have made and to resist temptation to relapse. Prochaska et al. (1992) maintained that people move from one stage to another in a spiral rather than a linear fashion, with several relapses that recycle people into a previous stage from which they again progress through the stages until they have completed their behavioral change. Thus, relapses are to be expected and can serve as learning experiences that help people recycle back through the stages.

Prochaska et al. suggested that people in each of these stages need different types of assistance in making changes. For example, change efforts aimed at people in the precontemplation stage will be unsuccessful because these people do not believe they have a problem. On the other hand, people in the preparation stage do not need to be convinced to change their behavior; they need specific suggestions about how to change. Those in the maintenance stage need help or information oriented toward preserving their changes.

Does the transtheoretical model apply equally to different problem behaviors? Prochaska and his colleagues (Prochaska, 1994; Prochaska, Velicer, et al., 1994) have looked at the model across 12 problem behaviors, including quitting smoking, controlling weight, practicing safe sex, and utilizing mammography screening. They found clear commonalities among the 12 problem areas in that people progress from precontemplation to action in each of these areas by weighing the pros and cons of behavior change.

Investigations by other researchers have also uncovered some value for the transtheoretical model. A study of women with a current or past diagnosis of **bulimia** (Levy, 1997) found, as expected, that preference for type of treatment matched closely with a woman's stage of change. This finding is important to therapists because it suggests that choice of therapy should be consistent with a person's readiness to change. Another study (Glanz et al., 1994) that applied the transtheoretical model to adopting healthy diets found, as one would expect, that people in the precontemplation, contemplation, and preparation stages tended to eat high-fat diets whereas those in the action and maintenance stages ate less fat and more vegetables. Although the stages-of-change variables predicted dietary intake better than either demographic variables or a measure of body mass, their ability to predict changes in eating habits was quite modest.

Critique of Health-Related Theories

In Chapter 2 we said that a useful theory should (1) generate significant research, (2) organize and explain observations, and (3) help the practitioner predict and change behaviors. How well do these health-related theories meet these three criteria?

First, the older theories—namely, the health belief model, the theory of reasoned action, and self-efficacy theory—have all produced substantial amounts of research, and the newer models show promise of stimulating additional research. In addition, all these models are able to do better than chance in explaining and predicting behavior, and they generally are more accurate than demographic factors in predicting health-related behaviors.

Despite some modest success of health-related theories, there is still a need for models that more accurately differentiate between people who will seek medical attention and those who will not in a variety of health-related situations. One review of the effectiveness of the health belief model, the theory of reasoned action, the theory of planned behavior, and self-efficacy theory as they applied to cardiovascular disease risk reduction found weaknesses in each of the models (Fleury, 1992). This review looked at 10 studies that used the health belief model and concluded that, at best, this model has yielded inconsistent results when attempting to predict or explain behavior of people diagnosed with heart disease. The review found somewhat more support for the theory of reasoned action and the theory of planned behavior, largely because both these theories include the concept of intention, which is a strong factor in predicting health-related behaviors. However, the subjective norm factor was only a weak predictor of behavior. The review also included 14 studies on self-efficacy and concluded that efficacy expectations can be important in a person's decision to initiate health-related behaviors, but its role in maintaining change is much less clear. Also, people may feel confident that they can change a behavior, as in giving up alcohol, but they may place more value on secondary benefits of drinking, such as visiting a favorite bar or drinking with friends. Self-efficacy theory does not weigh the differential values of drinking cessation and maintaining a risk-producing lifestyle.

Why are these theories somewhat less than adequate in explaining and predicting health-related behaviors? Several reasons exist. First, health-seeking behavior is determined by factors other than an individual's beliefs or perceptions. Rosenstock (1990) pointed out that interpersonal processes, institutional factors, community factors, and public policy (including law) all affect health-seeking behaviors. Rosenstock further commented that some health-related behaviors, such as cigarette smoking and dental care, can develop into habits that become so automatic that they are largely beyond the personal decision-making process. In addition, other health-producing behaviors, such as dietary changes, may be undertaken for the sake of personal appearance rather than health.

Another reason for the failure of theories to better predict health-seeking behaviors is that they must rely on consistent and accurate instruments to assess their various components, and such measures have not yet been developed. The health belief model, for example, might more accurately predict health-seeking behavior if valid measurements existed for each of its components. If a person feels susceptible to a disease, perceives his or her symptoms to be severe, believes that treatment will be effective, and sees few barriers, then logically, that person should seek health care. But each of these four factors is difficult to assess.

Also, a model may have some value for predicting health-seeking behaviors related to one disorder but not to another. Similarly, a theory may relate to health-seeking behavior but not to prevention behavior or to adherence to medical advice. No current theory is comprehensive enough to encompass all these areas. Also, the theories seldom consider that many people, such as children and some elderly persons, are often sent to health care professionals by someone else and have only limited choice in seeking care.

Finally, most of the models postulate some type of barrier or obstacle to seeking health care, and an almost unlimited number of barriers are possible. Often these barriers are beyond the life experience of researchers. For example, barriers for affluent European Americans may be quite different from those of poor Hispanic Americans or African Americans; thus, the health belief model, the theory of reasoned action, and self-efficacy theory may not apply to many Hispanic or African Americans (Cochran & Mays, 1993). These models tend to emphasize the importance of direct and personal control of behavioral choices. Little allowance is made for such barriers as racism and poverty. These and other barriers are rarely considered, much less accurately measured, by researchers testing the efficacy of health-related models.

In Summary

If and how people go about seeking medical attention when they feel unwell depends on several factors, many of which are included in one or more of the theories of health-seeking behaviors. Some of these determinants are (1) the characteristics of the symptoms being experienced, (2) the cost/benefit ratio of seeking help, (3) the perceived severity of the disease, (4) a person's intention to act, (5) a person's stage of readiness for change, and (6) multiple social and demographic factors.

People adopt health-related behaviors in order to stay healthy and to combat disease. Several theoretical models have been formulated in an effort to explain and predict health behaviors, and most of these theories have some value in predicting and explaining health-related behavior. However, all of them have some limitations, especially in their ability to predict the health-related behaviors of people who lack the financial resources necessary to pursue proper medical attention.

Current theories drawing the most interest among researchers include the health belief model, the theory of reasoned action, the theory of planned behavior, self-regulation theory, the precaution adoption process model, and the transtheoretical model. The health belief model includes the concepts of perceived severity of the disease, personal susceptibility, and perceived benefits of and barriers to health-enhancing behaviors. Research has shown that the health belief model has only limited success in predicting health-related behaviors.

The theory of reasoned action and the theory of planned behavior both include attitudes, subjective norms, and intention in an effort to predict and explain behavior. Moreover, the theory of planned behavior adds the person's perceived behavioral control. Research has found that the concepts of intention and perceived behavioral control are powerful predictors of health-seeking behaviors. Albert Bandura's self-regulation theory and its component self-efficacy have both generated volumes of research, only some of which relates to health-seeking behaviors. Although self-regulation theory has some validity in predicting behavior, people's motivation to adopt healthy behaviors must accompany their sense of self-efficacy. The precaution adoption process model of Neil Weinstein assumes that when people are faced with adopting health protective behaviors, they go through seven possible stages of belief about their personal susceptibility. Among these stages is the necessity of overcoming their optimistic bias; that is, their belief that although certain behaviors are dangerous, the danger pertains to other people and not to them. James Prochaska's transtheoretical model assumes that people progress through five stages in making changes in behavior—precontemplation, contemplation, preparation, action, and maintenance. As with each of the other models, more research is needed to establish the usefulness of the transtheoretical model. A further limitation of these models is their inability to accurately measure myriad social, ethnic, and demographic factors that also affect people's health-seeking behavior.

The balance of this chapter discusses issues involved in seeking medical attention, the problems of being in the hospital, and the preparations necessary to cope with stressful medical procedures.

Seeking Medical Attention

How do people know when to seek medical attention? How do they know whether they are ill or not? When Jeff injured his hand, he experienced pain that persisted for hours, yet he tried several alternatives before he sought medical attention. Those alternatives included home care and consulting nonexperts about his injury. Was Jeff unusually reluctant to seek medical care or was his behavior typical? Deciding when formal medical care is necessary is a difficult problem, compounded by personal, social, and economic factors. These issues come up later, but first a consideration of health, illness, and disease is in order.

Although the meaning of these three terms may seem obvious, their definitions have been elusive. Is health the absence of illness, or is it the attainment of some positive state? In the first chapter, we saw that the World Health Organization (WHO) defined health as positive physical, mental, and social well-being, and not merely as the absence of disease or infirmity. Unfortunately, this definition has little practical value for people trying to make decisions about their state of health or illness. Another difficulty for many people is the difference between illness and disease. These terms are often used interchangeably, but most health scientists make a distinction between illness and disease. Disease refers to the process of physical damage within the body, and this type of physical disorder can be identified through medical testing and diagnosis. Illness, on the other hand, refers to the experience of being sick, including discomfort and distress. People can be ill and have no identifiable disease. For example, people may feel bad and seek medical attention only to be told that nothing is wrong. On the other hand, people can have a disease and not be ill. For example, people with undiagnosed hypertension, HIV infection, or cancer all have a disease, but they may appear quite healthy and be completely unaware of their disease. Therefore, illness and disease may be separate conditions or they may overlap.

People frequently experience physical symptoms, but these symptoms may or may not indicate a disease. Symptoms such as a headache, a painful shoulder, sniffles, and sneezing would probably not prompt a person to seek medical care, but an intense and persistent stomach pain probably would. At what point should a person decide to seek health care? Errors in both directions are possible. People who decide to go to the doctor when they are not really sick feel foolish, must pay the bill for an office visit, and lose credibility with people who know about the error, including the physician. If they choose not to seek health care, they may get better, but they may remain uncomfortable from symptoms and become even sicker, thus making their disease more difficult to treat. In some cases, this behavior can seriously endanger their health or increase their risk of death. A prudent action would seem to be to chance the unnecessary visit, but research indicates that people are often reluctant to go to the doctor (Feldman, 1966).

Without a visit to a physician, one is not "officially" ill because in our culture, the physician is the gatekeeper to further health care; physicians not only *determine* disease by their diagnoses but also *sanction* it by giving a diagnosis. Hence, the person with symptoms is not the one who officially determines his or her health status. Instead, the practitioner makes the diagnosis that determines the disease. Jeff's case illustrates this process. The imaging center would not provide him with an X ray of his hand without a physician's referral—the gate to medical care was closed without a physician's permission to receive these services.

Dealing with symptoms occurs in two stages, which Stanislav Kasl and Sidney Cobb (1966a, 1966b) called illness behavior and sick role behavior. **Illness behavior** consists of the activities undertaken by people who experience symptoms but who have not yet received a diagnosis. That is, illness behavior occurs *before* diagnosis. These activities are oriented toward determining one's state of health and discovering suitable remedies. **Sick role behavior**, in contrast, is the term applied to the behavior of people after a diagnosis, either from a health care provider or a self-diagnosis. The activities of sick role behavior are oriented toward getting well. Jeff was engaging in illness behavior when he sought the opinion of his colleagues, when he went to the imaging center, and when he called his internist for a referral. All these actions took place before his diagnosis and were oriented toward receiving a diagnosis. He was exhibiting

sick role behavior when he got his broken hand put in a cast, kept his appointments to have his hand checked, stopped playing basketball for 6 weeks, and took care not to reinjure his hand. All these activities occurred after diagnosis and were oriented toward getting well. Diagnosis, then, is the event that separates illness behavior from sick role behavior.

Illness Behavior

Illness behavior takes place before one is officially diagnosed. It is directed toward determining health status in the presence of symptoms. People routinely experience symptoms that may signal disease. Symptoms are a critical element in seeking medical care, but the presence of symptoms is not sufficient to prompt a visit to the doctor (Cameron, Leventhal, & Leventhal, 1993). Given similar symptoms, some people readily seek help, others are reluctant, and others do not seek help. What factors affect the decision to seek professional care? Four factors may shape people's response to symptoms: (1) personal reluctance to seek care, (2) certain social and demographic factors, (3) the characteristics of the symptoms, and (4) one's personal view of illness.

Personal Reluctance   A discrepancy exists between what people recommend to others and what they report that they themselves would do about seeking health care. A national survey found that most people were willing to advise other people to see a doctor, but, with the same symptoms, they were less likely to go to the doctor themselves (Feldman, 1966). Indeed, many people said they would take care of even serious health problems without professional aid. This attitude is consistent with a general reluctance among many people to seek professional health care and a tendency to interpret any symptoms in a way that indicates the lowest level of threat.

Personal reluctance to seek health care may not be consistent for all disorders and for all people. Some research (Klonoff & Landrine, 1993) has explored the possibility that people think of

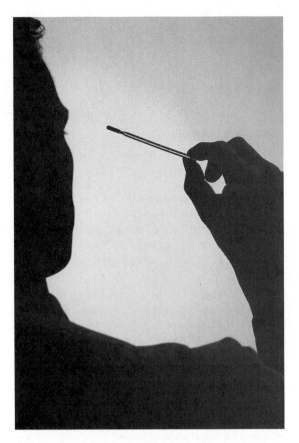

Illness behavior is directed toward determining health status.

different body parts in terms that affect their willingness to seek help when these body parts develop problems. College students rated different body parts along several dimensions, and their responses showed some differences in willingness to seek care. People viewed some body parts, such as the anus, as stigmatized and other body parts, such as the genitalia, as private, leading to reluctance in seeking medical care for such body parts than for those lower in stigma and privacy. In addition, people were more likely to seek help for body parts perceived as important and vulnerable, such as the heart and blood.

This reluctance may be especially strong for screening procedures, which are often oriented toward disease detection. Thinking about disease de-

tection may be more distressing than considering the adoption of health-promoting behaviors (Millar & Millar, 1995). This distress can contribute to personal reluctance and can provide a barrier for health screening for a variety of conditions. For many people, avoiding screening tests prevents the anxiety. This type of personal reluctance puts people at risk for the diseases that these screening procedures can identify.

Social and Demographic Factors   Aside from a general personal reluctance to go to the doctor, the tendency to seek professional care differs with several social and demographic variables. One is gender. Although women are more likely to use health care than men, the reasons for this difference are somewhat complex. James Pennebaker (1982) found that women report more symptoms than men and hypothesized that women are more sensitive to their internal body signals than men. This sensitivity makes women more likely to perceive and thus to report symptoms but does not make them sicker than men.

Social factors that shape gender roles also influence the gender difference in reporting symptoms (Waldron, 1997). Given the same level of symptoms, the female gender role allows women to seek many sorts of assistance whereas the male gender role teaches men to act strong and to deny pain and discomfort. In addition, men's social role permits them to take more risks, and failure to seek health care is among these risks. Men are more likely to need health care because of such risks as alcohol consumption and job hazards, but women are at greater risk through physical inactivity, unemployment, and stress. When all risk factors are controlled, the illness gap between men and women may be quite narrow, although men generally have worse chronic health than women (Verbrugge, 1989).

In addition to gender differences, socioeconomic factors relate to people's frequency of seeking medical care. People in higher socioeconomic groups experience fewer symptoms and report a higher level of health than people at lower socioeconomic levels (Pennebaker, 1982). Yet when higher income people are sick, they are more likely to seek health care. Nevertheless, poor people are overrepresented among the hospitalized, an indication that they are much more likely than middle- and upper-class people to become seriously ill. In addition, people in lower socioeconomic groups tend to wait longer before seeking health care, thus making treatment more difficult and hospitalization more likely. The poor also have less access to medical care, have to travel longer to reach health care facilities, and must wait longer once they arrive at those facilities.

Cultural and social factors also affect how people respond to symptoms. In some cultures, people are socialized not to react with strong emotion to illness, whereas in other cultures, a strong reaction is expected. David Mechanic (1978) reviewed several studies that reported varying attitudes toward illness in different ethnic groups. Jewish Americans, for example, were more likely to seek professional help, accept the sick role, and engage in preventive medical behavior; Mexican Americans tended to ignore some symptoms that physicians felt were serious and to inflate others that doctors regarded as minor; Irish Americans tended to deny pain stoically. These differences demonstrate the powerful effects of culture and context on the experience of illness and sick role behavior.

Age is yet another factor that influences people's willingness to seek medical care, with young and middle-aged adults showing the greatest reluctance. Children are more willing to seek help than adolescents, especially male adolescents (Garland & Zigler, 1994). As people age, they must make distinctions between symptoms of aging and those of disease, discriminating between what is normal and symptoms that signal problems. This distinction is not always easy, but people tend to interpret problems with a gradual onset and mild symptoms as resulting from age compared to those with sudden onset and severe symptoms (Leventhal & Diefenbach, 1991). People who are able to attribute their symptoms to age tend to delay in seeking medical care,

but older adults are not as strongly influenced by this tendency as the middle-aged (Leventhal & Diefenbach, 1991). Although older and middle-aged people did not differ in type of complaint or ease of access to health care, older people were quicker to seek medical care for symptoms that they could not identify. This difference may reflect a lack of tolerance for uncertainty in older adults and a desire to deny or minimize the severity of illness in middle-aged adults.

Stress is also a factor in people's readiness to seek care. People who experience a great deal of stress are more likely to seek health care than those under less stress, even with equal symptoms. Those who experienced concurrent and prolonged stress were more likely to seek care when the symptoms were ambiguous (Cameron, Leventhal, & Leventhal, 1995). When symptoms were clearly health threats, stress was not a factor. Many symptoms are unclear, presenting the possibility that stress sensitizes people to their symptoms and makes them more likely to seek health care.

Ironically, people under stress are less credible when they claim that they are ill. Patients who reported physical and psychological distress compromised their credibility (Skelton, 1991). When people complain to their friends and family about stress and pain, they are less likely to be judged to have a "real" disease than when their complaints center around physical symptoms. In addition, this lowered credibility extends to health care professionals, with nurses and physicians tending to discount the distress of patients who have many complaints. This tendency to discount symptom reports for people under stress may reflect the distinction between the physical and the psychological, with physical complaints having an organic basis and stress-related problems being psychological and thus not "real." The more psychological complaints people report, the less "real" patients' reports of physiological symptoms are considered to be.

Symptom Characteristics   In addition to personal and demographic factors, several symptom characteristics influence when and how people look for help. Symptoms themselves do not inevitably lead people to seek care, but certain characteristics are important in their response to symptoms. Mechanic (1978) listed four characteristics of the symptoms that determine one's response to disease.

First is the *visibility of the symptom*—that is, how readily apparent the symptom is to the person and to others. A study on intentions to adopt osteoporosis prevention (Klohn & Rogers, 1991) confirmed the importance of the visibility of symptoms. Young women who received messages about osteoporosis as a disfiguring condition were significantly more likely to say that they intended to adopt precautions against osteoporosis than young women who were not alerted to the disfiguring aspects of osteoporosis.

Mechanic's second symptom characteristic was *perceived severity of the symptom.* He contended that symptoms seen as severe would be more likely to prompt action than less severe symptoms. This point highlights the importance of personal perception and distinguishes between the perceived severity of a symptom and the judgment of severity by medical authorities. Indeed, patients and physicians differ in their perceptions of the severity of a wide variety of symptoms (Peay & Peay, 1998). Symptoms perceived as more serious produced greater concern and a stronger belief that treatment was urgently needed. Therefore, perceived severity of symptoms rather than the presence of symptoms is critical in the decision to seek care.

The third symptom characteristic mentioned by Mechanic was the *extent to which the symptom interferes with a person's life,* and some evidence (Suchman, 1965) indicates that the degree of incapacitation affected the person's action in seeking care. That is, the more incapacitated the person is, the more likely he or she is to seek medical care.

Mechanic's fourth hypothesized determinant of illness behavior is the *frequency and persistence of the symptoms.* Conditions that people view as requiring care tend to be those that are both severe and continuous, whereas intermittent symptoms

are less likely to generate illness behavior (Suchman, 1965). Severe symptoms prompt people to seek help, but even mild symptoms can motivate people to seek help if those symptoms persist (Prohaska, Keller, Leventhal, & Leventhal, 1987).

In Mechanic's description and subsequent research, symptom characteristics alone are not sufficient to prompt illness behavior. However, if symptoms persist or are perceived as severe, people are more likely to evaluate them as indicating a need for care. Thus, people are prompted to seek care on the basis of their interpretation of their symptoms, which relates to each person's view of illness.

Personal View of Illness   Despite a vast amount of knowledge in the fields of physiology and medicine, most people are largely ignorant of how their bodies work and how diseases develop. Even well-educated people and those who have had their disease fully explained to them tend to have inaccurate and incomplete conceptualizations, partly because when people gain information, they integrate it into their existing knowledge structure. If the new information seems incompatible with what they already "know," they may modify this new information to make it fit their preexisting knowledge rather than changing their knowledge to conform to the new information. This process may, of course, lead to substantial distortions.

One's personal view of illness depends on both knowledge of the disease and the structure of one's cognitions. An interest in how these cognitions develop has prompted a number of studies on disease conceptualizations. For example, children often have unrealistic beliefs about why people get sick and how they get well (Burbach & Peterson, 1986). Children's early concepts of disease can be organized by developmental stage (Bibace & Walsh, 1979). Childhood concepts of disease include a magical possibility of getting sick for no discernible reason. Later, children develop the concept of contagion, and even later they come to understand the mechanisms of how infectious diseases spread. With additional cognitive development, children begin to comprehend that they can do things to control their health. Finally, they form the idea that both psychological and physiological factors can influence health. A high level of cognitive development is probably required to integrate psychological and physiological factors into their concepts of disease.

Surprisingly, a group of college biology majors gave the same sort of explanations of disease as another group of college students who had taken no biology courses (Bibace & Walsh, 1979). Indeed, both groups gave explanations for catching a cold that were quite similar to those given by 7-year-old children. All three groups attributed their colds to such factors as cold weather, insufficient sleep, or not dressing warmly, even though the biology students knew that viruses cause colds. Although biology majors have been exposed to more accurate information about disease than most people, their inclusion of environmental and personal factors in the list of things that cause colds seems to reflect acceptance of the idea that disease has several causes—a personal version of the biopsychosocial model of health and illness.

In addition, many people hold beliefs in supernatural causes for disease, such as punishment from God, sinful thoughts, bad blood, and the evil eye (Landrine & Klonoff, 1994). Beliefs in the supernatural as a cause for disease appear more commonly among ethnic minorities than Whites in the United States. However, Whites too hold beliefs in supernatural causes of disease. For example, 30% of the White college students reported that a lack of faith was at least somewhat important as a cause of sickness (Landrine & Klonoff, 1994). The overall belief in supernatural causes of disease is low for all ethnic groups, but magical thinking concerning disease is not restricted to traditional societies. One study (Nemeroff, 1995) found that such thinking exists among contemporary U.S. college students who rated their lover's "germs" as less infectious than a disliked peer's "germs." Therefore, even people who have knowledge concerning disease processes may not apply that knowledge to their own lives.

Even disorders that are well understood medically may not be well understood by patients. Howard Leventhal and his colleagues (Benyamini, Leventhal, & Leventhal, 1997; Leventhal & Diefenbach, 1991; Meyer, Leventhal, & Gutman, 1985) have explored how people conceptualize various diseases. They have studied four components in the conceptualization of disease: (1) identity of the disease, (2) time line (the time course of both disease and treatment), (3) consequences of the disease, and (4) cause of the disease. Further research (Lau, 1997) has confirmed the factors identified by Leventhal and his colleagues in samples of healthy adults as well as adults with acute and chronic diseases.

The *identity of the disease,* the first component identified by Leventhal and his associates, is very important to illness behavior. A person who has identified his symptoms as a "heart attack" should react quite differently from one who labels the same symptoms as "heartburn." The presence of symptoms is not sufficient to initiate help seeking, but the labeling that occurs in conjunction with symptoms may be critical in a person's either seeking help or ignoring symptoms.

Labels provide a framework within which symptoms can be interpreted. People experience less emotional arousal when they find a label that indicates a minor problem (heartburn rather than heart attack). Initially, they will probably adopt the least serious label that fits their symptoms. For example, Jeff initially interpreted his broken hand as a bruise. To a large extent, a label carries with it some prediction about the time course of the disease, so if the time course does not correspond to the expectation implicit in the label, the person has to relabel the symptoms. When Jeff's hand failed to respond to the ice packs and the pain continued, he began to doubt the label he had applied. His friends told him he was foolish to ignore the swelling and pain out of a belief that these symptoms would disappear. However, the tendency to interpret symptoms as indicating minor rather than major problems is the source of many optimistic self-diagnoses, and Jeff's was no exception.

The second component in conceptualizing an illness is the *time line*. Even though the time course of an disease is usually implicit within the diagnosis, people's understanding of the time involved is not necessarily accurate. People with hypertension, a chronic disease, tended to conceptualize their disease as acute (Meyer et al., 1985); that is, these patients saw their disease as corresponding to the pattern of most temporary diseases, with the onset of symptoms followed by treatment, a remission of symptoms, and then a cure. This belief was frequent among patients who had been recently diagnosed as hypertensive, with 40% expressing a belief that they would be cured. It was much less common among those who had stayed in treatment for at least 3 months, with only 12% of these patients holding an acute concept of their disease.

The *consequences of a disease* are the third component in Leventhal's description of illness conceptualizations. Again, the consequences of a disease are implied by the diagnosis. However, an incorrect understanding of the consequences can have a profound effect on illness behavior. Many people view a diagnosis of cancer as a death sentence. Some neglect health care because they believe themselves to be in a hopeless situation. Women who find a lump in their breast sometimes delay making an appointment with a doctor (Champion & Miller, 1997), not because they fail to recognize this symptom of cancer but because they fear the possible consequences—surgery and possibly the loss of a breast, chemotherapy, radiation, or some combination of these consequences.

The last component of the personal view of illness is the *determination of cause*. For the most part, determining causality is more a facet of the sick role than of illness behavior because it usually occurs after a diagnosis has been made. But the attribution of causality for symptoms is an important factor in illness behavior. For example, if a person can attribute the pain in his hand to a blow received on the day before, he will not have to consider the possibility of bone cancer as the cause of the pain.

Attribution of causality, however, is often faulty. People may attribute a cold to "germs" or to the weather, and they may see cancer as caused by microwave ovens or by the will of God. The belief that God's will and sin play a role in disease is not unusual (Klonoff & Landrine, 1994), and these conceptualizations have important implications for illness behavior. People are less likely to seek professional treatment for conditions they consider to have emotional and natural causes. Even specific physical symptoms may not lead to the interpretation of a physical disease, and people are likely to ignore or use self-treatments for problems they do not consider physical. Therefore, people's conceptualizations of disease causality can influence their behavior.

The Sick Role

Kasl and Cobb (1966b) defined sick role behavior as the activities engaged in by those who believe themselves ill, for the purpose of getting well. In other words, sick role behavior occurs *after* a person has been diagnosed. The concept can be traced back to sociologist Talcott Parsons (1951, 1978), who contended that the sick role is based on three assumptions: (1) being sick is not the sick person's fault, (2) being sick relieves the sick person of normal responsibilities, and (3) a sick person will take steps to get well. This conception includes both rights and privileges for the sick person (Arluke, 1988), but it does not apply well to chronic diseases.

The first of Parsons's assumptions is that being sick is not the sick person's fault, but research has revealed a tendency to blame the victim for his or her misfortune (Ryan, 1971). This tendency extends to health care workers, who tend to blame patients for their illness (Janis & Rodin, 1979) and patients, who tend to blame themselves when they get sick (Lau & Hartman, 1983). In the case of chronic diseases such as heart disease and some cancers, this tendency may not be completely unfounded; these diseases have strong behavioral components, but the sick person is not completely to blame for those dis-

WOULD YOU BELIEVE . . . ?

Sick People Are Not Allowed to Feel Bad

Would you believe that sick people are not allowed to feel bad? Richard Lazarus (1984b) pointed out that both health care professionals and people in general have a tendency to "downplay the negative and accentuate the positive" (p. 126) to an extent that trivializes sick people's distress. For example, sick people are expected to be optimistic and cheerful and are not allowed to appear miserable or depressed. Although most people are distressed by illness, sick people are frequently discouraged from displaying their distress. Instead, they are encouraged to be brave and cheerful, even when they do not feel like it.

Healthy people encourage sick people to be optimistic, even when they know there is little basis for optimism. We admire stories about those who face catastrophic illness bravely, and such admiration conveys the expectation that courage is the way to behave in the face of adversity. Lazarus contended that this attitude is unfair to sick people, adding stress to their already stressful state of illness: "The tyranny of all this is that one cannot refuse to comply without appearing to be a misanthrope and an ingrate" (p. 126).

Lazarus argued that this attitude can have a negative effect on sick people. Rather than encouraging a positive attitude and productive coping efforts, the expectation of courage and optimism may produce a sense of failure in the sick person who finds it difficult to exhibit these admirable behaviors. In addition, the upbeat attitude of friends and family may lead the sick person to feel that honest opinions and feelings will not be welcomed, isolating the sick person from those who should be major sources of support. If a sick person cannot share true feelings, then he or she lacks meaningful social support.

Optimism and courage are excellent ways of facing adversity, including disease. Those patients who feel genuine optimism and a "fighting spirit" have advantages in coping with disease. However, pressure to exhibit these behaviors is not fair to those patients who do not feel optimistic or courageous. Although putting on a brave and cheerful face may make health care professionals, family, and friends feel better, the patient may feel isolated and abandoned. These feelings can interfere with coping and recovery.

Coping with disease is difficult, and distress is a common occurrence. Lazarus advocated broadened opportunities for coping, including emotion-focused as well as problem-focused efforts. He pointed out that medical care emphasizes the problem rather than the person, and the trivialization of distress discourages patients from focusing on their emotions. Focusing on emotions—even negative ones—can be useful, and Lazarus argued that patients should be allowed the full range of options for coping.

---

eases. The tendency to consider patients responsible for their disease suggests that lack of blame is not part of many illness episodes.

The second feature of the sick role in our society, according to Parsons, is the exemption of the sick person from normal social, occupational, and family duties. Sick people are usually not expected to go to work, school, or meetings; to cook, clean house, or care for children; to do homework or mow the lawn. Sick people are frequently allowed,

and often expected, to stay home and act sick (see the Would You Believe . . . ? box).

The desire to get well is Parsons's third component of the sick role. This component also applies more to acute than to chronic diseases. However, people with chronic diseases may think of their conditions as acute even though they will never be well. Research has confirmed the notion that most people believe disease is a temporary state, even when people have chronic diseases (Lau &

Hartman, 1983; Leventhal, Nerenz, & Steele, 1984). When people with hypertension believe they can discontinue treatment because they feel better, these beliefs threaten the treatment outcome.

Alexander Segall (1997) proposed an alternative sick role conceptualization that also includes three components: (1) the right to make decisions concerning health-related issues, (2) the right to be exempt from normal duties, and (3) the right to become dependent on others for assistance. This alternative includes duties as well as rights: (1) the duty to maintain health as well as to get well, (2) the duty to perform routine health care management and, (3) the duty to use a range of health care resources. This formulation expands the sick role concept to allow for conditions posed by chronic diseases as well as for the individual and social variation that occurs with different diseases.

Choosing a Practitioner

As part of their attempts to get well, sick people usually consult a health care practitioner. For most middle-class people in industrialized nations, the health care practitioner is a physician, but other types of health care practitioners exist. For example, midwives, nurses, physical therapists, psychologists, osteopaths, chiropractors, dentists, nutritionists, and herbal healers all provide various types of health care. Some of these sources of health care are considered "alternative" because they provide alternatives to traditional medicine. Almost a third of U.S. residents seek some form of alternative health care (Cowley, King, Hager, & Rosenberg, 1995). These alternative forms of health care exist not only among diverse ethnic groups but are also growing in acceptability among European Americans (Dressler & Oths, 1997). Moreover, insurance companies are beginning to cover some of the expenses for these treatments, which can be less expensive than traditional medical care.

The growing acceptability of alternative health care is but one of several changes taking place in the provision of health care. First, changes are oc-

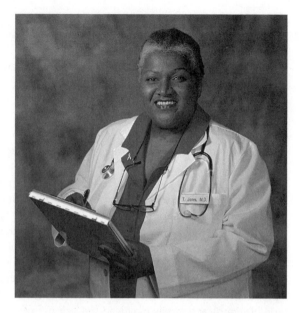

Patients are most pleased with health care providers who are friendly and willing to discuss health problems.

curring in the system of payment for health services. Currently, patients seldom pay the practitioner directly for services received. A second and related change is that the era of the solo practitioner is coming to an end. Third, the traditional authoritarian role of various health care providers is also changing, with physicians' authority and power diminishing. Younger people are particularly more likely to view patients as consumers of health care who, like any consumers, have choices in their selection of services and service providers (DiMatteo, 1997).

Satisfaction with medical encounters is most strongly related to the amount of information provided by the physician, and patients are most satisfied with physicians who are willing to interact with them regarding their health problems; talk about nonmedical topics; and display immediate, positive nonverbal behavior. In contrast, patients are most displeased with physicians who seem uninterested, who use an angry tone of voice, who act through power and authority, or who display anger in any way (Roter, 1988).

In Summary

No easy distinction exists between health and illness. The World Health Organization sees health as more than the absence of disease; rather health is the attainment of positive physical, mental, and social well-being. Curiously, the distinction between disease and illness is more clear. Disease refers to the process of physical damage within the body, whether or not the person is aware of this damage. Illness, on the other hand, refers to the experience of being sick; people can feel sick but have no identifiable disease.

Demographic factors of gender, socioeconomic level, and age influence the seeking of professional health care in the United States. In addition, cultural factors play a role in the experience of illness and also in when and how often people seek care. People whose cultural backgrounds teach the value of promptly seeking professional health care tend go to the doctor sooner than do people from cultures that do not hold this value. Life stress is also a factor in seeking help, with stress increasing the likelihood of seeking health care but decreasing the credibility of illness reports.

People tend to incorporate four components into their concept of disease: (1) the identity of the disease, (2) the time line of the disease, (3) the consequences of the disease, and (4) the cause of the disease. If a disease has been officially identified or diagnosed, then its time course and its consequences are implicit. However, people who know the name of their disease do not always have an accurate concept of its time course and consequences. For example, many people wrongly see chronic disease, such as hypertension, as having a short time course. Finally, people want to know the cause of their illness and will even accept faulty and irrational explanations.

Once people's symptoms are diagnosed and they believe themselves to be ill, they engage in sick role behavior in order to get well. People who are sick are relieved from normal responsibilities, but they have the added burden of trying to get well.

Many patients have begun to treat medical care as another type of service and have started to challenge the traditional authority of physicians. One aspect of this challenge has been the growth of alternate types of health care practitioners. Another has been patients' changing attitudes toward their health care providers; patients want them to be caring and reassuring as well as communicative. In addition, patients expect professional behavior and competence, and they want physicians to treat them with respect and to refrain from expressing anger in their questions or responses.

Being in the Hospital

The majority of health care occurs as self-care or on an outpatient basis, but sometimes people are hospitalized. The decision to be hospitalized is almost never a patient's decision: Patients initiate only 2% of hospitalizations (Greenley & Davidson, 1988), and physicians initiate the other 98%. Over the past 20 years, hospitals and the experience of being in the hospital have both changed (Weitz, 1996). Many types of surgery and tests that were formerly handled through hospitalization are now performed on an outpatient basis; hospital stays have become shorter; and an expanding array of technology is available for diagnosis and treatment. As a result of these changes, people who are not severely ill are not likely to be hospitalized. Therefore, people who are admitted to a hospital are more severely ill. Ironically, managed care directives have resulted in shorter hospital stays in the interest of controlling health care costs (but not always in the interest of the patient). Technological medicine has become more prominent in patient care, and personal treatment by the hospital staff has become less so. These factors can combine to make hospitalization a stressful experience (Weitz, 1996).

The Hospital Patient Role

The role of hospital patient is not the same as the sick role because sick people have many options in their care at home, but the hospital organization defines the patient role. Part of the sick role is to be a patient, and being a patient means conforming to the rules of the health care institution and complying with medical advice. Moreover, traditional hospital procedures can turn patients into "nonpersons."

Nonperson Treatment When people are hospitalized, all but their illness becomes invisible; frequently people lose the status of being human. Erving Goffman (1961) described this "nonperson" treatment as a process "whereby the patient is greeted with what passes as civility and said farewell to in the same fashion with everything in between going on as if the patient weren't there as a social person at all but only as some possession someone has left behind" (pp. 341–342). Although this statement is nearly 40 years old, it applies even more strongly today because of the growth of technology in medicine. The hospital staff tends to concentrate on the machinery rather than on the patient (Weitz, 1996).

Being referred to as "the multiple fracture in Room 458" may be both startling and annoying, but impersonal reference is not the extent of nonperson treatment. Not only are patients' identities ignored but their comments and questions may also be overlooked. During examinations or treatment, the depersonalization of patients is so blatant that they often are not spoken to directly (Zimbardo, 1969), and their comments may be totally ignored (Taylor, 1982). Practitioners frequently converse among themselves in the patient's presence, using technical jargon that the patient is unable to comprehend. This manner of conversing allows practitioners to convey a great deal of information to each other but leaves patients feeling anxious and helpless (Bennett & Disbrow, 1993). The hospital procedure focuses on the technical aspects of medical procedures but usually ignores patients' emotional needs, and patients treated as nonpersons, ignored, and deprived of information are less satisfied with their treatment than patients who are treated as persons and informed about their condition (Yarnold, Michelson, Thompson, & Adams, 1998).

The extent to which the hospital staff ignores the person extends to the experience of pain: Neither nurses nor physicians seem to perceive the pain of patients in the same manner that the patients view their own pain. Patients rate their own pain as more severe than the ratings given by nurses and much more severe than the ratings of doctors (Krokosky & Reardon, 1989). Perhaps this depreciation of patients' pain is part of their depersonalized treatment: Nonpersons should not feel much pain.

Lack of Information Hospitalized patients may experience a lack of information concerning their condition. The philosophy that physicians should decide how much patients ought to know has faded, and most physicians believe that patients should be fully informed about their conditions. However, for several reasons involving the hospital's organization, the ideal communication involving an open exchange of information between patient and practitioner is more likely to occur in a practitioner's private office than in the hospital (Weitz, 1996).

Hospitalized patients typically come in contact with nurses, technicians, and physicians. The nurses and technicians are hospital employees, but physicians may not be. Physicians in private practice admit their patients and retain responsibility for aspects of their care. Hospital policy may require that patients hear about their condition from their physicians, and patients who ask nurses or technicians for information may be told that they are not allowed to reveal the requested information. Patients' personal physicians may be in the hospital for only a brief time each day, limiting patients' access to information. This inaccessibility contributes to patients' lack of knowledge.

Patients may also lack information because that information is not available—that is, the patient may be admitted to the hospital for diagnostic testing. Patients in this situation are usually experiencing distressing symptoms, and their health care providers have been unable to make a diagnosis. Such patients are already stressed, and the exten-

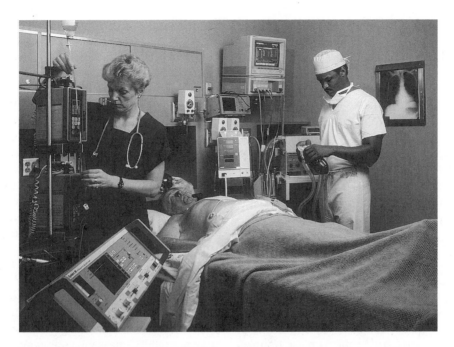

Hospitalized patients lack control of their lives and information about their conditions, resulting in increased distress.

sive and sometimes painful diagnostic testing adds to their anxiety. On the other hand, receiving a diagnosis may produce even more anxiety and does not exempt them from undergoing additional tests. The hospital staff may not explain the purpose or results of diagnostic testing, leaving patients without information and filled with anxiety.

Loss of Control   Hospitalized patients are expected to conform submissively to the rules of the hospital and the orders of their doctor, thus relinquishing much control over their lives. In her account of the impact of health organizations, Shelley Taylor (1979) argued that loss of control is patients' major complaint, and it can apply to three aspects of illness and hospitalization: (1) loss of normal control of one's body, (2) loss of typical activities such as work and leisure activities, and (3) loss of ability to predict what will happen.

First, illness and hospitalization can upset the control over body functions that people ordinarily

perform with little conscious effort. Second, the loss of control also extends to normal, everyday activities, such as what to wear, what and when to eat, when to sleep, who may touch (and even hurt) them, and when they can see their family and friends. Third, not being allowed to make decisions about even the simplest aspects of their lives is a psychological loss of control that reduces people's ability to take effective action concerning their health. This loss of control reduces people's ability to forecast the course of their disease or to predict what will happen to them. Once admitted to the hospital, patients relinquish much personal control and can do very little to restore it. Even leaving the hospital without another's consent is difficult.

This loss of control can be very stressful. Several experts (Bennett & Disbrow, 1993; Taylor, 1982) have proposed that research findings concerning loss of control can readily be applied to patients in hospital settings. For example, when exposed to uncontrollable, unpleasant stimulation, people experience more discomfort than they do when the situation is equally unpleasant but under their control (Glass & Singer, 1972). People tend to manifest heightened physiological responses and to react on a physical level to uncontrollable stimulation more strongly than they do when they can exert some control over the condition. Lack of control can decrease people's capacity to concentrate and can increase their tendency to report physical symptoms. These findings suggest that hospitalization can be a negative experience for both the staff and the patients.

"Good" Patients versus "Bad" Patients

To be a "good" patient from the viewpoint of hospital personnel, one must conform to a "nonperson" role. Good patients do not ask questions; they do as instructed and cooperate with requests. Above all, being a good patient means not making trouble for the staff. Conversely, "bad" patients make trouble; they ask questions and demand answers. They behave like consumers who have rights. Bad patients demand attention, and they complain.

Judith Lorber (1975) described these two patient roles and concluded that about 25% of patients exhibit "problem patient" behavior and about 75% conform to the "good patient" role. What are the consequences of each type of role? Which type of behavior is more conducive to a patient's recovery?

Consequences of Being a "Bad" Patient   The behavior of "bad" patients can be interpreted as an attempt to restore control (Taylor, 1979). Patients' problem behavior can be analyzed as an angry reaction to nonperson treatment and the loss of freedom associated with hospitalization. To assert control, patients may exhibit petty violations of hospital procedures, such as smoking, drinking, or flirting with the nurses, or they may fail to comply in more major ways that could endanger their health, such as failing to take medication or prematurely leaving the hospital. These angry behaviors exemplify **reactance**, a term borrowed from

the theory of psychological reactance (Brehm, 1966). According to this view, people who are deprived of personal freedom or threatened with loss of freedom react angrily and try to restore their control through a variety of strategies.

Physiologically, the anger and frustration experienced by the reactant patient stimulate the same physiological responses that other stressors do. Anger may therefore have negative effects on the patient's health, but is it always bad for the patient? Some possibility exists that being a bad patient may be healthier than being a good one, at least when being bad includes a questioning of medical care and developing an understanding of the treatment regimen.

Consequences of Being a "Good" Patient   Will a sick person benefit by being a good, compliant patient? Good patients receive more attention from the hospital staff, but good patient behavior may not reflect a peaceful acceptance of the situation (Taylor, 1979). Although good patients by definition are compliant and noncomplaining, they too may experience turmoil about their situation. What passes for acceptance of the patient role may actually be an expression of feelings of helplessness. These feelings are quite different from the anger experienced by reactant patients, but both may result from extreme frustration over the patient role.

Martin Seligman (1975) investigated the notion that extreme frustration can produce **learned helplessness**. He reported on studies demonstrating that some animal species learn to do nothing when put into stressful situations in which no control is possible. Because these animals have learned that nothing they did worked, they did nothing. They also failed to make appropriate responses when put into similar situations; that is, they generalized their learned helplessness. Seligman and his colleagues (Abramson, Garber, & Seligman, 1980) reviewed the research on learned helplessness as it applies to humans and found that the same sort of behavior observed in laboratory animals also occurs in humans in a variety of situations in which they experience (or perceive) loss of control.

The learned helplessness model can apply to hospitalized patients to explain the cognitive and emotional process of some "good" patients: They express helplessness as passivity, which is consistent with the good patient role (Taylor, 1979). This passivity extends beyond the lack of response expected by the hospital staff and may include the withholding of information important to treatment. This passivity is actually another form of "getting even" with the staff but can be indistinguishable from ideal patient behavior.

In addition, depression can result from learned helplessness (Abramson et al., 1980), which can apply to hospitalization. Depressed people are passive and uncommunicative. However, depression can lead to a depletion of norepinephrine and a suppressed immune system, reactions that make recovery more difficult.

Implications Loss of control, lack of information, and nonperson treatment may cause reactance or helplessness in hospitalized patients. Both these response patterns may be troublesome to the hospital staff, but both are patients' ways of coping with the stresses of hospitalization. Patients can react to stress in more constructive ways, but most people have no specific training or assistance in constructively coping with hospitalization. They also lack the extensive experience with hospitalization that might help them to develop effective coping strategies.

How can these problems be solved? The hospital staff could treat patients as people rather than as nonpersons. This solution would be ideal for the patients but perhaps not for the staff. Too much personal involvement on the part of health care workers can make the job of providing health care more stressful and can contribute to occupational "burnout" (Maslach, 1997). Providing personal care without personal involvement would, of course, be difficult.

For the efficiency of the organization, uniform treatment and conformity to hospital routine are desirable, even though they allow patients little personal control. Hospitals have no insidious plot to deprive patients of their freedom, but that is the result when hospitals impose their routine on patients. Restoring control to patients in any significant way would further complicate an already complex organization, but the restoration of small types of control may be effective. For example, many hospitals can allow patients some choice of foods and provide TV remote controls to give patients the power to select a program to watch (or not watch). These aspects of control are small, but a little control may go a long way toward combating feelings of helplessness (Langer & Rodin, 1976).

In Summary

Hospitalized patients often experience added stress as a result of being in the hospital. They are typically regarded as "nonpersons," receive inadequate information concerning their illness, and experience some loss of control over their lives. They are expected to conform to hospital routine and to comply with frequent requests of the hospital staff. Most do and are considered "good" patients. However, as many as 25% of patients complain, ask questions, and demand answers. These contentious people are regarded as "bad" patients because they insist on being treated differently than hospital procedures permit. Although these patients may be more of a nuisance to the hospital staff than "good" patients, such attitudes and behaviors may help these "bad" patients recover more quickly.

Preparing for Stressful Medical Procedures

Simply being in the hospital can be a stressful experience, but some patients encounter additional stress because they must undergo unpleasant medical procedures. In addition, a variety of outpatient procedures, such as dental visits, blood donation, and diagnostic tests can be stressful.

Patient anxiety ordinarily increases in anticipation of such painful medical procedures as surgery, **gastrointestinal endoscopy** (examining the gastrointestinal tract by inserting a tube through the esophagus or the rectum), and **cardiac catheterization** (inserting a tube into a vein and directing it to the heart, where dye is then injected to make a clear X ray possible). Chemotherapy for cancer is another stressful medical procedure, and most cancer patients anticipate this treatment with apprehension and anxiety. In all these cases, the anticipation may intensify the pain of the procedure, which becomes a serious problem for the patient and for health care providers.

Most patients cope with stressful and potentially painful medical procedures as well as they can, but health care providers, including psychologists, have devised support programs and specific training to help patients prepare. Efforts to prepare patients psychologically can be traced back to work by Irving Janis (1958), in a study comparing a group of patients who were psychologically prepared for surgery with a group given only the usual information provided by physicians and hospital staff. The preparation consisted of information about what would happen before, during, and after surgery. Janis found that the patients in the preparation group requested less medication for pain, made fewer demands on the staff, and were discharged earlier than those who received the usual information. These results were both promising and intriguing and have prompted many additional studies, most of which have confirmed the benefits of preparation.

One influential study (Shipley, Butt, Horwitz, & Farbry, 1978) involved patients waiting for a stressful endoscopy procedure. They either viewed a videotape of the endoscopy procedure three times, saw it once, or did not see the endoscopy tape but watched an irrelevant tape. In addition, all participants received extensive verbal information about the procedure. The results showed that patients who viewed the endoscopy tape three times were the least distressed, and those who did not see the tape were the most distressed.

In addition, researchers identified different coping styles, labeling patients as either Sensitizers or Repressors. Sensitizers tended to respond to stress with constant vigilance, overt anxiety, and sensitivity to cues of distress, whereas Repressors were overtly nonanxious, repressed distressful thoughts, and denied potential stress. The Sensitizers who watched the tape three times manifested the least stress, followed in order by those who saw it once and finally by those who did not see it. In contrast, the Repressors showed an inverted V-shaped relationship, with participants who viewed the tape once having much more distress than either the patients who never saw it or those who viewed it three times. This finding shows the importance of individual coping styles and hints that programs should be individually tailored to be most effective.

Techniques for Coping

Coping techniques can consist of at least three approaches: receiving accurate information; relaxation training; and modeling (watching others undergoing the procedure or viewing films of others). Patients can reduce the distress of preparing for stressful medical procedures with any one or a combination of these three activities, but individual coping styles influence which technique works best for each person.

Information   The sort of information that Janis provided was procedural; that is, patients received specific information about the procedures they would undergo. Another possible type of information presents the sensations that patients will experience during medical procedures. An early review of studies with these types of information (Kendall & Watson, 1981) indicated that sensory information is generally more valuable. A later meta-analysis (Johnson & Vögele, 1993) evaluated studies with a variety of outcome measures as well as studies that used sensory and procedural information as preparations for surgery. In general, research has substantiated the overall advantage for

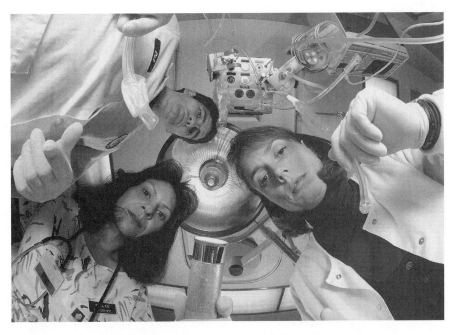

Preparation for surgery can ease the stress associated with such procedures.

procedural information, but both types of preparation can provide advantages.

Patients respond to information preparing them for stressful medical procedures with two different coping styles. Sensitizers, or vigilant copers, acknowledge the negative emotions that accompany such procedures whereas Repressors, or avoidance copers, deny thoughts about the negative aspects of the situation. People who use the active coping and the avoidance coping style are affected differently by preparatory information about surgery. The avoiders generally do not do as well postsurgically as the active copers, who acknowledge their negative feelings (Andrew, 1970). When given specific information about the procedures, the avoiders tend to do worse than when they are given no information or only general information. In contrast, active copers do better when given specific information, which suggests that coping style and type of information about the procedure interact.

However, both avoidant and active coping styles can be effective. Preparation for surgery that included information increased patients' feelings of control and produced better physical and psychological adjustments postsurgically (Anderson, 1987), demonstrating the effectiveness of active coping. In contrast, people who expected fewer problems experienced fewer problems in postsurgical adjustment (Kiyak, Vitaliano, & Crinean, 1988), which demonstrated the effectiveness of an avoidant coping strategy.

Different coping styles may each be effective with different medical procedures as well as for different patients. Avoidance coping through distraction was the most effective strategy for lowering anxiety during dental surgery (Wong & Kaloupek, 1986), and more active, vigilant coping might be maladaptive in medical situations requiring passivity. On the other hand, more active coping might be better in situations requiring action on the patient's part. Therefore, perhaps not only personal but also situational coping differences have an influence.

The research on providing information to prepare people for stressful medical procedures has yielded complex results. Specific information about a stressful medical procedure may help some patients cope. The success of the coping strategy depends partly on the type of information given to patients, with information about *sensations* being more helpful than information about *procedures*. In addition, patients' styles of coping interact with the information conveyed, so that only some patients do better when given information as a preparation for stressful medical procedures. Whereas some patients want and use information to help them cope, others prefer to avoid thoughts about the procedure, and this avoidance style helps them cope. An additional factor that predicts the success of information as a way of coping is the type of stressful medical procedure performed. Patients might be advised to adopt an avoidance coping style for procedures that require passivity and a vigilant style for procedures that require patient activity.

Relaxation Training   A second technique for coping with stressful medical procedures is relaxation training. An early review (Kendall & Watson, 1981) of several studies on relaxation training as an adjunct to surgery reported that the effects of relaxation are significant and positive for relatively minor medical procedures, such as dental surgery. With more serious procedures, the results of relaxation training are less dramatic but generally positive.

A meta-analysis of the effectiveness of surgical preparation (Johnson & Vögele, 1993) also indicated that behavioral instructions such as information about relaxation and cognitive coping instructions can be effective in preparing people for surgery, but hypnosis is less effective. In the studies in this meta-analysis, all techniques showed some effectiveness, but none were effective for all measures of improvement or in all studies.

Modeling   Finally, modeling—learning by watching others perform—is an effective technique for coping with unpleasant medical procedures. Modeling is often used with children who are facing surgery. The model appears on film in the same situation that the patient will soon encounter. An early study (Melamed, 1984) showed that the most effective models appeared anxious at first, even fearful, but in the end they successfully coped with the stress of the procedure. A necessary component of the filmed modeling seems to be the display of some initial anxiety, which the model then successfully overcomes. In addition, viewing the film more than once and with appropriate timing of the filmed presentation was important. A person's anxiety tends to increase immediately after viewing a filmed model coping with a stressful situation, but the anxiety decreases with time. Therefore, enough time must elapse between the presentation of the model and the procedure in order for the patient to make full use of the effect.

Modeling has also been a component in a program to reduce dental anxiety in adults (Law, Logan, & Baron, 1994). Not all patients benefited from viewing a film of an anxious patient who learns to cope through relaxing and communicating with the dentist. Those who wanted control but felt little control experienced decreased pain and stress whereas other patients did not. Once again, patients' style of coping interacts with the type of preparation, making modeling and other preparations for stressful procedures good choices for some patients. To be effective, preparations must allow for individual differences in coping style.

Children and Hospitalization

Hospitalization is a common experience for children as well as for adults. Few children negotiate childhood without some injury, disease, or condition that requires hospitalization, and the commonalities of the hospital experience are sources of stress and anxiety—separation from parents, an unfamiliar environment, diagnostic tests, administration of anesthesia, surgery, and postoperative pain (Routh & Sanfilippo, 1991).

Training children to cope with their fear of treatment presents special problems to health psychologists. First, young children's understanding of disease may not allow them to understand the reason for their disease or the necessity for the treatment (Bibace & Walsh, 1979). Although kindergarten-age children show signs of understanding the same dimensions that adults do (Goldman, Whitney-Saltiel, Granger, & Rodin, 1991), many adults fail to understand the tests and treatments that occur in hospitals.

Second, many life long treatment phobias are learned in childhood, making early prevention of unrealistic fears a critical goal for pediatric health psychology. A child's first experience with medical treatment should not be a traumatic one, because early unpleasant experiences tend to generalize. One study (Dahlquist et al., 1986) indicated that children 3 to 12 years old whose previous medical experiences had been negative demonstrated more distress during routine medical examinations than did children whose previous experiences had been either neutral or positive. The results with dental anxiety in children are parallel; previous aversive dental experiences related more closely to dental anxiety than did the children's general fearfulness (Liddell, 1990).

A third special problem in helping children prepare for stressful medical procedures comes from parents. Some interventions train parents to be less anxious and more informative. Also, parents can be trained to help their children learn various coping skills and thereby reduce their children's anxiety (Bush, Melamed, Sheras, & Greenbaum, 1986; Dahlquist et al., 1986).

However, parents' presence can either help or hurt their children's ability to cope with stressful medical procedures, depending on the parents' behavior (Manne et al., 1992). The time-honored parental technique of persistently reassuring a child facing medical treatment is not only ineffec-

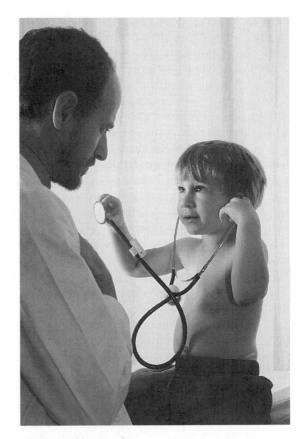

Allowing children to become comfortable with medical apparatus can ease distress.

tive but also tends to increase the child's feelings of distress (Bush et al., 1986). Distraction can be effective in helping children deal with a distressing medical procedure, but interestingly, adults are not necessarily helped by distraction (McCaul, Monson, & Maki, 1992). Like adults, children respond with less obvious distress when they are given some control over the medical procedures they must endure (Manne et al., 1992).

A fourth problem for children is their tendency to interpret their disease as a form of punishment for real or imagined misconduct (O'Brien & Bush, 1997). Guilt and anxiety often combine with hostility toward and fear of nurses and doctors to produce a complex of negative emotions in children. These problems are more prominent for children receiving treatment for chronic conditions such as cancer or burns.

A variety of psychological interventions, including some not used with adults, have been tried with children who are anticipating fear-provoking medical procedures. These approaches have been examined from the perspective of five themes or approaches (Elkins & Roberts, 1983). The first approach involves giving information to the child. A review of informational studies revealed that some reported positive results, but others found that preschool-age children may not always understand the information presented. A later study (Manne et al., 1992) confirmed that this strategy was not effective in reducing children's distress.

A second approach encourages emotional expression in children who are anxious about hospitalization. Children are given a chance to express their fears and anxieties by playing with puppets, doctors' kits, and other play materials and games. This type of play therapy shows mixed results (Elkins & Roberts, 1983) and even has the possibility of increasing rather than decreasing children's fears.

A third strategy centers on helping children establish a relationship of trust and confidence with members of the medical staff. This trust is typically achieved by using films, hospital tours, and books and by allowing parents to stay with the child in the hospital. Building a supportive relationship can be helpful, but by itself it is not sufficient to alleviate children's feelings of distress (Elkins & Roberts, 1983).

The fourth strategy involves the psychological preparation of parents whose children are facing hospitalization or other stressful medical procedures. Children of psychologically prepared parents are generally less anxious and better able to handle distressing hospital procedures (Elkins & Roberts, 1983). One study (Pinto & Hollandsworth, 1989) demonstrated reduction of emotional arousal in pediatric patients facing first-time elective surgery by showing them an informational videotape in the presence of their parents. A third of the children viewed an adult-narrated tape, a third saw a peer-narrated presentation, and a third were assigned to a control group who saw no videotape. Half the children in each group remained with their parents during the treatment and half were separated from their parents. Children who viewed the videotape with their parents and children who viewed the tape alone showed less preoperative arousal than children who did not view the tape. In general, children who were with their parents during psychological preparation experienced less emotional arousal than children who were separated from their parents. Moreover, the videotape also decreased parents' anxiety. Contrary to expectations, the researchers found no differences between adult-narrated and child-narrated videotapes; both were equally effective. The results of this study indicate an advantage for both the videotape presentation and the presence of parents during psychological preparation.

The fifth approach for helping children cope includes providing children with various coping strategies such as relaxation training, peer models, distraction, and instruction on self-talk techniques. Films and videotapes are commonly used for teaching all these techniques, and each has been used with some success. Such cognitive-behavioral interventions were successful with children who were receiving painful treatments for leukemia (Jay, Elliott, Woody, & Siegel, 1991), Indeed, this intervention was more successful in lowering distress, pain ratings, and pulse rates during treatment than no treatment and was also more successful than a drug treatment that included Valium. Thus, even though drugs are often considered an easier way to promote relaxation during stressful medical procedures, this research demonstrated the effectiveness of behavioral techniques.

In Summary

Patients facing invasive or painful medical procedures usually experience even more stress than other hospitalized patients. In recent years, health psychologists have helped these patients prepare for stressful medical procedures by using information, relaxation training, and modeling to help adults reduce their stress levels. With children they have used such interventions as play therapy and programs designed to prepare parents to help their children cope.

Answers

This chapter addressed four basic questions:

1. **Why do people adopt health-related behaviors?**

    Most people value good health and wish to avoid disease, but many fail to seek health care when necessary. Several theories attempt to explain health-related behavior. The *health belief model* was developed specifically to predict and explain health-related behaviors and includes the concepts of perceived severity of the disease, personal susceptibility, and perceived benefits and barriers of health-enhancing behaviors. Although recent research has demonstrated some utility for the original health belief model, other studies have introduced new concepts and have had only limited success in predicting health-seeking behavior.

    The *theory of reasoned action* and the *theory of planned behavior* are general behavior theories that have also been applied to health-related situations. Both theories include attitudes, subjective norms, and intention; in addition, the theory of planned behavior includes the person's perceived behavioral control. These two theories have not yet produced the volume of research generated by the health belief model, but some research suggests that the concepts of intention and perceived be-havioral control add to the predictive ability of theories of reasoned action and planned behavior.

    Bandura's concept of *self-efficacy,* a component of his *self-regulation theory* and similar to perceived behavioral control, has been found to relate positively to a number of health-related behaviors. However, research also suggests that some people may have the confidence to change health-related behaviors (high self-efficacy) but lack motivation to do so (low outcome expectancies).

    Weinstein's *precaution adoption process model* assumes that when people are faced with adopting health protective behaviors, they go through seven possible stages of belief about their personal susceptibility. Built into one stage is optimistic bias, a topic that has been heavily researched. However, most research on the total precaution adoption model has been limited to Weinstein and his colleagues. A limitation of each of these models is their inability to accurately assess various social, ethnic, and other demographic factors that also affect people's health-seeking behavior.

    Finally, Prochaska's *transtheoretical model* assumes that people progress through five stages in making changes in behavior—precontemplation, contemplation, preparation, action, and maintenance. Although cross-sectional studies show some promise for the transtheoretical model, more research is needed to establish its utility.

2. **What factors are related to seeking medical attention?**

    How people determine their health status when they don't feel well depends not only on social, ethnic, and demographic factors but also on the characteristics of their symptoms and their concept of illness. In deciding whether they are ill, people consider at least four characteristics of their symptoms: (1) the obvious visibility of the symptoms, (2) the perceived severity of the illness, (3) the degree to which the symptoms interfere with their lives, and (4) the frequency and persistence of the symptoms.

Once people are diagnosed as sick, they adopt the sick role. That role was proposed to include a lack of blame, but research has failed to support this component. The sick role involves relief from normal social and occupational responsibilities and the duty to try to get better.

3. **What is involved in the experience of hospitalization?**

Hospitalization is a stressful form of health care. Most patients conform to hospital routine and are considered "good" patients. A significant minority, however, complain, ask questions, and demand answers; they are therefore regarded as "bad" patients. "Problem" patients insist on exercising control in their daily lives, and their nonconforming behavior while in the hospital can be seen as an attempt to restore control. Even though these patients may not receive as much positive attention from the hospital staff as "good" patients, some evidence shows that such attitudes and behaviors may be helpful to them in restoring their health.

4. **How can people prepare for stressful medical procedures?**

Health psychology has a role to play in preparing patients for hospitalization and stressful medical procedures. Information, relaxation training, and modeling have helped adults, whereas interventions with children have also included play therapy and procedures designed to prepare parents to help their child cope. Psychological techniques can help children, parents, and adult patients cope with stressful and painful medical procedures by not only lowering their anxiety and enhancing their feelings of control, but even lowering their need for medication and shortening their hospital stays.

Glossary

bulimia An eating disorder characterized by periodic binging and purging, the latter usually taking the form of self-induced vomiting or laxative abuse.

cardiac catheterization A diagnostic procedure in which dye is injected into the circulatory system from a tube inserted into a vein.

gastrointestinal endoscopy An examination of the gastrointestinal tract performed by inserting a tube through the esophagus or rectum.

illness behavior Those activities undertaken by people who feel ill and who wish to understand their condition and what to do about it. Illness behavior precedes formal diagnosis.

learned helplessness The learned tendency to respond with passivity to a challenging situation because past experiences have instilled the belief that this situation cannot be controlled.

mammography An X-ray technique for detecting breast tumors before they can be seen or felt.

optimistic bias The belief that other people, but not one's self, will develop a disease, have an accident, or experience other negative events.

reactance In Brehm's theory, the angry state of reaction to loss of freedom and the attempt to restore personal control.

reciprocal determinism Bandura's model that includes environment, behavior and person factors as mutually interacting to determine conduct.

sick role behavior Those activities undertaken by people who have been diagnosed as sick in their efforts to get well.

Suggested Readings

Bennett, H. L., & Disbrow, E. A. (1993). Preparing for surgery and medical procedures. In D. Goleman & J. Gurin (Eds.), *Mind/body medicine: How to use your mind for better health* (pp. 401–427). Yonkers, NY: Consumer Reports Books.

Bennett and Disbrow discuss techniques and situations that help patients cope with surgery and stressful medical procedures and give practical advice on how such patients can design their own presurgical program.

Fleury, J. (1992). The application of motivational theory to cardiovascular risk reduction. *Image: Journal of Nursing Scholarship, 24,* 229–239.

In a review of studies using the health belief model, the theory of reasoned action, the theory of planned behavior, and self-efficacy theory as they have been applied to cardiovascular risk reduction, Fleury finds both strengths and weakness for each theory.

 Manczak, D. W. (1997, December). Hospitalization: Helping a child cope. *Clinical Reference Systems,* p. 1477.

This brief article gives specific suggestions to parents to help them prepare a child for the experience of being in the hospital. Although the suggestions are intended to help children, adults who face hospitalization can profit from considering the issues this article mentions. Available through InfoTrac College Edition by Wadsworth Publishing Company.

Prochaska, J. O., Norcross, J. C., & DiClemente, C. C. (1994). *Changing for good.* New York: Avon Books.

In this popular, easy-to-read book, the authors of the transtheoretical model offer many practical pointers for changing unhealthy behaviors. The book offers readers suggestions for recognizing their readiness to change and advice on how to accomplish change.

Strecher, V. J., & Rosenstock, I. M. (1997). The health belief model. In A. Baum, S. Newman, J. Weinman, R. West, & C. McManus (Eds.), *Cambridge handbook of psychology, health and medicine* (pp. 113–117). Cambridge, United Kingdom: Cambridge University Press.

This short article discusses the health belief model and reviews research that the model has generated.

CHAPTER 4

Adhering to Medical Advice

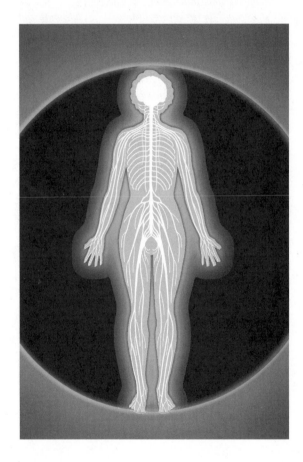

QUESTIONS

This chapter focuses on eight basic questions:

1. Why is adherence to medical advice an important issue?

2. What theoretical models have been used to explain adherence?

3. How can adherence be measured?

4. How frequent is nonadherence?

5. What factors predict adherence?

6. Why do some people fail to adhere to medical advice?

7. How can adherence be improved?

8. Does adherence pay off?

PAUL: DUTIFUL BUT NONCOMPLIANT

Two years ago, Paul, a 47-year-old European American, suffered a heart attack (myocardial infarction), and since that time he has been under treatment for coronary heart disease. After spending 3 weeks in a hospital, Paul felt well enough to go home, and soon afterward he returned to his job as a college professor. After his heart attack, Paul visited his physician on a regular basis and never missed a scheduled appointment. In addition, he strictly followed his doctor's orders concerning his prescribed medication. Despite these dutiful deeds, Paul was not a compliant patient. He continued to smoke a pack and a half of cigarettes a day, allowed himself to remain 60 to 70 pounds overweight, and refused to follow a regular exercise regimen. Paul knew that smoking, improper eating, and a sedentary lifestyle were associated with increased risk of a second heart attack, yet he continued to engage in these unhealthy behaviors. Why?

No completely satisfactory answer to this question is possible. However, some additional information may be illuminating. First, Paul had been smoking for 30 years and had never seriously tried to quit. Second, he had had a weight problem since he was about 25 and had tried several diets in years past, but none had been successful. Third, Paul had not exercised regularly since he played football in high school and college. For Paul, therefore, nonadherence to known healthy behaviors was simply a matter of continuing a lifestyle of long duration. There was a fourth factor involved in his nonadherence as well: His physician was himself a model for unhealthy behaviors. He smoked heavily, was considerably overweight, and did not exercise regularly. Moreover, he had never made clear to Paul what he should do to lower his risk of future coronary problem. Paul, who was divorced and lived alone, had little support or encouragement from family or physician to change his lifestyle.

The Importance of Adherence

For medical advice to benefit the health of patients, two contingencies must be met. First, the advice must be accurate. Second, patients must follow this good advice. Both conditions are essential. Ill-founded advice that patients strictly follow may introduce new health problems, which lead to disastrous outcomes for the compliant patient. On the other hand, excellent advice is essentially worthless if patients do not follow it.

Interestingly, inadequate treatment recommendations combined with low levels of patient adherence to that advice are probably less harmful than either adequate recommendations not followed or invalid advice closely heeded. Irving Janis (1984) suggested that as long as health care providers make mistakes, people are better off not adhering to certain aspects of their advice. Determining which advice is valid and which is not is an important health care problem but largely within the province of medicine; understanding why people adhere or fail to adhere to recommendations and finding ways to improve adherence entails behaviors that are mostly within the realm of psychology.

Paul had gone to considerable effort and expense to seek medical care only to undermine his own progress by neglecting to follow recommended medical regimens. Why do people engage in such self-defeating behavior? What theoretical models explain noncompliant behavior? Is nonadherence a matter of situational factors, such as money, convenience, and time, or do certain personality traits relate to adherence? How pervasive is the problem? How can adherence be measured? How can it be predicted? Does adherence pay off in better health? How can it be improved? This chapter addresses each of these questions, but first we ask a more basic question: What is adherence?

Traditionally, people in the medical profession have used the term *compliance* to refer to patient behaviors that conform to physicians' orders. But because the term compliance connotes reluctant obedience, many health psychologists and some physicians advocate the use of other words, and the terms *adherence, cooperation, obedience,* and

CHECK YOUR HEALTH RISKS

Check the items that apply to you.

☐ 1. I usually stop taking prescription medicine whenever I begin to feel better, even though some of the medication is still left.

☐ 2. If my prescription medicine doesn't seem to be working, I will stop taking it, even though some of the medication is still left.

☐ 3. I believe that faith will cure disease and heal injuries much more certainly than modern medicine.

☐ 4. I won't have a prescription filled if it costs too much.

☐ 5. Although my dentist tells me I should have regular checkups, I only make an appointment when I have a problem.

☐ 6. Often when I don't feel well, I take medication left over from a previous illness, or I borrow someone else's medication.

☐ 7. I am a woman who doesn't worry about breast cancer because I don't have any symptoms.

☐ 8. I am a man who doesn't worry about testicular cancer because I don't have any symptoms.

☐ 9. I sometimes fail to take prescribed medication because I don't want to become addicted to drugs.

☐ 10. I find prescription labels difficult or confusing to read.

☐ 11. People have advised me to stop smoking, but I have never been able to quit.

☐ 12. I frequently forget to take my medication.

☐ 13. If medication makes me feel bad or if it tastes bad, I won't take it.

☐ 14. The last time I was sick, the doctor gave me advice that I didn't completely understand, but I was too embarrassed to say so.

Each of these items represents a health risk from failure to follow medical advice. Although it may be nearly impossible to adhere to all good health recommendations (such as not smoking, eating a healthy diet, exercising, and having regular dental and medical checkups), you can improve your health by adhering to sound medical advice. Count your check marks to evaluate your health risks from failure to follow medical recommendations As you read this chapter, you will learn more about the health benefits of compliance.

---

collaboration have all been suggested as substitutes for compliance. Perhaps the most accurate term to describe the *ideal* relationship between physician and patient would be *cooperation*, a word that implies a relationship in which both the health care provider and the consumer are actively involved in the restoration and maintenance of the patient's health. However, because cooperation is neither a common practice nor an accepted label for this relationship, the terms *compliance* and *adherence* are still the most frequently used words, and many researchers employ these two words interchangeably to describe the patient's ability and willingness to follow recommended health practices.

What does it mean to be compliant? A classic definition of the term was presented by R. Brian Haynes (1979b) who called compliance "the extent to which a person's behavior (in terms of taking medications, following diets, or executing lifestyle changes) coincides with medical or health advice" (pp. 1–2). This definition expands the concept of compliance beyond merely taking medications to include maintaining healthy lifestyle practices, such as eating properly, getting sufficient exercise, avoiding undue stress, abstaining from smoking cigarettes, and not abusing alcohol. In addition, the concept of compliance or adherence includes making and keeping periodic medical and dental appointments, using seatbelts, and engaging in other behaviors that coincide with the best health advice available. Moreover, adherence is a complex concept, with people being compliant in one situation and noncompliant in another (Johnson, 1993). In other words, the noncompliant (or compliant) personality does not exist.

Theories of Adherence

Why do some people comply with medical advice while others fail to comply? Several theoretical models that apply to behavior in general have also been applied to the problem of adherence and nonadherence. Two of the most frequently used models are the behavioral model and the various cognitive learning theories, including self-efficacy theory, the theory of reasoned action, and the health belief model.

The Behavioral Model

The *behavioral model* of adherence is based on the principles of operant conditioning proposed by B. F. Skinner (1953). The key to operant conditioning is the immediate *reinforcement* of any response that moves the organism (person) toward the target behavior—in this case better compliance with medical recommendations. Psychologists have used reinforcement to strengthen compliant behavior. An example might be a monetary payment contingent on the patient's keeping a doctor's appointment. However, psychologists would seldom use **punishment** to lessen noncompliant behaviors. Whereas reinforcers strengthen behavior, the effects of punishment are limited and difficult to predict. At best, punishment will merely inhibit or suppress a behavior. At worst, it conditions strong negative feelings toward any persons or environmental conditions associated with it. Punishment, including threats of harm, are seldom useful in improving a person's compliance with medical advice.

Advocates of the behavioral model use cues, rewards, and contracts to reinforce compliant be-

haviors. Cues include written reminders of appointments, telephone calls from the practitioner's office, and a variety of self-reminders. Rewards can be extrinsic (money and compliments) or intrinsic (feeling healthier). Contracts can be verbal, but they are more often written agreements between practitioner and patient. Most adherence models recognize the importance of incentives in improving compliance.

Some research (Wysocki et al., 1997) shows that behavioral strategies are superior to support groups in reducing friction in families with adolescent diabetics—a serious problem in many households where an insulin-dependent adolescent resists complying to an unpleasant life-style. In addition, behavioral strategies may be at least as potent as more complex cognitive approaches in improving adherence in adult male hemodialysis patients (Hegel, Ayllon, Thiel, & Oulton, 1992).

Cognitive Learning Theories

Cognitive learning theories are based on many of the same learning principles that underlie behavioral models, but they include additional concepts, such as people's interpretation and evaluation of their situation, their emotional response, and their perceived ability to cope with illness symptoms. Many cognitive learning models exist, including self-efficacy theory, the theory of reasoned action, and the health belief model.

Self-Efficacy Theory Several researchers have used Albert Bandura's (1986) notion of *self-efficacy* as an explanation for adherence or nonadherence. Bandura has contended that people's beliefs concerning their ability to initiate difficult behaviors (such as an exercise program) predict their accomplishment of those behaviors. Self-efficacy is a situation-specific concept that refers to people's confidence that they can perform necessary behaviors to produce desired outcomes in any particular situation.

Self-efficacy theory has been used to predict adherence to a variety of health recommendations. For example, a study of sedentary, middle-aged participants with poor cardiorespiratory fitness and high percentages of body fat (McAuley, 1993) found that self-efficacy was a strong predictor of which participants would maintain a newly-begun exercise regimen over a 4-month follow-up. People who believed they could successfully complete the behaviors necessary to maintain an aerobic exercise program had an increased likelihood of adhering to such a program.

Another study (Borrelli & Mermelstein, 1994) examined the role of self-efficacy and goal setting among participants in a smoking cessation program and found that self-efficacy, or confidence in being able to quit smoking, accurately predicted which participants would be able to attain abstinence. Also, some evidence suggests that self-efficacy predicts compliance with dental regimens. For example, a study of adult dental patients (Tedesco, Keffer, & Fleck-Kandath, 1991) found that patients with high self-efficacy were more likely to brush and floss than were those patients low in self-efficacy. These studies indicate that self-efficacy predicts adherence to a variety of treatment programs.

The Theory of Reasoned Action   The *theory of reasoned action* (Ajzen & Fishbein, 1980; Fishbein & Ajzen, 1975) assumes that the immediate determinant of behavior is people's *intention* to perform that behavior. Behavioral intentions, in turn, are a function of (1) people's *attitudes* toward the behavior, which are determined by their beliefs that the behavior will lead to positively or negatively valued outcomes, and (2) their *subjective norm,* which is shaped by their perception of the value that significant others place on that behavior and by their *motivation* to comply with those norms (see Figure 3.1 in Chapter 3).

The theory of reasoned action has been used to predict adherence to a number of health-related behaviors, including exercising. A meta-analysis of studies on the usefulness of this model (Hausenblas, Carron, & Mack, 1997) found that both the theory of reasoned action and the theory of planned behavior have value in predicting who will adhere to an exercise program and who will not. More specifically, the analysis revealed a strong connection between attitude toward exercising and intention to exercise and a strong link between intention and exercise behavior. However, the relationship between subjective norms and intention was only moderate. (Refer again to Figure 3.1.) This study suggests that the theory of reasoned action has at least some value in predicting adherence to exercise behavior.

The Health Belief Model   The *health belief model* (Becker, 1979; Becker & Rosenstock, 1984) assumes that four interactive belief states influence compliance to health-related behaviors. These belief states, which have a cumulative effect for either increasing or decreasing compliant behavior, include (1) perceived susceptibility to the negative consequences of nonadherence, (2) perceived severity of these consequences, (3) the perceived costs/benefits ratio of performing compliant behaviors, and (4) the perceived barriers to incorporating adherence behaviors into one's lifestyle.

The health belief model has perhaps been *misused* more than most other health behavior models have been used (Strecher, Champion, & Rosenstock, 1997), and any evaluation of the health belief model is complicated by the number of different concepts in the model and the different ways the model has been tested. Consequently, some studies have failed to support the model, whereas others have found it to be useful in predicting compliant behaviors. For example, the health belief model suggests that patients who know most about a disease and its consequences should be more compliant than patients who are less knowledgeable. However, one recent study (Katz et al., 1998) found that dialysis patients who knew most about kidney disease were somewhat *less* likely to comply to established health practices than were patients with less knowledge of their disease. On a more positive note, a summary of earlier research (Strecher et al., 1997) revealed some support for the health belief model, with perceived barriers being the strongest and perceived severity of the disease the weakest predictor of all the dimensions.

In Summary

Adherence is the extent to which a person's behavior coincides with appropriate medical and health advice. When people do not adhere to sound health behaviors, they may risk developing serious health problems or even death. When participants in a health intervention study fail to comply, the results of the study may be seriously contaminated.

Several theoretical models attempt to predict and explain compliant and noncompliant behavior. The behavioral model uses contingency contracts and reinforcement for compliant behaviors; cognitive learning theories emphasize people's beliefs about illness and their ability to control their own health; the theory of reasoned action assumes that intentions, attitudes, subjective norms, and motivation predict adherence; and various health belief models may include perceived severity of the disease, perceived personal susceptibility, costs/benefits ratio, and perceived barriers to incorporating adherence behaviors into one's lifestyle. Although none of these models can account for all noncompliant behaviors, they all make some contribution toward a better understanding of reasons for adherence and nonadherence.

Assessing Adherence

The assessment of adherence raises at least two questions. First, how do researchers know the percentage of patients who fail to comply with their practitioner's recommendations? Second, how can noncompliant behaviors be identified? The answer to the first question is that compliance rates are not known with certainty, and that any reported percentage is usually only an estimate.

Second, at least five basic means of measuring patient compliance are available: (1) ask the clinician, (2) ask the patient, (3) ask other people, (4) count pills, and (5) examine biochemical evidence. The first of these methods, asking the clinician, is usually the poorest choice. Physicians generally overestimate their patients' compliance rates, and even when their guesses are not overly optimistic, they are usually wrong. In general, the accuracy of the estimates made by physicians and other health care practitioners is only slightly better than chance (Blackwell, 1997).

Asking patients themselves is a more valid procedure, but it is fraught with many difficulties. Self-reports are inaccurate for at least two reasons: First, patients may lie to avoid the disapproval of their health care provider; second, they may simply not know their own rate of compliance. Patients not only underreport poor adherence, but they also overreport good compliance. In addition, some patients take more medication than recommended, whereas others take less. Thus, self-report measures have questionable validity and should be supplemented by other assessment techniques.

One other technique is to ask hospital personnel and family members to monitor the patient, but this procedure also has at least two inherent problems. First, constant observation may be physically impossible, especially with regard to such regimens as diet and alcohol consumption. Second, persistent monitoring creates an artificial situation and frequently results in higher rates of compliance than would otherwise occur. This outcome, of course, is desirable, but as a means of assessing compliance, it contains a built-in error that makes observation by others inaccurate.

A fourth method of assessing compliance is to count pills. This procedure may seem ideal because very few errors would be made in counting the number of pills absent from a bottle or a drug dispenser. Unfortunately, this method also may be inaccurate. Even if the required number of pills are gone, the patient may not have been compliant. Once again, there are at least two possible problems with pill counts. First, the patient, for a wide variety of reasons, may have simply discarded some of the medication. Second, the patient may have taken all the pills, but in a manner other than the prescribed one.

Several investigators have developed automated devices that facilitate pill counting and determine whether patients take their medication at the prescribed time. One group of investigators (Cramer, Mattson, Prevey, Scheyer, & Ouellette, 1989) reported on a novel assessment technique in which a microprocessor in the pill cap recorded every bottle opening and closing and yielded information concerning the time of day that the bottle was opened. These researchers assumed that each bottle opening equaled one dose of medication. The procedure did not detect the number of pills removed with each opening, and although this procedure represents an improvement over the pill-counting technique, it too cannot ascertain whether patients are taking medication according to their doctor's recommendations.

Examination of biochemical evidence is a fifth method of measuring compliance. This procedure looks at the outcome of compliant behavior to find some biochemical evidence, such as analysis of blood or urine samples, to determine whether the patient has behaved in a compliant fashion. Indeed, research (Roth, 1987) suggests that blood and urine levels are more reliable measures of medicine intake than pill counts, but these measures are also more expensive and often not worth the cost. Other problems arise with using biochemical evidence as a means of assessing compliance. First, some drugs are not easily detected in blood or urine samples. Second, individual differences in absorption and metabolism of drugs can lead to wide variations among people who are equally compliant. Third, biochemical checks must be carried out frequently and regularly to assess compliance rates accurately. Fourth, biochemical methods do not measure the degree of compliance; the presence of a drug or drug marker merely reveals that the patient ingested some amount of the drug at some time and does not indicate that the patient took the proper amount at the proper time.

Computerized recording devices can also assess biochemical outcomes of adherence. One such automatic recording procedure is a *glucometer,* a device used with diabetic patients to record automatically both the occurrence and the results of each blood glucose test. However, use of the glucometer alone does not appear to increase the frequency of self-monitoring of blood glucose levels or to improve diabetic control. Over a relatively short period of time, the glucometer by itself is somewhat effective in increasing compliance, but over longer periods of time, it loses its effectiveness unless it is combined with a behavioral contract (Wysocki, Green, & Huxtable, 1989). This suggests that biochemical techniques alone do not appear to be adequate for assessing rates of compliance with medical recommendations.

In summary, no one of the five basic means of assessing compliance is both reliable and valid. However, with the exception of clinician judgment, most have some limited validity and usefulness. Therefore, when accuracy is crucial, it seems appropriate to use two or more of these basic measures for assessing patient compliance, a procedure that yields greater accuracy than reliance on a single assessment technique.

How Frequent Is Nonadherence?

How pervasive is the problem of nonadherence? The answer to this question depends in part on how nonadherence is defined, the nature of the illness under consideration, the demographic features of the population, and the methods used to assess compliance. In general the rate of noncompliance with medical or health advice is approximately 50% (Haynes, McKibbon, & Kanani, 1996). Robin DiMatteo (1994) reported that at least 38% of patients do not follow short-term treatment plans, and more than 45% fail to adhere to recommendations for long-term treatment. Moreover, as many as three-fourths of all people are unwilling or unable to stick to recommended healthy lifestyles, such as eating a low-fat diet, avoiding cigarette smoking, or exercising regularly.

In the late 1970s, David Sackett and John C. Snow (1979) reviewed more than 500 studies that dealt with the frequency of compliance and noncompliance. They eliminated studies with serious methodological flaws and summarized the results from the remainder. At that time about 75% of the

WOULD YOU BELIEVE...?

Noncompliant Health Care Professionals

Would you believe that health care professionals are as noncompliant as patients? Research on provider noncompliance is not nearly as extensive as studies on patients' failures to adhere to medical advice. However, Mary O'Brien (1997) reported on some research that indicates health care professions have many of the same problems with adherence as patients. Among health care providers, noncompliance consists of departures from guidelines for appropriate medical care and includes a wide variety of behaviors. Some of these failures to comply affect patients, whereas other compliance problems endanger health care providers.

Physicians fail to comply with appropriate medical care when they fail to provide patients with adequate information about their condition, fail to prescribe appropriate medication or order appropriate tests, fail to fulfill continuing education requirements, or fail to report suspected cases of child or spouse abuse. O'Brien found that a substantial percentage of physicians fails to comply with these procedures. About 50% of patients do not receive adequate information from their health care provider, and about 40% of physicians fail to provide themselves with adequate information as a result of not completing their continuing education requirements. Those physicians who comply with continuing education are more likely to order the appropriate screening tests. Physicians are less likely than nurses, ministers, or psychologists to report suspected child or spouse abuse.

Health care providers also endanger themselves through their noncompliance. A set of universal precautions guide hospital health care professionals to avoid infection. Although medical staff members believed that they were at risk, about half of medical students and hospital staff members failed to comply with procedures that would protect them from infections when working with HIV-positive patients. Noncompliance also extends to less serious infections such as influenza. Only 2% of nurses and physicians in one hospital received a flu vaccine, and over 75% of those who got the flu continued to work with patients while they were ill (O'Brien, 1997).

Why do health care professionals fail to comply with procedures that should improve their patients' health and safeguard their own? The reasons are similar to those of noncompliant patients: lack of knowledge, forgetfulness, inconvenience, and resistance to following orders. Physicians who understand the ease and benefits of screening tests are more likely to order such tests (O'Brien, 1997). Health care professionals who feel rushed are less likely to provide adequate information to patients. Increasing pressure on health care workers to provide more care to more patients decreases the chances that workers will comply with procedures that can control infection. In addition, health care workers who do not accept the rationale for hospital procedures are less likely to comply with those procedures.

Can health care workers' compliance be improved? As with patients, simply providing information is not very effective in changing compliance among health care professionals (O'Brien, 1997). However, behavioral strategies such as memory prompts, monitoring, and feedback about performance are more successful. The similarities in noncompliance for patients and health care providers highlight how pervasive and resistant these problems are.

---

patients kept their scheduled appointments when they had initiated them, but only about 50% kept appointments that had been scheduled by the health care professional. As expected, compliance rates were higher when treatment was to cure an illness than when it was to prevent an illness. For example, with reference to taking medication for a short time, 77% were compliant when the treatment was designed to cure a disease; only 63% complied when treatment was aimed at

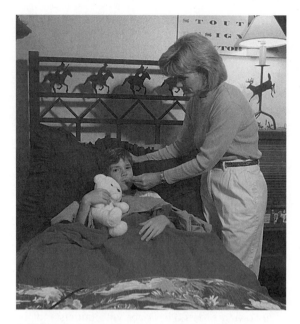

Parents follow medical advice for their sick children at a similar rate as for themselves—about 50%.

prevention. According to Sackett and Snow, when medication must be taken over a long period, compliance is around 50% for either prevention or cure. Compliance rates for dietary regimens ranged from 30% to 70%, again with a mean of about 50%. (See the Would You Believe . . . ? box.)

Unfortunately, little evidence exists that compliance rates have risen since this early review. Indeed, compliance rates have remained quite constant, with about half of all patients failing to comply with recommended medical programs (Dishman & Buckworth, 1997; Haynes et al., 1996; Monane et al., 1996). What factors determine who will be compliant and who will be noncompliant?

What Factors Predict Adherence?

If we assume that people always act in their own best interests, we may be at a loss to explain the factors that do and do not relate to adherence. For example, it may seem intuitively obvious that the amount of money invested in the treatment procedure would predict compliance. Intuition, however, does not always agree with the evidence. One study (Jamison & Akiskal, 1983) found that a third to half of the patients suffering from bipolar (manic-depressive) disorder stopped taking lithium, despite the very low cost of that drug and the potential disadvantages of noncompliance. An earlier study (Becker, Drachman, & Kirscht, 1972) reported that more than half the mothers who were giving penicillin to their children for middle ear infection stopped prematurely even though the medication was given to them at no cost. These mothers did what many noncompliant patients do—they simply stopped the medication when the symptoms disappeared.

Other than the disappearance of symptoms, what factors do or do not predict compliance? Possible predictors can be divided into four groups: characteristics of the disease, characteristics of the person, cultural norms, and characteristics of the relationship between the health care provider and the patient.

Illness Characteristics

Characteristics of the disease include the severity of the disease, the unpleasantness of the medication's side effects, the duration of treatment, and the complexity of treatment.

Severity of the Illness In general, people with a serious illness are no more likely than people with a mild illness to seek medical treatment or to comply with medical advice. Common wisdom might suggest that people with severe, potentially crippling or life-threatening illnesses will be highly motivated to adhere to regimens that protect them against such major catastrophes.

Interestingly, little evidence exists to support this logical hypothesis. Indeed, people sometimes seek health care not because they have a serious medical problem but because someone might casually mention that they looked bad. For example, Robin DiMatteo and Dante DiNicola (1982) reported a case study concerning a woman who had been hit by a baseball bat and had suffered some loss of vision in her left eye. The loss of vision, however, did not prompt her to go to a doctor. She sought treatment only after a friend casually commented that her eyelid drooped!

Indeed, studies on the relationship between compliance and severity of a disease reveal no consistent evidence that people are more likely to comply with treatment regimens for a serious illness than they are when the disorder is minor (Haynes, 1979a). Haynes summed up these studies by noting that "counter to common wisdom, not a single study has found that increasing severity of symptoms encourages compliance" (p. 51).

Although severity of symptoms as seen by the physician is not related to compliance, the severity of an illness as seen by the patient (Becker & Maiman, 1980) and the patient's experience with *pain* (Becker, 1979) both predict adherence. When people believe that their symptoms are serious and when they suffer great pain, they have strong motivation to comply to any treatment that might cure their illness or reduce their discomfort.

Research also indicates that compliance with regimens designed to treat or prevent major illnesses tends to be no higher than with those aimed at treating or preventing minor disorders. For example, a study of glaucoma patients (Vincent, 1971) reported that more than half did not follow simple instructions for using eyedrops. Even when people became legally blind in one eye, the rate of compliance remained below 60%. These findings suggest that about half of all people remain noncompliant even at the risk of a devastating disorder.

In summary, results of research on compliance and the severity of illness suggest two general conclusions. First, no direct relationship exists between the severity of an illness (as perceived by physicians) and a patient's probability of complying with recommended medical regimens, especially those prescriptions aimed at prevention. Second, if patients have experienced pain from a disorder, they are more likely to comply with their

physician's recommendations. Pain by itself, of course, is not a true indicator of the severity of an illness, but it may be one of several factors that help convince patients to cooperate in protecting their own health.

Why do people undermine their own health by not adhering to sound medical advice? One possible answer can be found in the parallel response model suggested by Howard Leventhal (Leventhal, 1970). The parallel response model assumes that when people perceive a dangerous situation, such as a severe illness, their appraisal of that threat produces two relatively independent processes—Danger Control and Fear Control. People primarily motivated by Danger Control ignore or overcome their fear by behaving adaptively—for example they seek medical care when symptoms first appear. On the other hand, people motivated largely by Fear Control behave in a manner aimed mostly at reducing their fear. Behaviors that reduce fear are negatively reinforcing, even those that are maladaptive—for example, drinking alcohol, using drugs, or ignoring illness symptoms. Leventhal believes that level of fear interacts with the perceived adequacy of a preventive measure to predict compliance. For example, if people believe that tetanus shots are completely reliable, that belief combined with a high level of fear should produce a high rate of compliance. Conversely, if people believe that a preventive program (such as dental hygiene) is less than adequate, then that belief combined with a high level of fear should produce a low level of compliance.

Leventhal's parallel response model suggests that at times, people are more strongly motivated to reduce their fear than to avoid the danger that accompanies a devastating and chronic disease. This may account for the poor relationship between severity of an illness and the rate of adherence to treatment.

Side Effects of the Medication   A second illness characteristic that might relate to adherence is the potential unpleasantness of the medication's side effects. One might guess that a drug with few or no unpleasant side effects will produce greater patient compliance, but the evidence in support of this position is not overwhelming. However, little evidence exists that unpleasant side effects are a major reason for discontinuing a drug or dropping out of a treatment program (Masur, 1981). This does not mean that side effects are completely unrelated to noncompliance but simply that most noncompliant people do not consider them a very important factor.

Duration of the Treatment   A third illness characteristic is the duration of the treatment. In general, the longer people must submit to treatment or preventive regimens, the more likely they are to drop out of treatment. Haynes (1976a) reviewed several studies that compared compliance rates to the length of treatment and concluded that in most cases, noncompliance increases as duration of therapy increases. However, most long-term treatment programs are for illnesses that have no symptoms, such as hypertension. Understandably, people are less motivated to continue a lengthy therapeutic regimen in the absence of unpleasant symptoms.

Complexity of the Treatment   A final illness characteristic is the complexity of the treatment. Are people less likely to comply as the treatment procedures become increasingly more complex? In general, the greater the variety of medications a person must take, the greater is the likelihood that people will not take pills in the prescribed manner. For example, one study (Cramer et al., 1989) found that as the number of pills per day increased from one to three, the rate of compliance decreased from 88% to 77%—a small but significant decline. However, patients who were prescribed four doses per day achieved only a 39% compliance rate. These data indicate that compliance drops dramatically when pills are to be taken more than three times a day.

The reason seems obvious. For most people, a day has one, two, or three prominent periods, and

medicine can be cued to each. For example, pills prescribed once a day can be taken early in the morning; those prescribed twice a day can be cued to early morning and late night; and those prescribed three times a day can be taken after each meal. Adherence to any of these three schedules is quite high. Schedules calling for medication to be taken four or more times a day create an unnatural division of the day for most people, resulting in low compliance rates.

In summary, the more complex the treatment, the lower the rate of compliance. After looking at the evidence, Philip Ley, who has studied adherence for more than 30 years, concluded that "the simpler the treatment schedule, and the shorter its duration, the greater is compliance" (Ley, 1997, p. 282).

Personal Characteristics

Researchers have investigated such individual characteristics as age, gender, social support, personality traits, and personal beliefs about health to determine their association with people's adherence to medical advice. Do any of these variables predict compliance?

Age   The relationship between adherence and age is complicated by several factors. Depending on the specific illness, the time frame, and the adherence regimen, studies show that compliance can either increase or decrease with age. For example, a study of adherence to an exercise program for 26- to 68-year-old-adults with high cholesterol initially revealed a positive correlation between age and adherence (Lynch et al., 1992). This might suggest that as people get older they become more concerned with their health and are more likely to comply with an exercise program designed to reduce cholesterol. However, as the program continued beyond 26 months, age was not significantly related to adherence, a finding that prompted the authors to suggest that older participants may have suffered some minor physical discomfort that interfered with exercise.

A later study (Thomas et al., 1995) added a further complication to this issue by finding a curvilinear relationship between age and compliance with colorectal cancer screening. In this large-scale, longitudinal study of both men and women, the best compliers were around 70 years old; the worst were below 55 or over 80. Perhaps after age 80 people simply do not regard screening for colorectal cancer to be important. Some evidence (Monane et al., 1996; Sherbourne, Hays, Ordway, DiMatteo, & Kravitz, 1992) suggests that among adults, adherence to regimens for diabetes, hypertension, and heart disease tends to increase as people get older. However, with young diabetic patients, age may be inversely related to compliance. One study of 10- to 19-year-old diabetics reported that as the patients' age increased, their compliance with their exercise program and insulin self-injection decreased (Bond, Aiken, & Somerville, 1992). A later study (Olsen & Sutton, 1998) found that as young adolescent diabetics grow into late adolescence, they feel more isolated from their family and tend to show greater noncompliance with an inconvenient health-protective regimen.

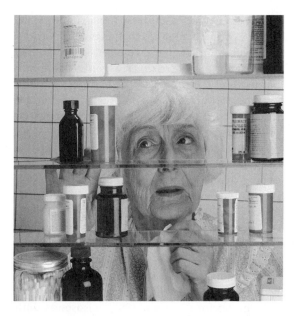

More complex treatments tend to lower compliance rates.

Gender   With regard to gender, researchers have found few differences between the overall adherence rates of women and men but some differences in adherence to specific recommendations. In general, men and women are about equal in dropping out or staying with an exercise program (Emery, Hauck, & Blumenthal, 1992) and in taking prescribed antihypertensive medication (Monane et al., 1996). However, women seem to be better at adhering to healthy diets with lots of vegetables (Laforge, Greene, & Prochaska, 1994) and at taking medication for a mental disorder (Sellwood & Tarrier, 1994).

Social Support   The introduction to this chapter presented the case of Paul, the coronary heart patient who faithfully adhered to his physician's prescriptions concerning medication but who was less compliant with regard to good health prac-

tices. Paul was divorced, lived alone, and enjoyed no close personal relationships. His case suggests an association between compliance and the support a patient receives from family and friends.

One of the strongest predictors of adherence is the level of social support one receives from friends and family, but even this factor is not invariably related to compliance. In general, people who are isolated from others are likely to be noncompliant; those whose lives are filled with close interpersonal relationships are more likely to follow medical advice. For example, compliance by hemodialysis patients increases when family members are neither emotionally distant nor emotionally overinvolved and when they have some understanding of the emotional effects of the illness (Sherwood, 1983).

Social support also increases rates of adherence to appointments in chronically ill patients. In an experimental design (Tanner & Feldman, 1997), low-income patients with no symptoms of their chronic illness were divided into four groups: (1) a control group that received only an exit interview; (2) an experimental group that received the interview plus social support counseling of the patient's significant other; (3) an experimental group that received the interview and counseling plus a postcard reminder; and (4) an experimental group that received the interview, counseling, and postcard plus a telephone call. Results revealed that social support counseling of the significant other led to significantly better adherence to appointment keeping than the interview and was at least as effective alone as it was when combined with the postcard and the telephone call.

Support of family and friends also increases compliance among heart patients. For example, strong social support is positively related to the likelihood that hypertensive patients will adhere to medical advice, including keeping appointments with the doctor (Stanton, 1987). Also, men with high cholesterol whose wives are highly supportive are more likely to adhere to their diet than men whose wives offer little support (Bovbjerg et al., 1995).

Emotional Support Some evidence suggests that *quality* rather than *quantity* of social support predicts diabetics' adherence to complex medical recommendations. The number of friends may be unrelated to a patient's compliance, but the quality of interpersonal relations is a significant predictor of adherence (Sherbourne et al., 1992). Similarly, emotional support may be a better predictor of compliance than marriage. One study (Kulik & Mahler, 1993) found that, although married men who had undergone artery bypass surgery were more likely than unmarried men to have followed their doctor's advice, the key to adherence was the level of emotional support they received from their wives rather than marriage itself.

Personality Traits Are certain personality types more likely than others to be noncompliant? Despite the belief among some doctors that the patient's "uncooperative personality" is the most likely explanation for nonadherence to medical ad-

vice, no research evidence has supported this supposition. Personality traits such as extraversion/introversion, authoritarianism, neuroticism, and impulsivity do not predict adherence. Neither do general personality disorders. One team of researchers (Pfohl, Barrash, True, & Alexander, 1989) administered the Personality Diagnostic Questionnaire (PDQ) to male hypertensive outpatients and found that more than a fifth of the patients met the criteria for at least one personality disorder. Nevertheless, they found no evidence that the PDQ was useful in identifying people who were at risk for noncompliance.

If personality traits did predict noncompliance, then the same people should be noncompliant in a variety of situations. Again, little evidence supports this conclusion. On the contrary, some indications exist that noncompliance is specific to the situation. For example, one study (Lutz, Silbret, & Olshan, 1983) exposed a group of people experiencing intense pain to five different pain relief regimens and found that compliance with one program was unrelated to compliance with the others. Another study (Orme & Binik, 1989) obtained similar results, finding that adherence to one diabetic treatment regimen was independent of adherence to others. Thus, the evidence suggests that noncompliance is not a global personality trait but is specific to a given situation.

Nevertheless, researchers have recently identified two personality traits—obsessive-compulsive disorders and cynical hostility—as possible predictors of compliance or noncompliance. Intuitively, it would seem that obsessive-compulsive individuals should be more compliant than other people, and some evidence supports this hypothesis. Using the Symptoms Checklist-90-R, Jon Kabat-Zinn and Ann Chapman-Waldrop (1988) found that scores on the obsessive-compulsive scale predicted which patients would adhere to an 8-week stress-reduction regimen and which ones would not. Obsessive-compulsive people, as one might guess, were more likely to complete the program. Kabat-Zinn and Chapman-Waldrop (p. 348) concluded that people who score low on the obsessive-compulsive scale "may be at a greater risk for ignoring or denying the importance of compliance."

The second personality trait that may be related to nonadherence is cynical hostility. A recent study (Christensen, Wiebbe, & Lawton, 1997) used the Cook-Medley Hostility (Ho) Scale to measure cynical hostility in hemodialysis patients. They found that high hostility scores were associated with poor dietary and medication adherence. People who score high on the Cook-Medley Hostility Scale are generally suspicious, mistrustful, and resentful of others and have frequent outbursts of anger, which may predispose them to reject or disregard the advice that health care professionals provide. (We discuss the Cook-Medley Hostility Scale and its relation to cardiovascular disease in Chapter 9.). In summary, although the noncompliant personality seems to be a myth, some evidence exists that obsessive-compulsiveness is positively related to good compliance, whereas cynical hostility is positively related to poor adherence.

Personal Beliefs Although few personality traits predict who will adhere to medical recommendations, some evidence suggests that patients' beliefs are related to compliance. We have seen that perceived self-efficacy, the theory of reasoned action, and the health belief model all have some ability both to predict and to explain adherence and nonadherence. In general, when patients believe that adherence to treatment recommendations will result in health benefits, they are likely to comply with those recommendations. During the past 20 years, some evidence has accrued suggesting that health beliefs might be a promising alternative to traditional personality traits in explaining adherence.

Martha Brownlee-Duffeck and her colleagues (Brownlee-Duffeck et al., 1987) examined health beliefs and their effects on adherence to diabetic treatment regimens for both adults and adolescents. For adults, the belief that compliance will benefit one's health predicted adherence. For adolescents, however, the perceived health benefits of compliance were not important. Young diabetic patients have notoriously low levels of compliance, and this study suggested that even when they see the long-range value of following treatment recommendations they are not very likely to comply. Factors that did predict adolescents' rate of adherence were financial costs, perceived severity of the illness, and their belief that they were susceptible to diabetic complications if they did not follow their treatment regimen. Brownlee-Duffeck et al. concluded that older diabetics are able to see the long-range benefits of adherence, whereas adolescent patients are more likely to adhere to their treatment regimen when they are experiencing immediate discomfort.

Some people cope with illness by denying personal vulnerability or by avoiding personal responsibility for taking actions that might restore health. These people use **avoidance coping** strategies to reduce the stress of being sick. They may smoke more, overeat, abuse alcohol or other drugs, or simply hope for a miracle. Such strategies are often effective for a short time, but in the long run they are usually hazardous to health. People who use avoidance coping are less likely than others to adhere to their doctor's advice, perhaps because they either deny the efficacy of such advice or because they reject responsibility for their own health care (Sherbourne et al., 1992).

On the other hand, people who believe they are personally responsible for their own health are more likely to adhere to medical advice. For example, one study (Helby, Gafarian, & McCann, 1989) found that diabetic patients who assumed responsibility for their health care were more likely than others to adhere to their treatment program. Similarly, hypertensive patients are more likely to adhere to their medical regimens when they believe that they exercise some personal control over both their blood pressure and their health (Stanton, 1987). In summary, people who believe they have little control over their own health tend to be noncompliant, whereas those patients believe that their own actions will bring about a health benefit are more likely to adhere to medical advice.

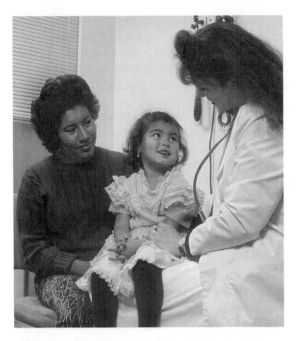

Patient compliance is high when practitioners convey information about the condition and reasons for treatment.

Cultural Norms

One factor that definitely relates to compliance is the patient's cultural beliefs and attitudes. DiNicola and DiMatteo (1984) suggested that people fail to comply not because they have basically uncooperative personalities, but because they live within a culture that holds beliefs and attitudes—which the patients share—that are not conducive to adherence to health regimens. For example, if one's family or tribal traditions include strong beliefs in the efficacy of tribal healers, it seems reasonable that the individual's compliance with modern medical recommendations might be low. A study of diabetic and hypertensive patients in Zimbabwe (Zyazema, 1984) found a large number of people who were not adhering to their recommended therapies. As might be expected, many of these patients still believed in traditional healers, and they had little faith in modern medical procedures. Another study (Ruiz & Ruiz, 1983) reported that Latino patients were more likely to comply with medical advice

when their physicians demonstrated some understanding of Hispanic cultural norms and practices. These findings have important implications for physicians and other health care providers whose clientele consists largely of people from many different cultural backgrounds.

The Practitioner-Patient Interaction

We have seen that both illness characteristics and personal characteristics are only minimally successful at predicting compliance with medical regimens. A more satisfactory group of predictors are those subsumed under the category of patient-practitioner interaction. Within this category are such factors as the verbal communication between health care provider and patient, the practitioner's perceived level of competence, the amount of time between referral and treatment, and the length of time patients must spend in the practitioner's waiting room.

Verbal Communication   Perhaps the most crucial factor in patient noncompliance is the insufficiency of verbal communication between the practitioner and the patient. Again, Paul's case illustrates this point. Because Paul recalled only vague and general information regarding diet and smoking, either his physician was remiss in detailing the precise healthful practices that Paul was to follow, or Paul was less than receptive to the information—or perhaps both.

The miscommunication can start when physicians ask patients to report on their symptoms and fail to listen to patients' concerns. What constitutes a concern for the patient may not be essential to the diagnostic process, and practitioners can seem unconcerned when they are, in fact, trying to elicit information relevant to making a diagnosis. However, patients may misinterpret the physician's focus as a lack of personal concern or as overlooking what patients consider important symptoms. After practitioners come to a diagnosis, they typically tell patients about that diagnosis. If the diagnosis is minor, patients are relieved and not highly motivated to adhere to (or even listen to) any instructions that may follow. If the verdict is grave, patients are likely to become anxious, and this anxiety may then interfere with their concentration on subsequent medical advice.

As already noted, physicians tend to overestimate the level of patient compliance and to assume that their directions will be heard, understood, and acted on. Little evidence exists, however, to support this assumption, and research indicates that misunderstanding and miscommunication in conveying information and instructions can adversely affect compliance.

Even when patients are both highly motivated and reasonably relaxed, they may not understand the information they hear. For a variety of reasons, physicians and patients frequently do not speak the same language. First, physicians operate in familiar territory. They know the subject matter, are comfortable with the physical surroundings, and are ordinarily calm and relaxed with procedures that have become routine to them. Patients, in contrast, may be unfamiliar with medical terminology; distracted by the strange environs; and distressed by anxiety, fear, or pain (Charlee, Goldsmith, Chambers, & Haynes, 1996). Differences in native language, educational level, ethnic background, or social class may also contribute to problems in communication. As a result, patients either fail to remember or misunderstand much of the information their doctors give them.

What types of verbal communication hinder patient adherence? Research suggests that patients are least likely to comply when they receive emotionally-toned information from a clinician. For example, a study of the effects of nurse-patient interactions (Rorer, Tucker, & Blake, 1988) on hemodialysis patients' compliance with their dietary regimen found a close relationship between emotionally negative responses by nurses and patient noncompliance. An emotionally negative response was defined as one that tended to make the nurse-patient relationship less cohesive or attractive to both nurse and patient. Interestingly, this study also found that emotionally positive verbal responses—those that made the nurse-patient relationship more cohesive—increased

noncompliance! In addition, these researchers found that more experienced nurses spent less time addressing the problem of patient noncompliance. Possibly, more experienced health care providers see the futility of providing information on treatment regimens and thus spend less time talking to patients about compliance.

Evidence also exists that physicians either fail to recommend good health practices or their patients fail to understand their communication. For example, data from the Stanford Five-City Project (Frank, Winkleby, Altman, Rockhill, & Fortmann, 1991) indicated that only 50% of smokers said that their doctors had ever advised them either to stop smoking or to smoke less. Moreover, fewer than 4% of ex-smokers reported that their physicians had helped them to quit, which indicates that the overwhelming proportion of people who stop smoking do so without the aid of their physicians.

How often do physicians offer patients health promotion advice during office visits? One study (Russell & Roter, 1993) found that doctors provided information or made suggestions about changes in patients' lifestyle and health behaviors in only about half the visits. The most frequent suggestions were about diet and weight control, but physicians also mentioned exercise, stress, smoking, and alcohol. Unfortunately, physicians tended not to use the most effective behavioral strategies for getting their patients to adopt the suggested changes, leading to the conclusion that physicians miss important opportunities to urge their patients to change unhealthy behaviors.

The Practitioner's Personal Characteristics A second aspect of the practitioner-patient interaction is the perceived personal characteristics of the physician. As might be expected, patients' compliance improves as confidence in their physician's technical ability increases (Becker, Drachman, & Kirscht, 1972; Gilbar, 1989). In addition, several physician personality variables—as perceived by the patient—are related to compliance. DiNicola and DiMatteo (1984) reported that people were more likely to follow the advice of doctors they

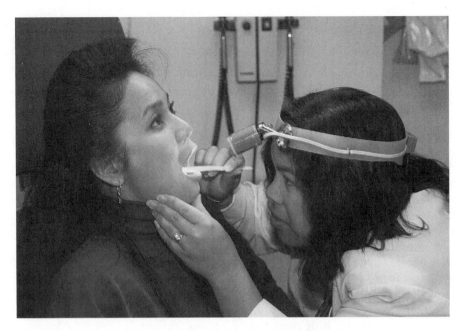

Female physicians encourage patient interaction, which can boost compliance rates.

saw as warm, caring, friendly, and interested in the welfare of patients. When physicians display a good bedside manner, such as making eye contact, smiling, leaning forward, and even joking and laughing, patient compliance improves.

Although patients are more likely to adhere to recommendations from competent and knowledgeable physicians, they become less eager to comply when the physician's expertise is expressed in an authoritarian fashion. Patients are more likely to remain noncompliant when they see their doctors as authoritarian and when they feel as though they are treated as inferiors in the decision-making process (Gastorf & Galanos, 1983). Also, doctors who take noncompliance personally and react defensively are more likely to have patients with low compliance rates (Heszen-Klemens, 1987). This evidence suggests that compliance could be enhanced by warm and caring physicians who take an interest in their patients' health and who regard patients as partners in the treatment and prevention processes.

The physicians' gender also may play a role in the exchange of information between doctor and patient. A study of both female and male physicians during patient visits (Hall, Irish, Roter, Ehrlich, & Miller, 1994) found that female physicians made more partnership statements, made more positive statements, and asked more questions than male physicians. In addition, patients talked to female physicians more than to male physicians, and the gender of both physician and patient contributed to the communication pattern during the visit.

Effective patient-physician interaction also encourages the patient to volunteer information. Although many patients merely respond to their physicians' questions, some research (Rost, Carter, & Innui, 1989) has found that compliance improved when patients both initiated information and provided it in answer to questions. This *bidirectional* information may contribute to a patient-doctor partnership that can arrive at meaningful treatment decisions.

In Summary

Adherence rates can be measured by (1) asking the physician, (2) asking the patient, (3) asking other people, (4) counting pills, and (5) examining biochemical evidence. Each has serious flaws. Assessing the frequency of nonadherence is complicated by the different definitions of the term, the nature of the illness, the population being studied, and the methods used to assess compliance. In general terms, however, the rate of nonadherence is about 50%.

Neither severity of the disease as seen by the physician nor severity of the side effects of the disease are reliable predictors of adherence. However, several conditions predict nonadherence: (1) long and complicated treatment regimens; (2) lack of social support for adherence; (3) patients' perception of the severity of their illness; (4) patients' cultural beliefs that modern medicine is ineffective; (5) patient's beliefs that their own behavior cannot benefit their health; (6) poor patient-practitioner communication; and (7) unfriendly, incompetent, or authoritarian physicians.

Factors with an inconsistent relationship to adherence include age, gender, and personality traits. Older adults are generally more compliant until they reach about age 80, whereas young diabetic patients become less compliant throughout adolescence. As for gender, women and men are about equal in their rates of adherence, although women do better at adhering to a healthy diet and taking some types of medication. Only two personality traits have been found to predict adherence: Obsessive-compulsive individuals are generally more compliant and cynically hostile people are less compliant. Table 4.1 summarizes the research on what factors do or do not predict adherence.

Problems of Adherence

We have surveyed several issues related to adherence, including examinations of theoretical models that might explain or predict compliance, techniques of measuring compliance, the frequency of compliance, and factors that do or do not relate to compliance. Now we look at three final questions: (1) Why are some people nonadherent? (2) Does adherence pay off? (3) How can adherence be improved?

Why Are Some People Nonadherent?

After his heart attack, Paul's physician told him, "Well, I guess we're going to have to get you off those damned weeds." This statement may have been meant as a requirement to quit smoking, but Paul interpreted it as a mere comment. Unfortunately, many patients leave the doctor's office still unclear about their instructions and with no specific plan for carrying out their medical regimen. Vagueness of physician advice is one of the communication problems between patient and physician, but it is only one of several reasons people fail to follow medical advice.

One reason for high rates of nonadherence is that the current definition of adherence demands certain difficult lifestyle changes. At the beginning of the 20th century, when the leading causes of illness and death were infectious diseases, compliance was simpler. Patients were compliant when they followed the doctor's advice with regard to medication, rest, diet, and so on. With health restored, patients could return to their former way of living. Adherence is no longer a matter of taking the proper pills and following short-term advice. The three leading causes of death in the United States—cardiovascular disease, cancer, and chronic obstructive lung disease—are all affected by unhealthy lifestyles. Thus compliance, broadly defined, currently includes adherence to healthy and safe behaviors as part of an ongoing lifestyle. To be compliant, people must now avoid cigarette smoking, use alcohol wisely or not at all, eat properly, and exercise regularly. In addition, of course, they must also make and keep medical and dental appointments, listen with understanding to the advice of health care providers, and finally, follow that advice. These requirements present a

Table 4.1 Predictors of patient adherence

	Findings	Studies
I. *Disease Characteristics*		
1. *Severity of medication's side effects*	No relationship	Masur, 1981
2. *Severity of illness*		
(as seen by the physician)	No relationship	Haynes, 1979a; Vincent 1971
(as seen by the patient)	Positive relationship	Becker & Maiman, 1980
3. *Duration of treatment*	Negative relationship	Haynes, 1976a
4. *Complexity of treatment*	Complexity leads to non-adherence, as does number of doses over 3	Cramer, 1989; Haynes, 1979a
II. *Personal Characteristics*		
1. *Age*		
Adults		
(exercise up to 6 months)	Positive relationship	Lynch et al., 1992
(exercise after 6 months)	No relationship	Lynch et al., 1992
(cancer screening)	Curvilinear relationship	Thomas et al., 1995
(hypertensive medication)	Positive relationship	Monane et al., 1996
(diabetes)	Positive relationship	Sherbourne et al., 1992
(heart disease)	Positive relationship	Sherbourne et al., 1992
Adolescents		
(diabetes)	Negative relationship	Bond et al., 1992
(diabetes)	Negative relationship	Olsen & Sutton, 1998
2. *Gender*		
(exercise)	Men and women equal	Emery et al., 1992
(hypertensive medication)	Men and women equal	Monane et al., 1996
(diet)	Women more compliant	Laforge et al., 1994
(medication)	Women more compliant	Sellwood & Tarrier, 1994
3. *Social support*	Positive relationship	Bovbjerg et al., 1995
(hemodialysis regimen)	Positive relationship	Sherwood, 1983
(appointment keeping)	Positive relationship	Tanner & Feldman, 1997
4. *Emotional support*		
(diabetes)	Positive relationship	Sherbourne et al., 1992
(heart regimen)	Emotional support better predictor than marriage	Kulik & Mahler, 1993
5. *Personality traits*		
(personality disorder)	No relationship	Pfohl et al., 1989
(obsessive-compulsive)	Positive relationship	Kabat-Zinn & Chapman-Waldrop, 1988
(cynical hostility)	Negative relationship	Christensen et al., 1997

Table 4.1   (continued)

	Findings	Studies
6. *Personal beliefs*		
(avoidance coping)	Negative relationship	Sherbourne et al, 1992
(personal control)	Positive relationship	Helby et al., 1989; Stanton, 1987
III. Cultural Norms		
(diabetic & hypertensive patients in Zimbabwe)	Cultural beliefs predict compliance	Zyazema, 1984
(Physician's knowledge of Hispanic culture)	Positive relationship	Ruiz & Ruiz, 1983
IV. Practitioner/Patient Interaction		
1. *Verbal communication*		
(emotional information)	Negative relationship	Rorer et al., 1988
(physician disinterest)	Negative relationship	Frank et al., 1991
(physician disinterest)	Negative relationship	Russell & Roter, 1993
2. *Practitioner's personal qualities*		
(friendliness)	Predicts compliance	DiNicola & DiMatteo, 1984
(gender)	Female doctors provide more information	Hall et al., 1994
(communication skills)	Positive relationship	Rost et al.,1989

complex array of requirements that are difficult to fulfill.

The second category of reasons for nonadherence includes all those problems inherent in hearing and heeding physicians' advice. Patients may reject the prescribed regimen as being too difficult, time-consuming, or expensive; or they may reject the practitioner as being incompetent, arrogant, or unfriendly. Also, many patients stop taking their medication when their symptoms disappear. Paradoxically, others stop because they begin to feel worse and thus believe the medication is useless. Still others, in squirrel-like fashion, save a few pills for the next time they get sick.

Responsibility for adherence rests with both the patient and the health care professional, and both contribute to patients' noncompliant behavior. Many patients don't understand their physician's criteria for specific adherence (Orme & Blink,

1989), and others stop taking their medication because adherence is simply too much trouble or it does not fit into the routine of their daily lives (Hunt, Jordan, Irwin, & Browner, 1989). Still other patients may make irrational choices about adherence because they have an **optimistic bias** that they will be spared the grave consequences of noncompliance (Brock & Wartman, 1990). Another suggestion is that some patients fail to follow medical advice because they hope for a miracle (Sherbourne et al., 1992). Other patients may be noncompliant because prescription labels are too difficult to read. For example, one study (Mustard & Harris, 1989) found that fewer than half of college students were able to correctly understand prescription labels that had been randomly selected from a pharmacist's records. Table 4.2 summarizes some of the reasons patients give for not complying with medical advice.

Table 4.2 **Reasons given by patients for not complying with medical advice**

"It's too much trouble."

"I won't get sick. God will save me."

"I just didn't get the prescription filled."

"The medication was too expensive."

"The medication didn't work very well. I was still sick, so I stopped taking it."

"The medication worked after only one week, so I stopped taking it."

"I have too many pills to take."

"I forgot."

"I want to remain sick."

"I don't want to become addicted to pills."

"If one pill is good, then two pills should be twice as good."

"I saved some pills for the next time I get sick."

"I gave some of my pills to my husband so he won't get sick."

"They're trying to poison me."

"This doctor doesn't know as much as my other doctor."

"The medication makes me sick."

"The medication tastes bad."

"Taking medication is just another bad habit."

"I was hoping for a miracle."

"I don't see any reason to take something to prevent illness."

"My doctor prescribes too many pills. I don't need all of them."

"I don't like my doctor. She thinks she knows everything."

"I didn't understand my doctor's instructions and was too embarrassed to ask him to repeat them."

"I don't like the taste of nicotine chewing gum."

"I won't get very sick anyway, so I don't need to take anything."

"I didn't understand the directions on the label."

How Can Adherence Be Improved?

Methods for improving compliance can be divided into educational and behavioral strategies. Educational procedures are those that impart informa-tion, sometimes in an emotion-arousing manner designed to frighten the noncompliant patient into becoming compliant. Included with educational strategies are such procedures as health education messages, individual patient counseling with various professional health care providers, pro-grammed instruction, lectures, demonstrations, and individual counseling accompanied by written instructions. Behavioral strategies, on the other hand, focus more directly on changing the person's behaviors involved in compliance. They include a wide variety of techniques, such as reducing eco-nomic barriers to compliance, using reward to re-inforce compliance, notifying patients of upcom-ing appointments, simplifying medical schedules, making home visits, and persistently monitoring and rewarding the patients' compliant behaviors.

When R. Brian Haynes (1976b) reviewed the lit-erature on educational, behavioral, and combined educational-behavioral strategies for improving compliance, he found educational techniques to be relatively ineffective. Of 16 studies reviewed, only 7 reported significant results. Interventions that threaten patients with disastrous consequences for noncompliance are only marginally effective in bringing about a meaningful change in their per-sonal behavior. Behavioral techniques proved to be more effective in improving patient compliance. Haynes (1976b) reviewed 20 studies that had em-ployed various behavioral strategies and found that 16 of them had reported a significant and positive effect on compliance. When he examined studies that had combined educational and behavioral ap-proaches, Haynes found that all eight had reported significant results. According to Haynes's review, therefore, both behavioral strategies and combina-tion approaches have an advantage over educa-tional procedures. Although Haynes's definition of behavioral strategies was quite broad, it appears from his review that techniques attempting to in-crease patient involvement and to encourage an ac-tive, ongoing relationship between patient and practitioner are most likely to improve patient compliance. Behavioral approaches had the advan-tage even though educational strategies increased patients' knowledge and improved their skill in taking medication. People, it seems, do not misbehave because they do not know better, but because proper behavior, for a variety of reasons, is less appealing.

Later, Haynes and his associates (Haynes, Wang, & da Mota Gomes, 1987) reviewed the literature on interventions designed to improve adherence and found only two well-designed studies that were able to increase compliance with short-term treatments (1 to 2 weeks in duration). These studies suggested that short-term compliance can be improved to some extent by reducing the prescribed dose to one or two times a day and by giving patients special pill packages and calendars that indicate when and how many pills they should take. Short-term compliance, of course, is easier to achieve than compliance that must continue over a long period.

In 1992, Haynes and his associates (Macharia, Leon, Rowe, Stephenson, & Haynes, 1992) searched the literature for articles on compliance and appointment keeping. They found 23 articles with "scientific merit" that also included an intervention for improving compliance. These studies used a variety of strategies to improve patients' compliance with keeping appointments, including letter and telephone prompts, computer-generated messages to the physician that identified patients who would be visiting the clinic, patient contracts, and educational information. Once again, education was not an effective means of improving adherence, but most of the other interventions were of limited value. For example, contracts improved compliance by about 14%, an increase very typical of the other interventions.

The ineffectiveness of educational and instructional procedures has instigated a growing interest in various behavioral and cognitive strategies for improving patient compliance. These interventions include self-monitoring, home visits, cues and rewards, and peer group discussions. Haynes et al. (1987) found that cues and rewards seem to be the most consistently effective means of improving compliance. Cues include using one's toothbrush or a completed meal as a signal to take one's medication. Rewards might include small sums of money given by the health care provider, or self-reinforcement, such as seeing a movie or treating oneself to a nice meal. Both cues and rewards have been shown to increase the chances that patients will take their prescribed medication.

DiMatteo and DiNicola (1982) recommended four behavioral strategies for improving adherence. First, various *prompts* can be used to remind patients to initiate health-enhancing behaviors. These prompts may be cued by regular events in the patient's life, such as taking medication before each meal, or they may take the form of telephone calls from a clinic to remind the person to keep an appointment or to refill a prescription. A second behavioral strategy, *tailoring the regimen,* involves fitting the treatment to habits and routines in the patient's daily life. Third, these authors suggested a *graduated regimen implementation* that reinforces successive approximations to the desired behavior. Such shaping procedures should be effective with exercise and diet, but of course they are not appropriate to the taking of medications. The final behavioral strategy listed by DiMatteo and DiNicola was a *contingency contract,* an agreement (usually written) between patients and the health care professionals that provides for some kind of reward to patients contingent on their achieving compliance. The ultimate goal of each of these approaches is self-regulation. However, before reaching this goal, patients often need help from others. This outside help, whether from family members or from professionals, ordinarily is given extensively at first and then is gradually withdrawn as patients begin to acquire more control over their health-related behaviors.

Cognitive-behavioral interventions are aimed at improving patients' knowledge of their disease and the consequences of nonadherence to treatment. They also attempt to enhance patients' social support and to increase their self-efficacy for ad-herence to healthy behaviors. Cognitive-behavioral strategies include training patients to monitor their health-related behaviors, to evaluate those behaviors against a predetermined criterion, and to use positive self-reinforcement

BECOMING HEALTHIER

You can improve your health by following sound health-related advice. Here are some things you can do to make adherence pay off.

1. Adopt an overall healthy lifestyle—one that includes incorporating safety into your life, not smoking, using alcohol in moderation or not at all, eating a diet high in fiber and low in saturated fats, and getting an optimum amount of regular physical activity. Procedures for adopting each of these health habits are discussed in *Becoming Healthier* boxes, Chapters 12 to 16.

2. Establish a relationship with your physician that is one of cooperation and not servile obedience. You and your doctor are the two most important people involved in your health, and the two of you should cooperate in designing your health practices.

3. Another important person interested in your health is your spouse, parent, friend, or sibling. Enlist the support of a significant person or persons in your life. Research shows that high levels of social support improve one's rate of adherence.

4. Before visiting a health-care provider, jot down some questions you would like to have an-

swered; ask the questions, and write down the answers during the visit. If you receive a prescription, ask the doctor about possible side effects—you don't want an unanticipated unpleasant side effect to be an excuse to stop taking the medication. Also, be sure you know how long you must take the medication—some chronic diseases require a lifetime of treatment.

5. If you feel that your physician gives you complex medical information that you don't comprehend, ask for clarification in a language that you can understand.

6. Remember that some recommendations (such as beginning a regular exercise program) should be adopted gradually. (If you run too far too fast the first day, you won't feel like exercising again the next day.)

7. Find a doctor who understands and appreciates your cultural beliefs, ethnic background, language, and religious beliefs.

8. Reward yourself for following your good health practices. If you faithfully followed your diet for a day or week, do something nice for yourself.

for any progress toward meeting the criterion. Several studies have demonstrated the effectiveness of cognitive-behavioral methods in improving patient compliance with a variety of health and medical regimens, including exercise (McAuley, 1993), lithium treatment for bipolar disorders (Cochran, 1984), and weight control for hemodialysis patients (Hegel et al., 1992).

In addition to behavioral and cognitive-behavioral strategies to improve compliance, several novel but simple interventions have shown promising results. Obtaining a *verbal commitment* from mothers increased their adherence to the

recommended medical regimen for their children (Kulik & Carlino, 1987). Also, the simple process of a *service fee* for missed appointments was effective in decreasing missed appointments at a college health center (Wesch, Lutzker, Frisch, & Dillon, 1987). *Hypnosis* can be effective in initiating and maintaining dental flossing by college students, increasing the rate from 15% to 67% of students who flossed daily (Kelly, McKinty, & Carr, 1988). Hypnosis can also improve compliance in adolescent diabetics who previously showed poor control of their blood glucose (Ratner, Gross, Casas, & Castells, 1990). Finally, an instructional audiotape helped undergraduate women improve their proficiency at breast self-examination (Jones et al., 1993). Although these studies generally used few participants and lacked rigorous controls, they point to potentially promising means of improving patient adherence.

Haynes et al. (1987) proposed several other means of improving adherence to medical recommendations. For all treatment regimens, they suggested that the prescription should be as simple as possible and that patients should receive clearly written instructions on the exact behaviors to follow. For long-term treatments, these authors recommended reminders, rewards, and social support. More specifically, they suggested that health care providers can increase compliance by (1) calling patients who miss an appointment, (2) providing medication that fits easily into a patient's daily schedule, (3) reinforcing the importance of adherence at each visit, (4) tailoring the number of visits to fit the patient's level of compliance, (5) verbally rewarding the patient's efforts to comply, (6) decreasing the frequency of visits as a reward for good adherence, and (7) involving the patient's spouse or other partner.

Despite these suggestions, little progress has been made in improving rates of compliance. In 1996, R. Brian Haynes and his colleagues (Haynes, McKibbon, & Kanani, 1996) once again reviewed the research on improving adherence and found serious flaws in most of the studies. Of more than 1500 studies, only 13 met the criteria of being randomized, controlled trials. Of these 13, only 7 were effective in improving compliance to medication, leading Haynes et al. to conclude that little evidence exists that adherence can be improved and also that complex and labor-intensive interventions are "not very effective despite the amount of effort and resources they consumed" (p. 386).

Does Adherence Pay Off?

We have seen that at least half of all patients do not fully follow their health care practitioner's advice and that patients give a variety of reasons for nonadherence. In addition, most health care

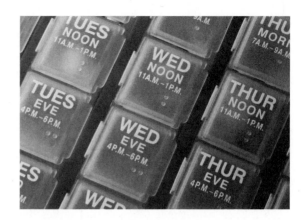

Finding ways to fit medication into patients' schedules can improve adherence rates.

providers view noncompliance as a serious problem and an obstacle to the prevention of disease and the restoration of health. Is such concern justified? Does adherence pay off?

Evidence for the efficacy of adherence is not clear-cut; some studies show that compliance pays off, whereas others suggest that it does not. Results of studies from the National Heart, Lung, and Blood Institute's Beta-Blocker Heart Attack Trial (Gallagher, Viscoli, & Horwitz, 1993) indicated that female heart patients who took their prescribed medication were less likely to have died from all causes than those patients who did not. In this study, women who were poor adherers were nearly two and a half times more likely to have died than women who were good adherers. The effect of compliance was independent of age, severity of the heart attack, congestive heart failure, marital status, smoking history, and other factors. Adherence also paid off for men who were part of the same study (Horwitz et al., 1990). Male heart patients who were low in compliance were more than 2.6 times as likely to have died than men high in adherence.

These two studies demonstrate a significant relationship between adherence and survival following a heart attack, but they do not prove that good adherence to the medical regimen prevented death from heart disease. Interestingly, the poor adherers in both studies had a greater risk of death whether they were in the heart medication group or in the placebo group. Women who took no heart medication but who were poor adherers to the placebo were 2.8 times more likely to have died than women in the placebo group who were good adherers. Noncompliant men in the placebo group were 2.5 times as likely to have died than compliant men in the placebo group. These findings suggest that noncompliance itself may contribute to all-cause mortality. Perhaps noncompliant people are not conscientious and have little regard for their own health. These two studies suggest that either the power of the placebo is much stronger than earlier studies indicated or that some heart patients do not protect themselves well from a variety of potentially fatal conditions.

Other studies have failed to show any strong positive association between faithful adherence and improved health. In the study cited above, Haynes and his associates (Haynes et al., 1996) conducted an exhaustive review of more than 1500 studies on adherence and found that compliance to medication generally does not pay off in improved health. Despite the extreme complexity of many of these studies, Haynes et al. concluded that the various interventions to improve compliance were not only ineffective, but they did not generally lead to better patient health.

Earlier, Ron Hays and his colleagues (Hays et al., 1994) had compared the health of compliant patients who suffered from a variety of disorders with the health of noncompliant patients. After 4 years, these researchers found that the compliant patients were not much more improved than the nonadherent patients. In this study, the relationships among health and adherence were complex and not always consistent with what the researchers hypothesized. The strongest positive relationship was between adherence to diet in insulin-using diabetics and subsequent ratings of positive health, but some negative relationships appeared between adherence and health. That is, the higher the compliance to their medication schedule, the lower the ratings of health for insulin-using diabetics and for depressed patients. It is possible that people with these disorders might have rated their health as worsening because of the side effects they experienced when they took their medication as prescribed. Hays et al. suggested four possible explanations for their finding of a generally poor relationship between adherence and improved health. First, their study relied on patient self-reports of adherence, so some errors may have existed in the assessment of compliance; second, physician advice may have been quite vague, a condition we discussed earlier; third, 4 years may not have been enough time to observe the results of continual noncompliance; and fourth, other factors, such as heredity or environmental conditions, may have affected the course of the illnesses. Somewhat pessimistically, these authors stated: "We cannot conclude from these data that assisting patients with these conditions to adhere to their physicians' recommendations will necessarily lead to better health over time" (Hays et al., 1994, p. 356). They added that adherence to unproved medical recommendations may be a questionable practice and concluded that "it may be time to turn the focus toward documenting what really works in medicine rather than spotlighting the failure of patients to follow recommendations that may or may not be therapeutic" (p. 357).

In Summary

Three important questions on adherence are: Why are some people nonadherent? Does adherence pay off? How can adherence be improved?

People are nonadherent for a variety of reasons, including the difficulty they face in altering lifestyles of long duration, incomplete practitioner-patient communication, and erroneous beliefs as to what advice they should follow. Effective programs to improve compliance rates frequently include clearly written instructions, simple prescriptions, follow-up calls for missed appointments, prescriptions tailored to the patient's daily schedule, rewards for compliant behavior, cues to signal the time for taking medication, and involvement of the patient's spouse or support network. Although many physicians regard nonadherence as a major detriment to people's health, research has failed to find a significant benefit to high levels of compliance.

Answers

This chapter addressed eight basic questions:

1. **Why is adherence to medical advice an important issue?**

   Adherence is the extent to which a person's behavior coincides with appropriate medical and health advice. For people to profit from medical advice, that advice first must be accurate and second, patients must follow that advice. When people do not adhere to sound health behaviors, they may risk developing serious health problems or even death. When participants in a health intervention study fail to comply, the results of the study may be seriously contaminated.

2. **What theoretical models have been used to explain adherence?**

   Several theoretical models attempt to predict and explain compliant and noncompliant behavior. These include the *behavioral model,* which relies on contingency contracts and reinforcement for compliant behaviors, and various *cognitive learning theories,* such as the *self-efficacy model,* which holds that people's beliefs that they can perform certain behaviors strongly predict what behaviors they will enact; the *theory of reasoned action,* which assumes that intentions, attitudes, subjective norms, and motivation predict adherence; and various *health belief models,* which typically include perceived severity of the disease, perceived personal susceptibility, costs/benefits ratio, and perceived barriers to incorporating adherence behaviors into one's lifestyle. Each of these models has some use in predicting and explaining compliance and noncompliance.

3. **How can adherence be measured?**

   There are at least five basic ways of measuring patient adherence: (1) ask the physician, (2) ask the patient, (3) ask other people, (4) count pills, and (5) examine biochemical evidence. Of these, physician judgment is the least valid, but each of the others also has serious flaws.

4. **How frequent is nonadherence?**

   Assessing the frequency of nonadherence is complicated by the different definitions of the term, the nature of the illness, the population being studied, and the methods used to assess compliance. In general terms, however, the rate of nonadherence has remained around 50% for the past 2 or 3 decades.

5. **What factors predict adherence?**

   Researchers have found little evidence that certain disease and personal characteristics predict adherence. Neither severity of the disease as seen by the physician nor severity of the side effects of the disease are reliable predictors of adherence. Also, personality traits are mostly unrelated to compliant behavior. Two exceptions are (1) obsessive-compulsive behaviors, which may be positively related to adherence and (2) cynical hostility, which seems to be positively related to nonadherence.

   Researchers have found some evidence for each of the following predictors of *nonadherence:* (1) long and complicated treatment regimens; (2) lack of social support for adherence; (3) patients' perception of the severity of their illness; (4) patients' cultural beliefs that modern medicine is ineffective; (5) patient's beliefs that their own behavior cannot benefit their health; (6) poor patient-practitioner communication; and (7) unfriendly, incompetent, or authoritarian physicians.

6. **Why do some people fail to adhere to medical advice?**

   There are probably as many reasons for nonadherence as there are noncomplying patients, and many of these reasons are difficult to determine with certainty. However, some relate to the difficulty of altering lifestyles of long duration. Others result from incomplete practitioner-patient communication, which leaves the patient with erroneous beliefs as to what course of action to follow.

7. How can adherence be improved?

Psychologists have suggested a variety of behavioral strategies to improve adherence, and a combination of these interventions usually increases compliance rates. Effective programs frequently include clearly written instructions, simple prescriptions, follow-up calls for missed appointments, prescriptions tailored to the patient's daily schedule, rewards for compliant behavior, cues to signal the time for taking medication, and involvement of the patient's spouse or support network.

8. Does adherence pay off?

Although many physicians regard nonadherence as a major detriment to people's health, research has failed to find a significant benefit to high levels of compliance.

Glossary

avoidance coping   Reacting to illness by the denial of threat and the use of such strategies as overeating, taking drugs, or hoping for a miracle.

optimistic bias   The belief that other people, but not one's self, will develop a disease, have an accident, or experience other negative events.

punishment   The presentation of an aversive stimulus or the removal of a positive one. Punishment sometimes, but not always, weakens a response.

Suggested Readings

Blackwell, B. (1997). From compliance to alliance: A quarter century of research. In B. Blackwell (Ed.), *Treatment compliance and the therapeutic alliance* (pp. 1–15). Amsterdam: Harwood Academic Publishers.

This concise overview of compliance addresses many of the basic issues in the field, including the meaning of compliance, its effectiveness, how it can be measured, and how it can be improved.

DiMatteo, M. R. (1994). Enhancing patient adherence to medical recommendations. *Journal of the American Medical Association, 271,* 79, 83.

In this brief report, DiMatteo reviews the frequency of nonadherence, looks at factors that determine noncompliance, and recommends a cooperative relationship between patient and health care provider.

Haynes, R. B., McKibbon, K. A., & Kanani, R. (1996). Systematic review of randomized trials of interventions to assist patients to follow prescriptions for medications. *Lancet, 348,* 383–386.

The latest of Haynes's reviews on various issues of adherence, this article presents a pessimistic look at interventions to improve either compliance or the health of people who are compliant.

Strecher, V. J., Champion, V. L., & Rosenstock, I. M. (1997). The health belief model and health behavior. In D. S. Gochman (Ed.), *Handbook of health behavior research I: Personal and social determinants* (pp. 71–91). New York: Plenum Press.

This chapter deals with many of the misuses of the health belief model and suggests how the model should be properly used, not only on issues of adherence but other health-seeking behaviors as well.

 USA Today Magazine. (1997, October). Clues that you may need a new doctor. *USA Today Magazine, 126*(2629), 1–2.

This brief article presents results from a survey on patient preferences in practitioners' behavior and attitudes, showing a preference for good communication skills. Available through InfoTrac College Edition by Wadsworth Publishing Company.

CHAPTER 5

Defining and Measuring Stress

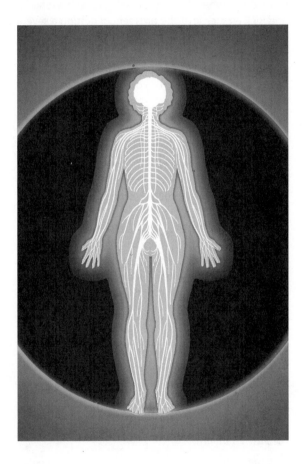

QUESTIONS

This chapter focuses on four basic questions:

1. What is the physiology of stress?

2. What theories explain stress?

3. What sources produce stress?

4. How has stress been measured?

RICK: DIVORCE, DEATHS, AND JOB STRESS

Three years ago, Rick's life was so filled with stress that he did not see how he was going to manage. When he was 28 years old, he separated and then divorced his wife and was involved in a bitter custody battle over his daughter. Both his father and a close friend died within weeks of each other. He lost his job and had to work at two and sometimes three jobs to meet his financial commitments.

His work was also a source of stress. Rick was in law enforcement, and his patrol duties and dealings with prisoners were sometimes dangerous and often difficult experiences. He also worked in a large discount store part time, and the constant activity and many demands of that work situation were quite difficult. Rick did not feel that he could cut back on the jobs because he needed the money.

His divorce and the death of his father and friend changed Rick's social life. According to Rick, his social network "fell apart," leaving him more isolated than he had ever been. In addition, he felt a great deal of animosity toward his ex-wife and her family. In the custody battle, his ex-wife and her family tried to alienate Rick from his daughter and keep him from seeing her. Rick was angry, but he felt that it was important not to lose control, so he suppressed his emotions.

Few facets of Rick's life were untouched. His diet became less healthy, and he abandoned his regular exercise program. He experienced problems in sleeping, and the headaches he had experienced for about 3 years became more severe and more frequent. Rick's headaches related to two neck injuries, but he also believed that stress played a major role in their developing into a chronic pain problem. There were times when his pain interfered with working, and Rick was tense at the prospect of getting a severe headache, a condition he knew made the headaches more likely.

For more than a year Rick experienced incessant, overabundant stress. To cope with the pressure and social isolation, he started college and became active in his church—activities that helped Rick build a new social life and career. Now, 3 years after his separation and the deaths of his father and his close friend, Rick experiences the "normal" stresses of taking tests and juggling work and school, but he views his life now as much less stressful than it was 3 years ago.

This chapter looks at what stress is and how it can be measured. Chapter 6 examines the question of whether stress, like Rick's, can cause illness or premature death, and Chapter 8 looks at ways of coping with stress. But first, we discuss the physiology of the peripheral nervous system and the neuroendocrine system.

 CHECK YOUR HEALTH RISKS

Social Readjustment Rating Scale (SRRS)

Check each of the items that have happened to you within the past 18 months.

Rank	Life event	Mean value	Rank	Life event	Mean value
❏ 1.	Death of spouse	100	❏ 8.	Fired at work	47
❏ 2.	Divorce	73	❏ 9.	Marital reconciliation	45
❏ 3.	Marital separation	65	❏ 10.	Retirement	45
❏ 4.	Jail term	63	❏ 11.	Change in health of family member	44
❏ 5.	Death of close family member	63	❏ 12.	Pregnancy	40
❏ 6.	Personal injury or illness	53	❏ 13.	Sex difficulties	39
❏ 7.	Marriage	50			

Rank	Life event	Mean value		Rank	Life event	Mean value
❑ 14.	Gain of new family member	39		❑ 33.	Change in schools	20
❑ 15.	Business readjustment	39		❑ 34.	Change in recreation	19
❑ 16.	Change in financial state	38		❑ 35.	Change in church activities	19
❑ 17.	Death of close friend	37		❑ 36.	Change in social activities	18
❑ 18.	Change to different line of work	36		❑ 37.	Mortgage or loan less than $10,000	17
❑ 19.	Change in number of arguments with spouse	35		❑ 38.	Change in sleeping habits	16
❑ 20.	Mortgage over $10,000	31		❑ 39.	Change in number of family get-togethers	15
❑ 21.	Foreclosure of mortgage or loan	30		❑ 40.	Change in eating habits	15
❑ 22.	Change in responsibilities at work	29		❑ 41.	Vacation	13
❑ 23.	Son or daughter leaving home	29		❑ 42.	Christmas	12
❑ 24.	Trouble with in-laws	29		❑ 43.	Minor violation of the law	11
❑ 25.	Outstanding personal achievement	28				
❑ 26.	Wife begins or stops work	26				
❑ 27.	Begin or end school	26				
❑ 28.	Change in living conditions	25				
❑ 29.	Revision of personal habits	24				
❑ 30.	Trouble with boss	23				
❑ 31.	Change in work hours or conditions	20				
❑ 32.	Change in residence	20				

Add the points for the items you checked. If your score is less than 150, your life events place you in a group that has experienced low levels of stress and no elevation of risk for stress-related disease. Individuals with scores between 150 and 300 have experienced more stressful life experiences, and those with scores over 300 may be at elevated health risk due to their levels of stress. Later in this chapter we examine this scale as well as other methods for measuring stress.

Source: From "The Social Readjustment Rating Scale," by T. H. Holmes and R. H. Rahe, 1967, *Journal of Psychosomatic Research II,* p. 216. Reprinted by permission of Pergamon Press and Thomas H. Holmes.

The Nervous System and the Physiology of Stress

The basic function of the nervous system is to integrate all the body's systems. Small, simple organisms do not need (nor do they have) nervous systems. In larger and more complex organisms, nervous systems provide internal communication and relay information to and from the environment.

The human nervous system contains billions of individual cells called **neurons.** The action of neurons is electrochemical. Within each neuron, electrically charged ions hold the potential for an electrical discharge. This discharge, a minute electrical current, travels the length of the neuron. The electrical charge leads to the release of chemicals called **neurotransmitters** that are manufactured within each neuron and stored at the ends of the neurons. The released neurotransmitters diffuse across the **synaptic cleft,** the space between neurons.

A number of different neurotransmitters have been identified; many more remain unidentified.

Of those that are understood, the chemical action is quite complex. Some neurotransmitters produce an excitatory action, which promotes the development of the neurons' electrical potential. Other neurotransmitters inhibit transmission, making neurons more difficult to activate. When a neuron is stimulated and releases its transmitter chemical, the excitatory and inhibitory messages have a cumulative effect. The next neuron's threshold must be exceeded for it to be activated. If the threshold is reached, then the next neuron "fires." If the threshold is not reached, then the next neuron will not be activated.

Neurons do not form an end-to-end chain; rather, they are more like a net, with each neuron having as many as several hundred synaptic connections. One neuron may form multiple connections with another neuron and, in addition, it may synapse with several other neurons. With the many avenues for communication among neurons, excitatory and inhibitory effects, and billions of neurons in each person's nervous system, great complexity in neural transmission is ensured.

The billions of neurons fall into three types. **Afferent neurons** (sensory neurons) relay information from the sense organs toward the brain. The action of **efferent neurons** (motor neurons) results in movement of muscles or stimulation of organs or glands. **Interneurons** connect sensory neurons to motor neurons.

The nervous system is organized hierarchically, with major divisions and subdivisions. The two major divisions of the nervous system are the **central nervous system (CNS)** and the **peripheral nervous system (PNS)**. The CNS is composed of the brain and the spinal cord, and the PNS consists of all other neurons. The divisions and subdivisions of the nervous system are illustrated in Figure 5.1.

The next section describes the nervous system from the bottom of its organizational hierarchy to the top—that is, beginning with the PNS and ending with the brain. This approach traces the path of information from the periphery of the nervous system to the brain.

The Peripheral Nervous System

The peripheral nervous system, that part of the nervous system lying outside the brain and spinal cord, is divided into two parts: the **somatic nervous system** and the **autonomic nervous system (ANS)**. The somatic nervous system has both sensory and motor components, primarily serving the skin and the voluntary muscles. The autonomic nervous system primarily serves internal organs.

The Somatic Nervous System   The somatic division of the peripheral nervous system serves muscles and skin. Sensory impulses begin with stimulation of the skin and muscles, and these neural impulses travel toward the spinal cord by way of sensory nerves in the somatic nervous system. Motor messages that originate in the brain travel down the spinal cord, are relayed to muscles, and initiate muscle movement. The motor nerves that activate muscles are part of the somatic nervous system.

Sensory and motor impulses in the head and neck region do not travel through the spinal cord. Instead, 12 pairs of cranial nerves enter and exit directly from the lower part of the brain. The cranial nerves are also part of the somatic nervous system. They function like the sensory and motor neurons that run through the spinal cord.

The Autonomic Nervous System   The term *autonomic* means "self-governing." It has been applied to this division of the peripheral nervous system because, traditionally, the autonomic nervous system has been considered outside the realm of conscious or voluntary control. Although the functions of the ANS do not require conscious thought, we now know it is possible for people to learn to exert conscious control over many ANS functions. Neal Miller's (1969) famous experiments with biofeedback demonstrated that rats could learn to accelerate or decelerate their heart rate, a function under autonomic control. Many types of biofeedback have been developed, and several have clinical ap-

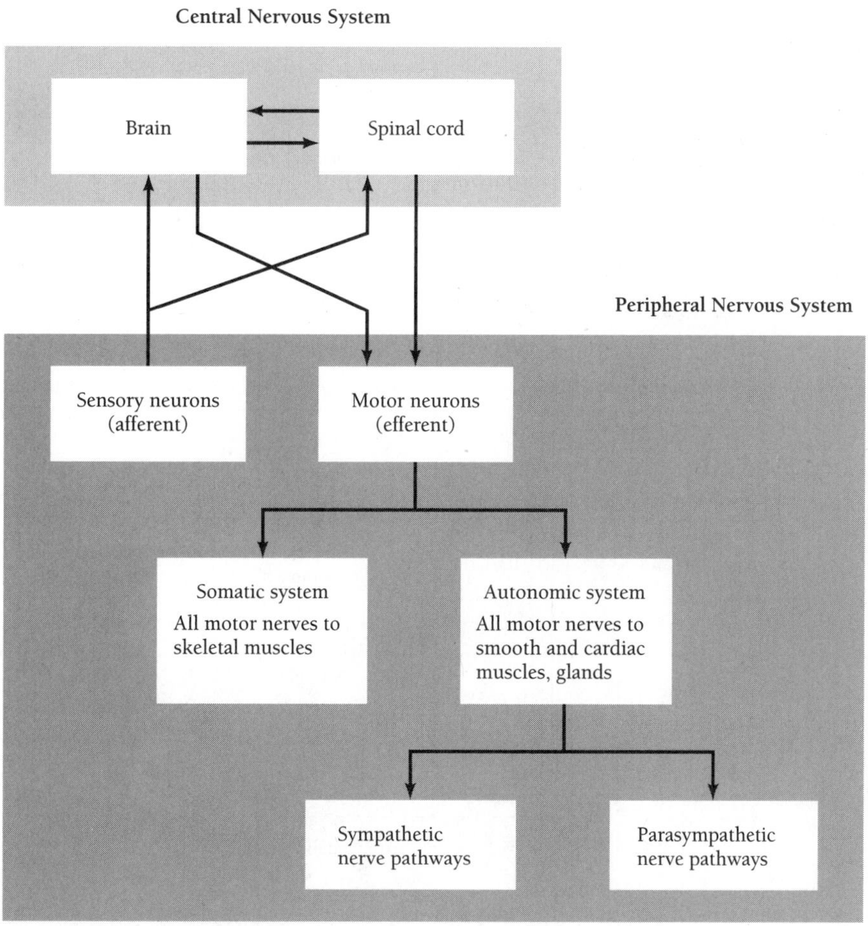

Central Nervous System

Figure 5.1   Divisions of the human nervous system.

plications in health psychology (as Chapter 8 explains). Learning to control autonomic functions requires both effort and training, but some control of the ANS is within the realm of human capability.

The ANS allows for a variety of responses through its two divisions: the **sympathetic nervous system** and the **parasympathetic nervous system**. These two subdivisions differ anatomically as well as functionally. They, along with their target organs, are shown in Figure 5.2.

The sympathetic division of the ANS mobilizes the body's resources in emergency, stressful, and emotional situations. Walter Cannon (1932) termed this configuration of responses the "fight or flight" reaction. Sympathetic activation prepares the body for intense motor activity, the sort necessary for attack, defense, or escape. The reactions include an increase in the rate and strength of cardiac contraction, constriction of blood vessels in the skin, a decrease of gastrointestinal activity, an increase in respiration, stimulation of the sweat glands, and dilation of the pupils in the eyes.

The parasympathetic division of the ANS, on the other hand, promotes relaxation and functions

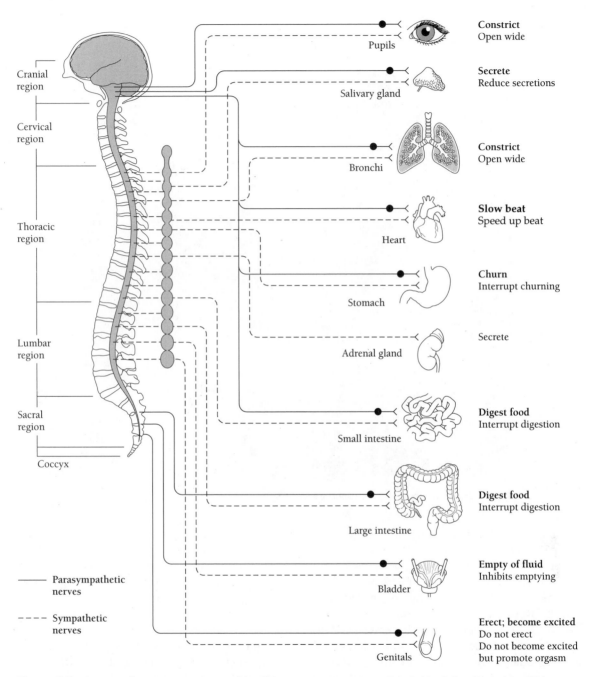

Figure 5.2 Autonomic nervous system and target organs. *Source:* From *Biological Psychology* (2nd ed., p. 18) by J. W. Kalat, 1984, Belmont, CA: Wadsworth Publishing Company. Reprinted by permission.

under normal, nonstressful conditions. The parasympathetic and sympathetic nervous systems serve the same target organs, but they tend to function reciprocally, with the activation of one increasing as the other decreases. For example, the activation of the sympathetic division reduces the secretion of saliva, producing the sensation of a dry mouth, whereas activation of the parasympathetic division promotes secretion of saliva.

As in other parts of the nervous system, neurons in the ANS are activated by neurotransmitters. Neurotransmission in the ANS is conducted mainly by two chemicals, **acetylcholine** and **norepinephrine,** which have complex effects. Each of these neurotransmitters has different effects in different organ systems because the organs contain different neurochemical receptors. In addition, the balance of these two main neurotransmitters, as well as their absolute quantity, is important. Therefore, even though there are only two major ANS neurotransmitters, they produce a wide variety of responses.

At its optimum, the autonomic nervous system adapts smoothly, rapidly mobilizing resources by sympathetic activation and adjusting to normal demands by parasympathetic activation.

The Neuroendocrine System

The **endocrine system** consists of ductless glands distributed throughout the body (see Figure 5.3). The **neuroendocrine system** consists of those endocrine glands that are controlled by the nervous system. Glands of the endocrine and neuroendocrine systems secrete chemicals known as **hormones,** which move into the bloodstream to be carried to different parts of the body. Specialized receptors on target tissues or organs allow hormones to have specific effects, even though the hormones circulate throughout the body. At the target, hormones may have a direct effect, or they may cause the secretion of another hormone.

The endocrine and nervous systems can work closely together because they have several similarities, but they also differ in important ways. Both systems share, synthesize, and release chemicals. In the nervous system these chemicals are called *neurotransmitters.* In the endocrine system they are called *hormones.* The activation of neurons is usually rapid and the effect is short term; the endocrine system responds more slowly, and its action persists longer. In the nervous system, neurotransmitters are released by stimulation of neural impulses, flow across the synaptic cleft, and are immediately either reabsorbed or inactivated. In the endocrine system, hormones are synthesized by the endocrine cells, are released into the blood, reach their targets in minutes or even hours, and have prolonged effects. The endocrine and nervous systems both have communication and control functions, and both work toward integrated, adaptive behaviors. The two systems are related in function and interact in neuroendocrine responses.

The Pituitary Gland   Located within the brain, the **pituitary gland** is an excellent example of the intricate relationship between the nervous and endocrine systems. The pituitary is connected to the hypothalamus, a structure in the forebrain. These two structures work together to regulate and produce hormones. The pituitary has been referred to as the "master gland" because it produces a number of hormones that affect other glands and prompts the production of other hormones.

Of the seven hormones produced by the anterior portion of the pituitary gland, **adrenocorticotropic hormone (ACTH)** plays an essential role in the stress response. When stimulated by the hypothalamus, the pituitary releases ACTH, which in turn acts on the **adrenal glands.**

The Adrenal Glands   The adrenal glands are endocrine glands located on top of each kidney. Each gland is composed of an outer covering, the **adrenal cortex,** and an inner part, the **adrenal medulla.** Both secrete hormones that are important in the response to stress. The **adrenocortical**

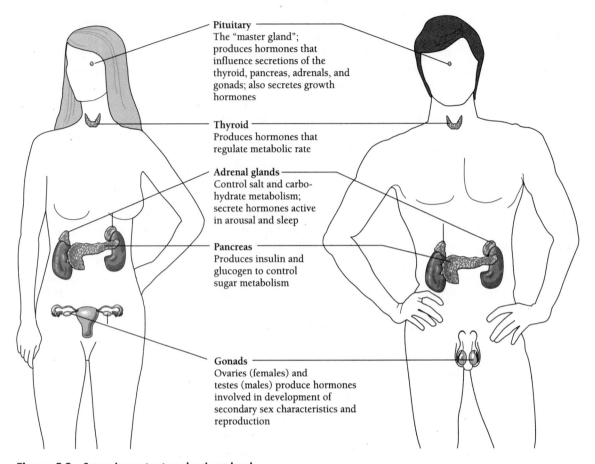

Pituitary
The "master gland"; produces hormones that influence secretions of the thyroid, pancreas, adrenals, and gonads; also secretes growth hormones

Thyroid
Produces hormones that regulate metabolic rate

Adrenal glands
Control salt and carbohydrate metabolism; secrete hormones active in arousal and sleep

Pancreas
Produces insulin and glucogen to control sugar metabolism

Gonads
Ovaries (females) and testes (males) produce hormones involved in development of secondary sex characteristics and reproduction

Figure 5.3 Some important endocrine glands.

response occurs when ACTH from the pituitary stimulates the adrenal cortex to release **glucocorticoids,** one type of hormone. **Cortisol** is the most important of these hormones and is capable of affecting every major organ in the body (Lovallo, 1997). This hormone is so closely associated with stress that the level of cortisol circulating in the blood can be used as an index of stress.

The **adrenomedullary response** includes activation of the adrenal medulla by the sympathetic nervous system, which prompts secretion of **catecholamines,** a class of chemicals containing **epinephrine** and norepinephrine. Epinephrine

(sometimes referred to as adrenaline) is produced exclusively by the adrenal medulla and accounts for about 80% of the hormone production of the adrenal glands. Norepinephrine is also a neurotransmitter and is produced in many places in the body besides the adrenal medulla. Both of these hormones act slower than other neurotransmitters and their action is more prolonged.

Physiology of the Stress Response

The sympathetic division of the autonomic nervous system controls mobilization of the body's resources in emotional, stressful, and emergency situations. Through the effects of various hormones, stress initiates a complex series of events within the neuroendocrine system. The anterior pituitary (the part of the pituitary gland at the base of the brain) secretes adrenocorticotropic hormone (ACTH), which stimulates the adrenal glands to secrete glucocorticoids, including cortisol. Its secretion mobilizes the body's energy resources, raising the level of blood sugar to provide energy for the cells. Cortisol also has an anti-inflammatory effect, giving the body a natural defense against swelling from injuries that might be sustained during a fight or a flight.

Activation of the adrenal medulla results in the secretion of catecholamines, the class of chemicals that includes norepinephrine and epinephrine. Norepinephrine, however, is also one of the neurotransmitters of the autonomic nervous system. Neurotransmitters work at the synapse whereas hormones circulate through the blood. Norepinephrine has both actions and is produced at many places in the body, not exclusively in the adrenal medulla.

Epinephrine, on the other hand, is produced exclusively in the adrenal medulla. It is so closely and uniquely associated with the adrenomedullary stress response that it is sometimes used as an index of stress. The amount of epinephrine secreted can be determined by assaying a person's urine, thus measuring stress by tapping into the physiology of the stress response. Such an index can be helpful because it does not rely on personal perceptions of stress and its use as a measure of stress can give an alternative perspective.

In Summary

The physiology of the stress response is extremely complex, and Figure 5.4 illustrates these nervous and endocrine responses. When a person perceives stress, the sympathetic division of the autonomic nervous system rouses the person from a resting state by way of stimulating the adrenal medulla, which produces catecholamines. The pituitary releases ACTH, which in turn affects the adrenal cortex. Glucocorticoid release prepares the body to resist the stress and even to cope with injury by the release of cortisol. The ANS activation is rapid, as is all neural transmission, whereas the action of the neuroendocrine system is slower. Together the two systems form the physiological basis for the stress response as well as the potential for illness.

An understanding of the physiology of stress does not completely clarify the meaning of stress. Thus, several models have been constructed in an attempt to better define and explain stress.

Theories of Stress

Despite a great deal of scientific research on the subject and the widespread use of the term in everyday conversation, *stress* has been defined in three different ways: as a stimulus, as a response, and as an interaction. When some people talk about stress, they are referring to an environmental *stimulus,* as in "I have a high-stress job." Others consider stress a physical *response,* as in "My heart races when I feel a lot of stress." Still others consider stress to result from the *interaction* between environmental stimuli and the person, as in "I feel stressed when I have to make financial decisions at work, but other types of decisions do not stress me."

These three views of stress also appear in the different theories of stress. The view of stress as an external event was the first approach taken by stress researchers, the most prominent of whom was Hans Selye. During the course of his research, Selye changed to a more response-based view of stress, concentrating on the biological aspects of the stress response. The most influential view of stress among psychologists has been the interactionist approach, proposed by Richard Lazarus. The next two sections discuss the views of Selye and Lazarus.

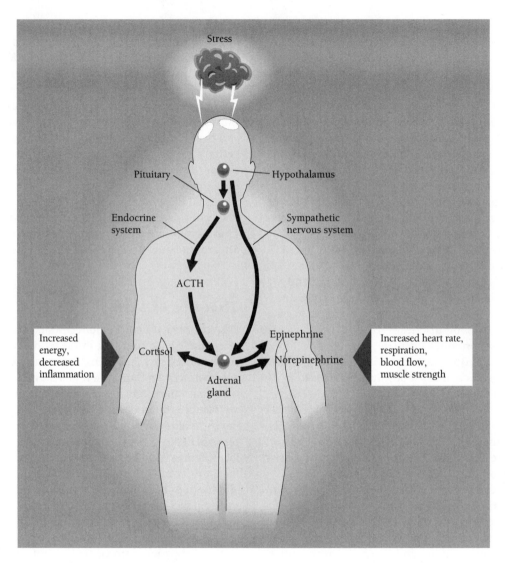

Figure 5.4 Physiological effects of stress.

Selye's View

Beginning in the 1930s and continuing until his death in 1982, Hans Selye (1956, 1976, 1982) researched and popularized the concept of stress, making a strong case for its relationship to physical illness and bringing the importance of stress to the attention of the public. Although he did not

originate the concept of stress, he researched the effects of stress on physiological responses and tried to connect these reactions to the development of illness.

Over the course of his career, Selye first considered stress to be a stimulus and later saw it as a response. His original position was that stress was a stimulus, concentrating on the environmental conditions that produced stress. In the 1950s, Selye started to use the term *stress* to refer to a response that the organism makes. To distinguish the two, Selye started using the terms *stressor* to refer to the stimulus and *stress* to mean the response.

Selye's contributions to stress research included a concept of stress and a model for how the body defends itself in stressful situations. Selye conceptualized stress as a nonspecific response, repeatedly insisting that stress is a general physical response caused by any of a number of environmental stressors. He believed that a wide variety of different situations could prompt the stress response, but that the response would always be the same.

The General Adaptation Syndrome The body's generalized attempt to defend itself against noxious agents became known as the **general adaptation syndrome (GAS).** This syndrome is divided into three stages, the first of which is the **alarm reaction.** During alarm, the body's defenses against a stressor are mobilized through activation of the sympathetic nervous system. This division activates body systems to maximize strength and prepares them for the "fight or flight" response. Adrenaline (epinephrine) is released, heart rate and blood pressure increase, respiration becomes faster, blood is diverted away from the internal organs toward the skeletal muscles, sweat glands are activated, and the gastrointestinal system decreases its activity. As a short-term response to an emergency situation, these physical reactions are adaptive, but many modern stress situations involve prolonged exposure to stress but do not require physical action.

Selye called the second phase of the GAS the **resistance stage.** In this stage the organism adapts to the stressor. How long this stage lasts depends on the severity of the stressor and the adaptive capacity of the organism. If the organism can adapt, the resistance stage will continue for a long time. During this stage, the person gives the outward appearance of normality, as Rick did following his father's death and during his divorce, but physio-

logically the body's internal functioning is not normal. Continuing stress will cause continued neurological and hormonal changes. Selye believed that these demands take a toll, setting the stage for what he described as *diseases of adaptation,* those diseases related to continued, persistent stress. Figure 5.5 illustrates these stages and the point in the process at which diseases develop.

Among the diseases Selye considered to be the result of prolonged resistance to stress are peptic ulcers and ulcerative colitis, hypertension and cardiovascular disease, hyperthyroidism, and bronchial asthma. In addition, Selye hypothesized that resistance to stress would cause changes in the immune system, making infection more likely.

The capacity to resist stress is finite, and the final stage of the GAS is the **exhaustion stage.** At the end, the organism's ability to resist is depleted, and a breakdown results. This stage is characterized by activation of the parasympathetic division of the autonomic nervous system. Under normal circumstances, parasympathetic activation keeps the body functioning in a balanced state. In the exhaustion stage, however, functioning is at an abnormally low level to compensate for the abnormally high level of sympathetic activation that has preceded it. Selye believed that exhaustion frequently results in depression and sometimes even death.

Evaluation of Selye's View Selye's early concept of stress as a stimulus as well as his later concentration on the physical aspects of stress have both been influential in researching and measuring stress. The stimulus-based view of stress prompted researchers to investigate the various environmental conditions that lead people to experience stress and also led to the construction of stress inventories. Such inventories ask people to check or list the events they have experienced in the recent past and measure the amount of stress by totaling these events. We consider both the environmental sources of stress and the life event approach to measuring stress later in this chapter.

In considering stress as a set of physical responses, Selye largely ignored psychological factors,

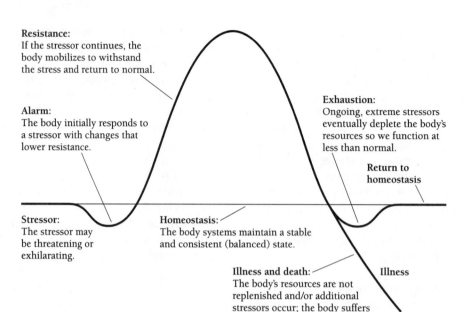

Figure 5.5   The three stages of Selye's General Adaptation Syndrome and their consequences.   *Source: From* An Invitation to Health *(7th ed., p. 40), by D. Hales, 1997, Pacific Grove, CA: Brooks/Cole. Copyright © 1997 by Brooks/Cole Publishing Company. Reprinted by permission of Wadsworth Publishing Co.*

including the emotional component and the individual interpretation of stressful events. John Mason (1971, 1975) criticized Selye for ignoring the element of emotion in stress and hypothesized that the consistency in the stress response is due to this underlying element of emotion.

Selye emphasized the physiology of stress and conducted most of his research on nonhuman animals. By downplaying the differences between humans and other animals, he neglected the factors that are unique to humans, such as perception and interpretation of stressful experiences. Selye's view has had a great influence on the popular conception of stress, but an alternative model formulated by psychologist Richard Lazarus has had a greater impact among psychologists.

Lazarus's View

In Lazarus's view, the interpretation of stressful events is more important than the events them-

selves. It is neither the environmental event nor the person's response that defines stress, but rather the individual's *perception* of the psychological situation. This perception includes potential harms, threats, and challenges as well as the individual's perceived ability to cope with them.

Psychological Factors   Lazarus's emphasis on interpretation and perception differs from that of Selye. Also, Lazarus has worked largely with humans rather than nonhuman animals. The ability of people to think about and evaluate future events makes them vulnerable in ways that other animals are not. Humans encounter stresses because they have high-level cognitive abilities that other animals lack.

According to Lazarus (1984a, 1993), the effect that stress has on a person is based more on that person's feelings of threat, vulnerability, and ability to cope than on the stressful event itself. For example, losing a job may be extremely stressful for someone who has no money saved or no confidence in finding another job. But to a person who has either another source of income or confidence in finding a new job, loss of a job may be far less stressful. In Lazarus's view, a life event is not what produces stress; rather, it is one's view of the situation that causes an event to become stressful. When Rick, our case study, lost his job he felt a high level of stress because he was involved in a divorce and needed extra money. He appraised this life event (job loss) as threatening to his career and financial position.

Lazarus and Susan Folkman defined psychological stress as *"a particular relationship between the person and the environment that is appraised by the person as taxing or exceeding his or her resources and endangering his or her well-being"* (1984, p. 19). You should note several important points in this definition. First, Lazarus and Folkman take an interactional or *transactional* position, holding that stress refers to a relationship between person and environment. Second, they believe that the key to that transaction is the person's appraisal of the psychological situation. Third, they believe the situation must be seen as threatening, challenging, or harmful.

Appraisal Lazarus and Folkman (1984) recognized that people use three kinds of appraisal to assess situations: primary appraisal, secondary appraisal, and reappraisal. **Primary appraisal** is not necessarily first in importance, but it is first in time. A person who first encounters an event, such as an offer of a job promotion, appraises it in terms of its effect on his or her well-being. An event may be viewed as irrelevant, benign-positive, or stressful. It is unlikely that an offer of a job promotion would be seen as irrelevant, but many environmental events, such as a snowstorm in another state, have no implications for a person's well-being. A benign-positive appraisal means that the event is seen as having good implications. A stressful appraisal can mean that the event is seen as harmful, threatening, or challenging. Each of these three—harm, threat, and challenge—is likely to generate an emotion. Lazarus (1993) defined *harm* as the psychological damage that has already been

done, such as an illness or injury; *threat* as the anticipation of harm; and *challenge* as a person's confidence in overcoming difficult demands. An appraisal of harm may produce anger, disgust, disappointment, or sadness; an appraisal of threat is likely to generate worry, anxiety, or fear; an appraisal of challenge may be followed by excitement or anticipation. It is important to remember that these emotions do not produce stress; instead, they are generated by the individual's appraisal of an event.

After a person's initial appraisal of an event, that person forms an impression of his or her ability to control or cope with harm, threat, or challenge, an impression called **secondary appraisal.** A person asks three questions in making secondary appraisals. The first is "What options are available to me?" The second is "What is the likelihood that I can successfully apply the necessary strategies to reduce this stress?" As an example, let's look at Jill, who has just lost her job. Her secondary appraisal would begin with an assessment of her ability to make a favorable impression that would lead to a job offer.

The third question a person asks is "Will this procedure work? That is, will it alleviate my stress?" Even if Jill believes that she makes a sufficiently good impression to get a job offer, she may not believe that a favorable impression will lead to another job. When people believe they can do something that will make a difference—when they believe they can successfully cope with a situation—stress is reduced.

The third type of appraisal is **reappraisal.** Appraisals change constantly as new information becomes available. Jill may recall some advice on writing an attractive letter of application or relaxing during a job interview and gain more confidence in her ability to cope, thereby reducing her stress. Or reappraisal may follow from an environmental source, as when Jill reads a newspaper article about the strong demand for employees with her training and experience. This new information may allow Jill to reappraise her employment situation and to turn her previously stressful appraisal into a benign-positive one.

Reappraisal does not always result in less stress; sometimes it increases stress. A situation previously assessed as benign or irrelevant can take on a threatening, harmful, or challenging aspect if the environment changes or the person begins to see the situation differently. For example, a husband who has been satisfied with his marriage for years may begin seeing his relationship with his wife as stressful when his wife begins college course work.

Vulnerability   Stress is most likely to be aroused when a person is vulnerable, when he or she lacks resources in a situation of some personal importance. These resources may be either physical or social, but their importance is determined by psychological factors, such as perception and evaluation of the situation. An arthritic knee, for example, would produce physical vulnerability in a professional athlete but would be a minor inconvenience to the professional life of someone who works behind a desk.

Lazarus and Folkman (1984) insisted that physical or social deficits alone are not sufficient to produce vulnerability. What matters is whether one considers the situation personally important. Vulnerability differs from threat in that it represents only the *potential* for threat. Threat exists when one perceives that his or her self-esteem is in jeopardy; vulnerability exists when the lack of resources creates a potentially threatening or harmful situation.

Coping   An important ingredient in Lazarus's theory of stress is the ability or inability to cope with a stressful situation. Lazarus and Folkman defined coping as "*constantly changing cognitive and behavioral efforts to manage specific external and/or internal demands that are appraised as taxing or exceeding the resources of the person*" (1984, p. 141). This definition spells out several important features of coping. First, coping is a process, constantly changing as one's efforts are evaluated as more or less successful. Second, coping is not automatic; it is a learned pattern of responding to

stressful situations. A response that is automatic (such as closing one's eyes to block out intense light) or which becomes automatic through experience (such as shifting one's weight while riding a bicycle) would not be considered coping. Third, coping requires effort. A person need not be completely aware of his or her coping response, and the outcome may or may not be successful, but effort must have been expended. Fourth, coping is an effort to *manage* the situation; control and mastery are not necessary. For example, most of us make an effort to manage our physical environment by striving for a comfortable air temperature. Thus we cope with our environment even though complete mastery of the climate is impossible.

How well people are able to cope depends on several factors. Lazarus and Folkman (1984) listed *health and energy* as one important coping resource. Healthy, robust individuals are better able to manage external and internal demands than are frail, sick, tired people. A second resource is a *positive belief*—the ability to cope with stress is enhanced when people believe they can successfully bring about desired consequences. This ability is related to the third resource: *problem-solving skills*. Knowledge of anatomy and physiology, for example, can be an important source of coping when a person is receiving information about her or his own health from a physician who is speaking in technical terms. A fourth coping resource is *social skills*. Confidence in one's ability to get other people to cooperate can be an important source of stress management. Closely allied to this resource is *social support*, or the feeling of being accepted, loved, or prized by others. (Chapter 8 presents information on the importance of social support in coping.) Finally, Lazarus and Folkman list *material resources* as an important means of coping. Having the money to get one's car repaired decreases the stress of having a transmission problem.

In Lazarus's transactional view, of course, material and social resources by themselves are not so important as one's personal belief about these resources. Perceiving that you can manage or alter a stressful environmental situation and feeling confident that you can regulate your own emotional distress are the two main ways to cope with stress. The ways people cope with stressful life events, including daily annoyances, play a leading role in stress-related illnesses.

In Summary

Two leading theories of stress are those of Hans Selye and Richard Lazarus. Selye, the first researcher to look closely at stress, first saw stress as a stimulus, but he later viewed it as a response. Whenever animals (including humans) encounter a threatening stimulus, they mobilize themselves in a generalized attempt to adapt to that stimulus, and this mobilization is called the general adaptation syndrome (GAS). The GAS has three stages—alarm, resistance, and exhaustion—and the potential for trauma or illness exists at all three stages.

In contrast, Lazarus holds a cognitively oriented, transactional view of stress and coping. Stressful encounters are dynamic and complex, constantly changing and unfolding, so that the outcomes of one stressful event alter the subsequent appraisal of new events. Individual differences in coping strategies and in the appraisal of stressful events are crucial to a person's experience of stress; therefore, the likelihood of developing any stress-related disorder also varies with individuals. The relationship between stressful events and subsequent health is complex, according to Lazarus, and any attempt to measure stress and a person's attempts to cope with it must also be complex.

Sources of Stress

Searching for sources of stress in the environment is consistent with the conceptualization of stress as a stimulus (Kasl, 1996). This view leads researchers to investigate factors that produce stress, to quantify those sources of stress, and to relate them to health outcomes.

Environment

Many people associate environmental sources of stress with urban life. They think of noise, pollution, crowding, fear of crime, and personal alienation as being associated with city living. However, adverse environmental factors are not limited to large metropolitan communities, although they are frequently more concentrated there. Rural life can also be noisy, polluted, hot, cold, humid, or even crowded, with many people living in a one- or two-room dwelling. The noise from farm machinery is often louder than any experienced by urban dwellers. And although air and water pollution usually originate in urban or industrial settings, they may then disperse to other parts of the world.

Therefore, environmental sources of stress are not limited to urban settings, but the crowding, noise, pollution, fear of crime, and personal alienation combine to produce an urban environment that is stressful to many city dwellers. Not only can each source of stress be considered separately, but the combination of these stressors occurs in a natural context.

Crowding Experiments with animals have revealed a variety of adverse effects from high-density living conditions (Calhoun, 1956, 1962), but research on human health is not as clear. When rats live in ideal conditions, they breed rapidly, and overcrowding occurs but does not progress to "standing room only." Rat behavior changes with population density: Male rats form dominance hierarchies, and the dominant rats become more territorial and aggressive. Infant mortality increases, and sexual behavior changes, resulting in a stable, high population level but with higher levels of violence and poorer social integration. Crowding causes social, emotional, and health changes in rats, but experiments to demonstrate similar effects in humans are not ethically acceptable. Therefore, many of the studies with humans have been short-term laboratory studies or naturalistic studies in crowded environments.

A distinction between the concepts of *population density* and *crowding* helps in understanding the effects of crowding on humans. In 1972, Daniel Stokols defined **population density** as a *physical* condition in which a large population occupies a limited space. **Crowding,** however, is a *psychological* condition that arises from a person's perception of the high-density environment in which that person is confined. Thus, density is necessary for crowding but does not automatically produce the feeling of being crowded. The crush of people in the lobby of a theater during intermission of a popular play may not be experienced as crowding, despite the extremely high population density. Conversely, however, a reclusive early American pioneer who migrated westward when a new resident came into his county would also not be crowded. He may have felt uncomfortable living within 10 miles of another person, but because the population was not dense, his experience would not meet Stokols's definition of being crowded. The distinction between density and crowding means that personal perceptions are critical in the definition of crowding.

Both density and crowding affect human behavior in negative ways, but the effect on mental well-being is clearer than the effect on health. A review of laboratory and field studies on crowding (Sundstrom, 1978) showed that density and crowding tended to increase aggression, lower performance on complex tasks, prompt withdrawal from interpersonal relations, and increase crime rates. Living in crowded conditions also leads to feelings of stress (Fuller, Edwards, Vorakitphokatorn, & Sermsri, 1996; Ruback, Pandey, & Begum, 1997) and a tendency to experience more physical symptoms (Ruback & Pandey, 1996).

One study that weighs directly on the issue of health and crowding was conducted within a prison environment (Paulus, McCain, & Cox, 1978). In addition to being crowded, prison inmates might find crowding particularly unpleasant because they have no control over the type and duration of their housing. The mortality rates in a prison psychiatric unit varied over a 16-year period during times of high- and low-density living conditions; Figure 5.6 shows nearly identical curves for the average yearly population and the death rate of inmates. As population rose, so did the rate of mortality, and as conditions became less crowded, the death rate dropped correspondingly.

Pollution   Pollution is a second environmental condition that may produce stress, but pollution exerts health effects directly as well as through increased stress. Although pollution of the environment has become an important concern, it is not a recent phenomenon. Both air and water pollution predate history (Eckholm, 1977). Modern technology has given us more pollutants and speeded their dispersion, but it did not originate the practice of adding harmful substances to the air, water, and soil.

Modern technology has increased not only the amount of pollution but also the potential for accidents in the storing or handling of dangerous nuclear or chemical pollutants. An accident with toxic chemicals could create extreme feelings of helplessness because such accidents are beyond the control of many of the affected people. Indeed, these accidents may occur quite randomly, as in a train derailment or a tank-car accident, and thus quite unpredictably. Furthermore, the fear of accidents may pervade entire neighborhoods near industries where dangerous chemicals are used or manufactured, providing long-lasting stress for residents (Baum, Gatchel, & Schaeffer, 1983; Moffatt, Phillimore, Bhopal, & Foy, 1995).

Studies on the psychological effects of pollution have implications for stress and health, and several of these studies deal with feelings of personal control and perceived severity of the pollution. According to an early study (Rankin, 1969), people who are concerned about air pollution in their community frequently do not complain because they believe their protests will do no good; that is, they feel helpless. Another study (Rotton, Yoshikawa, & Kaplan, 1979) investigated the effect of control over air quality on tolerance for frustration and found that the perception of control is more crucial than the level of pollution in making the experience stressful. In summary, pollution is a source of stress, but its health effects are mostly direct results of their toxic effects rather than indirect effects through increasing stress levels.

Noise   In addition to crowding and pollution, exposure to noise may produce stress. Noise is considered a type of pollution because it is a noxious, unwanted stimulus that intrudes into a person's environment. Evidence also shows a relationship between noise and health problems, but again, the health effects of noise might be direct influences of noise rather than indirect effects produced by increased stress. In addition, noise is quite difficult to define in any objective way. Definitions are invariably subjective, because noise is a sound that a person does not want to hear. Noise can be loud, soft, or somewhere between. One person's music is another person's noise.

Defined by the objective criterion of volume, noise can produce detrimental health effects. For example, workers exposed to high levels of noise reported more nausea, headaches, impotence, argumentativeness, and moodiness than workers exposed to less noise (Cohen, Glass, & Phillips, 1977). In a naturalistic study of the effects of noise on cognitive, physical, and emotional factors in children (Evans, Hygge, & Bullinger, 1995), results indicated that living in a high-noise area produced elevations of physiological responses associated with chronic stress. In addition, children living with high noise were less persistent in performing a challenging cognitive task and reported more annoyance with the noise in their community.

The importance of subjective attitude toward noise was illustrated by a study (Nivision & Endresen, 1993) that asked residents living beside a busy street about their health, sleep, anxiety level, and attitude toward noise. No relationship appeared between objective noise levels and either health or sleep. However, the study showed a strong association between residents' subjective view of noise and the number of their health complaints.

In laboratory studies of noise, like those for pollution, potential for control also seems to be a factor in perception of stress. When participants in a laboratory study (Glass & Singer, 1972) were

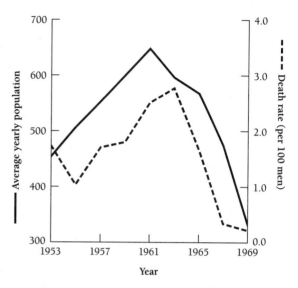

Figure 5.6   Total population and death rates per 100 men for a psychiatric prison.   *Source:* Adapted from "Death Rates, Psychiatric Commitments, Blood Pressure and Perceived Crowding as a Function of Institutional Crowding," by P. B. Paulus, G. McCain, & V. C. Cox, 1978, *Environmental Psychology and Nonverbal Behavior,* 3, p. 110. Copyright © 1978 by Human Science Press.

allowed the possibility of controlling a loud, distracting noise, they experienced less stress than a group not given this possibility. Although the group that could control the noise never exerted this control, having this possibility decreased the stress of the experience. The results indicated that personal control was an important factor in appraising the stressful effects of noise, acting as a buffer against the problems created by noise.

Urban Press   Crowding, pollution, and noise can occur in any social context, but these factors are a commonplace combination in the urban environment. Eric Graig (1993) used the term **urban press** to refer to the many environmental stressors that affect city living. Commuting hassles and fear of crime add to the urban dwellers' experience with crowding, pollution, and noise. Graig pointed out that the laboratory studies on crowding, noise, and pollution fall far short of capturing the experience of actually living with these stressors. Graig also noted that not only are all these sources of

WOULD YOU BELIEVE . . . ?

Declining Murder Rate

Would you believe that the murder rate in the United States is going down and is now much lower than it was 70 years ago? During the mid-1990s, former U. S. Surgeon General Joycelyn Elders named gun violence as the leading public health issue of our time. Her words have been echoed by almost daily reports from newspapers and television that feature stories on the escalating rise of murder and other crimes in the United States. Results from various opinion polls seem to show that crime is the most serious problem facing this country. How accurate are these perceptions? Just how rapidly are crime rates rising?

With regard to crime rates, popular perception diverges from reality. Although the *percentage* of murders by handguns increased from about 50% in 1990 to 54% in 1996, the *total number* of murders declined from more than 20,000 in 1990 to less than 16,000 for 1996. Moreover, the murder *rate* dropped by 14% from 1986 to 1996. During the 11-year period from 1986 to 1996, the United States experienced declining rates of all violent crimes except aggravated assault. During this period, aggravated assault rose by 12% while forcible rape declined by nearly 5% and robbery decreased by 10%. At the same time, property crime also dropped by 9%, with most of the drop due to a 30% decline in burglaries. The only property crime to increase was motor vehicle theft, which rose by less than 4%. In general, however, fewer people were touched by crime in 1996 than in 1990 (U.S. Bureau of the Census [USBC], 1998).

The patterns of homicide have changed, and young African American men are disproportionately affected. Although only about one in eight people in the United States is African American, as many African Americans as European Americans are murdered each year. Before the age of 10 and especially after the age of 35, murder victims are more likely to be white. However, of homicide victims from age 17 to 29, nearly 60% are African Americans (USBC, 1998).

Many people live in nearly constant fear of physical assault or murder, but their fears are not well justified. According to government statistics, less than one person per 10,000 will become a murder victim in any one year (USBC, 1998). As noted in the lead sentence, homicide rates have decreased substantially during the past 70 years. In 1930, the murder rate was 12.4 per 100,000, but by 1996 that rate had dropped to 7.4 (USBC, 1973, 1998), suggesting that the United States is a safer place to live now than it was in the 1930s.

Although crime, like any health problem, is a serious concern for those people directly affected, recent government figures tell us that the United States is not experiencing a rapid rise in murder, rape, robbery, burglary, or theft. Would you believe that the constant clamoring of politicians and the media over the escalating trends in crime does not reflect real risk?

---

stress combined in city life but that they tend to be beyond personal control. Laboratory studies on noise and pollution indicate that lack of control tends to make people feel stressed, which may apply to these factors in the urban environment.

Crime is not unique to urban life, but fear of crime has become part of the urban environment (Riger, 1985), and these fears can affect behavior, such as installing locks on the doors and bars on the windows and avoiding locations perceived as high-crime areas. Crime victimization is unlikely for any individual (see the Would You Believe . . . ? box), but the fear of crime is much more common than its actual occurrence.

One factor in the perception of the prevalence of crime is media coverage. Indeed, independent of demographic factors such as income and age, one study (Williams & Dickinson, 1993) found a significant positive correlation between people's fear of crime and newspaper reporting of crime information. Other research (Liska & Baccaglini, 1990) has shown more complex relationships between newspaper reports and people's fear of crime, but these researchers found that the information in official crime statistics was mediated through newspaper coverage. Such studies demonstrate the power of the press to increase or decrease the fear of crime.

When people fear victimization, their behavior changes, and some changes can lead people to withdraw from their communities (Taylor, Repetti, & Seeman, 1997). When people restrict activities that might take them into areas considered dangerous, they restrict their social interactions. For example, people who are concerned with increasing crime avoid walking alone at night (Forde, 1993). One study (Bazargan, 1994) showed that older African Americans limited their mobility out of fear of crime. Although giving up walking alone at night may not seem much of a sacrifice, it reflects the feeling of restriction that occurs in people's lives when they feel that they must think about their safety. When older people feel that they must limit how much they go out of their homes, this attitude reflects a distrust of others that can contribute to isolation (Krause, 1991).

The connection between fear of victimization and health appeared in the results of a survey of over 2,000 people varying in age from 18 to 90 years (Ross, 1993). People who were afraid of being assaulted, robbed, or physically injured reported worse health than people who had no such fears. One reason for this connection is that restriction from outdoor activities and exercise may contribute to poor health and fear of crime. Therefore, crime is not only a factor in the urban environment but fear of crime is also a stressor that can have indirect effects on health.

Occupation

Do business executives who must make many decisions every day suffer more from a high level of stress than do their employees who merely carry out those decisions? Most executives have jobs in

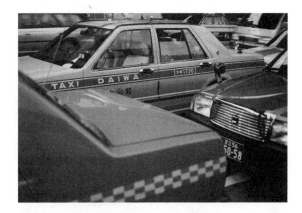

Traffic and crowding are factors that combine to make urban living stressful.

which the demands are high but so is their level of control, and research indicates that lack of control is more stressful than the burden of decision making. Lower-level occupations are actually more stressful than executive jobs (Smith, Colligan, Horning, & Hurrel, 1978). Using stress-related illness as a criterion, the jobs of construction worker, secretary, laboratory technician, waiter or waitress, machine operator, farm worker, and painter were among the most stressful. These jobs all share a high level of demand combined with a low level of control. Another highly stressful job is middle-level manager, such as foreman or supervisor. Middle managers must meet demands from two directions: their bosses and their workers. Thus, they have more than their share of stress and stress-related illnesses.

Several studies have confirmed that the combination of high demands and low control produces job stress and is also related to heart disease. For example, physicians, whose jobs include a very high level of demands but also a high degree of control, suffer less from stress than medical students, who are burdened with the undesirable combination of high demands and low control (Vitaliano et al., 1988). The more latitude men had in making decisions on the job, the lower was their death rate from coronary heart disease (Alterman, Shekelle, Vernon, & Burau, 1994). In addition, workers in high demand/low decision

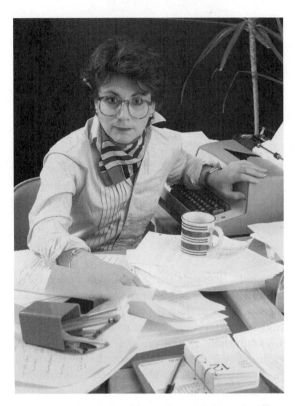

High job demands can produce stress, especially when combined with low levels of control.

jobs had an elevated risk of heart disease mortality, a risk that was greater for white-collar workers than for blue-collar workers.

Not only is the high demand-low control combination related to coronary heart disease (Karasek et al., 1988) but the social environment at work can increase or decrease risk for cardiovascular disease (Johnson & Hall, 1988) and hypertension (Schnall et al., 1990). Distressing interactions with supervisors or coworkers increase stress at work (Repetti, 1993b). In reviewing the research on the link between job demands and control and coronary heart disease, Rena Repetti (1993a) found strong evidence that jobs with the combination of high demand and low control constitute a risk factor for hypertension and heart disease. These conditions applied to Rick's job in law enforcement,

which was filled with occasional danger but almost constant demands from superiors as well as those who were arrested or victimized.

High demands and low control also combine with other workplace conditions to increase on-the-job stress. Neither noise nor danger of chemical exposure is sufficient to produce stressful work conditions (Cottington & House, 1987), but the combination of a noisy workplace and rotating shiftwork can produce a higher level of epinephrine excretion, a physiological index of stress. In addition, shiftwork can lead to a variety of physical complaints, including sleep and gastrointestinal problems, and rotating shifts can interfere with family life (Holt, 1993).

The conflict between work demand and family obligations affects both men and women, but the increase in employment for women has sparked more research on their potential sources of job stress. Contrary to what many people might assume, women who pursue careers are not at increased risk for coronary heart disease (Haynes, Feinleib, & Kannel, 1980). However, factors in their careers and home life may increase their stress, and women who have employment and child care obligations experience more stress than women without children (Luecken et al., 1997). However, employed women also experience more satisfaction and better health (Betz, 1993).

The positive or negative effects of work and family roles depend on the resources people have available (Taylor et al., 1997). For example, unmarried women with young children and a job show an elevated risk for poor health, (Verbrugge, 1983). However, married women with more support for their employment feel less stress. A good income, control, and support in family work are important in decreasing the stress of fulfilling multiple roles. Women are less likely than men to have jobs with good salaries and control (Brannon, 1999), and these factors might increase their vulnerability to stress and poor health. Do women who hold executive positions benefit from the high degree of control their jobs offer? The results of one study (LaRosa, 1990) indicated that they do. The female executives in this study had excellent physical health and reported greater life satisfaction than other employed women. Therefore, filling multiple obligations is not necessarily stressful for women, but low control and poor support for multiple roles can produce stress.

Personal Relationships

Personal relationships are another potential source of stress, but they can also buffer against stress; that is, people who have fewer personal relationships are at increased health risk compared to those with more relationships (Berkman & Syme, 1979; Hobfoll & Vaux, 1993). Relationships do not automatically provide benefits. As the research on social support at work suggests, problems in personal relationships can create stress, but supportive relationships can protect against stress. These effects are not unique to the workplace but apply to other relationships as well. In Rick's case, his relationship with his wife was a major source of stress, and the loss of a supportive wife and family added to his stress.

In a survey of college students (Ptacek, Smith, & Zanas, 1992), one third of the stress events involved relationships. The frequency of this source of stress should not be surprising considering the number of potential relationships—coworkers, supervisors, friends, and romantic partners as well as family relationships that include parents, children, spouses, aunts, uncles, and cousins. For the college students, nonfamily relationships were a more frequent source of stress than family relationships, but perhaps the social circumstances of college students tend to create more nonfamily interactions and stresses.

For married or cohabiting couples, relationships within the family are sources of stress that interact with other life circumstances. For example, the demands of employment and family life can create stress when these are in conflict (Aneshensel & Pearlin, 1987). Such stresses tend to differ for men and women, who occupy different roles and who are faced with different expecta-

tions within the family. Women often encounter stress because of the increased burden of doing the work associated with their multiple roles as employee, wife, and mother (Hochschild, 1989).

Husbands who do not support their wives' employment can create stress in the lives of both by failing to perform a fair share of household work and child care, leading to the perception of inequity that can escalate into conflict (Thompson & Walker, 1989). Although changes in gender roles have resulted in a more equitable distribution of household work, that equity disappears when the family includes children (Lundberg, 1998). Women carry out the great majority of child care responsibilities, making their work load larger than men. Indeed, disagreement over the inequitable distribution of household work is a point of conflict and stress for many couples, but men who do housework enjoy better physical health than men who do not (Gottman, 1991).

Many men are not completely supportive of their wives' employment because employed wives gain power in the marital relationship. In addition, husbands may feel that they are not receiving the care they believe wives should supply (Rosenfield, 1992). This attitude can contribute to more stress for husbands, which can lead to their failure to support their wives' efforts. Both wives and husbands who spend many hours devoted to their jobs and who feel a lack of support from their spouses tend to experience stress (Greenberger & O'Neil, 1993). To sum up, multiple commitments to employment and family can produce stress for both men and women, and this stress is increased by feelings of lack of support from spouses.

Marital interactions are a source of stress for both partners. Furthermore, couples whose interactions provoked the physiological responses associated with stress tended to have marriages that dissolved (Gottman, 1991). Thus, stress responses were a good predictor of marital stability. These physiological measures were 95% accurate in predicting which couples would stay together and which would separate. Research measuring neuroendocrine measures of stress showed that hostile

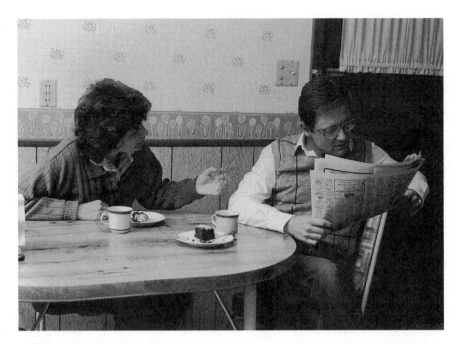

Personal relationships can be a source of stress, and physical stress reactions are related to marital instability.

marital interaction raised these indices in both recently married (Kiecolt-Glaser et al., 1996) and long-married (Kiecolt-Glaser et al., 1997) couples. These studies show that marital relationships can be a source of stress as well as a source of support.

Philip Blumstein and Pepper Schwartz's (1983) survey of couples showed that work, money, and sex were all potential sources of stress for married as well as cohabiting and gay and lesbian couples. Differing attitudes in any of these (or other) areas can lead to conflict, which can result in couples' failing to support each other. Lack of support increases feelings of stress and negates some of the benefits of personal relationships.

Sleep Problems

Sleep and stress interact: Stress is a common cause of sleep problems, and difficulties in sleeping are a source of stress for many people (Rosch, 1996).

The most common sleep-related problem is **insomnia,** the inability either to fall asleep or to stay asleep, but some people intentionally receive very little sleep in order to have more time to do other things. Whether voluntary or involuntary, sleep deprivation is associated with a variety of behavioral and health problems.

People who do not get sufficient sleep often feel tired, anxious, drowsy, weary, and fatigued; the number of people affected has been estimated at between 30% and 50% of the population (Hellmich, 1995). Adolescents often skip sleep to have more time to work, study, or socialize; and adults sometimes decrease their sleep time to do more work or to spend time with family. Additionally, many jobs require shift work and changes in workers' sleep schedules. Deprived of sleep, adolescents may fall asleep in class, and adults may be too fatigued to work efficiently. Sleep-deprived people have an increased risk for accidents resulting from fatigue, impaired coordination, and altered judgment.

Much of the knowledge about sleep deprivation comes from case studies and experimental studies in which people voluntarily go without sleep or reduce the amount of time they sleep. Most of the group experiments have prevented participants from sleeping for 60 to 120 hours and then measured their psychological and physiological responses, revealing that extreme sleep deprivation diminishes people's ability to perform physical tasks, impairs attention and concentration, and may produce hallucinations (Dinges, Pack, et al., 1997).

Although many people voluntarily decrease the amount of sleep they get, others have difficulty in getting to sleep or staying asleep long enough to feel rested. Both problems are typical of people classified as having *primary insomnia* (American Psychiatric Association, 1994). Stress and anxiety can be both a cause and an effect of such sleep problems (Fichten et al., 1995). Some of the other sources of stress—work, noise, and personal relationships—may interfere with sleep. Intrusive thoughts concerning work or interpersonal relationships and environmental factors such as noise, odors, or lights are common sources of sleep onset or sleep maintenance problems (Bennett, Goldfinger, & Johnson, 1987). Depression and other psychological disorders can also contribute to sleep problems (Benca, Obermeyer, Thisted, & Gillin, 1992). Changing these conditions or adopting other methods of coping with stress can improve sleep.

Another cause of sleep problems is a change in a person's normal sleep cycle. Such alterations can occur with rotating work schedules, travel across time zones, and weekend activities. The resulting sleep difficulty is labeled *circadian rhythm sleep disorder* (American Psychiatric Association, 1994). People who suffer from "Sunday night insomnia" can solve the problem by adhering to a regular sleep schedule, even on weekends. Travelers and shift workers, however, have greater difficulties in

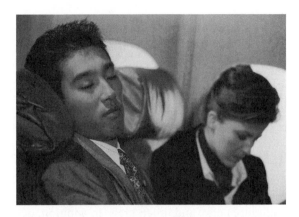

Travel across time zones can disrupt sleep patterns and produce difficulties in sleeping and effective functioning.

adjusting, and they not only exhibit sleep difficulties but also lose some ability to function effectively and safely. For shift workers, inattention and difficulty in concentrating has been associated with accidents (Åkerstedt, 1988), and shifting work schedules disrupt social and family life. Exposing shift workers to bright light during the night and complete darkness during the day can increase both their alertness and their cognitive performance (Czeisler et al., 1990). In addition, adjusting the timing of shifting schedules can allow workers to minimize the negative impact of unusual work schedules (Morgan, 1996).

A growing body of research indicates that sleep problems are associated with changes in the immune system and possibly with illness and death. Early research (Palmblad, Petrini, Wasserman, & Åkerstedt, 1979) indicated that certain immune system responses decreased during sleep deprivation; later research (Dinges et al., 1994) demonstrated that some immune system responses decrease and others increase during sleep deprivation. Even partial sleep deprivation can negatively affect immune system function (Irwin et al., 1994; Leproult, Copinschi, Buxton, & Van Cauter, 1997). These increases and decreases in immune function suggest a complex relationship between sleep deprivation and the immune system, allowing for the possibility that sleep loss may mobilize the immune system in a way similar to the effect of pathogens and yet depress other immune system responses. These changes present the possibility that sleep loss can lead to increased chances for illness, just as people commonly assume.

In Summary

In summary, stress has a number of sources, including such environmental factors as crowding, pollution, noise, and urban press. In addition, occupation, personal relationships, and sleep problems are all potential sources of stress.

Crowding, pollution, and noise are all related to the experience of stress. As environmental stimuli, these three conditions become stressful when people perceive that they have little or no control over them. Stress from crowding, pollution, and noise may combine in urban settings with commuting hassles and fear of crime to create a situation described as urban press. However, feelings of personal control can buffer these stressful conditions.

Personal control is also important in determining job-related stress. The most stressful jobs are those with high demands but low control. People who have some control over their work, such as executives of large corporations, have less stressful jobs than food service workers and middle-level managers. Personal relationships on the job offer the potential for stress or can provide a buffer against stress; this potential also applies to personal relationships with friends and family. Women with multiple roles and low social support from their husbands often have high levels of stress

Sleep deprivation can be both a cause and a result of stress, with effects on both psychological and physiological functioning. Some people voluntarily restrict their sleep, whereas others have trouble getting to sleep or staying asleep. Both may experience the negative effects of sleep deprivation. Health effects of sleep deprivation come from the increased risk of accidents and changes in immune system function.

Measurement of Stress

Several procedures have been developed for measuring stress. This section discusses some of the more widely used methods and addresses the problems in determining their reliability and validity.

Methods of Measurement

Researchers have used a variety of approaches to measure stress, but most fall into two broad categories: physiological measures and self-reports. Physiological measures are associated with the view that stress is a response, and concentrate on the biology of stress. Self-report measures are often used by health psychologists, who tend to take a transactional view of stress. Both approaches hold some potential for investigating the effects of stress on individuals' illness and health.

Physiological Measures   One method of measuring stress uses various physiological and biochemical measures. Physiological indexes include blood pressure, heart rate, galvanic skin response, and respiration rate, whereas biochemical measures include increased secretion of glucocorticoids such as cortisol and catecholamines such as epinephrine. These measures of stress have the advantage of being direct, highly reliable, and easily quantified.

A disadvantage of physiological measures is that the mechanical and electrical hardware and clinical settings that are frequently used may themselves produce stress. Physicians and nurses have long been aware that a person's blood pressure, for example, may rise as a result of the clinical setting in which blood pressure measures have traditionally been taken. Some measuring instruments have been miniaturized and used in settings away from the laboratory or clinic, making such measurements less intrusive (Carruthers, 1983). Neuroendocrine measures require blood, urine, or saliva samples, which can be intrusive or even uncomfortable to furnish, making their collection potentially stressful.

Life Events Scales   Since the late 1950s and early 1960s, researchers have developed a number of self-report instruments to measure stress. The most widely used of these self-report procedures is the Social Readjustment Rating Scale (SRRS), developed by Thomas H. Holmes and Richard Rahe in 1967. This scale appeared as Check Your Health Risk at the beginning of this chapter. The scale is simply a list of 43 life events arranged in rank order from most to least stressful. Each event carries an assigned value, ranging from 100 points for death of a spouse to 11 points for minor violations of the law. Respondents check the items they have experienced during a recent period, usually the previous 6 to 24 months. Adding each item's point value and totaling scores yields a stress score for each person. These scores can then be correlated with future events, such as incidence of illness, to determine the relationship between this measure of stress and the occurrence of physical illness.

Because the SRRS has a deceptively simple format, it has often been misused by people looking for an easily administered scale to predict future health or illness. Life events scales like the SRRS have sometimes appeared in the popular press with the implication that people should count their stress points and use care to avoid additional stress that might put them beyond some critical total, usually 300 points on the SRRS. This advice ignores the fact that many people accumulate far more than 300 points in a year and never become ill. Rick, in our case study, scored over 700 on the SRRS and his chronic headaches got substantially worse. He did not develop any major illnesses during the year following his assessment, but his physician believed that Rick was in danger and told him that he had to cut down on the number of hours he was working to decrease his stress.

Holmes and Rahe developed their scale by assuming that stress comes from events that people experience and that *change* in life adjustment is a key ingredient. Not all stressful life events result in undesirable changes. For example, marriage, outstanding personal achievement, and marital reconciliation are usually regarded as desirable or

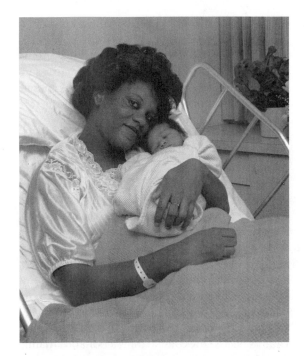

Positive life events can also be sources of stress that require adjustment.

positive changes, yet they appear on the SRRS. A number of other items, such as business readjustment and change in the number of arguments with one's spouse, could be either positive or negative. On the SRRS, however, either increasing or decreasing the number of arguments with one's spouse is worth the same number of points, and the experience of *change* is the critical factor in this view of stress.

Since the development of the Holmes and Rahe scale, considerable debate has arisen over the number and nature of items that should be included in life events scales. Holmes and Rahe began by observing which life events preceded the onset of disease in about 5,000 patients and came up with only 43 items. These life events were then weighted by a different group of people, who were asked to rate them according to the degree of readjustment each required (Holmes & Masuda, 1974). This "average person" scaling system gives each item a constant weight, with no consideration for an item's subjective meaning to a particular individual. For example, death of a spouse is weighted at 100 points for everyone, regardless of length of marriage, number of previous spouses, or degree of dependency. Some investigators (Lazarus & Folkman, 1984; Miller, 1996) have criticized any approach that does not permit individual subjective appraisal or the cultural context of the stressful situation.

Everyday Hassles Scales Richard Lazarus and his associates have pioneered an approach to stress measurement that looks at daily hassles rather than major life events. Daily hassles are "experiences and conditions of daily living that have been appraised as salient and harmful or threatening to the endorser's well-being." (Lazarus, 1984a, p. 376). Recall from the discussion of theories of stress that Lazarus views stress as a transactional, dynamic complex shaped by people's *appraisal* of the environmental situation and their *perceived capabilities to cope* with this situation. Consistent with this view, Lazarus and his associates insisted that measurement instruments must not conceptualize stress as an objective environmental stimulus but instead must allow for subjective elements such as personal appraisal, beliefs, goals, and commitments (Lazarus, DeLongis, Folkman, & Gruen, 1985).

As a consequence, Lazarus and his associates (Kanner, Coyne, Schaefer, & Lazarus, 1981) developed the original Hassles Scale, which consisted of 117 items of annoying, irritating, or frustrating ways in which people may feel hassled. A companion inventory, the Uplifts Scale, contained 138 items that might make a person feel good. These scales required respondents to check any hassle or uplifting experience that happened to them during the past month. Next, respondents indicated on a 3-point scale the degree to which each checked hassle or uplift was experienced. This second step was consistent with Lazarus's belief that an individual's *perception* of stress is more crucial than the objective event itself.

Does the original Hassles Scale measure the same kind of stress revealed by life events scales? A correlational study (Kanner et al., 1981) showed that hassles and life events were only modestly related. Lazarus (1984a) explained this slight overlap between life events and daily hassles as evidence that major life events have some effect on day-to-day routines but that many daily hassles are independent of life events. As a predictor of psychological health, the original Hassles Scale was more accurate than the life events scale. This finding suggests that the Hassles Scale supplements life events scales as a measure of stress and that the life events scale added little to the predictive value of the Hassles Scale.

Later, Anita DeLongis, Folkman, and Lazarus published a complete revision of the Hassles and Uplifts Scale (DeLongis, Folkman, & Lazarus, 1988). The revised Hassles and Uplifts Scale asks participants to think of how much of a hassle or uplift each of 53 items were to them that day. Respondents rate such items as "Your spouse" or "The weather" on a 4-point scale, ranging from *none* to a *great deal.* Each of the 53 items can be either a hassle or an uplift. The revised Hassles and Uplift Scale has an advantage over the original scales in that it is much simpler—participants respond to only 53 items rather than the 255 items on the original Hassles and Uplifts scales. Research on the revised Hassles Scale (Fernandez & Sheffield, 1996) indicated that this scale is superior to the Social Readjustment Rating Scale in predicting both the frequency and the intensity of headaches. This study also suggested that perceived severity of hassles is a stronger predictor of headaches than the number of hassles, once again supporting Lazarus's contention that perception of an event is more important than the event itself.

Another stress inventory that emphasizes perception is the Perceived Stress Scale (PSS) (Cohen, Kamarck, & Mermelstein, 1983). The PSS is a 14-item scale that attempts to measure the degree to which situations in people's lives are appraised as "unpredictable, uncontrollable, and overloading" (Cohen, et al., 1983, p. 387). The scale assesses three components of stress: (1) daily hassles, (2) major events, and (3) changes in coping resources. Respondents answer *never, almost never, sometimes, fairly often,* or *very often* to items that ask about their stressful situations during the past month. The PSS initially showed acceptable reliability but a low correlation between scores of a group of college students and their subsequent physiological ailments. Later research has shown greater ability of the PSS to predict symptoms, including psychiatric and physical symptoms (Hewitt, Flett, & Mosher, 1992; Pbert, Doerfler, & DeCosimo, 1992), changes in immune system function (Maes et al., 1997), and levels of cortisol (Harrell, Kelly, & Stutts, 1996). Its brevity combined with good reliability and validity have led to use of this scale in a variety of research projects.

Reliability and Validity of Stress Measures

The usefulness of stress measures rests on their ability to predict some established criterion consistently. For our purposes, that criterion is illness. To predict the future stress-related illness, these inventories must be both reliable and valid. Reliability is the consistency with which an instrument measures whatever it measures, and validity is the extent to which it measures what it is supposed to measure.

The *reliability* of self-report inventories is most frequently determined by either the paired-associate method or the test-retest technique. In the paired-associate method, close associates (usually a spouse) fill out the inventory, answering as if the item applied to their associate. Responses are then matched with those of the associate. The degree of agreement between the two associates is usually quite high for moderately or severely stressful events (Slater & Depue, 1981) but lower for less stressful experiences (Zimmerman, 1983).

The second approach to determining the reliability of self-report inventories is the test-retest technique, in which the same person completes the stress inventory at two different times. Inaccu-

racies in memory are the main reason for less than perfect agreement, and a review of test-retest reliability studies (Neugebauer, 1984) revealed that the relationship is far from perfect, even when participants were asked to recall the same time period. Studies that have asked people to report their stressful experiences over time has raised questions about the ability of self-report tests to demonstrate sufficient reliability (Klein & Rubovits, 1987; Raphael, Cloitre, & B. P. Dohrenwend, 1991). If self-reports of stress are not reliable, then they cannot validly predict illness—even if stress causes illness.

To consider the *validity* of self-report inventories, we must begin with the question "What are these instruments supposed to measure?" At least three approaches to answering this question are possible. First, the scales should accurately represent all of the life events experienced by the respondents. Second, these scales are supposed to measure stress. Thus scores on self-report inventories should correlate with some other measure of stress, such as judgments of a spouse or close associate or physical measurements of stress. Third, as they are most frequently used, self-report inventories are supposed to measure or predict the incidence of future illness. Let's consider these three approaches in more detail.

First, do self-report inventories accurately represent all experiences of stressful life events? Some investigators (Monroe, 1982) have suggested that many people tend to underreport (omit) life events, whereas other critics (Rabkin & Struening, 1976) contended that sick people overreport life events, providing a kind of justification for their illness. If people either overreport or underreport items on life events scales, then obviously the scales are not totally valid measures of life events.

The second approach asks how one can determine the degree to which a person is accurately reporting stressful events. One method is to compare reports from a spouse or close associate. But the result generally yields significant levels of disagreement between partners, especially when mildly distressful events are included. For example, one study (Yager, Grant, Sweetwood, & Gerst, 1981) found that the partners of psychiatric patients and nonpatients failed to confirm about two-thirds of all life events listed by the original reporter.

The third and most useful type of validity for stress inventories is the extent to which they predict future illnesses or disorders. If self-report scales can demonstrate predictive validity, then they will play a valuable role in determining who may be at risk for stress-related illnesses. One problem in measuring the relationship between stress inventories and illness is the confounding of items on the major life events scales with the presence of physical disorders. Being ill can be stressful, of course, but it can also lead to answers that have been included in the Social Readjustment Rating Scale, such as sex difficulties, revision of personal habits, change in sleeping habits, and change in eating habits. Therefore, a high score on the SRRS or other similarly constructed life events scales may be a consequence rather than a cause of illness. The next chapter reviews several studies dealing with the relationship between stress and illness, but conclusions from this research must be tempered by a consideration of reliability, validity, and confounding problems of the various measures of stress.

In Summary

Stress can be measured by several methods, including physiological and biochemical measures and self-reports of stressful events. The most popular life events scale is the Social Readjustment Rating Scale, which emphasizes *changes* in life events. Despite its popularity, the SRRS is not a good predictor of subsequent illness. Lazarus and his associates pioneered scales that measure daily hassles and uplifts. These inventories emphasize the *perceived* severity of importance of daily events. In general, the revised Hassles and Uplifts Scale is more accurate than the SRRS in predicting future illness.

Physiological and biochemical measures generally have acceptable levels of reliability, but their ability to predict illness has yet to be estab-

lished. Self-report inventories of stress have only moderate levels of reliability and low levels of validity, when validity is defined as the ability to predict illness.

Answers

This chapter addressed four basic questions:

1. **What is the physiology of stress?**

   The nervous system plays a central role in the physiology of stress. When a person perceives stress, the sympathetic division of the autonomic nervous system stimulates the adrenal medulla, producing catecholamines and arousing the person from a resting state. The pituitary gland releases adrenocorticotropic hormone (ACTH), which in turn affects the adrenal cortex. This release prepares the body to resist stress. The autonomic nervous system and the neuroendocrine system form the physiological foundation for both stress and illness.

2. **What theories explain stress?**

   Hans Selye and Richard Lazarus both proposed theories of stress. During his career, Selye defined stress first as a stimulus and then as a response. Whenever the body encounters a disruptive stimulus, it mobilizes itself in a generalized attempt to adapt to that stimulus. This mobilization is called the general adaptation syndrome. The GAS has three stages—alarm, resistance, and exhaustion—and the potential for trauma or illness exists at all three stages. Lazarus insisted that a person's perception of a situation is the most significant component of stress. To Lazarus, stress depends on one's appraisal of an event rather than the event itself. Whether or not stress produces illness is closely tied to one's vulnerability as well as to one's perceived ability to cope with the situation.

3. **What sources produce stress?**

   Several possible sources of stress have been suggested, but the level of stress people experience depends in large part on their perception of these sources and on their perceived ability to cope, adding a transactional component. Stressors can be either environmental or personal. One possible source of environmental stress is crowding, and the *feeling* of being crowded, which can be more stressful than population density itself. Lacking the means to avoid a crowded environment adds to the stress. The potential for accidents with toxic chemicals is another environmental stressor, and again, its effects are most severe when people feel that they have little or no control of the situation, which is often the case with a polluted environment. Noise can also be stressful, but the greatest health risk of loud noise is a direct effect—loss of hearing—rather than the indirect effect of stress. Stress from crowding, pollution, and noise may combine in urban settings with commuting hassles and fear of crime to create a situation described as *urban press.*

Some jobs are more stressful than others, but the number of decisions to be made on the job is not a valid indicator of stress. People who have some control over their work, such as executives of large corporations, have less stressful jobs than those who don't, such as food service workers and middle-level managers. Personal relationships on the job can increase stress or can provide a buffer against it; this potential also applies to personal relationships with friends and family. Surveys of stressful experiences list personal interactions as an important source of stress. Family relationships and the multiple roles that both women and men fulfill can be sources of stress, especially when people feel that their partners are not supportive.

Sleep problems may cause stress, and stress may cause problems in sleep. Some people voluntarily limit their sleep, whereas others have difficulty going to sleep or staying asleep. Either cause of sleep deprivation can limit a person's ability to function, increasing the risk of accidents. In addition, a growing body of research indicates that sleep deprivation affects the immune system in complex ways, suggesting that sleep problems adversely affect health.

4. **How has stress been measured?**

Stress has been assessed by several methods, including physiological and biochemical measures and self-reports of stressful events. Most life events scales are patterned after Holmes and Rahe's Social Readjustment Rating Scale. Some of these instruments include only undesirable events, but the SRRS and other self-report inventories are based on the premise that any major *change* is stressful. Lazarus and his associates have pioneered scales that measure daily hassles and uplifts. These scales, which generally have better validity than the SRRS, emphasize the severity of the event as *perceived* by the person.

Physiological and biochemical measures have the advantage of good reliability, but self-report inventories of stress pose more problems in demonstrating reliability and validity. Although most self-report inventories have acceptable reliability, their ability to predict illness remains to be established. For these stress inventories to predict illness, two conditions must be met: First, they must be valid measures of stress; second, stress must be related to illness. Chapter 6 takes up the question of whether stress causes illness.

Glossary

acetylcholine   A neurotransmitter in the autonomic nervous system.

adrenal cortex   The outer layer of the adrenal glands; secretes glucocorticoids.

adrenal glands   Endocrine glands that are located on top of each kidney and that secrete hormones and affect metabolism.

adrenal medulla   The inner layer of the adrenal glands; secretes epinephrine and norepinephrine.

adrenocortical response The response of the adrenal cortex, prompted by ACTH and resulting in release of cortisol.

adrenocorticotropic hormone (ACTH) A hormone produced by the anterior portion of the pituitary gland that acts on the adrenal gland and is involved in the stress response.

adrenomedullary response The response of the adrenal medulla, prompted by sympathetic nervous system activation and resulting in release of epinephrine.

afferent neurons Sensory neurons that relay information from the sense organs toward the brain.

alarm reaction The first stage of the general adaptation syndrome (GAS), in which the body's defenses are mobilized against a stressor.

autonomic nervous system (ANS) The part of the peripheral nervous system that primarily serves internal organs.

catecholamines A class of chemicals containing epinephrine and norepinephrine.

central nervous system (CNS) All the neurons within the brain and spinal cord.

cortisol A type of glucocorticoid that provides a natural defense against inflammation and regulates carbohydrate metabolism.

crowding A person's perception of discomfort due to a high-density environment.

efferent neurons Motor neurons that convey impulses away from the brain.

endocrine system That system of the body consisting of ductless glands.

epinephrine A chemical manufactured by the adrenal medulla that accounts for much of the hormone production of the adrenal glands; sometimes called *adrenalin.*

exhaustion stage The final stage of the general adaptation syndrome (GAS), in which the body's ability to resist a stressor has been depleted.

general adaptation syndrome (GAS) The body's generalized attempt to defend itself against stress; consists of alarm reaction, resistance, and exhaustion.

glucocorticoids Hormones secreted by the adrenal cortex that increase the concentration of liver glycogen and blood sugar.

hormones Chemical substances released into the blood and having effects on other parts of the body.

insomnia The inability either to fall asleep or to stay asleep.

interneurons Neurons that connect sensory neurons to motor neurons; association neurons.

neuroendocrine system The system pertaining to the influence of the neural and endocrine systems and hypothesized to be the mechanism underlying the relationship between stress and illness.

neurons Nerve cells.

neurotransmitters Chemicals that are released by neurons and that affect the activity of other neurons.

norepinephrine One of two major neurotransmitters of the autonomic nervous system.

parasympathetic nervous system A division of the autonomic nervous system that promotes relaxation and functions under normal, nonstressful conditions.

peripheral nervous system (PNS) The nerves that lie outside the brain and spinal cord.

pituitary gland An endocrine gland that lies within the brain and whose secretions regulate many other glands.

population density A physical condition in which a high level of population is confined in a limited space.

primary appraisal One's initial appraisal of a potentially stressful event (Lazarus and Folkman's term).

reappraisal One's nearly constant reevaluation of stressful events (Lazarus and Folkman's term).

resistance stage The second stage of the general adaptation syndrome (GAS), in which the body adapts to a stressor.

secondary appraisal One's perceived ability to control or cope with harm, threat, or challenge (Lazarus and Folkman's term).

somatic nervous system The part of the PNS that serves the skin and voluntary muscles.

sympathetic nervous system A division of the autonomic nervous system that mobilizes the body's resources in stressful, emotional, and emergency situations.

synaptic cleft The space between neurons.

urban press The many environmental stressors that affect city living, including noise, crowding, crime, and pollution.

Suggested Readings

Graig, E. (1993). Stress as a consequence of the urban physical environment. In L. Goldberger & S. Breznitz (Eds.), *Handbook of stress: Theoretical and clinical aspects* (2nd ed., pp. 316–332). New York: Free Press.

Graig discusses the many stressful conditions associated with living in large urban areas. These conditions include noise, pollution, commuting problems, and fear of crime.

Kasl, S. V. (1996). Theory of stress and health. In C. L. Cooper (Ed.), *Handbook of stress, medicine, and health* (pp. 13–26). Boca Raton, FL: CRC Press.

Kasl reviews the diverse theoretical conceptualization of stress, dividing these views into three categories: stress as a stimulus, as a response, or as a transaction. He also summarizes critical points in evaluating stress research and gives suggestions for methodology for future research.

Lazarus, R. S., & Folkman, S. (1984). *Stress, appraisal, and coping.* New York: Springer.

A comprehensive treatment of Lazarus's views of stress, cognitive appraisal, and coping, this book discusses Lazarus's psychological model of stress and the relevant literature.

 Taylor, S. E., Repetti, R. L., & Seeman, T. (1997). Health psychology: What is an unhealthy environment and how does it get under the skin? *Annual Review of Psychology, 48,* 411–447.

This lengthy review includes a consideration of factors in the physical and social environment that may be unhealthy and discusses some ways that these stressors can affect people's health. Available through InfoTrac College Edition by Wadsworth Publishing Company.

CHAPTER 6

Understanding Stress and Disease

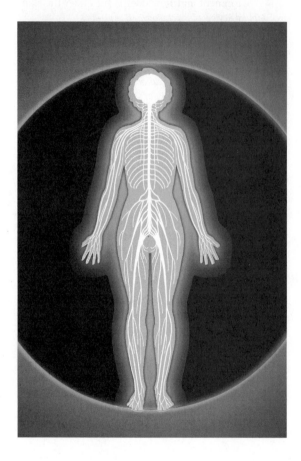

CASE STUDY
How Stress Affects Rick's Body

CHAPTER OUTLINE

Questions

Physiology of the Immune System

Psychoneuroimmunology

Does Stress Cause Disease?

Personality Factors Affecting Stress and Disease

Answers

Glossary

Suggested Readings

QUESTIONS

This chapter focuses on four basic questions:

1. How does the immune system function?

2. How does the field of psychoneuroimmunology relate behavior to disease?

3. Does stress cause disease?

4. What personality factors affect stress and disease?

138

HOW STRESS AFFECTS RICK'S BODY

Chapter 5 introduced Rick, who had undergone a period of extreme stress because of the deaths of his father and a close friend; he had also experienced a bitter divorce and custody dispute. As a consequence of these problems, Rick was left without family and social support, felt alienated from people at work, believed that he needed to hold at least two jobs to pay his bills, and began to have trouble sleeping. Did all these changes in lifestyle, most of which are negative, place Rick at risk for stress-related diseases?

This chapter reviews the evidence relating to stress as a possible cause of disease and follows Rick to see whether his high levels of stress place him at an elevated risk for disease or death. If stress, a psychological factor, can influence physical disease, some mechanism must exist to allow this interaction. We begin with a discussion of the immune system, which protects the body against stress-related diseases and could provide the mechanism for stress to cause disease.

Physiology of the Immune System

The immune system consists of tissues, organs, and processes that protect the body from invasion by foreign material, such as bacteria, viruses, and fungi. In addition, the immune system performs housekeeping functions by removing worn-out or damaged cells and patrolling for mutant cells. Once the invaders and renegades are located, the immune system activates processes to eliminate them.

Organs of the Immune System

Rather than being a centralized system like the heart or the brain, the immune system is spread throughout the body in the form of the **lymphatic system**. The tissue of the lymphatic system is **lymph**; it consists of the tissue components of blood except red cells and platelets. In the process of vascular circulation, fluid and *leukocytes* (white blood cells) leak from the capillaries. These blood components routinely escape from the circulatory system in the process of capillary diffusion. In addition, fluid is also secreted from body cells. This tissue fluid is referred to as *lymph* when it enters the lymph vessels, which circulate lymph and eventually return it to the bloodstream.

The structure of the lymphatic system (see Figure 6.1) roughly parallels the circulatory system for blood. Lymph also circulates, but it does so by entering the lymphatic system and then reentering the bloodstream rather than staying exclusively in the lymphatic system. In its circulation, all lymph travels through at least one **lymph node**. The lymph nodes are round or oval capsules spaced throughout the lymphatic system that help clean lymph of cellular debris, bacteria, and even dust that has entered the body.

Lymph gets its name from the **lymphocytes**, a type of white blood cell found in lymph. There are several types of lymphocytes, the most fully understood of which are T-lymphocytes, or **T-cells**; B-lymphocytes, or **B-cells**; and **natural killer (NK) cells**. Lymphocytes arise in the bone marrow, but they mature and differentiate in other structures of the immune system. In addition to lymphocytes, two other types of leukocytes exist, granulocytes and monocytes/macrophages. These leukocytes are involved in the nonspecific response of the immune system, whereas lymphocytes are involved in specific immune system responses (discussed more fully below).

The **thymus**, which has endocrine functions, secretes a hormone called **thymosin**. This hormone seems to be involved in the maturation and differentiation of the T-cells. Interestingly, the thymus is largest during infancy and childhood and then atrophies during adulthood. Its function is not entirely understood, but the thymus is clearly important in the immune system because its removal impairs immune function. Its atrophy also suggests that the immune system's production of T-cells is more efficient during childhood and that aging is related to lowered immune efficiency. The **tonsils** are masses of lymphatic tissue

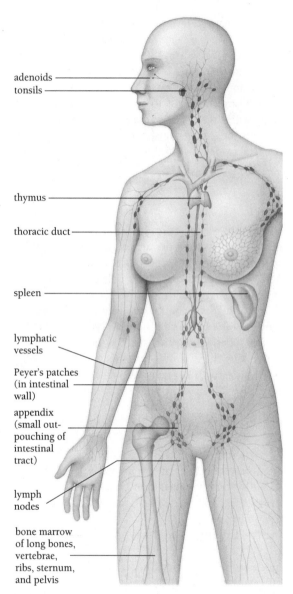

adenoids
tonsils

thymus

thoracic duct

spleen

lymphatic
vessels

Peyer's patches
(in intestinal
wall)

appendix
(small out-
pouching of
intestinal
tract)

lymph
nodes

bone marrow
of long bones,
vertebrae,
ribs, sternum,
and pelvis

Figure 6.1 **Lymphatic system.** *Source: From Introduction to Microbiology (p. 407), by J. L. Ingraham & C. A. Ingraham, 1995, Belmont, CA: Wadsworth. Copyright © 1995 by Wadsworth Publishing Company. Reprinted by permission.*

located in the throat. Their function seems to be similar to that of the lymph nodes: trapping and killing invading cells and particles. The **spleen**, an organ near the stomach in the abdominal cavity, is one site of lymphocyte maturation. In addition,

it serves as a holding station for lymphocytes as well as a disposal site for worn-out blood cells.

The surveillance and protection that the immune system offers is not limited to the lymph nodes but takes place in other tissues of the body that contain lymphocytes. Therefore, the organs of the immune system may be considered all those structures that manufacture, differentiate, store, and circulate lymph; but immune function relies on more than these structures and is not confined to the lymphatic system. To protect the entire body, immune function must occur in all parts of the body.

Function of the Immune System

The immune system's function is generally to protect against injury and specifically to maintain vigilance against foreign substances that the body has encountered. The immune system must be extraordinarily effective to prevent 100% of the invading bacteria, viruses, and fungi from damaging our bodies (R. J. Glasser, 1976). Few other body functions must operate at 100% efficiency, but the immune system must perform at that level for people (and other animals) to remain healthy.

Invading organisms have many ways to enter the body, and the immune system has a means to combat each type of entry. In general, immune system responses to invading foreign substances are of two types: general (nonspecific) and specific responses.

Nonspecific Immune System Responses Intact skin and mucous membranes are the first line of defense against foreign substances, but some invaders regularly bypass them and enter the body. Those that do face two general (nonspecific) mechanisms. One is **phagocytosis**, the attack of foreign particles by cells of the immune system. Two types of leukocytes perform this function. **Granulocytes** contain granules filled with chemicals. When these cells come into contact with invaders, they release their chemicals, which attack the invaders. **Macrophages** perform a variety of immune functions, including scavenging for worn-out cells and debris, assisting in the initiation of specific immune responses, and secreting a variety of chemicals involved in the immune response. Several chemical substances, called *complement,* are involved in breaking down the cell membranes of the invaders. Therefore, phagocytosis, which is part of the nonspecific immune system response, involves several mechanisms that can quickly result in the destruction of invading bacteria, viruses, and fungi. However, some invaders escape this nonspecific action.

Inflammation is a second type of nonspecific immune system response. Inflammation works to restore tissues that have been damaged by invaders. When an injury occurs, blood vessels in the area of injury contract temporarily. Later they dilate, increasing blood flow to the tissues and causing the warmth and redness that accompany inflammation. The damaged cells release enzymes that help destroy invading microorganisms; these enzymes can also aid in their own digestion, should the cells die. Both granulocytes and macrophages migrate to the site of injury to battle the invaders. Finally, tissue repair begins. Figure 6.2 illustrates the process of inflammation.

Specific Immune System Responses Two types of lymphocytes, T-cells and B-cells, carry out specific immune responses—that is, an immune response that is specific to one invader. When a lymphocyte encounters a foreign substance for the first time, both the general response and a specific response are initiated. Invading microorganisms are killed and eaten by macrophages, which present fragments of these invaders to T-cells that have moved to the area of inflammation. This contact sensitizes the T-cells; they acquire specific receptors on their surfaces so they can recognize the invader. An army of *cytotoxic T-cells* forms through this process, and it soon mobilizes a direct attack on the invaders. This process is referred to as *cell-mediated immunity* because it occurs at the level of the body cells rather than in the bloodstream. Cell-mediated immunity is especially effective against fungi, viruses that have already entered the cells, parasites, and mutations of body cells.

The other variety of lymphocyte, the B-cells, mobilizes an indirect attack on invading microorganisms. With the help of one variety of T-cell (the *helper T-cell*), B-cells differentiate into **plasma cells** and secrete **antibodies.** Each antibody is specifically manufactured in response to a specific invader. Foreign substances that provoke antibody manufacture are called **antigens** (for *anti*body *gen*erator). Antibodies circulate, find their antigens, bind to them, and mark them for later destruction. Figure 6.3 shows the differentiation of T- and B-cells.

The specific reactions of the immune system constitute the *primary immune response.* Figure 6.4 shows the development of the primary immune response and depicts how subsequent exposure activates the *secondary immune response.* During initial exposure to an invader, some of the sensitized T-cells and B-cells replicate, and rather than going into action, they are held in reserve. These *memory lymphocytes* form the basis for a rapid immune response on second exposure to the same invader. Memory lymphocytes can persist for years. They will not be activated unless the antigen invader reappears. If it does, then the memory lymphocytes initiate the same sort of direct and indirect attacks that occurred at the first exposure, but much more rapidly. This specifically tailored rapid response to foreign microorganisms that occurs with repeated exposure is what most people consider **immunity.**

This system of immune response through B-cell recognition of antigens and their manufacture of antibodies is called **humoral immunity,** because it happens in the bloodstream. The process is especially effective in fighting against bacterial invaders and viruses before they enter the cells—that is, while they are still circulating in the blood.

Creating Immunity One widely used method to induce immunity is **vaccination.** In vaccination, a weakened form of a virus or bacterium is introduced into the body, stimulating the production of antibodies. These antibodies then confer immunity

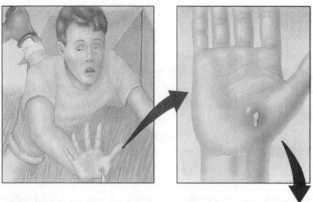

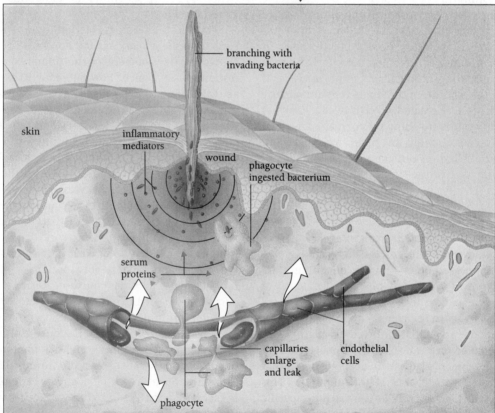

Figure 6.2 Acute inflammation is initiated by injury or infection. Inflammatory mediators are produced at the site of the stimulus. They cause blood vessels to dilate and increase their permeability; they also attract phagocytes to the site of inflammation and activate them.   *Source:* From *Introduction to Microbiology* (p. 386), by J. L. Ingraham & C. A. Ingraham, 1995, Belmont, CA: Wadsworth. Copyright © 1995 by Wadsworth Publishing Company. Reprinted by permission.

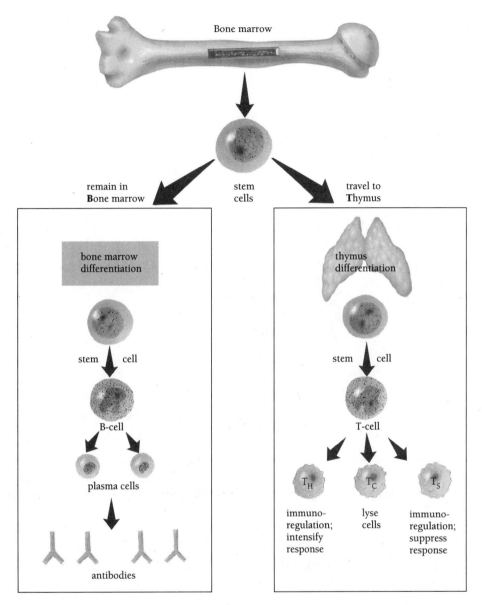

Figure 6.3 **Origins of B-cells and T-cells.** *Source:* From *Introduction to Microbiology* (p. 406), by J. L. Ingraham & C. A. Ingraham, 1995, Belmont, CA: Wadsworth. Copyright © 1995 by Wadsworth Publishing Company. Reprinted by permission.

for an extended period. Smallpox, which once killed thousands of people each year, has been eradicated through the use of vaccination. Now smallpox is a scientific curiosity confined to labora-

tory cultures. Other vaccines exist for a variety of diseases. They are especially useful in the prevention of viral infections. However, immunity must be created for each specific virus, and thousands of

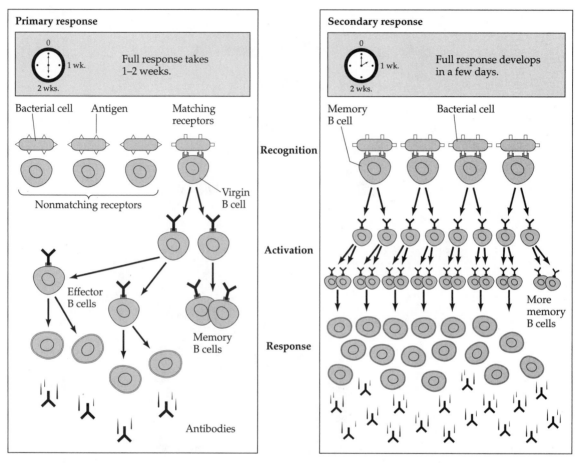

Figure 6.4   Primary and secondary immune pathways.   *Source:* From *Introduction to Microbiology* (p. 414), by J. L. Ingraham & C. A. Ingraham, 1995, Belmont, CA: Wadsworth. Copyright © 1995 by Wadsworth Publishing Company. Reprinted by permission.

viruses exist. Even viral diseases that produce similar symptoms, like the common cold, may be caused by many different viruses. Therefore, immunity for colds would require many vaccinations, and the development of these has not yet proven practical.

Immune System Disorders

Immune deficiency, an inadequate immune response, may occur for several reasons. For example, it is a side effect of most chemotherapy drugs used to treat cancer. Immune deficiency also occurs naturally. Although the immune system is not fully functional at birth, infants are protected by antibodies they have received from their mothers through the placenta, and infants who breastfeed receive antibodies from their mother's milk. These antibodies offer protection until the infant's own immune system develops during the first months of life.

In rare cases, the immune system fails to develop, leaving the child without immune protection. Physicians can try to boost immune function, but the well-publicized "children in plastic bubbles" still show the results of immune deficiency. Exposure to any virus or bacterium can be fatal to these children. They are sealed into sterile quarters to isolate them from the microorganisms that are part of the normal world.

An even more publicized type of immune deficiency is **acquired immune deficiency syndrome (AIDS).** This disease is caused by a virus, the human immunodeficiency virus (HIV), which acts to destroy the T-cells and macrophages in the immune system (O'Leary, 1990). Those who are infected with HIV are thus vulnerable to a wide range of bacterial, viral, and malignant diseases. The disease is known to be contagious but not easily transmitted from person to person. The highest concentrations of the virus are found in blood and in semen. Blood transfusions from an infected person, injection with a contaminated needle, and sexual intercourse seem to be the most common routes of infection. Treatment consists of the management of the diseases that develop because of immune deficiency. As of 1999, the only direct treatment for the AIDS virus consisted of administering drugs that affect viral infections, a treatment that slows the progress of the disease but does not cure it.

Allergies constitute another immune system disorder. An allergic response is an abnormal reaction to a foreign substance that normally elicits little or no immune reaction. People with allergies are hypersensitive to certain substances. A wide range of substances cause allergic reactions, and the severity of the reactions also varies widely. Some allergic reactions may be life threatening, whereas others merely cause runny noses. Some cases of allergy are treated by introducing regular, small doses of the allergen. This process desensitizes the person to the allergen, alleviating the allergic response. Other cases of allergy are treated by teaching allergic individuals to recognize and avoid their allergens.

Autoimmune diseases occur when the immune system attacks the body, for reasons not well understood. Part of the function of the immune system is to recognize foreign invaders and mark them for destruction. In some people, the person's own body cells are marked for destruction. In these cases, the immune system appears to have lost the ability to distinguish the body from an invader, and it mounts the same vicious attack against itself that it would against an intruder. Lupus erythematosus and rheumatoid arthritis are autoimmune diseases, and multiple sclerosis may also be.

Transplant rejection is not really an immune disorder, but it is a problem caused by the immune system's activity. When working efficiently, the immune system has the ability to detect foreign substances. With the exception of identical twins, no two humans have the same biochemistry. Therefore, the immune system normally recognizes any foreign tissue as an invader. A transplanted heart, liver, or kidney will be recognized as foreign tissue because the biochemical markers from its donor differ from those of its host. Thus the host's immune system will try to destroy the transplant. In an effort to prevent this reaction, drugs are administered that suppress immune system function. This strategy often works, but unfortunately the suppression is not specific to the transplanted organ. The entire immune response is affected, leaving the person vulnerable to infection. Currently, people who have received successful organ transplants must adapt their lifestyles to minimize the risk of infection due to their weakened immune system. Modification of lifestyle and compliance with medical regimens are topics of interest to health psychologists and other health professionals who use them in the treatment of organ transplant patients.

According to the **immune surveillance theory,** cancer is also the result of an immune system dysfunction. This view holds that the cellular mutations that initiate cancer occur quite frequently, but that these mutations are normally identified and killed by the T-cells in the immune system. Cancer develops when the immune system fails to identify and destroy mutant cells. Researchers who are investigating this theory are interested in discovering methods of stimulating immune system function as a treatment for cancer. If this theory is supported by future research, a vaccine against cancer may be possible. As in the case of smallpox, cancer could someday become an object of laboratory study rather than the killer of thousands.

In Summary

If stress can cause a disease, it can do so only by affecting biological processes. The most likely candidate for this interaction is the immune system, which is made up of tissues, organs, and processes that protect the body from invasion by foreign material such as bacteria, viruses, and fungi. The immune system also protects the body by eliminating damaged cells. Immune system responses can be either specific or nonspecific. Specific responses attack one particular invader, whereas nonspecific immunity is capable of attacking any invader. Immune system problems can stem from several sources, including organ transplants, allergies, drugs used for cancer chemotherapy, and immune deficiency. Acquired immune deficiency syndrome (AIDS) is a type of immune deficiency that gradually destroys the immune system and leaves the person vulnerable to a variety of viral and malignant diseases.

Psychoneuroimmunology

The previous section examined the function of the immune system as well as its tissues, structure, and disorders. Physiologists have traditionally taken a similar approach, studying the immune system as separate and independent of other body systems. About 25 years ago, however, evidence began to accumulate suggesting that the immune system interacts with the central nervous system (CNS) and the endocrine system and that the CNS, endocrine system, and immune system can be affected by psychological and social factors. In addition, immune function can affect neural function, providing the potential for the immune system to alter behavior and thought (Maier, Watkins, & Fleshner, 1994). This recognition has led to the founding and rapid growth of the field of **psychoneuroimmunology**, a multidisciplinary field that focuses on the interactions among behavior, the nervous system, the endocrine system, and the immune system.

History of Psychoneuroimmunology

George Solomon and Rudolph Moos first used the term *psychoneuroimmunology* in a publication in 1964. In that article and in his research in the 1960s, Solomon laid the groundwork for the field of psychoneuroimmunology (Kiecolt-Glaser & Glaser, 1989).

An event that dramatically shaped the field of psychoneuroimmunology was the 1975 publication of an article by Robert Ader and Nicholas Cohen on classical conditioning of the immune system. This research demonstrated how the nervous system, the immune system, and behavior could interact. Ader and Cohen conditioned rats to associate a novel, conditioning stimulus (CS)—a saccharine and water solution—with an unconditioned stimulus (UCS) that naturally produces an unconditioned response (UCR). In Ader and Cohen's procedure, a drug that suppresses the immune system was the UCS. The rats were allowed to drink the saccharin solution and then were injected with the drug. The response was the expected suppression of the immune system. However, the rats later showed immune suppression when they were given the saccharin solution alone. That is, their immune systems had been conditioned to respond to the saccharin solution in much the same manner that it reacted to the drug. This type of conditioning is not so surprising when one recalls Pavlov's classical experiment in which dogs learned to associate ringing bells with meat powder. But Ader and Cohen demonstrated that the immune system was subject to the same type of associative learning as other body systems.

Until Ader and Cohen's 1975 report, most physiologists believed that the immune system and the nervous system did not interact, and their results were not immediately accepted (Kiecolt-Glaser & Glaser, 1989, 1993). After many replications of their findings, physiologists now believe that the immune system and other body systems are interdependent. This belief has spurred researchers to explore the physical mechanisms by which behavior might affect the immune system.

Despite difficulties, psychoneuroimmunology research grew rapidly during the 1980s. Many psychologists became interested in research in the area, but few had the required knowledge of immunology and the resources to conduct the immunological assays that are necessary to measure immune system function (Kiecolt-Glaser & Glaser, 1989). On the other hand, advances in the field of immunology excited many researchers, and the AIDS epidemic focused public attention (and federal funding) on how behavior influences the immune system and therefore health. The vitality of the new field of psychoneuroimmunology was demonstrated by the appearance in 1987 of a journal, *Brain, Behavior, and Immunity,* devoted to reporting psychoneuroimmunology research.

Research in Psychoneuroimmunology

"The long-range goal of this research is to provide a comprehensive understanding of the role that behavior might play in promoting health and provoking illness" (Ratliff-Crain, Temoshok, Kiecolt-Glaser, & Tamarkin, 1989, p. 747). To reach this goal, researchers must establish a connection between psychological factors and changes in immune function and also establish a relationship between impaired immune function and changes in health status. Ideally, research should include all three components—psychological distress, immune system malfunction, and development of disease—in order to establish the connection between stress and disease (Keller, Shiflett, Schleifer, & Bartlett, 1994). This task is difficult for several reasons.

Not all people whose immune systems malfunction become ill (Cohen, 1996). Disease is a function of both the immune system's competence and the person's exposure to pathogens, the agents that produce illness. Also, the development of disease can be investigated only through longitudinal studies that follow people for a period of time after they have experienced a decline in immunocompetence resulting from stress. Only a few studies have included all three psychoneuroimmunology components, and most have been restricted to nonhuman animals.

The majority of research in psychoneuroimmunology has focused on the relationship between various stressors and altered immune system function. Also, most studies measure the immune system's function by testing blood samples rather than by testing immune function in people's bodies (Cohen & Herbert, 1996). Some research has concentrated on the relationship between altered immune system function and the development of disease or spread of cancer, but such studies are in the minority. Furthermore, the types of stressors, the species of animals, and the facets of immune system function studied have varied, resulting in a variety of findings (Ader & Cohen, 1993).

Some researchers have manipulated short-term stressors, such as electric shock, loud noises, or complex cognitive tasks, in a laboratory situation; others have used naturally occurring stress in people's lives to test the effect of stress on immune system function. Laboratory studies allow researchers to investigate the physical changes that accompany stress, and such studies have shown correlations between sympathetic nervous system activation and immune responses (Cohen & Herbert, 1996). This research suggests that sympathetic activation may be a pathway through which stress can affect the immune system.

The naturally occurring stress of school exams provided an opportunity to study immune function in medical students (Kiecolt-Glaser, Malarkey, Cacioppo, & Glaser, 1994). A series of studies showed differences in immunocompetence measured by numbers of natural killer cells, percentages of T-cells, and percentages of total lymphocytes. A longitudinal assessment of these medical students revealed a trend toward more symptoms of infectious disease before and after exams.

Exam stress is typically a short-term stress, but chronic stress has also been related to decreases in immune competence. Relationship conflict has been shown to relate to immune system suppression for couples who experience marital conflict (Kiecolt-Glaser et al., 1996; Kiecolt-Glaser et al., 1997), for women who had recently separated (Kiecolt-Glaser et al., 1987), and for men whose wives had recently died (Schleifer, Keller, Camerino, Thorton, & Stein, 1983). In addition, stressful living conditions can affect immune system function. For example, residents who lived near the Three Mile Island nuclear plant at the time of a major accident at that facility had fewer B-cells, T-cells, and natural killer cells than matched controls (McKinnon, Weisse, Reynolds, Bowles, & Baum, 1989).

Chronic stress can also come from caring for someone with Alzheimer's disease (see Chapter 11 for more about the disease and the stress of caregiving). Janice Kiecolt-Glaser and her colleagues (Esterling, Kiecolt-Glaser, Bodnar, & Glaser, 1994; Kiecolt-Glaser, Dura, Speicher, Trask, & Glaser, 1991; Kiecolt-Glaser, Marucha, Malarkey, Mercado, & Glaser, 1995) have studied a group of Alzheimer's caregivers over a period of years. These researchers found that, compared to a control group who were not caregivers for someone with a chronic illness, Alzheimer's caregivers had poorer psychological and physical health, longer healing times for wounds, and lowered immune function. Furthermore, the death of the Alzheimer's patient did not improve the caregivers' psychological health or immune system functioning. Both caregivers and former caregivers were more depressed and showed lowered immune system functioning, suggesting that this stress continues after the caregiving is over. Thus, chronic stress can affect not only immune system function but also physical and psychological health.

Chronic stress can also influence immune system reaction to acute stressors. For example, one study (Pike, Smith, Hauger, Nicassio, & Irwin, 1994) presented a laboratory stressor to young men who either were or were not chronically stressed and measured their distress as well as several measures of endocrine and immune function. The results indicated that the participants who were under chronic stress at the time of the laboratory stress reacted much more strongly to the laboratory stressor. These results suggest that chronic stress sensitizes people so that their responses to other stressors are exaggerated.

After conducting a meta-analysis of studies on stress and immunity, Tracy Herbert and Sheldon Cohen (1993b) concluded that substantial evidence exists for a relationship between stress and decreased immune function. This meta-analysis showed that many types of immune system function are related to stress and that immune suppression varies with the duration and intensity of the stressor.

Some of the psychoneuroimmunology research that has most clearly demonstrated the three-way link among stress, immune function, and disease has used rats as subjects. In one such study (Ben-Eliyahu, Yirmiya, Liebeskind, Taylor & Gale, 1991), researchers injected stressed rats with tumor material and observed the resulting change in natural killer cell activity and tumor metastases. The results showed that stress increased the metastases when the rats received the tumor material and experienced the stress within 1 hour of each other but not when a 24-hour gap occurred between the stress and the exposure to the malignancy. Thus, this study demonstrated that stress affected both immune function and a disease-related condition. Research using a different disease (herpes simplex virus) and a different laboratory stressor showed similar results of immune system inhibition (Bonneau, Sheridan, Feng, & Glaser, 1991).

This research has not been limited to rats; a study using human participants has also demonstrated the link among stress, immune function, and disease (Marucha, Kiecolt-Glaser, & Favagehi, 1998). This experimental study measured healing time after receiving a standardized wound either during vacation or during exams; thus, the stress component varied. Immune system function was measured during the two time periods, and the time for healing provided a physical outcome measurement. The results indicated that students under exam stress showed a decline in a specific immune function related to wound healing and that they healed 40% slower than the same students during vacation. Thus, some research on human as well as nonhuman subjects has demonstrated that stress can affect immune function and disease processes.

Physical Mechanisms of Influence

"Psychosocial factors do not influence disease in some mystic fashion. Rather, the physiological status of the host is altered in some way" (Plaut & Friedman, 1981, p. 5). The previous section presented studies showing that such influence occurs but did not explore the physiology underlying that influence.

Immunosuppression may be either part of the body's response to stress or a result of the effects of the stress response (Baum, Davidson, Singer, & Street, 1987). In other words, it may be either a direct or an indirect effect of stress. The effects of stress can occur through the relationship of the nervous system to the immune system through two routes—the peripheral nervous system and the secretion of hormones.

Evidence exists for connection through both routes (Maier et al., 1994). The connection between the nervous system and the immune system occurs through the peripheral nervous system, which has connections to immune system organs such as the thymus, spleen, and lymph nodes. The brain can also communicate with the immune system through the production of releasing factors, hormones that stimulate endocrine glands to secrete hormones. These hormones travel through the bloodstream and affect target organs, such as the adrenal glands. (Chapter 5 included a description of these systems and the endocrine component of the stress response.) T-cells and B-cells have receptors for the glucocorticoid hormones, and lymphocytes have catecholamine receptors.

When the sympathetic nervous system is activated, the adrenal glands release several hormones. The adrenal medulla releases epinephrine and norepinephrine, and the adrenal cortex releases cortisol. The modulation of immunity by epinephrine and norepinephrine seems to come about through the autonomic nervous system rather than through a direct link with the immune system (Hall & Goldstein, 1981).

The release of cortisol from the adrenal cortex results from the release of adrenocorticotropic hormone (ACTH) by the pituitary in the brain. Another brain structure, the hypothalamus, stimulates the pituitary to release ACTH. Elevated cortisol is associated with a number of physical and emotional distress conditions (Baum et al., 1987), and it exerts an anti-inflammatory effect. Cortisol and the glucocorticoids tend to depress immune responses, phagocytosis, and macrophage activation (Cunningham, 1981).

The brain might modulate the immune response through the activity of the hypothalamus (Stein, Schleifer, & Keller, 1981) or through its secretion of neurochemicals (MacLean & Reichlin, 1981). Lymphocytes have receptors for beta-endorphin, one of the brain's opoid peptides that has been shown to relate to immunosuppression (Jemmott & Locke, 1984). Moreover, the release of the opoid peptides occurs through the same stimuli—stress and distress—that trigger the release of hormones in the interaction between the pituitary and adrenal glands (Baum et al., 1987). The similarity of the situations that prompt release and the of physical mechanisms for reception suggests that neurochemicals are a possible mechanism by which the brain influences the immune response.

As can be seen, the relationship between the nervous and immune systems is complex and still far from fully understood. The nervous system can influence the immune system through either the sympathetic nervous system or through neuroendocrine response to stress. In addition, the physical mechanisms of influence may also act in the other direction: The immune system has the power to alter behavior through its effect on the nervous system.

The response to immune system activation is equivalent to the peripheral nervous system's stress response. Thus, the interrelationship between nervous system and immune system allows possibilities for influence of each on the other.

Therapeutic Effects

Most studies in psychoneuroimmunology have demonstrated that immune system activity decreases following distress. A basic assumption of many psychoneuroimmunologists is that increases in psychological distress lead to immunological changes and that these changes lead to disease (Keller et al., 1994). If this reasoning is correct, then the field of psychoneuroimmunology can spell out conditions that produce disease. But is it possible to *boost* immunocompetence through changes in behavior? Would such an increase enhance health? A few studies have suggested that therapeutic uses of psychoneuroimmunology may be possible but that boosting immune function above normal functioning is probably not possible (Kiecolt-Glaser & Glaser, 1993). However, through infection or through distress, many people have compromised immune system function, and improvements could make a difference for them.

Dealing with troubling experiences can help immune function. A study (Pennebaker, Kiecolt-Glaser, & Glaser, 1988) with healthy college students demonstrated this possibility. One group of healthy college students wrote about troubling experiences, and the other group wrote about superficial topics. The rationale for the comparison was that writing about troubling experiences would constitute a confrontation with them. The results suggested that college students benefited from confronting traumatic experiences simply by writing about them. These college students showed increased cellular immune system function and reported fewer visits to the health center.

People who are HIV-positive would also benefit from boosts in immune system function, and researchers have attempted to formulate behav-ioral interventions that enhance immunocompetence. A series of studies with infected and at-risk individuals (Antoni, 1993; Antoni et al., 1990; Antoni et al., 1991) included several components for a healthy lifestyle, such as aerobics training and stress management. The purpose was to determine whether such a psychosocial intervention could boost immune function in these at-risk individuals or delay the onset of AIDS symptoms in infected men. Although complex, results from this program of research suggest that the intervention positively affected immune system function, holding some potential that such interventions could slow the progress of HIV infection to full-blown AIDS.

Another potential application involves depression of immune system function. In 1975, Ader and Cohen demonstrated that immune function could be classically conditioned, and in a subsequent study (Ader & Cohen, 1982), showed that conditioned immunosuppression could be used therapeutically. Their subjects consisted of mice that were genetically prone to lupus erythematosus, an autoimmune disease. This disease can be controlled with a drug that suppresses the immune system, slowing the body's attack on itself. Using the same procedure as in their 1975 study, Ader and Cohen conditioned the mice to respond to a saccharin solution with immunosuppression; the saccharin solution was the conditioning stimulus, the immunosuppressant drug was the unconditioned stimulus—and immune suppression was the unconditioned response. The magnitude of the immune system suppression from the conditioning alone was not sufficient to produce therapeutic effects. However, administering the saccharin solution *and* a low dose of the drug (which would not have produced therapeutic effects by itself) brought about sufficient immunosuppression to produce therapeutic effects. Ader and Cohen were able to demonstrate that conditioned immune suppression allowed a lower dose of a drug to have therapeutic effects. This provocative result suggests that behavioral treatments may have a role in the management of autoimmune diseases.

In Summary

Researchers in the field of psychoneuroimmunology have demonstrated that various functions of the immune system respond to both short-term and long-term psychological stress. The field of psychoneuroimmunology has therefore made progress toward linking psychological factors, immune system function, and disease, but few studies have included all three elements.

Some research has been successful in linking immune system changes to changes in health status; this link is necessary to complete the chain between psychological factors and disease. In addition to establishing links between psychological factors and immune system changes, theorists and researchers in the field of psychoneuroimmunology have attempted to specify the physical mechanisms through which these changes occur. The possibilities for the mechanisms include direct connections between nervous and immune systems and an indirect connection through the neuroendocrine system; evidence exists for both. The promise of psychoneuroimmunology is that it may yield not only an understanding of the relationships among behavior, the nervous system, and the immune system but also therapeutic applications in the form of behavioral interventions for people whose immune systems are not functioning effectively.

Does Stress Cause Disease?

Disease is caused by many factors, and stress may be one of those factors. In any consideration of the association between disease and major life events or daily hassles, it is well to remember that most people at risk from stressful experiences do *not* develop a disease. Furthermore, in contrast to other risk factors—such as having high cholesterol levels, smoking cigarettes, or drinking alcohol—the risks conferred by life events are usually temporary. As one of the authors of the Social Readjustment Rating Scale expressed it, "Most individuals with high recent life-change totals do not remain at such levels for more than a year or two before returning to baseline levels which connote far less risk" (Rahe, 1984, p. 49).

In this section, we review the evidence concerning the link between stress and several diseases, including headache, infectious disease, cardiovascular disease, diabetes mellitus, premature birth, asthma, and rheumatoid arthritis. In addition, stress shows some relationship to negative moods and mood disorders such as depression and anxiety disorders.

Stress and Disease

What is the evidence linking stress to disease? Which diseases have been implicated? What physiological mechanism might mediate the connection between stress and disease?

Selye's concept of stress (see Chapter 5) included suppression of the immune response, but until recently no evidence existed to support this hypothesis. Now a growing body of evidence suggests interactions among the nervous, endocrine, and immune systems. This interaction is similar to the responses hypothesized by Selye and provides strong evidence that stress could cause a variety of physical ailments. Figure 6.5 shows some of these possible effects.

There are several possible pathways through which stress could produce disease (Herbert & Cohen, 1994). Direct influence could occur through the effects of stress on the nervous and endocrine systems as well as on the immune system. Because any or all of these systems can create disease, there are sufficient physiological foundations for a link between stress and disease. In addition, indirect effects could occur through changes in health practices that increase risks; that is, stress tends to be related to increases in drinking, smoking, drug use, and sleep problems, all of which can increase the risk for disease. Thus, possibilities exist for both direct and indirect effects

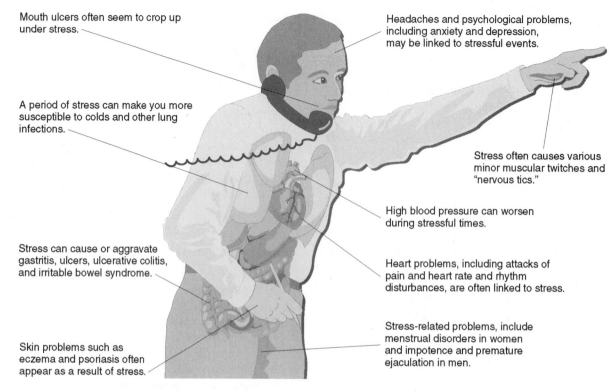

Mouth ulcers often seem to crop up under stress.

A period of stress can make you more susceptible to colds and other lung infections.

Stress can cause or aggravate gastritis, ulcers, ulcerative colitis, and irritable bowel syndrome.

Skin problems such as eczema and psoriasis often appear as a result of stress.

Headaches and psychological problems, including anxiety and depression, may be linked to stressful events.

Stress often causes various minor muscular twitches and "nervous tics."

High blood pressure can worsen during stressful times.

Heart problems, including attacks of pain and heart rate and rhythm disturbances, are often linked to stress.

Stress-related problems, include menstrual disorders in women and impotence and premature ejaculation in men.

Figure 6.5 **Effects of long-term stress.** *Source:* From *An Invitation to Health* (7th ed. p. 58), by D. Hales, 1997, Pacific Grove, CA: Brooks/Cole. Copyright © 1997 by Brooks/Cole Publishing Company. Reprinted by permission of Wadsworth Publishing Co.

of stress on disease. Does the evidence support these hypothesized relationships?

Headaches For most people, headaches are a minor problem that require no more than over-the-counter medication, but headache is also one of the most frequent causes of visits to physicians (Hatch, 1993). Headache can signal serious medical conditions, but most often the pain associated with the headache is the problem. The majority of people who seek medical assistance for headaches are plagued by the same sorts of headaches as those who do not; the difference stems from the frequency and severity of the headaches or from personal factors involved in seeking assistance.

Although over 100 types of headaches exist, distinguishing among them has become controversial, and the underlying causes for the most common types remain unclear (Hatch, 1993). Nevertheless, diagnostic criteria have been devised for several types of headaches. The most frequent type of headache is *tension headache,* usually associated with increased muscle tension in the head and neck region. Tension is also a factor in vascular headache, and many tension headaches have a vascular component. The most notorious of the vascular headaches are *migraine headaches,* hypothesized to be caused by changes in constriction of the vascular arteries and associated with throbbing pain localized in one side of the head.

Stress is recognized as a factor in both tension and vascular headaches (Rasmussen, 1993). However, the type of stress associated with headaches tends not to be traumatic life events but rather small daily hassles (Fernandez & Sheffield, 1996). People with tension and mixed headaches were more likely than those with migraines to report more daily hassles as well as more intense daily hassles. In addition, stressful events precede periods of headache more often than they precede times with no headache, and stress during a headache intensified the attack (Marlowe, 1998).

Like most people, Rick had always experienced occasional headaches, but several years before his divorce, his headaches became more frequent and more severe. He traces this change to a neck injury, but he also believes that tension is the basis for his headaches and that they are exacerbated by stress. Indeed, headaches were a major problem during the 18 months in his life when he was under exceedingly high levels of stress.

Infectious Disease Are people who are under stress more likely than nonstressed individuals to develop infectious diseases such as the common cold? Research suggests that the answer is yes. An early study (Stone, Reed, & Neale, 1987) followed married couples who kept diaries on their own and their spouse's desirable and undesirable daily life experiences. Results indicated that participants who experienced a decline in desirable events or an increase in undesirable events developed somewhat more infectious diseases (colds or flu) 3 and 4 days later. The association was not strong, but this study was the first prospective design to show a relationship between daily life experiences and subsequent disease.

Later studies used a more direct approach: intentionally inoculating healthy volunteers with common cold viruses to see who would develop a cold and who would not. In one such study (Stone et al., 1992), students who developed colds reported significantly more positive and negative major life events during the previous year, suggest-

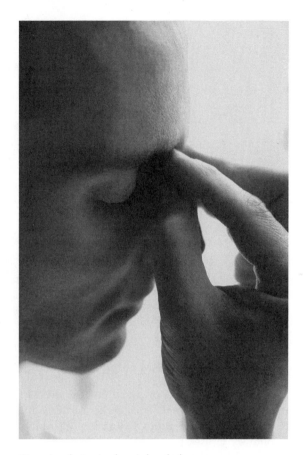

Stress is a factor in chronic headaches.

ing that a high level of life events (either positive or negative) may lead to the development of colds.

Sheldon Cohen and his colleagues (Cohen et al., 1998; Cohen, Tyrrell, & Smith, 1991, 1993) have also intentionally exposed healthy volunteers to various common cold viruses. Cohen et al. (1991) used three measures of psychological stress: (1) number of major stressful life events during the past year; (2) perception that demands exceed a person's ability to cope; and (3) current level of negative affect—that is, a person's self-ratings on 15 emotional states, such as hostile, scared, and angry at self. The experimenters combined the three stress measures into a single stress index and

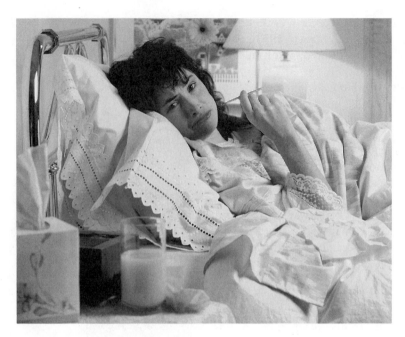

Research has shown that stress can influence development of infectious disease.

then assessed the level of psychological stress in nearly 400 healthy male and female participants. Next, they gave nasal drops containing one of five respiratory viruses to people in an experimental group and placebo saline nasal drops to people in a control group. They found that the degree of psychological stress was related in a dose-response manner to the number of both respiratory infections and clinical colds the participants developed. In other words, the higher the person's stress, the more likely it was that he or she would become ill. The associations were similar for all five viruses and could not be explained by other health-related habits or personal qualities. Later, Cohen and his colleagues (Cohen et al., 1993) analyzed the relationship between the common cold and the same three individual measures of stress. Each of the three measures independently predicted a person's risk of developing a cold.

More recently, Cohen et al. (1998) used the same inoculation procedure to see what types of stressors induce cold symptoms in people exposed to a cold virus. They found that duration of a stressful life event was more important than severity. Acute severe stress of less than 1 month did not lead to the development of colds, but severe chronic stress (more than 1 month) led to a substantial increase in colds. This association between stress and cold symptoms could not be explained by increases in epinephrine, norepinephrine, or cortisol or by such factors as social support, personality, or health practices.

The findings of these studies suggest that stress may be a more important contributor to the common cold than diet, lack of sleep, or even white cell count. To develop a cold, one must be exposed to a cold virus, but exposure alone cannot predict who will develop a cold and who will not. Psychological stress seems to be an important predictor.

Cardiovascular Disease   Cardiovascular disease (CVD) has a number of behavioral risk factors, some of which are related to stress. Chapter 9 examines these behavioral risk factors in more detail; in this section we look only at stress as a contributor to CVD. Although some people assume that stress is a major cause of heart disease, the available evidence is less clear.

Studies from the 1970s seemed to support the notion that stress leads to heart disease; their findings indicated that people who died of a sudden heart attack had experienced more stressful life events in the 6 months preceding the attack than did those who survived (Rahe, Romo, Bennett, & Siltanen, 1974). In addition, specific stresses such as bereavement, loss of prestige, and loss of employment have been found to be risks for heart attack (Kavanagh & Shepard, 1973). A later study (Gullette et al., 1997) found that stress can serve as a trigger for heart attacks. This study looked at negative emotions of outpatients with coronary heart disease during the hour immediately preceding a heart attack and discovered that feelings of sadness, frustration, or tension can more than double the risk for heart attack. Results of this last study, of course, do not apply to people with no coronary heart disease.

Does stress contribute to cardiovascular disease in healthy individuals? Studies have generally yielded inconsistent results. Only a modest relationship appeared between stress and coronary artery disease (CAD) in one study of middle-aged men (Rosengren, Tibblin, & Wilhelmsen, 1991). This study followed men with no prior history of heart disease for 12 years and noted different rates of coronary artery disease for six different levels of stress. Men in the lowest categories differed from those in the higher categories in CAD risk, but the difference was significant only for the extremes, suggesting that only *substantial* psychological stress contributes to coronary artery disease.

In a study (Karasek et al., 1988) on job strain (defined as jobs low in decision latitude and high in psychological work load), a modest risk of heart attack appeared. Using the same definition of job strain, a later study in Sweden found a 70% increase in all-cause mortality for men with jobs low in control and high in psychological demand (Falk, Hanson, Issacsson, & Ostergren, 1992). The

study indicated that high job strain combined with a weak social network and low social support resulted in an increase of relative risk that was more than four times the rate of men who had low job strain and adequate social supports. Thus, it appears that job strain may have a synergistic effect with a weak social network and low social support to contribute to death rates. (A **synergistic effect** means that the total impact exceeds the sum of two or more individual effects; that is, the combination of job strain, a weak social network, and low social support would have a much higher risk than their separate risks added together.)

This increased risk, however, does not hold for all groups. In the Honolulu Heart Program (Reed, LaCroix, Karasek, Miller, & MacLean, 1989), no significant relationship appeared between job strain (high psychological demands and low job control) and coronary heart disease (CHD) in men of Japanese ancestry in Hawaii. For the men who had adopted a more Westernized lifestyle, there was a slight inverse trend; that is, men high in job strain had slightly lower CHD.

These somewhat inconsistent results suggest that individual factors such as social support and a traditional lifestyle may interact with job strain either to buffer the risk for heart disease and all causes of mortality or to contribute to them. Also, physical fitness may moderate the effects of stress on disease (Brown, 1991). Thus, the link between stress and heart disease risk is not as strong as many people assume.

Hypertension "Contrary to the implication of its name, hypertension is not a high level of nervous tension, in terms either of its causes or its manifestations" (Jenkins, 1998, p. 604). Although high blood pressure would seem to be the result of stress, no simple relationship exists between stress and blood pressure. Situational factors such as noise can elevate blood pressure, but most studies have shown that blood pressure returns to normal when the situational stimulus is removed. Chronic exposure to noise, in contrast, may play a role in the development of hypertension (Talbott et al., 1985).

Another possible link between hypertension and stress is sodium retention. Stress situations are capable of inducing kidney retention of salt in greater amounts in rats that developed high blood pressure and in humans whose sympathetic nervous systems respond strongly to stress situations (Light, Kopke, Obrist, & Willis, 1983). This finding suggests that stress can cause sodium retention in a particular type of person, and further research (Miller et al., 1998) showed that hostility is also a factor. Men high in hostility tended to consume more salt than men lower in hostility. A review of research on stress and sodium intake (Haythornthwaite, 1992–93) showed that both factors can affect blood pressure and that the two may have a synergistic effect in combination. In studies using both human and nonhuman animals, the combination of stress and sodium in the diet has resulted in elevations in blood pressure.

In summary, the relationship between stress and temporary increases in blood pressure is stronger than the evidence for stress as a factor in chronic hypertension. Some evidence exists showing that chronic stress may be related to hypertension, but other factors, such as sodium intake or hostility, may interact with stress to raise the risk for hypertension.

Reactivity   The idea that some people react more strongly to stress than other people has received considerable attention in recent years. This response, called *reactivity,* may be an important stress-related factor in the development of cardiovascular disease. For reactivity to play a role in the development of cardiovascular disease, the response must be relatively stable within an individual and be prompted by events that occur frequently in the individual's life. Researchers have investigated the stability of reactivity and have also tried to discover those events that prompt it. Exercise, competition, cigarette smoking, cold temperatures, video games, and arguments are some of the situations that have been considered as possible stressors. In addition, researchers have measured an array of cardiac responses, including diastolic blood pressure, systolic blood pressure, heart rate, and catecholamine excretion as indices of reactivity.

With such a variety of independent and dependent variables, unambiguous results would be surprising. A factor analysis of stress-related measures of reactivity (Kamarck, Jennings, Pogue-Geile, & Manuck, 1994) revealed two factors, vascular reactivity and cardiac reactivity. This research showed that the patterns of responses for these factors were stable over time for the same people and for similar tasks on different people. This research demonstrated one of the necessary conditions for a relationship between reactivity and cardiovascular disease: a stable pattern of responding to similar stresses over time for the same individual.

Individual factors also play a role in reactivity. Hostility is one such factor in men (Suarez, Kuhn, Schanberg, Williams, & Zimmermann, 1998), and aggression, anxiety, and locus of control are others (Houston, 1986). Gender and ethnicity are also factors of substantial interest in reactivity. Because men develop cardiovascular disease at a younger age than women, researchers expected to find gender differences in reactivity, and research (Voegele, Jarvis, & Cheeseman, 1997) has shown this gender difference. Other research (Light, Turner, Hinderliter, & Sherwood, 1993a) revealed some variability in the tasks that elicit different cardiovascular reactions for women and men, but men showed greater overall blood pressure increases and slower recovery times than women. Blood pressure changes in the workplace are also related to reactivity (Light, Turner, Hinderliter, & Sherwood, 1993b). These gender differences appear during childhood (Treiber et al., 1993) and persist over time from childhood to adolescence (Murphy, Stoney, Alpert, & Walker, 1995). In summary, boys and men seem to show higher reactivity than girls and women, and these gender-related differences may relate to the development of cardiovascular disease.

The higher rates of cardiovascular disease for African Americans compared to European Americans has led researchers to examine differences in reactivity between these two ethnic groups. The results generally confirm the differences in the expected direction. Beginning during childhood and continuing to adolescence, African Americans showed greater reactivity than European Americans (Murphy et al., 1995), and such differences appeared among children as young as 6 years of age (Treiber et al., 1993). In addition, African American children with a family history of cardiovascular disease showed significantly greater reactivity than any other group of children in the study.

The ethnic and gender differences in reactivity are intriguing but not explanatory. The agreement between the demographics of cardiovascular disease and differences in reactivity among various groups suggests that reactivity plays a role in the development of disease. As Norman Anderson (1993) pointed out, the underlying nature of those differences remains to be explained. Knowing that African Americans are higher in both reactivity and in rates of cardiovascular disease does not tell us *why* African Americans are more likely to develop cardiovascular problems. The research on reactivity demonstrates a potential link between stress and the development of heart disease, but it does not yet reveal the mechanisms through which reactivity might produce cardiovascular disease.

Risky Behaviors In addition to affecting physiological responses in ways that promote disease, stress may alter health-related behaviors and produce an indirect effect on health (Herbert & Cohen, 1994). Stress may interact with risky behaviors to increase people's risk for heart disease. For example, people under stress may smoke more cigarettes, drink more alcohol, use illicit drugs, and change their eating habits. Each of these behaviors can affect the development of cardiovascular disease. The tendency to drink (Berger & Adesso, 1991) and use drugs (Tavris, 1992) as a way of coping with negative experience is more common among men than among women. Women, however, are more likely to use food as a

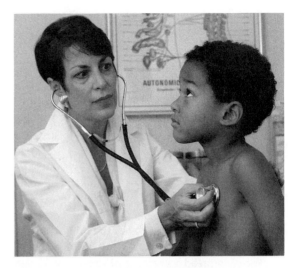

Beginning during childhood, African Americans show higher cardiac reactivity than other ethnic groups, which may relate to their higher levels of cardiovascular disease.

means of personal comfort, which can result in unhealthy eating habits (Tavris, 1992).

Other Physical Disorders Besides headache, infectious disease, and cardiovascular disease, stress has been linked to several other physical disorders, including diabetes, premature delivery for pregnant women, asthma, and rheumatoid arthritis.

Diabetes mellitus is a chronic disease that may be related to stress. Two kinds of diabetes mellitus are Type I or insulin dependent diabetes mellitus (IDDM) and Type II or noninsulin dependent diabetes mellitus (NIDDM). IDDM is also called juvenile-onset diabetes, because it begins in childhood and requires insulin injections for its control. NIDDM usually appears during adulthood and can most often be controlled by dietary changes. (The lifestyle adjustments and behavioral management required by diabetes mellitus are discussed in Chapter 11.)

Stress may contribute to the development of both types of diabetes through several routes (Cox & Gonder-Frederick, 1992). First, stress may

WOULD YOU BELIEVE . . . ?

Stress and Ulcers

Would you believe that stress is not a major factor in the development of ulcers? During the 1980s, two Australian researchers, Barry Marshall and J. Robin Warren, proposed that ulcers were the result of a bacterial infection rather than stress (Alper, 1993). At the time, their hypothesis seemed somewhat unlikely because most physicians believed that bacteria could not live in the stomach environment with its extreme acidity. Researchers had searched for a bacterium that caused ulcers but had failed to find it, concluding that no bacteria could grow in the stomach.

The widespread acceptance of stress as an underlying factor in ulcers was an additional barrier to the search for an alternative cause; Marshall (1995) reported that he had trouble receiving funding to research the possibility of a bacterial basis for ulcers. Marshall and Warren hypothesized that the *Helicobacter pylori* bacterium was responsible for ulcers. With no funding for his research and the belief that he was correct, Marshall infected himself with the bacterium to demonstrate its gastric effects. He developed severe gastritis and took antibiotics to cure himself, providing further evidence that this bacterium has gastric effects.

Beginning with the premise that the *Helicobacter pylori* bacterium was responsible for ulcers, Marshall and Warren set up a clinical trial in which half the patients received antibiotics and half received the traditional treatment—an acid suppressant (Alper, 1993). Results of this study revealed that stomach ulcers returned in 50%–95% of patients who received the acid suppressant, but only 29% of the patients treated with antibiotics experienced a recurrence of ulcers. *Helicobacter pylori* is also implicated in duodenal and gastric ulcers among children. Macarthur, Saunders, and Feldman (1995) reviewed 45 studies dealing with this bacterium in children with gastroduodenal disease and found that for children under 18 with duodenal ulcer, an overwhelming majority also had the bacterium; and for children with gastric ulcer, a smaller but still substantial number had this bacterium. Not all occurrence of ulcers is due to *Helicobacter pylori*. Some people with ulcers are not infected with the bacterium, and some people who are infected do not develop ulcers. *Helicobacter pylori*, however, may also be a factor in gastric cancer and other gastric diseases (Alper, 1993).

Even with the dramatic improvement from antibiotic treatment, many physicians were reluctant to accept the bacterial cause of ulcers (Alper, 1993; Marshall, 1995). Part of that reluctance was the continued belief that stress was involved in ulcer formation. This belief is more common among the general public than among physicians; 60% of a sample of U.S. residents believed that stress is the major cause of ulcers, but 90% of physicians accepted bacterial infection as the major cause of ulcers (Novelli, 1997).

This increased knowledge among physicians has led to changes in treatment for ulcers. Antibiotic regimens have become more common as a treatment, but physicians continue to prescribe antisecretory drugs rather than antibiotics for 50% of ulcer patients (Novelli, 1997). The tendency among both physicians and people in general to link ulcers with stress is a tribute to the strength of this belief but a sad situation for people with curable ulcers.

---

contribute directly to the *development* of insulin-dependent diabetes through the disruption of the immune system. In general, retrospective studies have found that insulin-dependent diabetics had somewhat more stressful life events than nondiabetics. However, prospective investigations of this issue are extremely difficult to conduct on humans. Second, stress may contribute directly to NIDDM through its effect on the sympathetic nervous system; and third, stress may contribute to

NIDDM through its possible effects on obesity. Research on stress and noninsulin-dependent diabetics has shown that stress can be a triggering factor and thus play a role in the age at which people develop adult-onset diabetes.

In addition, stress may affect the *management* of diabetes mellitus through its direct effects of raising blood glucose (Wylie-Rosett, 1998) and through the indirect route of hindering people's compliance with controlling glucose levels (Herschbach et al., 1997). Indeed, compliance is a major problem for this disorder, as discussed in Chapter 4.

Stress during pregnancy has been the topic of research for both human and nonhuman subjects (Dunkel-Schetter & Lobel, 1998). Research with nonhuman subjects has conclusively demonstrated that stressful environments relate to lower birthweight and developmental delays in the infants of stressed mothers. Research with human participants cannot experimentally manipulate stress, so the results are not as conclusive, but a review of studies on stress during pregnancy (Adler & Matthews, 1994) revealed a tendency for stress to make preterm deliveries more likely and to result in babies with lower birth weights. Both factors are related to a number of problems for the infants. The importance of type and timing of stress remains unclear, but there is some indication that chronic stress may be more damaging than acute stress, and stress late in pregnancy is more risky than earlier stress (Dunkel-Schetter & Lobel, 1998).

Asthma is a respiratory disorder characterized by difficulty in breathing due to reversible airway obstruction, airway inflammation, and increase in airway responsiveness to a variety of stimuli (Creer & Bender, 1993). The prevalence and mortality rate of asthma have increased in recent years for both European American and African American women, men, and children, but poor African Americans living in urban environments are disproportionately affected.

Stress can be among the stimuli that are associated with asthma attacks, including emotional events, physical stressors such as pain, and the belief that an allergen is present (Bieliauskas, 1982).

Even though asthma's symptoms are physical, the events that trigger attacks can be emotional and may follow stressful events, either immediately or after a delay. In addition, controlling the conditions that can precipitate an attack can be stressful, adding to the problems of management (Schmaling, 1998).

Rheumatoid arthritis, a chronic inflammatory disease of the joints, may also be related to stress. Rheumatoid arthritis is believed to be an autoimmune disorder in which a person's own immune system attacks itself (Young, 1993). The attack produces inflammation and damage to the tissue lining of the joints, resulting in pain and loss of flexibility and mobility.

A growing body of evidence (Zautra, 1998) indicates that stress can make arthritis worse by increasing pain sensitivity, reducing coping efforts, and possibly affecting the process of inflammation itself. Direct effects of stress on inflammation could occur through neuroendocrine responses to stress. Because the disorder is not completely understood, the role of stress in the development of this disorder remains unclear. However, the stress that results from rheumatoid arthritis brings about negative changes in people's lives and requires extensive coping efforts.

Stress and Negative Mood

The relationship between stress and negative mood seems obvious—stress puts people in a bad mood. Being in a bad mood can change immune function. One group of researchers (Futterman, Kemeny, Shapiro, & Fahey, 1994) investigated the effect of mood change on immune function by inducing positive and negative mood states in a group of actors and measuring their immune function afterward. They found that mood changes of both types affected immune function. Thus, even daily normal mood swings can influence the function of the immune system.

Negative mood, however, may mean to a stable way of looking at the world as well as to a temporary bad mood. *Negative affectivity* is a general tendency to experience distress and dissatisfaction in a variety of situations. Individuals high in negative affectivity focus on the negative aspects of self, others, and situations; the result is a pessimistic view of life. They complain about their health even when they are not sick.

Earlier, we saw that Sheldon Cohen and his colleagues inoculated healthy people with cold viruses to learn of the effects of stress on the common cold. Cohen et al. (1995) also measured negative affectivity in these volunteers and found that those high in negative affectivity who got sick complained more than those lower in negative affectivity, even though they were not objectively more sick. Thus, people with negative affectivity feel worse than other people when they are ill. In addition, the tendency for people high in negative affectivity to overreport stress and to see themselves as being in poor health makes them subject to depression and anxiety disorders.

Depression   The evidence that stressful life events cause depression is less than overwhelming. In general, research suggests a slight tendency for stressful life events to be a factor in depressive symptoms (Kessler, 1997). The ability to cope and coping resources, however, are more closely associated with depression: People who can cope effectively are able to avoid depression. Again, the factor of negative affectivity may exacerbate stress, making people complain of health problems more prone to poor coping and to increased depression (Nolen-Hoeksema, 1994).

Depressed people are more likely than nondepressed individuals to have experienced major stressful life events preceding the onset of depression (Rabkin, 1993). Although the correlations between life events and depression are typically quite small, some life events have been shown to relate to depression. One such life event is the experience of chronic disease, either as a person with the disease or as a caregiver. Heart disease (Holahan, Moos, Holahan, & Brennan, 1995), cancer (Telch & Telch, 1985), AIDS (Fleishman & Fogel,

1994), and Alzheimer's disease (Rabins, 1989) have all been related to increased incidence of depression. In addition, some research (Bodnar & Kiecolt-Glaser, 1994) indicates that the depression of caring for an Alzheimer's patient persists even after the caregiving has ended with the patient's death. In general, caregivers are two to three times more likely than other people to become depressed (Wright, 1997). Also, the incidence of depression seems to be directly proportional to amount of caregiving; that is, wives have the greatest burden for caregiving, and caregiving wives have the highest rates for depression, followed by caregiving daughters, sons, and husbands in that order (Wright, 1997).

However, stressful life experiences themselves may be less important than people's appraisal of an event, their vulnerability, and their perceived ability to cope with stress. Richard Lazarus and his colleagues (Kanner et al., 1981; Lazarus & DeLongis, 1983; Lazarus & Folkman, 1984) regard stress as the combination of an environmental stimulus plus the person's appraisal, vulnerability, and perceived coping strength. According to this theory, people become ill not merely because they had too many stressful experiences but because they evaluate these experiences as threatening or damaging, because they are physically or socially vulnerable at that time, or because they lack the ability to cope with the stressful event.

Research has found some support for the hypothesis that depression results from a complex of interrelated factors. One study (Persons & Rao, 1985) found no significant relationship between depression and life events, but when the these researchers looked at the interaction between stressful events and such cognitive factors as irrational beliefs and attribution of personal responsibility, small but significant results began to emerge. In addition, they found some indication that depressed people are more likely to attribute positive life events to external factors; nondepressed people tend to attribute them to internal causes. For example, a depressed student might attribute good test performance to making lucky guesses, whereas a nondepressed student might recognize a high grade as the result of long and hard study.

Lazarus's view that stressful events interact with vulnerability and perceived coping ability to bring about or worsen depression has received some research support in a study of occupational stress among family physicians (Revicki & May, 1985). As with studies that looked exclusively at life events, this study reported small but statistically significant relationships between stress and depression, but this relationship was moderated by family (but not peer) support and the physicians' beliefs that they could control important aspects of their lives. This finding partially confirmed Lazarus's belief that the effects of stress are moderated both by social support and by the expectation that one can deal with the stressful event.

A review of the literature (Brown & Harris, 1989) found that although stress may be related to depressive symptoms, other factors also played an important role in the etiology of depression. Some of these psychosocial factors included low self-esteem, lack of social support, feelings of hopelessness, and loss of a sense of self-control—all common to those with negative affectivity. The results of these studies tend to support the hypothesis that stress may increase depression but that cognitive and other psychosocial factors interact with stressful events to affect subsequent levels of depression.

The relationship between stress and depression is complex, but depression has a relationship to immune function (Herbert & Cohen, 1993a). Depression that meets the diagnostic criteria for clinical depression (American Psychiatric Association, 1994) is associated with several measures of immune function, with larger effects for older and for hospitalized patients. In addition, the more severe the depression, the greater will be the alteration of immune function. However, this relationship may not be directly due to stress but may be mediated through changes in health-related behaviors that occur in depressed people. Research (Cover & Irwin, 1994) has suggested that sleep disturbances were more strongly related to the changes in immune function than to other behavioral changes among depressed patients.

Anxiety Disorders   Anxiety disorders include a variety of fears and phobias, often leading to avoidance behaviors. Included in this definition are such conditions as panic attack, **agoraphobia**, generalized anxiety, obsessive-compulsive disorders, and posttraumatic stress (American Psychiatric Association, 1994). This section looks at stress as a possible contributor to anxiety states.

One anxiety disorder that, by definition, is related to stress is **posttraumatic stress disorder (PTSD)**. The *Diagnostic and Statistical Manual of Mental Disorders* (4th ed.) (American Psychiatric Association, 1994) defines PTSD as "the development of characteristic symptoms following exposure to an extreme traumatic stressor involving direct personal experience of an event that involves actual or threatened death or serious injury" (p. 424). PTSD can also stem from experiencing threats to one's physical integrity; witnessing another person's serious injury, death, or threatened physical integrity; and learning about death or injury to family members or friends. The traumatic events often include military combat, but sexual assault, physical attack, robbery, mugging, and other personal violent assaults can trigger posttraumatic stress disorder.

Symptoms of PTSD include recurrent and intrusive memories of the traumatic event, recurrent distressing dreams that replay the event, and extreme psychological and physiological distress. Events that resemble or symbolize the original traumatic event as well as anniversaries of that event may also trigger symptoms. People with posttraumatic stress disorder attempt to avoid thoughts, feelings, or conversations about the event and to avoid any person or place that might trigger acute distress.

A review of several studies on PTSD (Friedman, Clark, & Gershon, 1992) found support for the underlying assumption of the posttraumatic stress disorder; that is, PTSD symptoms are triggered by

BECOMING HEALTHIER

As James Pennebaker (1990, 1997a) has demonstrated, writing about difficult or traumatic experiences can improve your physical as well as mental health. The technique is simple but powerful: Write about an event or experience that has caused you pain. Pennebaker's research indicated that writing about trivial events has little or no benefit. He asked people to write about the most traumatic event in personal terms. Therefore, choose an event that is personally meaningful and painful.

If you have a trauma in your life that has been a problem, choose that event. If there is no big trauma that has posed problems, write about something that is currently stressful or an ongoing problem.

Write for 20 minutes, and keep writing as constantly as you can. Don't worry about spelling or punctuation; just concentrate on writing. This ex-

perience will not be pleasant and may well be painful. Keeping thoughts bottled up takes emotional energy that exerts physical effects. Writing releases this energy, and the experience can be overwhelming at first. Don't expect to feel better when you write for the first time. Indeed, you may feel bad during the process, but the experience will help you understand and deal with the problem or trauma.

To get the full benefit, write each day for 4 days. Additional benefits can come from being able to talk about what you write, but talking is not necessary; writing itself provides benefits. Writing allows you to express anger and frustrations, but the process does much more than "let off steam." Writing allows you to get in touch with your past and release those problems, dealing with them in a productive way that can diminish their power over you.

---

stressful events. Research has confirmed that exposure to crime and violence is related to the development of PTSD. Prevalence of PTSD in the general population is only around 1% (Helzer, Robins, & McEvoy, 1987), but 3.5% of civilians exposed to physical attack as well as Vietnam veterans who were not wounded showed symptoms of PTSD. In contrast, 20% of wounded veterans had PTSD symptoms. Participants in Operation Desert Storm during the Persian Gulf War also had an elevated risk for PTSD. About 2% of the Air National Guard reservists who served at home and about 7% of those who served in combat were diagnosed with PTSD (Holmes, Tariot, & Cox, 1998).

An investigation of the relationship between crime victimization and PTSD in a sample of female crime victims (Resnick, Kilpatrick, Best, & Kramer, 1992) found that 35% of women involved in high crime stress (defined as life threats and physical injury) showed PTSD, whereas only 13%

of victims of low crime stress did so. Both figures are much higher than in the general population, and all these figures demonstrate the negative impact of stress produced by violence and victimization. A later study (Roth, Newman, Pelcovitz, van der Kolk, & Mandel, 1997) reported that physically abused women had an elevated rate of PTSD, but women who were both physically and sexually abused were much more likely to suffer from posttraumatic stress.

The relationship between stress and other anxiety disorders is less clear. In retrospective investigations in which phobic patients are asked whether they identify any stressful event as the trigger for their anxiety disorder, most patients implicate one or more stressful events. Rabkin (1993) found that about two-thirds of phobic patients reported some precipitating stressor. However, these subjective claims fall far short of proving that stress causes anxiety disorders. In her review of the literature, Rabkin (1993) reached a generally negative view of the possible connection between stress and anxiety or phobic reactions, concluding that "despite both clinical and lay expectations that phobic disorders are triggered, if not caused, by a particular stressor, investigators have not found a strong association" (p. 486). However, she noted that well-designed studies on the relationship between phobic disorders and stress remain to be conducted.

In Summary

Much evidence points to a relationship between stress and disease, but claims that stressful life events and daily hassles cause various somatic disorders are still premature. In general, stress is a moderate risk factor for several physical disorders, including headache and infectious disease. The evidence for a relationship between stress and heart disease is complex, with the possibility that stress may be involved in hypertension. Differential reactivity to stress plus gender differences in response to stress may also contribute. Stress is also a factor in other diseases, including diabetes, asthma, and rheumatoid arthritis, as well as some premature deliveries.

The concept of negative affectivity relates both to a person's tendency to report negative life events and to a style of perceiving and dealing with stress that increases psychological problems. People with a pessimistic view of life and the tendency to ruminate over their problems increase their chances of becoming depressed, and the heightened sensitivity to negative aspects of life can increase their anxiety. Furthermore, their pessimistic outlook decreases their ability to cope actively, heightening their vulnerability to stressful events.

Contrary to the commonsense belief that stress is a major contributor to psychological disorders, little evidence exists that a stressful life event, or even an accumulation of events, contributes significantly to the onset of depression or anxiety disorders, except, of course, posttraumatic stress disorder.

Personality Factors Affecting Stress and Disease

Why does stress affect some people, apparently causing them to get sick, while leaving others unaffected? The relationship between stress and illness is far from perfect, and some high-stress individuals become sick while others remain healthy. Then, too, some low-stress people develop a disease while others do not. Why do some people fall ill from stress while other people stay well? This section looks at two possible explanations for this question. First, the *diathesis-stress model* suggests that some people are more inherently vulnerable to the effects of stress; and second, the *hardy personality model* holds that psychologically healthy individuals are buffered against the harmful effects of stress.

The Diathesis-Stress Model

The **diathesis-stress model** suggests that some individuals are vulnerable to stress-related diseases because either genetic weakness or biochemical imbalance inherently predisposes them to those diseases (Gatchel, 1993). The diathesis-stress model has a long history in psychology, particularly in explaining the development of psychological disorders. During the 1960s and 1970s, the concept was used as an explanation for the development of psychophysiological disorders (Levi, 1974) as well as schizophrenic episodes, depression, and anxiety disorders (Zubin & Spring, 1977).

Applied to either psychological or physiological disorders, the diathesis-stress model holds that some people are predisposed to react abnormally to environmental stressors. This predisposition (diathesis) is usually thought to be inherited through biochemical or organ system weakness, but some theorists (Zubin & Spring, 1977) also have included acquired propensities as components of vulnerability. Whether inherited or acquired, the vulnerability is relatively permanent. What varies over time is the presence of environmental stressors, which may account for the waxing and waning of illnesses.

Thus, the diathesis-stress model assumes that two factors are necessary to produce disease. First, the person must have a relatively permanent predisposition to the disease and second, that person must experience some sort of stress. Diathetic individuals respond pathologically to the same stressful conditions with which most people can easily cope. For those people with a strong predisposition to a disease, even a mild environmental stressor may be sufficient to produce an illness episode. The disease does not flow from an interaction between personality and stress but from the interaction of *personal physiology* and stress (Cotton, 1990).

Does perfectionism make people more vulnerable to stress-related illness? Some research has indicated that perfectionism may interact with other factors to contribute to illness. One study (Flett, Hewitt, Blankstein, & Mosher, 1995) found that college students who demanded perfection from themselves were more likely than other students to react to stress from major life events with symptoms of depression. Another study of female college students and female college graduates (Joiner, Heatherton, Rudd, & Schmidt, 1997) investigated the interaction of perfectionism and perceived weight status (a potential stressful condition) to see if this combination was related to symptoms of bulimia. This study found that perfectionistic women who believed they were overweight were at risk for bulimia, but no such risk occurred for perfectionistic women who did not see themselves as overweight. Interestingly, actual weight did not interact with perfectionism to produce bulimic symptoms. These two studies generally support the notion that perfectionism (a personality trait) may interact with stress to produce illness symptoms.

The diathesis-stress model may explain why life event scales (see Chapter 5) are so inconsistent in predicting illness. The number of points accumulated on the Holmes and Rahe's Social Readjustment Rating Scale is only a weak predictor of illness. The diathesis-stress model holds that a person's diathesis (vulnerability) must be considered along with stressful life events in predicting who will get sick and who will stay well (Monroe & Simons, 1991).

The Hardy Personality Model

The converse of the diathesis-stress model would hold that psychologically healthy people are buffered against levels of stress that might lead to an illness in less healthy individuals. In 1977, Suzanne Kobasa and her mentor Salvatore Maddi proposed the notion of the hardy personality as an explanation for why stress relates to illness in some people but not others. The **hardy personality model** grew out of existential personality theory, which emphasizes the idea of an authentic person in control of his or her life. Kobasa and Maddi (1977) hypothesized that hardiness buffers the harmful effects of stress and thus protects the hardy personality from stress-related illness. In her original study, Kobasa (1979) looked at middle-aged, mostly White Protestant executives who had filled out Holmes and Rahe's Social Readjustment Rating Scale. She followed these middle- and upper-level managers for 3 years, monitoring both their level of stress and their incidence of illness. As a result, she was able to identify two groups: high-stress/low-illness executives and high-stress/high-illness executives.

Kobasa used the term *hardiness* to describe those people who were able to withstand stress and not succumb to disease. Hardy executives differed from those who became sick in three important ways. First, they expressed a stronger sense of *commitment* to self; second, they demonstrated an internal locus of *control* over their lives; and third, they were more likely to view necessary readjustments as a *challenge* rather than a stress. These three factors—commitment, control, and challenge—separated the hardy executives from those who became ill even though both groups experienced equal amounts of stress. Those who became ill were characterized by external locus of control or the belief that important factors in their lives are beyond their personal control, a sense of nihilism or meaninglessness of life, a feeling of powerlessness, alienation from self, and a lack of vigor or active involvement with their surroundings. These findings suggest that hardiness may act as a buffer against the harmful effects of stress.

Later, Kobasa and her colleagues (Kobasa, Maddi, & Courington, 1981; Kobasa, Maddi, & Kahn, 1982) investigated the hypothesis that hardy people are able to fend off the effects of stress and thus avoid subsequent disease. Again using male executives, these investigators found that hardiness—defined as commitment, control, and challenge—was related to a decrease in illness, thus suggesting that hardiness protected high-stressed executives against illness.

Can hardiness protect health care workers against job burnout? Recent studies have reported mixed support for hardiness as a buffer against job-related stress. Health care workers in cancer and AIDS wards are especially prone to burnout, and one study (Constantini, Solano, Di-Napoli, & Bosco, 1997) found that nurses working in these wards who scored high on the Kobasa Hardiness Scale were less likely to later show emotional exhaustion and job burnout. Another study of more than 1500 geriatric nurses found that those who scored high on the hardiness scale were better able than low scorers to reduce stress and avoid burning out (Duquette, Kerouac, Sandhu, Ducharme, & Saulnier, 1995). However, another study (Rowe, 1997) found that hardiness—independent of temperament and coping skills—was only weakly associated with burnout among health care professionals.

The notion that some people possess personal traits that help protect them against the harmful effects of stress is an appealing one. Nevertheless, Kobasa's conception of hardiness has been widely criticized. Some researchers (Schmied & Lawler, 1986) have criticized the concept as not being applicable to a large range of people. Others (Benishek, 1996) have suggested the three factors of commitment, control, and challenge do not constitute the essence of hardiness. Still others (Benishek & Lopez, 1997) have found that, contrary to Kobasa's conception, frequency of stress was not as important as perceived severity of stress. In addition, hardiness does not appear to be a unitary construct, because some research (Hull, Van Treuren, & Virnelli, 1987; Williams, Wiebe, & Smith, 1992) has found that commitment and control are more significant than challenge in predicting which people are most likely to use adaptive coping behaviors in response to stress. Control and commitment may have a direct rather than a buffering effect on health because lack of control and lack of commitment are themselves psychologically stressful. Also, the use of self-reports to assess disease is a potentially serious methodological weakness in Kobasa's studies, as people who score low on the hardiness scales have a tendency to see themselves as having numerous physical symptoms, even when they are not sick (Funk, 1992).

However, Kobasa (who has also published under the names S. C. Ouellette and S. C. Ouellette Kobasa) has pointed out that many of the inconsistent findings on hardiness are the result of different measures of the hardy personality (Ouellette, 1993). She contended that many investigators have attempted to extend the concept to inappropriate populations—for example, college undergraduates. Hardiness, with its origins embedded in existential philosophy and psychology, is probably most applicable to people who are searching for a sense of meaning or purpose in life, who are motivated by responsibility and freedom, who view subjective experience as reality, and who believe that they are capable of significantly shaping society (Ouellette, 1993).

In Summary

Two personality models, the diathesis-stress model and the hardiness concept, may help explain why some people are adversely affected by stress whereas others remain free from illness. Both models adopt a biopsychosocial approach, which assumes that psychological, social, and biological factors interact to contribute to illness. The diathesis-stress model holds that some people, by reason of an inherent diathesis, are more vulnerable to stress than other people. Conversely, Kobasa's hardiness concept suggests that some people possess a hardy personality that helps protect them against any potential adverse affects of stress. To Kobasa, hardiness consists of three factors—commitment, control, and challenge—which she believes can buffer top-level executives and perhaps others against stress. At present, however, neither of these models offers a satisfactory explanation for why some people develop stress-related diseases while others stay well.

Answers

This chapter addressed four basic questions:

1. **How does the immune system function?**

   The immune system consists of tissues, organs, and processes that protect the body from invasion by foreign material such as bacteria, viruses, and fungi. The immune system marshals both a nonspecific response capable of attacking any invader and a specific response tailored to specific invaders. The immune system can also be a source of problems when it is deficient (as in AIDS) or when it is too active (as in allergies and organ transplants).

2. **How does the field of psychoneuroimmunology relate behavior to disease?**

   The field of psychoneuroimmunology relates behavior to illness by finding relationships among behavior, the immune system, the central nervous system, and the endocrine system. Psychological factors can depress immune function, and some research has linked these factors with immune system depression and severity of physiological symptoms.

3. **Does stress cause disease?**

   Research indicates that stress and illness are related. Stress is a moderate risk factor for headache and infectious disease. The role of stress in heart disease is not clear, but reactivity to stress may be involved in hypertension. Stress is one of the many factors that contribute to negative mood and mood disorders. Negative affectivity describes a pessimistic life outlook that is related to stress and health problems.

4. **What personality factors affect stress and disease?**

   The diathesis-stress model predicts that vulnerability to disease varies, with some individuals predisposed to disease. In such cases, even low levels of stress could produce illness in vulnerable individuals. A sense of control, commitment, and challenge characterizes the hardy personality, but little research support exists for the buffering effects of this configuration.

Glossary

acquired immune deficiency syndrome (AIDS)   An immune deficiency caused by viral infection and resulting in vulnerability to a wide range of bacterial, viral, and malignant diseases.

agoraphobia   An anxiety state characterized by fear about or avoidance of places or situations from which escape might be difficult.

allergy   An immune system response characterized by an abnormal reaction to a foreign substance.

antibodies   Protein substances produced in response to a specific invader or antigen, marking it for destruction and thus creating immunity to that invader.

antigens   Substances that provoke the immune system to produce antibodies.

asthma   A respiratory disorder characterized by difficulty in breathing.

autoimmune diseases   Disorders that occur as a result of the immune system's failure to differentiate between body cells and foreign cells, resulting in the body's attack and destruction of its own cells.

B-cell   A variety of lymphocyte that attacks invading microorganisms.

diabetes mellitus   A disorder caused by insulin deficiency.

diathesis-stress model   A theory of stress that suggests that some individuals are vulnerable to stress-related illnesses because they are genetically predisposed to those illnesses.

granulocytes A type of lymphocyte that acts rapidly to kill invading organisms.

hardy personality model The theory that suggests some people are buffered against the potentially harmful effects of stress due to their hardy personality.

humoral immunity Immunity created through the process of exposure to antigens and production of antibodies in the blood stream.

immune surveillance theory A theoretical model suggesting that cancer is the result of an immune system dysfunction.

immunity A response to foreign microorganisms that occurs with repeated exposure and results in resistance to a disease.

inflammation A general response that works to restore damaged tissue.

lymph Tissue fluid that has entered a lymphatic vessel.

lymphatic system System that transports lymph through the body.

lymph nodes Small nodules of lymphatic tissue spaced throughout the lymphatic system that help clean lymph of debris.

lymphocytes White blood cells that are found in lymph and that are involved in the immune function.

macrophages A type of lymphocyte that attacks invading organisms.

natural killer (NK) cells A type of lymphocyte that attacks invading organisms.

phagocytosis The process of engulfing and killing foreign particles.

plasma cells Cells that are derived from B-cells and that secrete antibodies.

posttraumatic stress disorder (PTSD) An anxiety disorder caused by experience with an extremely traumatic event and characterized by recurrent and intrusive re-experiencing of that event.

psychoneuroimmunology A multidisciplinary field that focuses on the interactions among behavior, the nervous system, the endocrine system, and the immune system.

rheumatoid arthritis An autoimmune disorder characterized by a dull ache within or around a joint.

spleen A large organ near the stomach that serves as a repository for lymphocytes and red blood cells.

synergistic effect The combined effect of two or more variables that exceeds the sum of their individual effects.

T-cells The cells of the immune system that produce immunity.

thymosin A hormone produced by the thymus.

thymus An organ located near the heart that secretes thymosin and thus processes and activates T-lymphocytes.

tonsils Masses of lymphatic tissue located in the pharynx.

vaccination A method of inducing immunity in which a weakened form of a virus or bacteria is introduced into the body.

Suggested Readings

Adler, N., & Matthews, K. (1994). Health psychology: Why do some people get sick and some stay well? *Annual Review of Psychology, 45,* 229–259.

Two leaders in health psychology look at stress as a possible explanation for why some people get sick and others stay well.

Baum, A., Davidson, L. M., Singer, J. E., & Street, S. W. (1987). Stress as a psychophysiological process. In A. Baum & J. E. Singer (Eds.), *Handbook of psychology and health: Vol. 5. Stress* (pp. 1–24). Hillsdale, NJ: Erlbaum.

In this review of the physiological responses to stress, the authors organize and present difficult material in a way that integrates the physiology and psychology of stress.

 Cohen, S., & Herbert, T. B. (1996). Health psychology: Psychological factors and physical disease from the perspective of human psychoneuroimmunology. *Annual Review of Psychology, 47,* 113–142.

Cohen and Herbert review research in psychoneuroimmunology as it applies to human disease. This lengthy article includes a presentation of the possibilities for interactions between the nervous and immune systems to produce disease as well as the evidence for psychological factors in several diseases. Available through InfoTrac College Edition by Wadsworth Publishing Company.

Kiecolt-Glaser, J. K., & Glaser, R. (1993). Mind and immunity. In D. Goleman & J. Gurin (Eds.), *Mind/body medicine: How to use your mind for better health* (pp. 39–61). Yonkers, NY: Consumer Reports Books.

In this readable review, two important researchers discuss the growing field of psychoneuroimmunology, including an explanation of the immune system and the basic findings of the field.

Maier, S. F., Watkins, L. R., & Fleshner, M. (1994). Psychoneuroimmunology: The interface between behavior, brain, and immunity. *American Psychologist, 49,* 1004–1017.

This review is oriented toward psychologists who may be unfamiliar with the field. In addition to a description of the field and some review of research, Maier and his colleagues explain the reciprocal relationship between nervous and immune systems and speculate on the adaptive advantages of such an arrangement.

CHAPTER 7

Understanding Pain

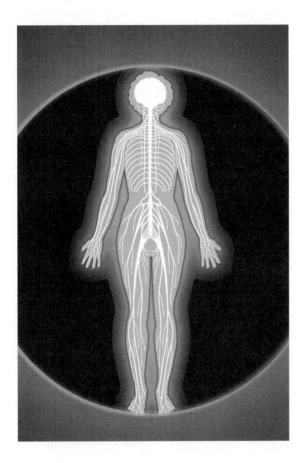

QUESTIONS

This chapter focuses on five basic questions:

1. How does the nervous system register pain?

2. What is the meaning of pain?

3. How can pain be measured?

4. How can pain be prevented?

5. What are the leading physical treatments for pain?

BARB'S PAIN

Barb was 24 when she sustained a back injury in a serious automobile crash. Her injuries included a ruptured disc in her spinal column and torn muscles. Her physician recommended back surgery, but she was afraid of such surgery and did not consent. Her treatment consisted of pain medication and physical therapy to allow her to regain the use of her muscles. After several months, Barb's pain was not so bad, and she didn't experience pain every day.

Barb got a job in a factory on an assembly line. This job required some lifting, which led to another back injury. This injury ruptured three discs and left her unable to walk or stand. After 9 months, she agreed to undergo back surgery to treat the damaged discs and nerves that were causing her pain. The surgery was only partially successful. She was in terrible pain and walked with a noticeable limp. Barb went through several physical therapy programs. The one that worked best helped her to develop muscle tone and improve her walking. During the 2 years after her surgery, Barb took prescription drugs to control her almost constant pain. She didn't know how to cope with her pain, so in addition to the prescription drugs, she drank alcohol. But then Barb began having hallucinations. When she asked her doctor to help her get off the drugs, the doctor referred her to a pain specialist who put her in a program that included a variety of behavioral techniques to help manage her pain. Barb was successful in this program: She discontinued the drugs and got control of her pain.

Now, 10 years after her accident, Barb still has bad days during which hot, shooting pains course up her back and down her legs, but she strictly limits her medication so that she does not take a drug for more than 3 days. When she decided that her pain was permanent, she found ways to cope. Barb has made some changes in her life to adapt to more limited physical ability—she no longer plays softball—but she has found ways to do most of the things she wants to do.

Barb's experience is all too common. Chronic pain is a serious health problem in all countries (Gureje, Von Korff, Simon, & Gater, 1996), with as many as 20% of the people suffering from some type of persistent pain. These pain experiences account for lost work days and diminished productivity, with financial costs in the billions of dollars each year. Additionally, financial costs to the individual include money spent for surgery, loss of income, medication, hospitalization, disability payments, and litigation settlements (Turk & Nash, 1993). Personal suffering as well as family and relationship distress are additional costs with no dollar estimates.

Although pain can affect people of any age, older people complain of more pain than younger ones do. One survey (Mobily, Herr, Clark, & Wallace, 1994) of rural people 65 and older revealed that nearly all of them reported some type of pain in the year prior to the interview. In addition, more than half had multiple pain complaints. As might be expected with an older population, joint pain, leg pain, and back pain were the most frequently reported pains. Interestingly, respondents 85 and older were *less* likely to report pain than were younger ones.

Pain and the Nervous System

All sensory information begins with sense receptors on or near the surface of the body. These receptors change physical energy—such as light, sound, heat, and pressure—into neural impulses. We can feel pain through any of our senses, but most of what we think of as pain originates as stimulation to the skin and muscles.

Neural impulses that originate in the skin and muscles are part of the peripheral nervous system (PNS); all neurons outside the brain and spinal cord, the central nervous system (CNS), are part of the PNS. Neural impulses that originate in the PNS travel toward the spinal cord and brain. Therefore, it is possible to trace the path of neural impulses from the receptors to the brain. Tracing this path is a way to understand the physiology of pain.

The Somatosensory System

The **somatosensory system** conveys sensory information from the body to the brain. The word *soma* means body in Greek; the somatic division of the PNS exists in and serves the body. All the PNS neurons that reach the skin's surface and serve muscles are part of the somatic nervous system. The interpretation of this information results in a person's perception of sensations about his or her body and its movements. The somatosensory system consists of several senses, including touch, light and deep pressure, cold, warmth, tickling, movement, and body position.

Sensory input from the skin and muscles makes its way toward the spinal cord by way of the somatic nervous system. For example, a neural impulse that originated in the right index finger would travel through the somatic nervous system to the spinal cord. At that point the impulse would be in the central nervous system. The CNS relays this information to the brain.

If the processing of information in the brain led to the decision to move that finger, a motor impulse would be initiated in the brain. That impulse would travel down the spinal cord. When it crossed into the body from the spinal cord, it would once again be in the somatic division of the PNS. That motor impulse would finally reach the muscles of the finger, and the finger would move.

A complex web of nerves carries sensations and motor impulses. The spinal cord gives rise to 31 pairs of spinal nerves, each nerve containing both sensory and motor neurons. These nerves branch into a finer and finer network covering the entire body below the neck. Sensory and motor functions of the head and neck are provided by the 12 cranial nerves emanating from the brain. The cranial nerves do not go through the spinal cord, but they carry the messages in the head and neck region that are equivalent to the information carried by the spinal nerves. The cranial nerves are also part of the somatic nervous system.

Afferent Neurons   Afferent neurons are one of the three types of neurons. *Afferent (sensory) neurons* relay information from the sense organs toward the brain. The action of *efferent (motor) neurons* results in the movement of muscles or the stimulation of organs or glands. *Interneurons* connect sensory to motor neurons.

The sense organs contain afferent neurons, called **primary afferents,** with specialized receptors that convert physical energy into neural impulses. By way of these receptors, we gain information about the world in the form of neural impulses. Afferent neurons convey this information to the spinal cord and then to the brain, where that information is processed and interpreted.

The action of neurons is partly electrical and partly chemical. An electrical impulse forms in the receptors when the sense organs are stimulated. Sufficient stimulation will result in the formation of an **action potential,** or electrical discharge, and the neuron will "fire." But the stimulation must exceed the neuron's threshold to create an action potential. The action of each individual neuron is simple: Each neuron is sufficiently stimulated either to fire or not. However, the events that lead up to the firing (or failure to fire) are not simple. The number of afferent neurons and the pattern of their responses is what permits them to relay enormously complex information.

Involvement in Pain   The skin is the largest of the sense organs, and its numerous receptors provide sensation for the skin. Some are covered with **myelin,** a fatty substance that acts as insulation. Myelinated afferent neurons are called A fibers. A fibers conduct neural impulse faster than the unmyelinated **C fibers** do. In addition, neurons differ in size, and larger ones conduct impulses faster than smaller ones. Two types of A fibers are important in pain perception—the large **A-beta fibers** and the smaller **A-delta fibers.** The large,

---

SCALE YOUR PAIN

Pain is practically a universal experience but not a uniform one. The following questions allow you to understand the role pain plays in your life. To complete the exercise, think of the most significant pain that you have experienced within the past month, or if you have chronic pain, make your ratings with that pain problem in mind.

1. How long did your pain persist? _____ hours and _____ minutes

2. If this pain is chronic, how often does it occur?

❏ less than once a month   ❏ about once a week

❏ once a month   ❏ several times a week

❏ several times a month   ❏ daily

❏ throughout most of every day

3. What did you do to alleviate your pain? (Check all that apply.)

❏ took a prescription drug   ❏ took an over-the-counter drug

❏ tried to relax   ❏ tried to ignore the pain

❏ did something to distract me from the pain

4. Place a mark on the line below to indicate how serious your pain was.

Not at all   Unbearable

0	10	20	30	40	50	60	70	80	90	100

5. Place a mark on the line below to indicate how much this pain interfered with your daily routine.

Not at all   Completely disrupted

0	10	20	30	40	50	60	70	80	90	100

6. During your pain, what did people around you do? (Check all that apply)

❏ gave me a lot of sympathy   ❏ ignored me

❏ did my work for me   ❏ relieved me of my normal responsibilities

❏ complained when I could not fulfill my normal responsibilities

Completing this assessment will show you something about your own pain experience. Some of the items on this assessment are similar to those on some of the standardized pain scales that are described in "The Measurement of Pain" later in the chapter.

---

myelinated A-beta fibers conduct impulses over 100 times faster than small, unmyelinated C fibers (Melzack, 1973). A-beta fibers are easily stimulated to fire, whereas C fibers require more stimulation. C fibers are much more common, however, with over 60% of all sensory afferents being C fibers (Melzack & Wall, 1982). Having two types of fibers involved in pain might account for some of the variations in people's experience of pain. The fast action of the A-delta fibers might account for the fast, sharp feeling of pain, whereas stimulation of the C fibers might result in slower, more diffuse aching.

The stimulation of A and C fibers creates neural impulses and starts the sensory message on its path to the brain. If the sensory information originates in the head and neck region, it will go to the brain by way of the cranial nerves. If the impulses originate in the rest of the body, the information will travel to the brain by way of the spinal cord.

The Spinal Cord

Protected by the vertebrae, the spinal cord is an avenue for sensory information traveling toward the brain and motor information coming from it. The spinal cord also produces the spinal reflexes. However, the most important role of the spinal cord is to provide a pathway for ascending sensory information and descending motor messages.

Damage to the spinal cord may interrupt the flow of sensory information or motor messages or both. The type and extent of the loss of function depends on the extent and location of damage. If the cord is completely cut, incoming sensory messages cannot reach the brain for interpretation. The region of the body below the break loses feeling. Motor impulses from the brain are also blocked when the cord is cut, resulting in paralysis from the point of injury downward, yet the function of the spinal cord above and below the injury may remain intact. For example, the spinal reflexes (such as the patellar reflex) still occur, but the same movements cannot be made voluntarily.

The afferent fibers group together after leaving the skin, and this grouping forms a nerve. Nerves may be entirely afferent, entirely efferent, or a mixture of both. Just outside the spinal cord, each nerve bundle divides into two branches (see Figure 7.1). The sensory tracts, which funnel information toward the brain, enter the dorsal (toward the back) side of the spinal cord. The motor tracts, which come from the brain, exit the ventral (toward the stomach) side of the cord. On each side

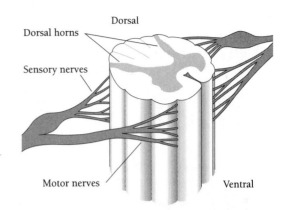

Figure 7.1 Cross-section through the spinal cord. *Source:* From *Biological Psychology* (2nd ed., p. 89), by J. W. Kalat, 1984, Belmont, CA: Wadsworth. Copyright © 1984 by Wadsworth Publishing Company. Reprinted by permission.

of the spinal cord, the dorsal root swells into a dorsal root ganglion, which contains the cell bodies of the primary afferent neurons. The neuron fibers extend into the **dorsal horns** of the spinal cord. In the spinal cord, some afferent neurons connect to other neurons, called *secondary afferents* or **transmission cells,** and others continue to the lower part of the brain (Graham, 1990).

The dorsal horns contain several layers, or **laminae.** Each lamina receives incoming messages from afferent neurons. In general, the larger fibers penetrate more deeply into the laminae than the smaller fibers do (Melzack & Wall, 1982). The cells in laminae 1 and 2 receive information from the small A-delta and C fibers, and these two laminae form the **substantia gelatinosa.** Ronald Melzack and Peter Wall (1965) hypothesized that the substantia gelatinosa modulates sensory input information, an hypothesis that seems reasonable because many afferent neurons from the skin terminate in it, and it receives projections from lower laminae. Other laminae also receive projections from A and C fibers as well as fibers descending from the brain and fibers from other laminae. Such reciprocal connections would allow for elaborate interactions between sensory input and the central processing of neural information.

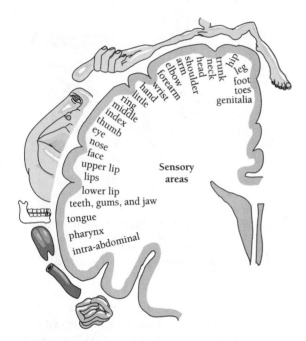

little
ring
middle
index
thumb
eye
nose
face
upper lip
lips
lower lip
teeth, gums, and jaw
tongue
pharynx
intra-abdominal

hand
wrist
forearm
elbow
arm
shoulder
head
neck
trunk
hip

leg
foot
toes
genitalia

Sensory
areas

Figure 7.2   Somatosensory areas of the cortex.

Information from the body is relayed toward the brain through three spinal cord pathways that cross from one side of the body to the opposite side of the brain; few neurons carry information from one side of the body to the same side of the brain. For the majority of information, stimuli impinging on the right hand would enter the spinal cord and cross over to the left side of the brain for interpretation. However, not all the neurons cross to the opposite side of the brain at the same level. Some cross while still in the spinal cord, and others do not cross until they reach the brain. But most cross over at one or the other level.

The Brain

The **thalamus** receives information from all three of the afferent systems in the spinal cord, although a different part of the thalamus receives input from each system. After making connections in the thal-

amus, the information is relayed to other parts of the brain.

Neural impulses go to the **somatosensory cortex** in the cerebral cortex, which is on the surface of the brain. The *primary somatosensory cortex* receives information from the thalamus that allows the entire surface of the skin to be mapped onto the somatosensory cortex. However, not all areas of the skin are equally represented. The top part of Figure 7.2 shows the area of the primary somatosensory cortex allotted to various regions of the body. Areas that are particularly rich in receptors occupy more of the somatosensory cortex than those areas that are poorer in receptors. For example, the hands take up more of the somatosensory cortex than the back does. Even though the back has more skin, the hands have more receptors, and therefore more area of the brain is devoted to interpreting the information these receptors supply. This abundance of receptors also means that the hands are more sensitive; hands are capable of sensing stimuli that the back cannot.

The *secondary somatosensory cortex* is next to the primary somatosensory cortex. This area also receives information from the thalamus, but it is not mapped in the same well-organized way as the primary somatosensory cortex. No clear map of the skin's surface occurs in this cortex. In addition, the neurons are not arranged by the types of stimulation to which they are sensitive because these neurons tend to be sensitive to various types of stimulation. The neurons in the secondary somatosensory cortex may not react to pressure on the skin but rather to active manipulation of an object (Graham, 1990). In short, the primary and secondary somatosensory cortices are different in location, organization, and possibly function.

Not all sensory information enters the brain by way of the spinal cord. Sensory information from the head and neck regions enters the brain directly through the cranial nerves. These nerves serve a function similar to that of the afferent pathways that go through the spinal cord, but the cranial nerves enter the brain directly at the level of the **medulla**, a structure in the lower part of the brain. In the brain, the afferent impulses from the skin of the head and neck go to the thalamus, as do the tracts coming from the spinal cord.

The person's ability to localize pain on the skin's surface is more precise than it is for internal organs. The viscera are not mapped in the brain in the same way as the skin. Internal stimulation can also give rise to sensations, including pain, but localizing internal sensation is much harder. In fact, intense stimulation of internal organs can result in the spread of neural stimulation to the pathways serving skin senses. Thus visceral pain may be perceived as originating on the skin's surface. For example, a person who feels pain in the upper arm may not associate this sensation with the heart, but that type of pain is commonly produced by a heart attack.

Neurotransmitters and Pain

Neurotransmitters are chemicals that are synthesized and stored in neurons. The release of neurotransmitters carries neural impulses across the synaptic cleft, the space between neurons. The electrical action potential causes the release of neurotransmitters from the ends of neurons. After flowing across the synaptic cleft, neurotransmitters act on other neurons by occupying specialized receptor sites. Sufficient amounts of neurotransmitters will prompt the formation of an action potential in the stimulated neuron. Many different neurotransmitters exist, and each one is capable of causing an action. Each occupies a specialized receptor site in the same way that a key fits into a lock. Without the proper fit, the neurotransmitter will not affect the neuron.

In the 1970s, researchers (Pert & Snyder, 1973; Snyder, 1977) demonstrated that the neurochemistry of the brain plays a role in the perception of pain. Receptors in the brain are sensitive to opiate drugs, and some neurons have receptor sites that opiate drugs are capable of occupying. This discovery explained how opiates reduce pain. Although the opiates are foreign substances, they apparently fit into receptors in the brain. There they stimulate neurons and produce pain relief.

The discovery of opiate receptors in the brain raised another question: Why does the brain respond to the resin of the opium poppy? In general, the brain is selective about the types of molecules that it allows to enter; only substances similar to naturally occurring neurochemicals can enter the brain. Researchers soon began to supply an answer to this question (Goldstein, 1976; Hughes, 1975). They found that a naturally occurring substance has properties similar to those of the opiate drugs. This discovery prompted a flurry of research that identified more neurochemicals with opiate-like effects, such as the **endorphins**, the *enkephalins*, and *dynorphin*.

Research has not yet revealed exactly how the body's own opiates affect pain perception. However, these neurochemicals seem to be one of the brain's mechanisms for relieving pain. One type of endorphin seems stronger than morphine in its ability to relieve pain. Whereas the enkephalins are weaker than morphine, dynorphin is 200 times more powerful. The pain-relieving properties of drugs like morphine may be coincidental. Perhaps they are effective only because the brain contains its own system for pain relief, which the opiates stimulate.

Neurochemicals also seem to be involved in producing pain. The neurotransmitters *serotonin* and *substance P* as well as the chemicals *brandykinin* and *prostaglandins* sensitize or excite the neurons that relay pain messages (Grunau & Craig, 1988). Brandykinin, a chemical composed of a string of amino acids, is released by body cells when damage occurs. If brandykinin is injected into an animal, the animal's experience of pain worsens. The prostaglandins share some properties of hormones (they are secreted by a variety of cells) and have some properties of neurotransmitters (they are released by neurons). But the prostaglandins are classified as neither because they are not secreted by a gland and are secreted by cells that are not neurons. Prostaglandins are released in the case of injury and have a role in the inflammation response of the immune system.

The Modulation of Pain

Research directed toward finding the brain structures involved in pain led to the discovery that one area of the brain, the **periaqueductal gray**, is involved in modulating pain. This brain structure is in the midbrain, close to the center. If it is stimulated, pain is relieved, and the relief continues after stimulation of the area ceases (Graham, 1990). Neurons in the periaqueductal gray run down into the medulla, where they connect to neurons in the **nucleus raphe magnus**. These neurons descend into the spinal cord and make connections with neurons in the substantia gelatinosa. The result is that the dorsal horn neurons are kept from carrying pain information to the thalamus.

The inhibition of transmission also involves some familiar neurotransmitters. Endorphin acts in the periaqueductal gray, where it initiates activity in this descending inhibitory system. The substantia gelatinosa contains synapses that use enkephalin as a transmitter. Indeed, neurons that contain enkephalin seem to be concentrated in the same parts of the brain that contain substance P, the transmitter that activates pain messages (McLean, Skirboll, & Pert, 1985).

These elaborate physical and chemical systems are the body's way to modulate the neural impulses of pain. They exist naturally in the brain, and drugs happen to produce pain relief by mimicking their action. Researchers have traditionally concentrated on developing more drugs that produce pain relief, believing that drugs (and surgery) were the only ways to relieve pain. Discovery of the body's own opiates and the brain structures that modulate pain have indicated that pain control may be possible without drugs. Researchers are now exploring the possibility of enlisting the brain's own mechanisms to relieve pain.

The circumstances that prompt the production of endorphins is not completely understood. One

review (Sherman & Liebeskind, 1980) found evidence that the release of endorphins is influenced by expectation, length of pain stimulation, timing of painful stimuli, ability to cope with the pain, and previous pain experience. This review also considered the possibility that nondrug methods of pain control may work because they prompt the release of endorphins. If environmental and psychological circumstances can cause the release of endorphins, voluntary control of pain seems within reach.

In Summary

The activation of receptors in the skin results in neural impulses that move along afferent pathways to the spinal cord by way of the dorsal root. In the spinal cord, the afferent impulses proceed along one of three systems to the thalamus in the brain. Impulses from two of the three systems arrive in the somatosensory cortex in the cerebral cortex. Impulses from the third system also reach the cerebral cortex, but by a less direct route. The somatosensory cortex has two parts. The primary somatosensory cortex includes a map of the skin, with more cortex devoted to areas of the body richer in skin receptors, but the organization of the secondary somatosensory cortex is not so straightforward. Some types of nerve fibers, the A-delta and C fibers, are involved in pain, and the spinal cord is important in the perception of pain. However, pain perception is not specific to any one type of afferent neuron, nor is pain relayed to the brain by only one spinal system.

The brain also contains mechanisms for modulating sensory input and thereby affecting the perception of pain. One mechanism is through the naturally occurring neurochemicals that relieve pain and mimic the action of opiate drugs. These neurochemicals exist in many places in the central and peripheral nervous systems. The second mechanism is a system of descending control through the periaqueductal gray and the nucleus raphe magnus. This system affects the activity of the spinal cord and provides a descending modulation of activity in the spinal cord.

The Meaning of Pain

Pain has been called "perhaps the most universal form of stress" (Turk, Meichenbaum, & Genest, 1983, p. 73). Yet pain differs from stress in that it is usually experienced as an unwanted physical stimulus located in a specific anatomical region. Like stress, it often has a strong psychological component.

Until about 100 years ago, pain was most frequently considered a direct consequence of physical injury, and its intensity was generally thought to be proportional to the degree of tissue damage. Near the end of the 19th century, C. A. Strong (1895) and others began to think of pain in a new light. Strong hypothesized that pain was due to two factors: the sensation and the person's reaction to that sensation. In other words, psychological factors and organic causes were of equal importance. This view received some support when Henry Beecher (1946) reported that soldiers wounded at the Anzio beachhead during World War II reported very little pain despite serious battle injuries. These men had been removed from the front and thus from the threat of death or further injury. Under these conditions, the wounded soldiers were in a cheerful, optimistic state of mind.

Additional confirmation for the notion that a person's reaction to the physical sensation of pain strongly influences the degree of suffering came 10 years later from another study by Beecher (1956). In this report, injured civilians were found to have experienced more pain and requested more pain-killing drugs than did the wounded World War II soldiers, even though the civilians' injuries were less severe. These findings prompted Beecher (1956) to conclude that "the intensity of suffering is largely determined by what the pain means to the patient" (p. 1609) and that "the extent of wound bears only a slight relationship, if any (often none at all), to the pain experienced"

(p. 1612). Finally, Beecher (1957), in a statement reminiscent of Strong, described pain as a two-dimensional experience consisting of both a sensory stimulus and an emotional component. Despite the methodological shortcomings of Beecher's studies, his view of pain as a psychological and physical phenomenon came to be accepted by others working in this field.

Most investigators now agree that personal perception mediates the experience of pain. Melzack (1973) listed such individual variables as anxiety, depression, suggestion, prior conditioning, attention, evaluation, and cultural learning as possible contributors to one's experience of pain. This multidimensional view has also been incorporated into the definition of pain offered by the International Association for the Study of Pain (IASP). The IASP Subcommittee on Taxonomy (1979, p. 250) defined pain as "an unpleasant sensory and emotional experience associated with actual or potential tissue damage, or described in terms of such damage."

John Loeser (1989) has proposed a model for understanding and evaluating pain that includes four components. The first level is *nociception,* which Loeser defined as the experience of tissue damage and the activation of A-delta and C fibers. *Pain* is the second level, which includes the perception of tissue damage. The third level is *suffering,* the negative emotional response to tissue damage, and the fourth level is *pain behavior,* actions that reflect the presence of tissue damage.

This model's four levels highlight the separate processes of sensing and perceiving as well as the emotional and behavioral components of pain. A person can have nociception (the experience of tissue damage) without pain if something happens to block that perception. For example, anesthesia can block pain even in the presence of serious tissue damage. Suffering is connected to tissue damage but not necessarily proportional to it; that is, people may suffer a great deal with relatively minor tissue damage, or very little even with a great deal of tissue damage, as Beecher's soldiers did. The behaviors that reflect the experience of pain

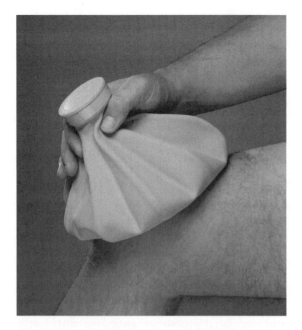

Acute pain is typically the result of injury and does not progress to the stage of chronic pain.

and suffering vary according to many factors, but the stage of the pain experience is an important aspect.

The Stages of Pain

Pain is not a single entity, but it can be seen according to various stages or types. Francis J. Keefe (1982) has identified three stages of pain: acute, prechronic, and chronic. **Acute pain** is ordinarily adaptive; it signals the person to avoid further injury. It usually lasts less than 6 months, and includes pains from cuts, burns, surgery, dental work, childbirth, and other injuries. **Prechronic pain** is experienced between the acute and the chronic stages. According to Keefe, this period is critical because the person either overcomes the pain at this time or develops the feelings of helplessness that lead to chronic pain. **Chronic pain** endures beyond the time of healing. "For the individual experiencing chronic pain, there is a continuing quest for relief that often remains elusive

and leads to feelings of demoralization, helplessness, hopelessness, and outright depression" (Turk, 1997, p. 148). Chronic pain is more or less constant and is often self-perpetuating; that is, chronic pain frequently leads to behavior that is designed to elicit reward and comfort, which results in more pain behavior. Chronic pain is frequently experienced in the absence of any detectable tissue damage.

Chronic pain is often associated with some type of psychopathology. People with severe chronic pain are much more likely than other people to suffer from some type of psychopathology, but the direction of the cause and effect is not always clear (Gatchel, 1996). Patients suffering from chronic pain are more likely to be depressed, to abuse alcohol and other drugs, and to suffer from personality disorders. For Barb, alcohol was a way to cope with her pain, and she abused alcohol and her prescription drugs. Although some chronic pain patients develop these disorders as a result of their chronic pain, others had some form of psychopathology prior to the inception of pain (Kinney, Gatchel, Polatin, Fogarty, & Mayer, 1993).

John J. Bonica (1990) contended that psychological or environmental factors play a central role in chronic pain but are rarely involved in acute pain. In other words, acute pain is caused by tissue damage, whereas chronic pain is a result of tissue damage plus one's experience of being rewarded for pain behaviors. Bonica agreed with most pain experts that acute pain is ordinarily beneficial, because it warns that something is wrong and usually prompts the person to seek health care. But he disagreed with those who set 6 months as an arbitrary time to designate pain as chronic. To wait 6 months to term pain as chronic, he insisted, increases the chances that the pain will become irreversible. Instead he defined chronic pain as "pain that persists a month beyond the usual course of an acute disease or a reasonable time for an injury to heal or that is associated with a chronic pathologic process that causes continuous pain or the pain recurs at intervals for months or years" (Bonica, 1990, p. 19). Chronic pain never has a biological benefit, and it "often imposes se-

WOULD YOU BELIEVE...?

Life without Pain

Would you believe that a life with pain is preferable to one without pain? Although pain is always unpleasant, a person who feels no pain has anything but a pleasant life.

Some people might imagine that a life without pain would be pleasant, and that feeling no pain would be preferable to feeling pain. These people have not thought through the consequences of the inability to feel pain. Medical science has identified very few people who have been unable to feel pain, but studying those people shows that a life without pain is not enviable.

A young western Canadian woman, Miss C, was described by Ronald Melzack (1973) as unfamiliar with the experience of pain. The daughter of a physician, she was an intelligent young woman who attended college at McGill University in Montreal. Her father alerted his colleagues in Montreal about her condition, and these physicians studied her inability to feel pain.

Miss C was apparently normal in all respects except that she had never reported feeling pain. Once as a child she sustained third-degree burns because she had climbed on a hot radiator to look out of a window. Without the ability to feel pain, she was unaware of the damage that she was doing to her knees and legs. She could not remember ever sneezing or coughing. The gag reflex was difficult to elicit from her, and the corneal reflex that protects the eye was absent.

The physicians who tested her in Montreal subjected her to various stimuli that would have been horrible for a normal person. They administered electric shock to different parts of her body, applied hot water, immersed her limbs in cold water for prolonged periods, pinched tendons, and injected histamine under her skin. She felt no pain. In addition, her heart rate, blood pressure, and respiration remained normal throughout these tortures.

Without pain to alert her, Miss C sustained many injuries and failed to protect damaged tissues, thus making them worse. Her insensitivity to pain caused serious medical problems, especially in the joints and spine. Melzack and Peter Wall (1982) explained that insensitivity to pain can lead people to remain in one position too long, causing inflammation of the joints. Even worse, the failure to feel pain leads one to neglect injuries and thus healing is obstructed. Injured tissue can easily become infected, and these infections are very difficult to treat if they extend into bone.

Miss C died when she was only 29 years old, and her death was from a failure to bring massive infections under control. During the last month of her life, Miss C finally complained of pain, which was relieved with aspirin. Although she felt practically no pain during her life, neither did she gain the benefits of feeling pain. Her insensitivity to pain directly contributed to the infections that killed her.

The story of Miss C provides ample evidence that a life without pain is not preferable to one with pain, and that pain provides us with a useful signal that we should take action to avoid potentially life-threatening damage to our bodies.

---

vere emotional, physical, economic, and social stresses on the patient and on the family" (p. 19).

Pain Syndromes

Pain can also be categorized according to location or syndrome. Headache and low back pain are the two most frequently treated types of pain but people also seek treatment for several other common pain syndromes.

Headache Pain   Although many different kinds of headache have been identified, the most common are migraine and tension headaches. **Migraine headaches** are generally considered *vascular* in origin, although some authorities have questioned

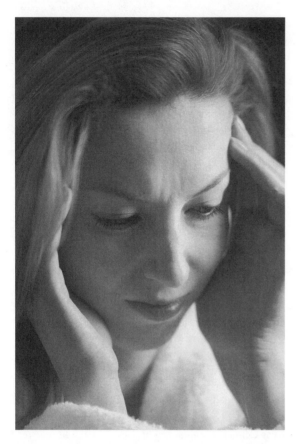

Headache is a frequent pain syndrome, accounting for substantial loss of work days and decreased effectiveness.

any distinction between migraine and tension headaches (Hatch, 1993). Migraine headaches are characterized by recurrent attacks of pain that vary widely in intensity, frequency, and duration. The attacks often are associated with loss of appetite, nausea, vomiting, and exaggerated sensitivity to light. Migraine headaches also often involve sensory, motor, or mood disturbances. The two most frequent kinds are migraine with aura and migraine without aura. Migraine with aura is characterized by identifiable sensory disturbances that precede the headache pain; migraine without aura has a sudden onset and an intense throbbing on one side of the head.

Women are much more likely than men to have migraine headaches. About 18% of women

but only about 7% of men in the United States suffer at least one migraine per year (Stewart, Lipton, Celentano, & Reed, 1992). For both men and women, migraine headaches occur most frequently between ages 35 and 45, with most migraine patients experiencing their first headache before age 30. However, no age group is exempt (Pearce, 1994). Children can have migraines, with a third of these patients below the age of 10. Few patients have a first migraine after age 40, but people who have migraines continue to do so, often throughout their lives. Also, low-income people have significantly more migraines than people in the highest income brackets, and women 30 to 49 from low-income households have the greatest risk for migraine headache. However, disability from migraines is not related to gender, age, income, or urban/rural background (Stewart et al., 1992).

Tension headaches are *muscular* in origin and are characterized by sustained contractions of the muscles of the neck, shoulders, scalp, and face. They are characterized by a gradual onset; sensations of tightness; constriction or pressure; highly variable intensity, frequency, and duration; and a dull, steady ache on both sides of the head. Over 38% of the general population experiences tension headaches (Schwartz, Stewart, Simon, & Lipton, 1998), and people with this pain syndrome reported lost workdays and decreased effectiveness at work, home, and school because of their pain.

A third type of headache is the **cluster headache**, a type of severe headache that occurs in daily clusters for 4 to 16 weeks (Pearce, 1994). Some symptoms are similar to migraine, including severe pain and vomiting, but cluster headaches are much briefer, rarely lasting longer than 2 hours. The headache is localized on one side of the head, and often the eye on the other side becomes bloodshot and waters. In addition, cluster headaches are much more common in men than women, with a ratio of 10:1. These headaches appear in a cluster and disappear, only to recur every year or two.

Low Back Pain   Low back pain is also very common, with as many as 80% of people in the

United States experiencing this type of pain at some time (Deyo, 1998). More than 2.6 million men and women incur back injuries at work and another 4.5 million develop low back pain from performing repeated job activities (Behrens, Seligman, Cameron, Mathias, & Fine, 1994). Barb is a good example of the millions of people who sustain injuries at work. Even more people experience back pain from activities not associated with work, making the problem extensive but not necessarily serious: Most injuries are not permanent, and people recover quickly.

Although many physiological factors have been implicated in low back pain, a good deal of mystery still surrounds this disorder (Deyo, 1998). Low back pain has many potential causes, including infections, degenerative diseases, and malignancies, but the most frequent cause is probably injury or stress resulting in musculoskeletal, ligament, and neurological problems in the lower back. Aging is another factor in back pain, because the fluid content and elasticity of the intervertebral disks decrease as one grows older. In addition, stress and psychological factors may play roles in back pain. These many potential causes, combined with problems in diagnosis, result in many back pain patients without a definite diagnosis for the physical cause of their pain.

Many people experience back pain, but only a small percentage of these people develop chronic low back pain (Deyo, 1998). At any specific time, as few as 1% of U. S. workers are disabled by back pain. The high percentage of people who experience back pain and the low percentage of chronic disability points to the large number of people who recover from acute back pain. Those who do not recover have a poor prognosis. Many seek a variety of treatments, and like Barb, still experience pain.

Arthritis Pain   Another common pain syndrome is arthritis. The term *arthritis* literally means joint inflammation, but of the more than 100 arthritic conditions, only some involve inflamed joints (Achterberg-Lawlis, 1982). **Rheumatoid arthritis** is an autoimmune disorder characterized by

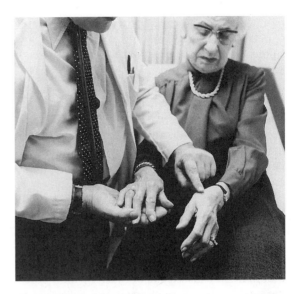

Arthritis is a source of pain and disability for over 20 million Americans.

swelling and inflammation of the joints as well as destruction of cartilage, bone, and tendons. These changes alter the joint, producing direct pain, and the changes in joint structure lead to change in movement, which may result in additional pain through this indirect route (Young, 1993). The symptoms of rheumatoid arthritis are extremely variable, with some people experiencing steady progression of increasing symptoms and most facing remissions and intensifications. In contrast, **osteoarthritis** is a progressive inflammation of the joints affecting mostly older people and characterized by a dull ache, exacerbated by movement, in the joint area.

The various forms of arthritis affect about 38 million residents of the United States (Wisocki, 1998). Osteoarthritis is the most common form of arthritis. A majority of those over age 60 experience some arthritic condition, and older women make up a disproportionate number of those affected. Arthritis is one of the primary causes of disability in the elderly.

Cancer Pain   Cancer pain can come either from a malignancy or from treatment for the disease

(Bonica, 1980). Cancer is the second leading cause of death in the United States (see Chapter 10), and studies have shown that pain is present in about 30% to 40% of all cancer cases and 60% to 90% of all terminal cancer cases (Fife, Irick, & Painter, 1993). Cancer pain afflicts more than one million Americans annually (Bonica, Ventafridda, & Twycross, 1990), and cancer patients adapt to pain in much the same way as do other chronic pain patients (Turk et al., 1998). Some cancers are much more likely than others to produce pain. About 85% of patients suffering from bone and cervix cancer experience pain, but only about 5% of leukemia patients experience pain (Bonica, 1980). Not infrequently, cancer patients suffer from two or more sources of pain at the same time. The tumor itself may cause pain, but such medical procedures as surgery, chemotherapy, and radiation can also be painful (Benedetti & Bonica, 1984).

Phantom Limb Pain   Just as injury can occur without producing pain, pain can occur in the absence of injury. One such type of pain is **phantom limb pain**, the experience of chronic pain in an absent body part (Loeser, 1990). Amputation removes the nerves that produce the impulses leading to the experience of pain. Despite removal of the physical basis for pain, phantom limb pain is not an unusual experience for amputees.

Estimates of the proportion of amputees who experience phantom limb pain have varied. Until the 1970s, phantom pain was believed to be rare, with less than 1% of amputees experiencing a painful phantom limb, but more recent research has indicated that the percentage may be as high as 80% (Sherman, Katz, Marbach, & Heermann-Do, 1997). Most commonly, amputees feel sensations from their amputated limbs soon after surgery. These sensations often start as a tingling sensation and then develop into other sensations that resemble actual feelings in the missing limb. Nor are the sensations of a phantom limited to limbs. Women who have undergone breast removal also perceive sensations from the amputated breast, and people who have had teeth

pulled sometimes continue to experience feelings from those teeth.

Amputees who experience unpleasant sensations from their amputated limbs may feel that the phantom limb is of an abnormal size or in an uncomfortable position (Melzack & Wall, 1982). Phantom limbs can also produce painful feelings of cramping, shooting, burning, or crushing. These pains vary from mild and infrequent to severe and continuous. The pain may start shortly after amputation or not begin until years later. Melzack and Wall (1988) reported that 72% of amputees have pain in their phantom limb 8 days after their surgery, 65% have pain 6 months afterward, and 60% have pain 2 years later. The severity and frequency of the pain tend to decrease over time.

The underlying cause of phantom limb pain has been the subject of bitter controversy (Melzack, 1992; Melzack & Wall, 1982, 1988). Because surgery rarely relieves the pain, some have hypothesized that phantom limb pain has an emotional basis. Melzack (1992) argued that phantom limb sensation arises within the brain as a result of the generation of a characteristic pattern of neural activity, which he called a *neuromatrix*. Melzack contended that this brain activity constituted "a characteristic pattern of impulses indicating that the body is intact and unequivocally one's own" (p. 123). This neuromatrix pattern continues to operate, even if the neurons in the peripheral nervous system do not furnish input to the brain. Melzack believes that this brain activity is the basis for phantom limb sensations, which may include pain.

Relief from phantom limb pain can come from a variety of interventions, but not all cases of phantom pain respond to treatment (Sherman, 1997). One therapeutic approach uses local anesthesia on peripheral nerves; this treatment can provide relief of pain for days or months after the anesthesia has worn off. Relief from increased stimulation can come through massage or through the application of electrical stimulation to the skin, a technique called transcutaneous electrical nerve stimulation (TENS). An experimental technique involving destruction of spinal cells that receive sensory messages from the stump has been more successful than other surgical interventions (Melzack, 1992). However, many of these treatments provide temporary rather than permanent relief from phantom pain (Sherman, 1997).

Theories of Pain

Pain consists of several stages and a multitude of syndromes. How people experience pain, however, is the subject of a number of theories. Of the several models of pain, two capture the divergent ways of conceptualizing pain: the specificity theory and the gate control theory.

Specificity Theory Specificity theory explains pain by hypothesizing that specific pain fibers and pain pathways exist, making the experience of pain virtually equal to the amount of tissue damage or injury. The view that pain is the result of transmission of pain signals from the body to a "pain center" in the brain can be traced back to Descartes, who in the 1600s proposed that the body works mechanically. This mechanistic action of the body is consistent with the notion that transmission of pain signals is a relaying of information about body damage. Descartes hypothesized that the mind works by a different set of principles, and body and mind interact in a limited way. According to Melzack (1993), Descartes's view influenced not only the development of a science of physiology and medicine but also the view that pain is a physical experience largely uninfluenced by psychological factors.

Working under the assumption that pain was the transmission of one type of sensory information, researchers tried to determine which type of receptor conveyed what type of sensory information (Melzack, 1973, 1992). For example, they tried to determine which type of receptor relayed information about heat, about cold, about pain, and so forth. The attempt to tie specific somatic sensations to specific types of receptors did not succeed. Researchers found that some parts of the body (like the cornea of the eye) contain only one type of receptor, yet those areas feel a full range of sensations. Some receptors seem specialized to react to specific types of stimulation, but these specialized receptors can also respond to other types of stimuli as well. The specificity of skin receptors is therefore limited, and any simple version of specificity theory is not valid.

Specificity does exist in the different types of receptors and nerve fibers. The different types of receptors in the skin allow us to sense light touch, pressure, itching, pricking, warmth, and cold. In addition, we can perceive texture, shape, and vibration and can localize the source of these stimuli on the surface of the skin. We can also sense pain, but pain can come through any of these stimuli rather than from another specific type of receptor.

The A and C fibers convey messages from the skin to the spinal cord, and other specific nerve tracts convey information to the brain. Some pain authorities (Melzack, 1973; Wall & Jones, 1991) have argued against the interpretation that these two fibers are exclusively pain fibers. Although these fibers relay messages that are interpreted as pain, not every neural impulse initiated in these fibers will receive this interpretation. Specific nerve fibers, such as the A and C fibers, play a role in the perception of pain, and some (Perl & Kruger, 1996) have argued for the existence of some specific pain fibers. Others (Wall & Jones, 1991) have argued against labeling any type of fiber as an exclusive pain fiber. Melzack (1993) has opposed interpreting any nerve tract as exclusively devoted to pain and cited the failure of severing nerve tracts through surgery to control chronic pain as evidence supporting this point. Even when nerve tracts are surgically severed, pain relief is usually temporary, and the chronic pain that prompted the drastic measure of surgery typically returns within weeks or months.

Specificity theory fails to integrate the variability of the experience of pain with the physiology of the somatosensory system. Even if specific skin receptors are devoted to relaying pain, the existence of pain without injury (phantom limb pain),

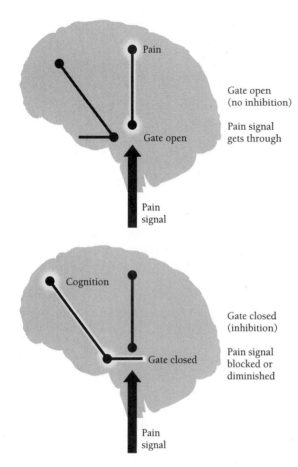

Figure 7.3 Gate control theory of pain.

injury without pain (as experienced by the soldiers at Anzio beach), and the failure of surgical treatments for pain make a simple, physiological theory of pain untenable. Contemporary theorists who believe in the specificity of pain acknowledge that specificity is limited and that pain is a complex, multidimensional phenomenon.

The Gate Control Theory In 1965, Ronald Melzack and Peter Wall formulated a new theory of pain, which suggests that pain is *not* the result of a linear process that begins with sensory stimulation of pain pathways and ends with the experi-

ence of pain. Rather, pain perception is subject to a number of modulations that can influence the experience of pain. These modulations begin in the spinal cord.

Melzack and Wall hypothesized that structures in the spinal cord act as a gate for the sensory input that is interpreted as pain. Melzack and Wall's theory is thus known as the **gate control theory** (see Figure 7.3). It is based on physiology but explains both sensory and psychological aspects of pain perception.

Melzack and Wall (1965, 1982, 1988) pointed out that the nervous system is never at rest, and the patterns of neural activation constantly change. When sensory information from the body reaches the dorsal horns of the spinal cord, that neural activation enters a system that is already active. The existing activity in the spinal cord and brain influences the fate of incoming sensory information, sometimes amplifying and sometimes decreasing the incoming neural signals. The gate control theory hypothesizes that these complex modulations in the spinal cord and in the brain affect the perception of pain.

According to the gate control theory, neural mechanisms in the spinal cord act like a gate that can either increase or decrease the flow of neural impulses. Figure 7.3 shows the results of opening and closing the gate. With the gate open, impulses flow through the spinal cord toward the brain, neural messages reach the brain, and the person feels pain. With the gate closed, impulses are inhibited from ascending through the spinal cord, messages do not reach the brain, and the person does not feel pain. Moreover, sensory input is subject to modulation, depending on the activity of the large A-beta fibers, the small A-delta fibers, and the small C fibers that enter the spinal cord and synapse in the dorsal horns.

The dorsal horns of the spinal cord are composed of several layers (laminae). Two of those laminae make up the substantia gelatinosa, which is the hypothesized location of the gate (Melzack & Wall, 1965; Wall, 1980). Both the small A-delta and C fibers and the large A-beta fibers travel through the substantia gelatinosa, which also re-

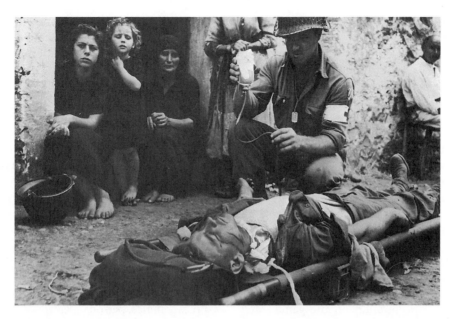

The experience of pain varies with the situation. Wounded soldiers removed from front lines may feel little pain despite extreme injuries.

ceives projections from other laminae (Melzack & Wall, 1982, 1988). This arrangement of neurons provides the physiological basis for the modulation of incoming sensory impulses.

The gate control theory hypothesizes that information enters the dorsal horns of the spinal cord by way of primary afferent neurons. This information passes through the substantia gelatinosa, where the information is modulated by the activity of that structure, affecting the activity of the transmission cells. The transmission cells relay the modulated information toward the brain.

Melzack and Wall (1982) proposed that activity in the small A-delta and C fibers causes prolonged activity in the spinal cord. This type of activity would promote sensitivity, which produces pain. Activity of these small fibers would thus open the gate. On the other hand, activity of the large A-beta fibers produces an initial burst of activity in the spinal cord, followed by inhibition. Activity of these fibers closes the gate.

The gate may be closed by activity in the spinal cord and also by messages that descend from the brain. Melzack and Wall (1965, 1982, 1988) proposed the concept of a **central control trigger** consisting of nerve impulses that descend from the brain and influence the gating mechanism. They hypothesized that this system consists of large neurons that conduct impulses rapidly. These impulses from the brain affect the opening and closing of the gate in the spinal cord and are affected by cognitive processes. That is, Melzack and Wall proposed that the experience of pain is influenced by beliefs and prior experience, and they also hypothesized a physiological mechanism that would account for such factors in pain perception. According to the gate control theory then, pain not only has sensory components but also motivational and emotional components.

The gate control theory explains the influence of cognitive aspects of pain by hypothesizing central control mechanisms that affect sensory input as well as being affected by it. Anxiety, worry, depression, and focusing on an injury can increase pain by affecting the central control trigger, thus opening the gate. Distraction, relaxation, and positive emotions can cause the gate to close, thereby decreasing pain.

Many personal experiences with pain are consistent with the gate control theory. When you accidentally hit your finger with a hammer, many of the small fibers are activated, opening the gate. An emotional reaction accompanies your perception of acute pain. You may then grasp your injured finger and rub it. According to the gate control theory, rubbing stimulates the large fibers that close the gate, thus blocking stimulation from the small fibers and decreasing pain.

The gate control theory also explains how injuries can go virtually unnoticed. If sensory input is sent into a heavily activated nervous system, then the stimulation may not be perceived as pain. A tennis player may turn an ankle during a game but not notice the acute pain because of excitement and concentration on the game. After the game is finished, however, the player may notice the pain because the nervous system is functioning at a different level of activation and the gate is more easily opened.

Although it is not universally accepted, the gate control theory is the leading theory of pain. It is seen as an advance over simplistic sensory views of pain, including the view that pain is relayed by specific pain fibers. Melzack and Wall proposed the gate control theory before the discovery of the body's own opiates or of the descending control mechanisms through the periaqueductal gray and the nucleus raphe magnus. These structures have been shown to modulate the experience of pain, much as the gate control theory proposed, and other experimental evidence is consistent with this theory (Humphries, Johnson, & Long, 1996). The gate control theory has been and continues to be successful in spurring research and generating interest in the psychological and perceptual factors involved in pain.

Melzack (1993) has proposed an extension to the gate control theory called the neuromatrix theory, which places a stronger emphasis on the brain's role in pain perception. He hypothesized a network of brain neurons that he called the neuro-matrix, which is "distributed throughout many areas of the brain, comprises a widespread network of neurons which generates patterns, processes information that flows through it, and ultimately produces the pattern that is felt as a whole body" (p. 623). Normally, the neuromatrix acts to process incoming sensory information, including pain, but the neuromatrix acts even in the absence of sensory input, such as with phantom limbs. Melzack's neuromatrix theory extends gate control theory but maintains that pain perception is part of a complex process affected not only by sensory input but also by activity of the nervous system and by experience and expectation.

In Summary

Although extent of damage is important in the pain experience, personal perception is also important. Pain can be classified as acute, prechronic, or chronic, depending on the length of time that the pain has persisted. Acute pain is usually adaptive and lasts for less than 6 months. Chronic pain continues beyond the time of healing, often in the absence of detectable tissue damage. Prechronic pain occurs between acute and chronic pain. All of these stages of pain appear in pain syndromes such as headache pain, low back pain, arthritic pain, cancer pain, and phantom limb pain.

Several models have been proposed to explain pain, but specificity theory does not capture the complexity of the pain experience. The gate control theory is currently the most influential model of pain. This theory holds that pain can be increased or diminished by mechanisms in the spinal cord and the brain. Since its formulation, increased knowledge of the physiology of the brain and spinal cord has supported this theory.

The Measurement of Pain

We have seen that pain has physical and psychological elements, both of which can be quantified and measured. The measurement of pain is important because it allows clinicians to quantify their patients' pain and allows researchers to evaluate different pain-reducing techniques. Numerous techniques have been used to measure pain, but these generally fall into three major categories: (1) physiological measures, (2) behavioral assessment, and (3) self-reports (Syrjala & Chapman, 1984).

Physiological Measures

Because pain produces an emotional response and because strong emotional arousal affects the autonomic nervous system as well as other physiological conditions, one might assume that a number of organic states would be highly correlated with the experience of pain (Nigl, 1984). Research on this hypothesis, however, generally has not produced positive results. The physiological variables that have been investigated as potential measures of pain include muscle tension and autonomic indices (Syrjala & Chapman, 1984). Unfortunately, none of these measures show strong, consistent relationships to other measures of pain.

Electromyography (EMG) has been used to measure the level of muscle tension experienced by patients suffering from low back pain. Although EMG can reveal abnormal patterns of muscle activity, these patterns do not consistently correlate with reported severity of the pain, and EMG levels can be either elevated or reduced in pain patients (Wolf, Nacht, & Kelly, 1982). Research (Andrasik, Blanchard, Arena, Saunders, & Barron, 1982) with headache patients and a variety of physiological measures found no consistent results to suggest that level of muscle tension is an accurate predictor of headache pain. These studies failed to support the notion that muscle tension, as measured by electromyography, is a reliable and valid index of pain.

Researchers have also attempted to assess pain through several autonomic indices, including such involuntary processes as hyperventilation, blood flow in the temporal artery, heart rate, hand surface temperature, finger pulse volume, and skin resistance level. Again, most of these attempts have met with only limited success. One exception to these generally negative results has been the use of thermography to measure skin temperature (LeRoy & Filasky, 1990). Thermographic instruments measure minute changes in skin temperature and provide an estimate of autonomic nervous system functioning. This procedure has demonstrated some success in measuring some types of pain, but pain is only one of many factors contributing to changes in skin temperature (Nigl, 1984). In conclusion, although intense pain may affect autonomic functions, the devices used to measure these changes have not yet yielded satisfactory results.

Behavioral Assessment

A second major approach to pain measurement is observation of patients' behavior. More than 25 years ago, Wilbert Fordyce (1974) reported that people in pain often groan, grimace, rub, sigh, limp, miss work, remain in bed, or engage in other behaviors that signify to observers that they may be suffering from pain. Other observable behaviors include lowered levels of activity, use of pain medication, body posture, and facial expressions (Keefe & Block, 1982). Each of these behaviors has potential reward value; that is, pain patients are frequently reinforced by some sort of disability compensation, avoidance of responsibility, and sympathy and attention from other people. Fordyce (1976, 1990b) has pointed out that these types of environmental reinforcers increase the tendency for pain behaviors to recur and for their prominence to increase. The use of operant conditioning techniques to decrease these learned behaviors is discussed in Chapter 8.

Methods of assessing pain can be divided into (1) observations made by significant others and (2) observations made by trained personnel in either a clinic or a laboratory setting.

Observations by Significant Others   Spouses and others close to the pain patient can be trained to make careful observations of pain behaviors without

further reinforcing these behaviors. For example, Fordyce (1976) has trained significant others by first asking them to list 5 to 10 items indicating that the patient is in pain. This list might include such behaviors as requesting medication, moaning, or verbalizing pain. Fordyce recommends a list of this length because more than 10 items might prompt too much attention to pain behaviors and fewer than 5 items would probably not be enough to make reliable observations. Once the list is complete, the significant other is asked to record the amount of time the patient spends exhibiting each of these behaviors. Next, the significant other records his or her own behaviors immediately following the patient's pain behaviors.

This system has been modified and refined (Turk, Meichenbaum, & Genest, 1983) with the development of both a spouse diary and a significant-other pain questionnaire. The spouse diary asks the husband or wife to note the time, date, and location of behaviors that express unusually severe pain. Next, the spouse's subsequent feelings and actions are recorded. Then the spouse estimates the effectiveness of such actions along a 6-point scale from "did not help at all" to "seemed to stop the pain completely." The significant-other pain questionnaire is made up of 30 items inquiring about the patient's severity of pain and its effect on such areas as work, recreation, and family relations. Some questions deal with the significant other's feelings and responses toward the patient and the pain situation. These two assessment devices can be compared with the patient's own diary and pain questionnaire over the same period.

Clinical and Laboratory Observations   Some researchers have relied on trained observers in a clinic or laboratory to assess such pain behaviors (Fordyce, 1990a; Keefe, 1982; Keefe & Block, 1982). Investigators have used both direct observations (carried out surreptitiously) and videotape recordings, and both techniques have demonstrated acceptable reliability and validity.

One study (Keefe & Block, 1982) used two trained observers to independently view and record videotapes of patients with low back pain. The two observers had very high categories of agreement on each of five nonverbal pain behaviors: sighing, grimacing, rubbing, bracing, and guarding, indicating strong reliability for this technique. Patients also rated their intensity of pain, thus allowing a validity check of the observers' ratings. For all behaviors except grimacing, the correlation was significant, a result suggesting that the ratings of trained observers have some validity. Moreover, the frequency of pain behaviors tended to decrease with behaviorally oriented treatment and these decreases in pain behaviors correlated with changes in pain ratings. In addition, the five behaviors differentiated pain patients from normal people and also from pain-free depressed patients.

These results indicate that a number of pain behaviors can be reliably measured. Raters independently agree when pain patients are guarding their movements, bracing, rubbing, grimacing, emitting pain sounds, and restricting their movements. Moreover, a number of these behaviors can distinguish between patients known to be in pain and those who are pain free.

Self-Reports

The third approach to pain measurement is the use of self-reports. Self-reports include simple rating scales, standardized pain inventories, and standardized personality tests. These types of pain assessment are the most common approach clinicians use with pain patients.

Rating Scales   One of the oldest pain measures, the self-report scale, is still widely used. On the simplest rating scales, patients are asked to rate their intensity of pain on a scale from 1 to 10 or 1 to 100, with 100 being the most excruciating pain possible, and 1 being the lowest level of pain detectable. A similar technique is the Visual Analog Scale (VAS), which is simply a line anchored on the left by a phrase like "no pain" and on the right by a phrase like "worst pain imaginable."

Both the VAS and the numerical rating scales are easy to use, and both have acceptable reliability ratings (Kremer, Atkinson, & Ignelzi, 1981). However, they have been criticized as sometimes being confusing to patients not accustomed to quantifying their experience and for allowing the underreporting of pain for those who are reluctant to admit to pain (D. A. Williams, 1996).

Pain Questionnaires Melzack (1975b, p. 278) was referring to the multidimensional nature of pain when he stated that "the word 'pain' refers to an endless variety of qualities that are categorized under a simple linguistic label, not to a specific, single sensation that varies only in intensity." He contended that describing pain on a single dimension was "like specifying the visual world only in terms of light flux without regard to pattern, color, texture, and the many other dimensions of visual experience" (p. 278). In an attempt to rectify this weakness in single-dimensional measurement scales, Melzack (1975b) developed the McGill Pain Questionnaire (MPQ).

The McGill Pain Questionnaire provides a subjective report of pain and categorizes it in three dimensions: sensory, affective, and evaluative. *Sensory* qualities of pain are its temporal, spatial, pressure, and thermal properties; *affective* qualities are its fear, tension, and autonomic properties; *evaluative* qualities are the subjective overall intensity of the pain experience.

The MPQ has four parts. Part 1 consists of front and back drawings of the human body. Patients mark on these drawings the areas where they feel pain. Part 2 consists of 20 sets of words describing pain, and patients draw a circle around the one word in each set that most accurately describes their pain. These adjectives are ordered from least to most painful—for example, *nagging, nauseating, agonizing, dreadful,* and *torturing.* Part 3 asks how patients' pain has changed with time. Part 4 measures the intensity of pain on a 5-point scale from *mild* to *excruciating.* This fourth part yields a Present Pain Intensity (PPI) score. As might be expected, the PPI has been found to correlate

highly with the Visual Analog Scale (Walsh & Leber, 1983).

The MPQ is the most frequently used pain questionnaire (Piotrowski, 1998). It has been used to assess pain relief in a variety of treatment programs and has demonstrated some validity in assessing cancer pain (Dudgeon, Raubertas, & Rosenthal, 1993), headache (Hunter & Philips, 1981), and several other pain syndromes (Chapman & Syrjala, 1990; Dubuisson & Melzack, 1976; Melzack, 1975b). The MPQ shows considerable promise as a multidimensional pain assessment inventory, but it has a difficult vocabulary and lacks a standard scoring format (Syrjala & Chapman, 1984). A short form of the McGill Pain Questionnaire (Melzack, 1987) preserves the multidimensional assessment and correlates highly with scores on the standard MPQ.

The West Haven-Yale Multidimensional Pain Inventory (MPI) is another assessment tool specifically designed for pain patients (Kerns, Turk, & Rudy, 1985). The 52-item MPI is divided into three sections. The first rates (1) pain severity, (2) pain's interference with patients' lives, (3) patients' dissatisfaction with their present functioning, (4) patients' view of the support they receive from others, (5) patients' perceived life control, and (6) patients' negative mood states. The second section rates the patients' perceptions of the responses of significant others, and the third measures how often patients engage in each of 30 different daily activities.

Using this scale allowed researchers (Kerns et al., 1985) to develop 13 different scales that captured different dimensions of the lives of pain patients. Further studies (Turk & Rudy, 1988; Rudy, Turk, Zaki, & Curtin, 1989) have used the statistical technique of cluster analysis to group pain patients according to the pattern of their responses on the MPI. The pain patients fell into three clusters, labeled dysfunctional, interpersonally distressed, and active copers. Patients in the dysfunctional cluster tended to report higher levels of pain, greater psychological distress, lower perceived control, greater interference with their lives, lower levels of activity, and lower levels of perceived control over their lives. These patients experienced many problems attributable to their pain. The second cluster of patients perceived that their families and significant others did not support them, so this group was called *interpersonally distressed*. The people in this profile had problems because they perceived that those around them were failing to provide necessary support. The researchers called people in the third cluster *adaptive copers*. These individuals reported lower levels of pain severity, lower interference with their lives, lower personal distress, and higher levels of activity and control. These patients were less troubled by their pain and appeared to be coping with it.

Other research (Rudy et al., 1989; Turk et al., 1998; Walter & Brannon, 1991) has obtained similar clusters using different populations of pain patients. The MPI assesses many aspects of psychological and physical functioning and could provide a comprehensive assessment of the lives of pain patients. The researchers involved with the development of the MPI have validated it against many standardized tests, including the McGill Pain Questionnaire and the Minnesota Multiphasic Personality Inventory.

Many kinds of pain questionnaires have been developed for general use and for specific uses such as for children, specific pain syndromes, fear of pain, and pain behaviors. However, the McGill Pain Questionnaire and the Multidimensional Pain Inventory are the pain assessments most commonly used by clinical practitioners treating pain patients (Piotrowski, 1998). In addition, clinicians also use a variety of standardized psychological tests in assessing pain patients.

Standardized Psychological Tests Another approach to pain measurement is the use of standardized psychological tests. The most commonly used such test is the Minnesota Multiphasic Personality Inventory (MMPI) (Piotrowski, 1998). This instrument was not originally designed to assess pain but to measure such clinical diagnoses as hypochondriasis, depression, paranoia, schizophrenia, and other psychopathologies. Research from the early 1950s (Hanvik, 1951) found that different types of pain patients could be differentiated on several MMPI scales. Since that time, other researchers have used this inventory for pain measurement. Research has indicated that high scores on the hypochondriasis scale (a measure of preoccupation with body functions) correlate with pain (Sternbach, 1978). Other researchers have found that clusters of three or four MMPI scales reliably predict pain in clinical populations (Bradley, Prokop, Gentry, Van der Heide, & Prieto, 1981; Bradley & Van der Heide, 1984). The so-called neurotic triad— a cluster of elevated scores on hypochondriasis, depression, and hysteria—consistently relate to reports of pain.

The MMPI is the standardized psychological test that is most commonly used among clinicians who assess pain patients (Piotrowski, 1998), but the Beck Depression Inventory (Beck, Ward, Mendelson, Mock, & Erbaugh, 1961) and the Symptom Checklist-90 (Derogatis, 1977) are used almost as often. The Beck Depression Inventory is a short self-report questionnaire that assesses depression, and the Symptom Checklist-90 measures symptoms related to various types of behavioral problems. The widespread use of standardized psychological tests for pain patients reflects the diversity of symptoms that chronic pain may create.

A comparative analysis of nine commonly used self-report measures of chronic pain (Mikail, DuBreuil, & D'Eon, 1993) revealed five core dimensions tapped by these inventories. These factors were (1) general affective distress, (2) coping, (3) support, (4) pain description, and (5) functional capacity. This analysis also revealed that the McGill Pain Questionnaire, the Multidimensional Pain Inventory, and the Beck Depression Inventory measured the pain experience with very little overlap, a result suggesting that each of these three has something unique to offer. Thus, the strategy of using various standardized psychological tests in combination with pain inventories seems to be warranted in the assessment of pain.

In Summary

Pain measurement techniques can be grouped into physiological measures, behavioral assessment, and self-reports. Physiological measures include muscle tension and autonomic indices; this approach has shown limited success. Observations of pain-related behavior show some reliability and validity, but self-reports are a more common strategy of measurement. Self-reports include (1) rating scales; (2) pain questionnaires, such as the McGill Pain Questionnaire and the Multidimensional Pain Inventory; and (3) standardized objective tests, such as the Minnesota Multiphasic Personality Inventory, the Beck Depression Inventory, and the Symptom Checklist-90. Clinicians who treat pain patients often use a combination of assessments, relying most often on self-report inventories.

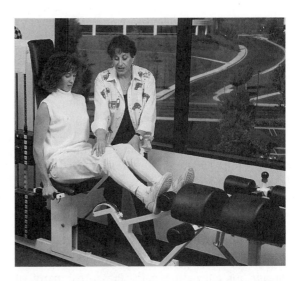

Physical activity can help to diminish pain and prevent injury from becoming chronic pain.

Preventing Pain

Pain can be prevented by avoiding injury or by medical or psychological treatment for pain. The next section looks at medical treatments for pain, and Chapter 8 discusses psychological treatments, but physicians and psychologists would agree that preventing chronic pain is preferable to treating it once it occurs. Two strategies exist for preventing chronic pain: minimizing injury and deterring acute pain from becoming chronic pain.

Several programs have targeted the prevention of low back pain, the type of pain that most often causes lost work days. An educational program called Back to Balance (Donaldson, Stanger, Donaldson, Cram, & Skubick, 1993) has attempted to minimize work-related back injuries. Participants of this study were nursing aides, orderlies, and other employees at a health care facility who had a very high rate of lost work time due to chronic repetitive lifting injuries to the back. The Back to Balance procedure consists of an easy-to-read booklet that contains information on the anatomy of the back and guidelines on how to keep the back balanced while engaging in repetitive lifting.

After 3 months, the employees in the control also participated in the educational program.

Results from this study indicated that the treatment group reported significantly less pain (as measured by the McGill Pain Questionnaire) than the controls at 3- and 12-month follow-up periods. Moreover, participants generalized their knowledge to the home. Most important for the facility, wages and relief costs were reduced to less than 25% of previous rates. Although most educational programs are not effective in changing behavior, the results indicated that this one was, offering a way to prevent back injuries at work.

A second approach involves treating injured people to prevent them from developing chronic pain. A review of such programs (Linton & Bradley, 1996) indicated that the time since injury is an important factor. For those who have been injured recently and whose pain is still acute, limited bed rest and analgesics combined with a rapid return to normal activities was an effective strategy. A study in Finland (Malmivaara et al., 1995) indicated that back pain patients who continued their ordinary activities as well as they could recovered better than patients who had complete bed rest or who did special back exercises.

For those whose injuries are several months old and who are still experiencing pain, more complex programs are required (Linton & Bradley, 1996). Such programs include exercise, training in safe lifting procedures, and behavioral components designed to boost problem-solving and coping skills. To sum up, early attention and treatment are important in preventing injury from developing into chronic pain.

Physical Treatments for Pain

For centuries, physicians have used a variety of means for alleviating pain. Presently, many of these procedures are supplemented by psychological or behavioral procedures so that patients receive both physical and behavioral treatments for the same disorder at the same time (Eisenberg et al., 1993). Behavioral treatments are discussed in the next chapter; this section looks at physical treatments for pain.

Evaluation of physical treatments for pain is complicated by disagreements between patients and health care professionals about the experience of pain. One study (Krokosky & Reardon, 1989) used the shortened form of the McGill Pain Questionnaire to assess pain in patients who were recuperating from surgery and then administered the questionnaire to the patients' nurses and physicians to measure their perception of each patient's pain. A comparison of the three sets of pain scores revealed many discrepancies. The correlations between the patients' ratings of their pain and the nurses' ratings of the patients' pain failed to show a statistically significant relationship, as did the correlation between physicians' and patients' ratings. The lack of correlation shows that neither nurses nor physicians perceived the amount and duration of their patients' pain. Both nurses and physicians generally underestimated the pain their patients experienced.

These results indicate that patients who are in pain may not be perceived to be in pain by those who are caring for them or that patients' pain may be perceived as less severe by professionals than by the patients themselves. These differing perceptions of pain can create problems both in the treatment of acute pain and in the management of chronic pain.

Physical treatments have traditionally been chosen according to the type and source of pain. Acute pain is usually treated with drugs, but their use in treating chronic pain is controversial. Both acute and chronic pain have been treated by stimulation to the skin, either electrical impulses (transcutaneous electrical nerve stimulation) or needles (acupuncture) or pressure (acupressure or massage). Chronic pain that has not responded to other methods of management is sometimes treated by surgery.

Drugs

Analgesic drugs relieve pain without causing loss of consciousness. Hundreds of different analgesic drugs are available, but almost all fall into two major groups: the opiates and the non-narcotic analgesics (Polatin, 1996). Both types exist naturally as derivatives of plants, and both have many synthetic variations. Of the two, the opium type is stronger and has a longer history of use.

The non-narcotic analgesics include aspirin, the nonsteroidal anti-inflammatory drugs (NSAIDs), and acetaminophen. *Aspirin* comes from an extract of willow bark. The active component is salicin, a compound isolated in 1827 (Melzack & Wall, 1982). The Bayer Company used the name aspirin as a trade name beginning in 1899. In addition to having analgesic properties, aspirin acts against inflammation and fever.

NSAIDs, such as ibuprofen and naproxen sodium, appear to block the synthesis of prostaglandins (Winter, 1994), a class of chemicals released by damaged tissue and involved in inflammation and the sensitization of neurons that increase pain.

BECOMING HEALTHIER

One technique that helps people manage and minimize pain is guided imagery. This technique involves creating an image and being guided (or guiding yourself) through it. The process can be helpful in dealing with both chronic pain and acute pain such as medical or dental procedures. Those who are not experienced at guided imagery will benefit from putting the guided imagery instructions on an audiotape.

To practice guided imagery, choose a quiet place where you will not be disturbed and where you will be comfortable. Prepare for the experience by placing the tape player where you can turn it on, seating yourself in a comfortable chair, and taking a few deep breaths. Turn on the tape, close your eyes, and follow the instructions you have recorded.

The tape should include a description of a special place, one that you either imagine or have experienced, where you feel utterly safe and at peace. Tailor the place to fit with your life and experiences—one person's magic place may not be so attractive to another person, so think about what will be appealing to you. Many people enjoy a beach scene, but others like woods, fields, or spe-

cial rooms. The goal is to imagine somewhere that you will feel relaxed and at peace.

Put instructions on your tape concerning this place and its description. Spend time in this place and experience it in detail. Pay attention to the sights and sounds, but do not neglect the smells and skin senses associated with the place. Spend time imagining each of these sensory experiences, and include instructions to yourself about the feelings. You should feel relaxed and peaceful as you go though this scene. Linger over the details and aim to allow yourself to become completely absorbed in the experience.

Include some instructions for relaxed breathing in your tour of your special place. Your goal is to achieve peace and relaxation that will replace the anxiety and pain that you have felt. As you repeat the guided imagery exercise, you may want to revise the tape to include more details. The tape should include at least 10 minutes of guided instructions, and you may want to re-do the tape into a longer version as you become more proficient in the exercise. Eventually, you will not need the tape, and you will be able to take this technique with you wherever you go.

These drugs act at the site of injury instead of crossing into the brain and changing neurochemical activity in the nervous system. As a result, NSAIDs do not alter pain perception when no injury is present, as in laboratory situations with people who receive experimental pain stimuli.

Aspirin and the NSAIDs have many uses in pain relief. Because these drugs appear to work by influencing the effects of injury, they are especially useful for pain in which injury has occurred. This description takes in a wide variety of pain, including minor cuts and scratches as well as more severe injuries such as broken bones. But pain that

occurs without inflammation is not so readily relieved by NSAIDs, and some gastric problems are worsened by the irritation that these drugs cause.

Another of aspirin's side effects is the alteration of blood clotting time, a condition that can be either an advantage (as in patients who are at risk for forming internal blood clots) or a disadvantage (as in patients who are candidates for surgery). This side effect makes aspirin unsuitable for some people who are in pain. Aspirin and other NSAIDs are also toxic in large doses and can cause damage to the liver and kidneys. People who take an overdose of these drugs sometimes do

WOULD YOU BELIEVE...?

Pain Varies by Culture

Would you believe that pain varies from one culture to another? Although pain itself is a consistent experience around the world, cultural background and social context can affect the experience, expression, and treatment of pain (Gureje et al., 1996). These differences come from varying meanings that different cultures attach to pain and from stereotypes associated with various cultural groups.

Cultural expectations for pain are apparent in the pain women experience during childbirth (Streltzer, 1997). Some cultures hold birth as a dangerous and painful process, and women in these cultures reflect these expectations by experiencing great pain. Other cultures expect quiet acceptance during the experience of giving birth, and women in those cultures tend not to show much evidence of pain.

Since the 1950s, studies have compared pain expression for people from various ethnic backgrounds (Streltzer, 1997). Some studies have shown differences whereas others have not, but the studies all suffer from the criticism of stereotyping. For example, Italians are stereotyped as people who show a lot of emotion. Consistent with this stereotype, studies have found that Italian Americans express more distress and demand more pain medication than "Yankees" (White Anglo-Saxons who had lived in the United States for generations), who have the reputation for stoically ignoring pain. These variations in pain behaviors among different cultures may reflect behavioral differences in learning and modeling. Alternatively, the perceived differences might come from observers' stereotypical expectations concerning pain behaviors and the lack of objective measurements of pain behaviors.

More recent studies have been more methodologically sound, and some of those studies have also shown cultural variations in the experience of pain. For example, Europeans consider pain to be a common experience for cancer patients, and pain experts in those countries believe that this type of pain is undertreated (Streltzer, 1997). Experts from China, on the other hand, consider cancer pain as less of a problem. These varying attitudes lead to differences in treatment: About 70% of patients in Europe receive opiates to manage the cancer pain, whereas only about 4% of Chinese cancer patients receive such drugs. The variations may be more in physicians' beliefs than in patients' pain, but the interaction of patient and physician may moderate the experience of pain.

Ethnicity does influence the amount of analgesic medication that patients receive. African American and Hispanic American patients received significantly less postoperative medication than White Americans (Ng, Dimsdale, Shragg, & Deutsch, 1996). This difference may have been due to the medical staff's perceptions of need or to the patients' pain behaviors. In either case, the result was differential treatment and possibly needless pain for ethnic minority patients.

---

so by taking a combination of over-the-counter analgesics without recognizing the similarity of many of them (Winter, 1994).

Acetaminophen, another non-narcotic analgesic, is not one of the NSAIDs. It has no anti-inflammatory properties but has a pain-relieving capability that is similar to aspirin but somewhat weaker. Under brand names like Tylenol, acetaminophen has become the most frequently used drug for pain relief (DeNitto, 1993). Acetaminophen does not have the gastric side effects of aspirin, so people who cannot tolerate aspirin find it a good substitute. Despite the lack of gastric effects, acetaminophen is not harmless. Large quantities of acetaminophen can be fatal, but even nonlethal doses can do serious damage to the liver, especially when combined with alcohol (Winter, 1994).

The most powerful analgesics are of the *opium* type. The extract of the opium poppy has been in use for at least 5,000 years, and its analgesic properties were known to the ancient Romans (Melzack & Wall, 1982). In 1803, morphine was isolated. Many synthetic compounds have structures and actions similar to those of morphine, and several neurotransmitters produce analgesia in the same way that the opiates do (Pert & Snyder, 1973). This mechanism is responsible for the pain-relieving effect of opiates and explains why these drugs can alleviate even strong pain.

Because morphine is so powerful, many physicians are reluctant to prescribe it in amounts strong enough to reduce intense pain, and many patients fear the possibility of addiction and are reluctant to take sufficient doses to obtain relief. Thus, many acute pain patients and people with chronic cancer pain do not receive sufficient relief. However, one physician, C. Stanton Hill (1995), contended that all types of pain are inadequately treated and that patients should begin to demand adequate pain relief. Hill also condemned health care workers for overtly or covertly conveying the message that patients who request pain medication are drug abusers. This problem was not part of Barb's experience. Instead, Barb's physician continued for several years to prescribe opiates, which Barb (unwisely) combined with alcohol. This pattern of drug use posed problems, and Barb finally discontinued opiates as a way to manage her pain.

One procedure that has overcome the undermedication problem is a system of self-paced administration. Patients can activate a pump attached to their intravenous lines and deliver a dose of medication whenever they wish (Moyer, 1989). Such systems began to appear in the late 1970s and have since gained wide acceptance. The initial fears that patients would overmedicate if allowed free access to self-administered opiate analgesics has proven unfounded. In fact, the average amount of medication consumed is often lower than with the traditional type of delivery. Because an intravenous line is necessary for this system of drug

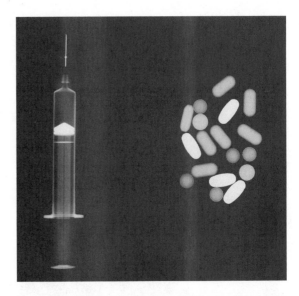

Drugs offer effective treatment for acute pain but are not a good choice to treat chronic pain.

delivery, it is most common in postsurgical patients. The system has also been used with success for burn patients (Moyer, 1989) and cancer patients (Sheidler, 1987).

How realistic are the fears of drug abuse as a consequence of prescribed opiate drugs? Do patients become addicted while recovering from surgery? What about the dangers to patients with terminal illnesses? According to one study (Porter & Jick, 1980), the risk of addiction is less than 1%. Several authorities have even questioned the risk of problems due to tolerance in cancer patients, contending that tolerance occurs for only the first few days of administration and does not continue to escalate (Elliott & Elliott, 1992; Melzack & Wall, 1982).

Like all drugs, the opiates have side effects. They alter a person's perception, usually by decreasing anxiety or clouding judgment. They affect the digestive system, producing constipation and sometimes nausea. They also depress the respiratory system and can cause death by respiratory failure. Pain activates the central nervous system, however, making the threat of respiratory failure

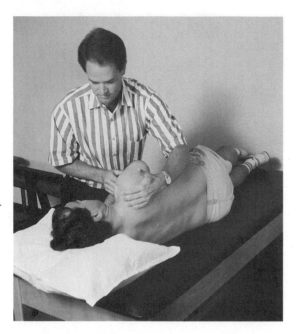

Manipulating muscles is one of the alternative therapies that can be effective in relieving pain.

more likely in recreational users than in pain patients (Polatin, 1996).

The advantages of opiate drugs outweigh their dangers. No other type of drug produces more complete pain relief. However, their potential for abuse and their side effects make them more suitable for treating acute pain than for managing chronic pain. The opiate drugs remain an essential part of pain management for the most severe, acute injuries, for recovery from surgery, and for terminal illnesses.

Skin Stimulation

As Melzack and Wall (1982) pointed out, skin stimulation is one of the activities that can close the gate that relays pain impulses. Several techniques furnish such stimulation, including electrical stimulation of nerves, acupuncture, acupressure, application of heat and cold, and massage. Manipulations of the skin to relieve pain have a long and successful history (Field, 1998).

Transcutaneous electrical nerve stimulation (TENS), however, has a short history, dating only to the early 1970s (McCaffery, 1979). Electrical stimulation, which affects all nerves within about 4 centimeters of the skin's surface, can be accomplished by placing an electrode on the surface of the skin. The TENS system typically consists of electrodes that attach to the skin and are connected to a unit that supplies electrical stimulation. Many of these units are portable, and run on rechargeable batteries (McCaffery, 1979). Patients can vary the strength of the stimulation to suit their needs. Usually, pain decreases during the stimulation (Melzack & Wall, 1982), and the relief can persist for hours after the stimulation has ceased. Patients with both chronic and acute pain can use TENS units to achieve pain relief.

Acupuncture is an ancient Chinese form of analgesia that consists of inserting needles into specific points on the skin and continuously stimulating the needles (Melzack & Wall, 1982). The stimulation can be accomplished electrically or by twirling the needles. **Acupressure** is the application of pressure rather than needles to the points used in acupuncture. Inherent in the use of acupuncture and acupressure is a philosophy of the body and illness not accepted by many Westerners. Acupuncture has been used as an anesthetic for surgery, and some patients in China have undergone surgery with acupuncture as their only anesthetic. Melzack and Wall (1992) reported that acupuncture is more effective than a placebo in producing pain relief in both humans and nonhuman animals.

The U.S. National Institutes of Health convened a panel that found acupuncture to be effective in the treatment of some conditions, including postoperative pain and low back pain (Morey, 1998). In addition, acupuncture is not as likely to produce side effects as drug therapy. About 10,000 licensed acupuncturists practice in the United States; the treatment is among a variety of alternative treatments seeing an increase in use (Rosenfeld, 1998).

Considered a luxury a few years ago, massage is another alternative therapy now used to control pain (Bower, Rubik, Weiss, & Starr, 1997). Several different types of therapeutic massage can be applied to a variety of pain problems. Benefits come from direct manipulation of soft tissue as well as from relaxation and stress relief (Field, 1998). This therapy can decrease muscle tension, ease muscle pain, disperse fluid to decrease swelling, and relieve anxiety. Massage can be useful in easing not only muscle pain but cancer pain and a variety of other pains.

In summary, a variety of therapies involve manipulation of the skin to relieve pain. A growing body of research indicates that these therapies can be effective, and an increasing number of people seek such therapies.

Surgery

Surgery is the most extreme form of treatment for pain and is usually used only when other treatments have failed. The most common use of surgery for pain management is to alleviate chronic low back pain. Not all patients experience analgesia from surgery, and of course, surgery has its own dangers and possibilities for complications. Both the recommendation for surgery and its failure to control pain were reflected in Barb's experience. Her two back surgeries were only partially successful in repairing damage and not very successful in controlling her pain.

Surgery to control pain can occur at any level of the nervous system. The least radical surgery involves destroying the peripheral nerves close to the site of the pain (Carson, 1987). This type of surgery is recommended only if the pain is localized well enough to allow limited destruction of nerves and if this destruction is likely to produce relief. The best approach is first to use a local anesthetic on the nerves so the patient can experience the effects of nerve destruction. Some patients prefer the pain to the complete loss of sensation that surgery confers. Another consideration is that, in most cases, the peripheral nerves include both sensory and motor fibers. Thus, surgery will cause not only loss of sensation but also loss of movement. Because nerves in the peripheral nervous system regenerate, the entire nerve section

must be destroyed; otherwise, the pain will recur when the nerves regenerate.

Another possible site for surgery is the dorsal root ganglion, just outside the spinal cord. Nerves split into the dorsal and ventral branches before entering the spinal cord. Because the dorsal branch is entirely sensory, severing it will produce only sensory loss and leave motor functioning unaffected. The complete loss of sensation can be distressing, and some patients develop phantom limb-type sensation and even pain as a result of this surgery.

Other possible sites for surgical intervention to control pain include the spinal cord and the brain itself. The most common of the surgeries to the spinal cord involve severing the spinothalamic tract (Melzack & Wall, 1982). This surgery initially produces a complete loss of sensation for the area of the body below the damage. However, patients often experience a return of an unpleasant sensation, which typically starts as a tingling and often progresses to a serious pain. Therefore, spinal cord surgery is usually performed on people with terminal conditions who would benefit from a relief of pain for the remainder of their lives.

Pain control through surgery to the brain is possible but rare. Brain surgery, of course, is very serious, because lesions to the brain can produce many effects in addition to pain relief. Interestingly, prefrontal lobotomies produce pain relief in the form of a decreased concern with pain, but this surgery produces no sensory deficit; it merely causes patients to be so little concerned with the sensation that they do not report pain. Surgery to the thalamus and the somatosensory cortex are dangerous and have not proven to be effective in relieving pain.

Limitations of Physical Treatments

Drugs, skin stimulation, and surgery can all be effective means of controlling pain. However, all these physical treatments have limitations.

One limitation of opiate drugs is the tolerance and dependence they produce in patients. *Tolerance* occurs when a larger and larger dose of a drug is required to bring about the same effect. *Dependence* occurs when the drug's removal produces withdrawal symptoms. Because opiates produce both tolerance and dependence, they are potentially dangerous and subject to abuse. As a result, health care professionals are reluctant to prescribe these drugs, and the public is afraid to use them, even when they could relieve intractable pain (Donovan, 1989; Melzack & Wall, 1982).

Because of these concerns, patients are often undermedicated and do not receive sufficiently large or frequent doses of medication to produce relief. The average dose of opiate drugs is often below the therapeutic level, and many patients take only a fourth to a third of the medication that their physicians had ordered (Donovan, 1989). Physicians also hold misconceptions about the use of opiates (Elliott & Elliott, 1992), making their patients more likely to suffer needlessly as a result.

Whereas undermedication may be a problem for cancer pain patients, overmedication is often a problem for patients suffering from low back pain. Barb's physician continued to prescribe opiates for her back pain and referred her to a pain specialist only when Barb requested help in getting off the drugs. One team of investigators (Von Korff, Barlow, Cherkin, & Deyo, 1994) grouped primary care physicians into low, moderate, and high frequency of prescribing pain medication and bed rest for back pain patients. A 1- and 2-year follow-up found that patients who took less medication and who remained active did just as well as back pain patients who were told to take more medication and to rest. (Barb's current experience is consistent with this finding. She says that remaining active is the best way to avert pain; when she rests, her back hurts more.) In addition, patients with the least medication were the most satisfied with their treatment. Moreover, patients whose physicians rated low in prescription of medication and bed rest spent only about half as much money on treatment as patients whose doctors rated high on medication and bed rest.

All forms of skin stimulation also have limitations. Transcutaneous electrical nerve stimulation (TENS), despite some promising early results, has not proven to provide long-term relief for chronic pain patients (Finsen et al., 1988). Barb's many treatments for pain included TENS, which she believes provided relief by distracting her from her pain rather than through the nerve stimulation. Like drug treatment, massage does not continue to provide pain relief once the therapy is discontinued (Field, 1998). In addition, massage is not suitable for arthritis or other pain problems related to joints (Bower et al., 1997). Acupuncture and acupressure do not work for everyone. Only about 10% of surgery patients experience sufficient analgesia from acupuncture (Melzack & Wall, 1982). Its effects are not instantaneous, and the needles must be stimulated for about 20 minutes to produce analgesia. Moreover, the stimulation must be fairly intense and continuous.

Surgery, too, has limitations as a pain analgesia. First, the surgery does not always repair damaged tissue, and second, not all patients receiving surgery experience sufficient pain relief. Surgery is not a successful treatment for many people with chronic back pain (Deyo, 1998). Despite the popularity of surgical interventions, back pain patients often fail to obtain relief from surgery, or their pain returns, making this approach an expensive but unreliable approach to controlling this pain syndrome. Also, surgery has its own potential dangers and possibilities for complications. These limitations of surgery as a treatment for pain were reflected in Barb's experience. Her two back surgeries were only partially successful in repairing tissue damage and not very successful in controlling her pain.

In Summary

A variety of medical treatments for pain have demonstrated uses but also limitations. Analgesic drugs offer pain relief for acute pain and can be of use for chronic pain. These drugs include non-narcotic and opiate drugs. Non-narcotic drugs include aspirin, nonsteroidal anti-inflammatory drugs (NSAIDs), and acetaminophen. These drugs are effective in managing mild to moderate acute pain and have some uses in managing chronic pain. Opiates are effective in managing severe chronic pain, but their tolerance and dependence properties pose problems for use by chronic pain patients. Indeed, both health care professionals and patients are so cautious concerning the use of opiates that physicians are reluctant to prescribe and patients are reluctant to use these drugs in sufficient doses to achieve adequate pain control.

Other medical treatments include skin stimulation such as transcutaneous electrical nerve stimulation (TENS), acupuncture and acupressure, and massage. TENS may be useful for short-term but not long-term pain relief. Acupuncture and massage therapy are among the alternative medical approaches that are increasing in popularity and recognition. Surgery can alter either peripheral nerves or the central nervous system. Surgical procedures are often done as a last resort in controlling chronic pain, and unfortunately, surgical procedures often provide only temporary relief.

Answers

This chapter addressed five basic questions.

1. **How does the nervous system register pain?**

   Receptors near the skin's surface react to stimulation, and the nerve impulses from this stimulation relay the message to the spinal cord. The spinal cord includes laminae (layers) that modulate the sensory message and relay it toward the brain. The somatosensory cortex in the brain receives and interprets sensory input, and neurochemicals and the periaqueductal gray can also modulate the information and change the perception of pain.

2. **What is the meaning of pain?**

   Pain is difficult to define, but it can be classified as acute (resulting from specific injury and lasting less than 6 months), prechronic, or chronic (continuing beyond the time of healing). Pain can also be defined in terms of syndromes that include headache pain, low back pain, arthritic pain, cancer pain, and phantom limb pain; the first two are the most common sources of chronic pain. The meaning of pain can also be understood through theories, the gate control theory of pain being the leading model. This view proposes that both physical and psychological factors influence the experience of pain.

3. **How can pain be measured?**

   Pain can be measured physiologically by assessing muscle tension or autonomic arousal, but these measurements do not have high validity. Observations of pain-related behaviors (such as limping, grimacing, complaining) have some reliability and validity. Self-reports are the most common approach to pain measurement and include rating scales, pain questionnaires, and standardized psychological tests.

4. **How can pain be prevented?**

   Pain can be prevented by avoiding injury or by stopping acute pain from becoming chronic pain. Several effective programs address each approach.

5. **What are the leading physical treatments for pain?**

   Analgesic drugs are used to control acute pain, but fears about addiction to opiates prevent their use for controlling chronic pain. In addition to drugs, other approaches to pain control exist. Skin stimulation techniques include transcutaneous electrical nerve stimulation (TENS), acupuncture, acupressure, and massage. TENS has limited effectiveness, but acupuncture and massage can be effective for some types of pain. Surgery is often used when other methods have failed and is most successful for pain associated with terminal illness. For other types of chronic pain, surgery is not an effective approach to the alleviation of pain.

Glossary

A-beta fibers   Large fibers in the spinal cord that inhibit the transmission of pain.

acupressure   The application of pressure rather than needles to the points used in acupuncture.

acupuncture   An ancient Chinese form of analgesia that consists of inserting needles into specific points on the skin and continuously stimulating the needles.

action potential   An electrical discharge.

acute pain   Short-term pain that results from tissue damage or other trauma.

A-delta fibers   Small fibers that facilitate the transmission of pain.

analgesic drugs   Drugs that decrease the perception of pain.

central control trigger   A nerve impulse that descends from the brain and influences the perception of pain.

C fibers   Small-diameter nerve fibers that provide information concerning slow, diffuse, lingering pain.

chronic pain   Pain that endures beyond the time of normal healing; frequently experienced in the absence of detectable tissue damage.

cluster headache   A type of severe headache that occurs in daily clusters for 4 to 16 weeks. Symptoms are similar to migraine, but duration is much briefer.

dorsal horns   The part of the spinal cord away from the stomach that receives sensory input and that may play an important role in the perception of pain.

endorphins   Naturally occurring neurochemicals whose effects resemble those of the opiates.

gate control theory   A theory of pain holding that structures in the spinal cord act as a gate for sensory input that is interpreted as pain.

laminae   Layers of cell bodies.

medulla   The structure of the hindbrain just above the spinal cord.

migraine headache   Headache pain caused by constriction and dilation of the vascular arteries.

myelin   A fatty substance that acts as insulation for neurons.

nucleus raphe magnus   A group of neurons in the medulla that send inhibitory signals to neurons in the spinal cord; part of the descending control system for pain.

osteoarthritis   Progressive inflammation of the joints.

periaqueductal gray   An area of the midbrain that, when stimulated, decreases pain.

phantom limb pain   The experience of chronic pain in an absent body part.

prechronic pain   Pain that endures beyond the acute phase but has not yet become chronic.

primary afferents   Sensory neurons that convey impulses from the skin to the spinal cord.

rheumatoid arthritis   An autoimmune disorder characterized by a dull ache within or around a joint.

somatosensory cortex   The part of the brain that receives and processes sensory input from the body.

somatosensory system   The part of the nervous system that carries sensory information from the body to the brain.

substantia gelatinosa   Two layers of the dorsal horns of the spinal cord.

tension headache   Pain produced by sustained muscle contractions in the neck, shoulders, scalp, and face.

thalamus   Structure in the forebrain that acts as a relay center for incoming sensory information and outgoing motor information.

transcutaneous electrical nerve stimulation (TENS)   Treatment for pain involving electrical stimulation of neurons from the surface of the skin. This stimulation blocks other sensory input, providing pain relief.

transmission cells   Afferent neurons that connect to other neurons; also called secondary afferens

Suggested Readings

 Brownlee, S., & Schrof, J. M. (1997). The quality of mercy: Effective pain treatments already exist. Why aren't doctors using them? *U.S. News & World Report, 122*(10), 54–61.

This article presents the puzzle of chronic pain but also criticizes the treatment that patients typically receive. The authors assert that treatments are available but that physicians and patients both fear overusing drugs that can be helpful. Available through InfoTrac College Edition by Wadsworth Publishing Company.

Fordyce, W. E. (1990). Learned pain: Pain as behavior. In J. J. Bonica (Ed.), *The management of pain* (2nd ed., pp. 291–299). Malvern, PA: Lea & Febiger.

One of the foremost authorities on pain discusses the influence of learning on pain behavior. Fordyce points out that the consequences of pain behaviors are often reinforcing to the pain patient.

Melzack, R. (1992, April). Phantom limbs. *Scientific Amer-*

ican, 266, 120–126.

This article includes a review of the gate control theory and a description of Melzack's neuromatrix theory, which he formulated as a result of the failure of the gate control theory to explain phantom limb sensation and pain.

Morris, D. B. (1994, Autumn). Pain's dominion: What we make of pain. *Wilson Quarterly,* pp. 8–33.

Morris concentrates on the cultural meaning of pain in the historical context. His review is easy to read and provides information on the personal difficulties of dealing with pain in a medical establishment that tends to find the concept troublesome.

Turk, D. C. (1996). Biopsychosocial perspective on chronic pain. In R. J. Gatchel & D. C. Turk (Eds.), *Psychological approaches to pain management: A practitioner's handbook* (pp. 3–32). New York: Guilford Press.

Turk reviews theoretical and practical issues related to pain along with research in the field.

CHAPTER 8

Coping with Stress and Pain

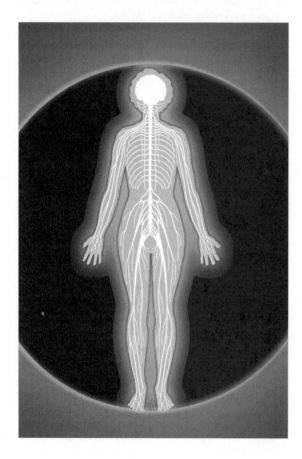

QUESTIONS

This chapter focuses on eight basic questions:

1. How does social support influence coping?

2. How does personal control influence coping?

3. How effective is relaxation training in coping with stress and pain?

4. How effective is hypnotic treatment in coping with stress and pain?

5. How effective is biofeedback in coping with stress and pain?

6. How effective is behavior modification in coping with stress and pain?

7. How effective is cognitive therapy in coping with stress and pain?

8. How effective are multimodal approaches in coping with stress and pain?

RICH AND BARB: HOW CAN THEY COPE WITH STRESS AND PAIN?

In Chapter 5 we met Rick, the college student who had lost his job, experienced a divorce and the loss of his father and close friend, and faced financial problems. Rick was feeling an unusually high level of stress as a result of the myriad life events that befell him. We learned that Rick tried to cope with his stress by isolating himself and working two and sometimes three jobs. These strategies, of course, were not beneficial to his overall health. He also decided to begin college and to become more involved in church activities. Were any of these choices good alternatives for managing his problems? What other methods were avail-able to Rick? Would those alternatives have been more helpful?

In Chapter 7 we considered the case of Barb, a young woman experiencing chronic pain. Barb had received physical treatment for pain control, including surgery, opiate drugs, transcutaneous electrical nerve stimulation, and physical therapy. When Barb found herself taking the prescription opiates and drinking alcohol as her only coping strategy, she sought alternatives, which included a pain treatment program with biofeedback and relaxation training. This program helped Barb find alternative ways to cope and to control her pain. In this chapter, we reconsider the problems of Rick, Barb, and the millions of other Americans who suffer from elevated stress and chronic pain.

 CHECK YOUR HEALTH RISKS

Check the items that apply to you.

☐ 1. I live alone.

☐ 2. If I needed a favor, I wouldn't have anyone to call.

☐ 3. I would like to talk to someone about my personal problems, but I don't have anyone I can trust to keep a secret.

☐ 4. I feel isolated from my family.

☐ 5. My job offers little or no opportunity to make any meaningful decisions.

☐ 6. I believe strongly in fate—whatever will be will be.

☐ 7. I feel responsible for nearly everything that happens around me.

☐ 8. I have a lot of stress in my life, but I don't know how to reduce it.

☐ 9. When I feel too much stress, I turn to alcohol as a way of reducing that stress.

☐ 10. I suffer from chronic pain and believe that pain-killing drugs are the only way to control it.

☐ 11. When I'm in pain, I find that alcohol is a good way to forget about it.

☐ 12. I suffer from back pain, and when it becomes too intense, I stay in bed for a couple of days.

Each of these items represents an attitude, situation, or behavior that may increase your risk for a stress-related illness or lead you to unhealthy or ineffective ways of coping with stress and pain. Count your check marks to evaluate these risks. As you read this chapter, you will see the advantages of adopting other attitudes or behaviors to minimize your chances of developing a stress-related illness and to enhance your health and well-being.

Personal Resources That Influence Coping

Stress and chronic pain are common conditions for humans—common but not normal. The normal tendency is toward health, and any inclination away from health sets up a state of "disease." People fight against distress and disease in a variety of ways. One way is through the immune system, the body's natural protection from invasion by foreign material, as discussed in Chapter 6. People sometimes adjust to pain through medical treatments, such as drugs and surgery, which are discussed in Chapter 7. Still other ways of seeking relief from stress and chronic pain include taking recreational drugs, overeating, abusing alcohol, smoking, and exercising. Exercising usually promotes health, but the other behaviors are ultimately unhealthy, and even exercise can be carried to an unhealthy extreme. The health-related effects of smoking, drinking, eating, and exercising are discussed in Chapters 13 through 16.

This chapter looks at several psychological strategies for coping with stress and chronic pain. These strategies are used in programs oriented toward helping people cope with stress and pain problems. Such formal programs offer help to people who seek treatment, but personal resources, such as social support and feelings of personal control, help everyone to cope.

Social Support

Some people react better than others to stress and chronic pain, and they tend to be the ones who have greater personal resources for coping. One of the most beneficial personal resources appears to be social support from family members, friends, and health care providers. This section discusses the meaning of social support and suggests possible reasons why social support seems to protect against disease and death.

The Meaning of Social Support   What is social support? Although social support has been widely researched, no single definition of the concept has emerged (Sarason & Sarason, 1994), and researchers have used dozens of inventories to measure social support, many of them with questionable reliability and validity (Kaplan, 1994). The term **social support** refers to a variety of material and emotional supports a person receives from others. The related concepts of **social contacts** and **social network** are sometimes used interchangeably, and both refer to the number and kinds of people with whom one associates. The opposite of social contacts is **social isolation**, which refers to an absence of specific meaningful interpersonal relations. People with a high level of social support ordinarily have a broad social network and many social contacts; socially isolated people have neither.

Social support may be measured in terms of either the structure or the function of social relationships (Wills, 1998). Structural support includes the number of social relationships and the structure of interconnections among these relationships. Functional support includes emotional support, information or advice, and companionship, as well as assistance with financial or material needs. These two measures are not strongly related to each other, but both are related to health.

The Link between Social Support and Health
Stress researchers generally agree that a link exists between social support and health; people who receive high levels of social support are usually healthier than those who do not. Evidence from studies done in California, Georgia, Michigan, and Scandinavia (Wills, 1998) demonstrates that people with higher levels of social support have lower rates of mortality and better health than people with lower levels of support.

The Alameda County Study (Berkman & Syme, 1979) was the first to establish a strong link between social support and longevity. This study indicated that lack of social support was as strongly linked to mortality as cigarette smoking and a sedentary lifestyle. Figure 8.1 shows that women in all age groups had lower mortality rates than men (as indicated by the height of the bar in the graph). However, for both men and women, as the number of social ties decreased, the death rate in-

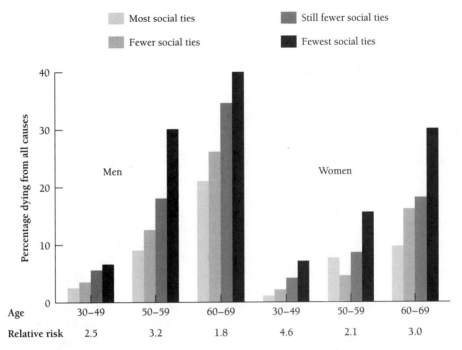

Figure 8.1 **Social isolation and 9-year mortality in Alameda County, California, 1965–1974.** *Source:* From "Social Networks, Host Resistance, and Mortality: A Nine-Year Follow-up of Alameda County Residents," by L. F. Berkman & S. L. Syme, 1979, *American Journal of Epidemiology,* 109, p. 190. Copyright © 1979 by the Johns Hopkins University School of Hygiene and Public Health. Reprinted by permission of the publisher and the senior author.

creased. In general, participants with the fewest social ties were two to four times more likely to die than participants with the most social ties. This trend was most pronounced from age 30 to 49, and it extended to both men and women.

Marriage, Gender, Ethnicity, and Social Support

Marriage (or at least happy marriage) would seem to provide excellent social support for both partners, but the benefits of marriage are not equal for women and men. The studies in the United States and Scandinavia that demonstrated the advantages of social support also showed that marriage benefits men more than women (Chesney & Darbes, 1998). The mechanisms of this advantage are not clear, but women's role as caregiver may be the key. Women tend to provide more care than they receive and may ignore their own health in taking care of their spouses and children.

For older people, marriage may not be as important as having a confidant. A survey of men and women age 65 and older (Oxman, Berkman, Kasl, Freeman, & Barrett, 1992) showed that the more social support these older people experienced, the lower were their levels of depression. Emotional support provided more protection against depression than tangible support, such as a visit from a friend. The older people who never had a confidant were more likely to become depressed than were those who had never been married, and long-standing confidants were more protective than those gained in more recent years.

The health benefits of having a wife would lead to the prediction that husbands would be more affected by the death of their spouse than would wives. This prediction is correct (Martikainen & Valkomen, 1996); death of a spouse increased mortality risk for the surviving spouse, but men were at greater risk than women. The risk was higher not only for men but also for younger persons of either gender. In addition, the risk was higher during the 6 months following the spouse's death. Death from heart disease and cancer increased, but the greatest mortality risks were from accidental and violent deaths, especially suicide. Again, these risks may relate to typical gender roles in which men depend on their wives for support, but women cultivate a larger social network of family members and friends and are thus more likely to receive support after the death of a husband.

Although men gain more from marriage, women gain more from social support, at least up to a point. In the Alameda County Study (Berkman & Syme, 1979), women with few social ties had a substantially higher relative risk for mortality than comparable men (see Figure 8.1). A meta-analysis (Schwarzer & Leppin, 1989) confirmed this finding, revealing that for women the overall correlation between social support and good health was about .20, but for men the correlation was only .08. Many social contacts do not extend (and may decrease) women's advantage (Orth-Gomér, 1998). A possible explanation for this finding is that women with many social contacts are overextended, receiving demands for support that may add to rather than detract from their stress.

Does ethnic background play a role in social support? African American and Hispanic American families have traditions of close extended family relationships that can provide stronger social support than those of many European American families. Analyses of African American (Neighbors, 1997) and Mexican American (Castro, Coe, Gutierres, & Saenz, 1996) families indicated that these relationships can be sources of stress as well as support. Indeed, the people who provide support at one time are those who cause problems at other times. An analysis of network characteristics among various ethnic groups (Pugliese & Shook, 1998) revealed only small differences in size of social networks. This study confirmed earlier findings (Berkman, 1986) concerning White men's tendency to have smaller social networks and to use social support less than others but revealed some interactions be-

tween gender and ethnicity. For example, White men tended to have smaller social networks when they were employed, but employment was not a factor in network size for men from other ethnic groups or for women. The findings from this study suggested that the structure and use of social networks are complex and influenced by a number of factors, including marriage, gender, and ethnicity.

How Does Social Support Contribute to Health?
If stress causes illness, then social support may offer some buffer against stress-related illnesses. Evidence suggests that this buffering effect is especially strong for European American men but also applies to other people. What does social support provide that is helpful? What is stressful, even life-threatening, about social isolation? Answers to these questions are still not clear, but several possible routes exist for social support to affect health (Wills, 1998). One route is through health-related behaviors, another is through appraisal and coping, and a third is through moderation of physiological responses to stress.

People who are isolated are less likely to have friends and acquaintances who encourage them to protect their health or who insist that they go to the doctor when they are sick. One study (Broman, 1993) showed that social isolation led to unhealthy coping responses such as smoking and abusing alcohol, which can negatively affect health. In addition, people who were more socially involved were more likely to use seat belts, indicating that integration into a social network can increase safety behaviors as well as decrease risk behaviors. Thus, social support networks can encourage people to behave in healthy ways. This explanation may contribute to the relationships between social support and health, but an increased number of healthy practices is not the only explanation for the link. In the Alameda County study, for instance, health practices were taken into account, and lack of social support still had an independent association with mortality. Suggestions and encouragement from friends may enhance healthy behaviors, but they are not the only answer.

People with strong support networks know that assistance is available, so when they experience stress, they may appraise the stressor as less threatening than people who have fewer coping resources (Wills, 1998). Indeed, knowledge of the availability of support (even if that support is not used) can reduce the magnitude of the stress response (Uchino & Garvey, 1997). Support may also directly change coping strategies such that people with more sources of support are better able to gain information, solve problems, and implement solutions.

Social support may also alter the physiological responses to stress (Chesney & Darbes, 1998). This view is referred to as the *buffering hypothesis,* which suggests that social support lessens or eliminates the harmful effects of stress and therefore protects against disease and death. Some laboratory research has shown that people react less strongly to stressors when social support is available. Thus, people who have less social support may react more strongly to stress, showing higher levels of neurohormones and more physical damage than people with strong social support networks.

Losing his father, his friend, and his family resulted in Rick's social support system "falling apart." In addition, he began to have trouble getting along with his colleagues at work. Being isolated and feeling alone was one of the aspects of the situation that Rick found most distressing. This lack of a social support system added to his stress. Rick managed to construct another support system through beginning college and becoming more involved in church activities, a strategy that was wise and probably beneficial.

Mobilizing Social Support If social support provides health advantages, can people improve their social support through specific efforts? Perhaps so, but increasing social support is not as easy as increasing the number of social contacts. People who are high in hostility receive less social support than those who are lower in hostility (Hardy & Smith, 1988), and increasing the number of social contacts would probably not increase social support for people who are unpleasant or difficult to be-

friend. (See the Would You Believe . . . ? box for an interesting alternative.)

One hint concerning increased social support comes from the gender difference in social support: Women tend to have larger and more active support networks than men. The reason for this difference can be seen in women's friendship style, which tends to rely on emotional sharing, cooperation, and positive nonverbal signals (Argyle, 1992). Indeed, both men and women prefer to have women as confidants, but women are more likely than men to fulfill this preference. Therefore, women's tendency to form such networks gives them an advantage in social support. Men can gain the advantages of a large, active social support network when they form such networks.

Are people who are lacking in social support destined to remain so? Two strategies exist to improve social support (Gottlieb, 1996). One strategy involves enhancing existing support sources and the other creates support networks in the form of support groups. Professionals are typically the agents who advise people about restructuring networks to enhance support for families with chronic stress. For example, restructuring might be useful to those caring for a family member with a chronic illness such as Alzheimer's disease. Support groups are constructed networks consisting of people with similar stressful circumstances. Meeting with others in similar circumstances can give people many valuable experiences, including emotional support, information, and practical help. A huge variety of support groups exist to serve people with a variety of conditions and to help their families cope. In summary, there are several ways to boost social support, including making changes to allow the formation of more intimate personal relationships, enhancing existing support structures, and joining a support group.

Personal Control

A second factor that may affect a person's ability to cope with stressful life events is a feeling of personal control. Many investigators believe that people who feel that they have some control over the events of

WOULD YOU BELIEVE...?

Pets Can Be Sources of Support

Would you believe that pets can provide humans with healthy social support? Many people love animals and include pets in their lives, treating them almost like one of the family. In addition to providing enjoyment, the companionship that pets offer may provide health benefits to their owners, according to some research.

Although companion animals cannot offer the equivalent of material support, they can provide companionship and emotional support. Indeed, people form attachments with their pets that share characteristics with the types of attachments they form with other people (Collis & McNicholas, 1998). People seek the company of their pets, talk to them, play with them, and care for the pets' needs. In addition, pets offer tactile comfort, are more available than humans, and are not as judgmental as friends and family may be. Most people can maintain a relationship with a companion animal more easily than with a human companion. These factors can make pets good and easily available sources of support.

The availability factor may be especially important for older people who have experienced decreased social contacts due to losses of family and friends. Loneliness can be a devastating problem for such people, and loneliness and attachment to a pet were found to be higher in older people who had no human confidant (Keil, 1998). The importance of animal companionship may extend to physical as well as mental health and quality of life. Older pet owners who experienced stress made fewer visits to physicians than equally stressed older people who had no

pet (Siegel, 1990). This result suggests that forming a relationship with a pet may have the same type of stress buffering effects that come from human social support. In addition, a pet (especially a dog) can help people make contact with other humans, increasing the potential for support from the pet as well as from people.

The health benefits of relationships with pets extend to the leading cause of death—cardiovascular disease and include lower systolic blood pressure and plasma triglycerides (Jennings et al., 1998). Although these differences are small, considering the number of people who have pets, the decreased risk is large enough to have an impact on community health. Whether the advantages are due directly to alterations of physical responses or to some other factor that pet owners have in common, several risk factors for cardiovascular disease are lower in pet owners. Indeed, the potential routes for these effects are the same possibilities that exist for the benefits of social support from humans.

Should people acquire pets to improve their health? This strategy may be effective, at least for some people. People who do not like animals, of course, would not only make poor companions for their animals but would also fail to form the attachment that is probably a necessary component for gaining support. Those who like animals and would enjoy a companion animal may profit. To sum up, many people, particularly older people, may improve the quality of their lives and health through nonhuman social support.

---

their lives are better able to cope with stress than are people who feel that their lives are determined by forces outside themselves. Rick felt that the events that happened to him were beyond his control, and he was accustomed to feeling in control.

Research in the area of personal control was given an impetus in 1966 when Julian Rotter published a scale for measuring internal and external control of reinforcement. Rotter hypothesized that people can be placed along a continuum according to the extent to which they believe they are in control of the important events in their lives. Those who believe they control their own lives score in the direction of *internal locus of control* whereas those people who believe that luck, fate, or the acts of others are the determinants of their lives score high on *external locus of control.*

Psychologists have applied the locus of control concept to health problems in order to learn if a sense of personal control can help people adopt a healthy lifestyle. For example, one study (Jih, Sirgo, & Thomure, 1995) studied locus of control and drinking behavior in college and high school students and found that students high in external control tended to drink more in a variety of situations, both pleasant and unpleasant. Other studies have supported the relationship between external or internal control and drinking behavior. One study (Clements, York, & Rohrer; 1995) showed a direct relationship between external scores and degree of alcoholism, and another study (Koski-Jannes, 1994) reported that high internal scores predicted an abstinence from drinking for alcoholics attending treatment programs.

A classic example of the effects of personal control was reported by Ellen Langer and Judith Rodin (1976) in a study that demonstrated the importance of a sense of personal control for health. These researchers studied older nursing home residents, some of whom were encouraged to assume more responsibility and control over their daily lives and some of whom had decisions made for them. The type of control was fairly minor: rearranging their furniture, choosing when and whom to visit in the home, deciding what leisure activities to pursue, and so on. In addition, these residents were offered a small plant, which they were free to accept or reject and to care for as they wished. A comparison group of residents received information that emphasized the responsibility of the nursing staff, and each received a plant.

The two groups of residents were approximately equal in age, gender, physical and psycho-

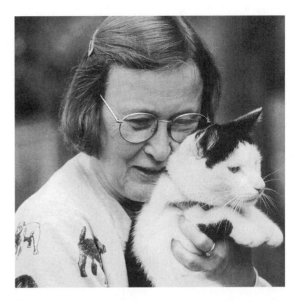

Caring for a pet can provide a sense of control, and people can receive social support from pets.

logical health, and prior socioeconomic status. The main difference was in the amount of control they had, and that factor made a substantial difference in health. Residents in the responsibility-induced group were happier, more active and more alert; they had a higher level of general well-being. In just 3 weeks, most of the comparison group (71%) had become more debilitated, whereas nearly all the responsibility-induced group (93%) showed some overall mental and physical improvement.

An 18-month follow-up of these same residents (Rodin & Langer, 1977) showed that residents in the original responsibility-induced group retained their advantage. They were more healthy, active, sociable, vigorous, and self-initiating than residents in the original comparison group. In addition, the mortality rate in the original responsibility-induced group was lower than expected and also lower than that for the original comparison group. The significance of these findings is obvious: Older people (and perhaps others as well) seem to thrive on personal control and responsibility.

How much control does a person need in order to feel in control? The Langer and Rodin studies suggest that control over relatively minor matters can have major consequences in the life of the individual. People need to be able to make choices and to assume responsibility for these choices.

In Summary

Humans have a natural tendency toward health and away from distress, disease, and pain. When "dis-eases" become part of our lives, we attempt to cope with them in order to restore our health. Some attempts at coping, such as self-medication with alcohol and drugs, have long-term disadvantages rather than benefits, but other methods of coping provide ways to manage these problems.

Some people cope successfully with stress and chronic pain because they possess sufficient personal resources such as social support and a strong feeling of being in control of their lives. Social support, defined as the emotional quality of one's social contacts, is inversely related to disease and death. In general, people with high levels of social support, compared to those with low levels, are only about half as likely to die within a designated period of time. These findings are most pronounced for European American men, but other groups also show some benefit from a network of quality relationships. People with adequate social support probably receive more encouragement and advice regarding good health practices, have advantages in coping, and may react less strongly to stress than people who are socially isolated. All of these factors can contribute to greater health and lower mortality.

Adequate feelings of personal control also seem to enable people to cope better with stress and illness. People who believe that their lives are controlled by fate or outside forces have greater difficulty changing health-related behaviors than do those who believe that the locus of control resides with themselves. The classic study by Langer and Rodin (1976) demonstrated that when people are allowed to assume even small amounts of personal control and responsibility, they seem to live longer and healthier lives.

Techniques for Coping with Stress and Pain

Both social support and personal control seem to enhance one's ability to cope with stress and pain. In addition to these two personal resources, an increasing number of nonmedical interventions are being used by health professionals to help people cope with pain and stress. Among these are relaxation training, hypnotic techniques, biofeedback, behavior modification, cognitive therapy, and various combinations of these techniques—that is, multimodal approaches.

Relaxation Training

Relaxation training is perhaps the simplest and easiest to use of all psychological interventions. The therapeutic uses of relaxation methods predate modern psychology, with ancient Egyptians, Hebrews, Tibetans, and others using some form of rhythmic breathing or chanting for the purpose of healing (Lavey & Taylor, 1985). Modern uses of relaxation training are usually traced to Edmond Jacobson (1934, 1938) who termed this method *progressive relaxation*. In progressive muscle relaxation, people learn to relax one muscle group at a time, progressing through the body's entire range of muscle groups until the whole body is relaxed.

What Is Relaxation Training? Progressive muscle relaxation is only one of several types of relaxation techniques; others include meditative relaxation and guided imagery. For *progressive muscle relaxation,* patients are first given a rationale for the procedure, including an explanation that their present tension is mostly a physical state resulting from tense muscles (Jacobson, 1938). While reclining in a comfortable chair, often with eyes closed and with no distracting lights or sounds, patients first breathe deeply and exhale slowly.

BECOMING HEALTHIER

Progressive muscle relaxation is a technique that you may be able to use to cope with stress and pain. Although some people may need the help of a trained therapist to master this approach, others are able to train themselves. To learn progressive muscle relaxation, recline in a comfortable chair in a room with no distractions. You may wish to remove your shoes and either dim the lights or close your eyes to enhance relaxation. Next, breathe deeply and exhale slowly. Repeat this deep breathing exercise several times until you begin to feel your body becoming more and more relaxed. The next step is to select a muscle group (for example, your left hand) and deliberately tense that group of muscles. If you begin with your hand, make a fist and squeeze the fingers into your hand as hard as you can. Hold that tension for about 10 seconds and then slowly release the tension, concentrating on the relaxing, soothing sensations in your hand as the tension gradually drains away. Once the left hand is relaxed, shift to the right hand and repeat the procedure, while keeping your left hand as relaxed as possible. After both hands are relaxed, go through the same tensing and relaxing sequence progressively with other muscle groups, including the arms, shoulders, neck, mouth, tongue, forehead, eyes, toes, feet, calves, thighs, back, and stomach. Then repeat the deep breathing exercises until you achieve a deep feeling of relaxation. Focus on the enjoyable sensation of relaxation, restricting your attention to the pleasant internal events and away from irritating external sources of pain or stress. You will probably need to practice this procedure several times to learn to quickly place your body into a state of deep relaxation.

After this, the series of deep muscle relaxation exercises begins, a process described in the box, Becoming Healthier. Therapists frequently encourage patients to focus on the pleasant feeling of relaxation, a condition that directs attention away from external sources of anxiety, pain, and stress. Patients can rate their level of relaxation on a scale of 1 to 10, or they can signal the therapist by raising their index finger whenever they experience increasing levels of pain, discomfort, or distress.

Once patients learn the relaxation technique, they may practice independently at home. If independent practice is too difficult, prerecorded audiotapes are available that allow patients to listen to the soothing voice of a professional instructor without returning to the clinic. Length of relaxation training programs varies, but 6 to 8 weeks and about 10 sessions with an instructor are usually sufficient to allow patients to easily and independently enter a state of deep relaxation (Blanchard & Andrasik, 1985).

Another frequently used relaxation technique is *meditative relaxation,* developed by Herbert Benson and his colleagues (Benson, 1974; Benson, Beary, & Carol, 1974). This approach derives from various religious meditative practices, but as used by psychologists, it has no religious connotations. Bensonian relaxation combines muscle relaxation with a quiet environment, comfortable position, repetitive sound, and passive attitude. Participants usually sit with eyes closed and muscles relaxed. They then focus attention on their breathing and repeat silently a sound, such as "om" or "one" with each breath for about 20 minutes. Repetition of the single word prevents distracting thoughts and sustains muscle relaxation. Meditation involves conscious intention to focus attention on a single thought or image along with effort not to be distracted by other thoughts.

Mindfulness meditation is another type of meditation that has its roots in ancient Buddhist practice but has implications for anyone suffering from

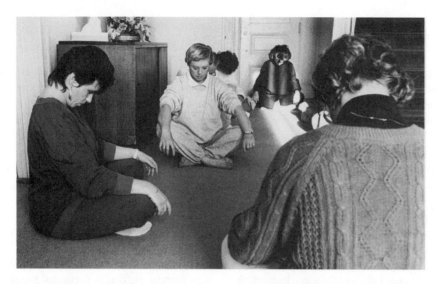

Meditation is one relaxation technique that can help people cope with a variety of stress-related problems.

stress, anxiety, or pain (Kabat-Zinn, 1993; Kabat-Zinn, Lipworth, & Burney, 1985). In mindfulness meditation, people do not try to ignore unpleasant thoughts or sensations by focusing on their breathing or on a single sound. Rather, they take the opposite approach, focusing on any thoughts or sensations as they occur. However, they are asked to observe these thoughts nonjudgmentally. By noting thoughts objectively as they occur, people can gain insight into how they see the world and what motivates them. "Observing without judging, moment by moment, helps you see what is on your mind without editing or censoring it, without intellectualizing it or getting lost in your own incessant thinking" (Kabat-Zinn, 1993, p. 263).

Guided imagery has some elements in common with meditative relaxation, but it also has important differences. In guided imagery, patients conjure up a calm, peaceful image such as the repetitive rhythmic roar of an ocean or the quiet beauty of a pastoral scene. Patients then concentrate on that image for the duration of a painful or anxiety-filled situation. The assumption underlying guided imagery is that a person cannot concentrate on more than one thing at a time. Therefore, the patient

must imagine an especially powerful or delightful scene—one so pleasant or powerful that it averts attention from the painful experience.

In addition to progressive muscle relaxation, meditative relaxation, mindfulness meditation, and guided imagery, many health psychologists have used hypnotic-induced relaxation and biofeedback-induced relaxation to alleviate pain and stress. Combining two or more interventions frequently leads to increased rates of success, but this strategy yields less information about the effectiveness of each individual intervention. We discuss these and other multimodal approaches later in this chapter.

How Effective Is Relaxation Training?

Like other psychological inventions, relaxation can only be regarded as effective if it proves more powerful than a placebo. Research (Cox, Freundlich, & Meyer, 1975; Turner & Chapman, 1982a) indicates that relaxation techniques are generally more effective than placebos. In addition, relaxation is at least equal to biofeedback in reducing pain and alleviating stress and it may be an essential part of both biofeedback and hypnotic therapies.

Relaxation techniques have been used successfully to treat both tension and migraine headaches. An early review (Turner & Chapman, 1982a) looked at the research on the efficacy of relaxation procedures and biofeedback on tension headache. All the studies reviewed reported at least some benefit for relaxation training, and the authors concluded that relaxation methods were superior to placebos and equal to EMG biofeedback in controlling tension headache pain. A later meta-analysis (Hermann, Kim, & Blanchard, 1995) found that when progressive muscle relaxation was added to thermal biofeedback, the combination was superior to psychological and drug placebos and more effective than medication in controlling migraine headache in children.

Progressive muscle relaxation can be an effective treatment for such stress-related disorders as migraine and tension headache, depression, hypertension, low back pain, and the stressful effects of cancer chemotherapy. A meta-analysis of studies (Carlson & Hoyle, 1993) found that an abbreviated form of progressive muscle relaxation was generally helpful in coping with each of these disorders, although the effect size varied substantially from study to study. This variation was due partially to differences in procedures: Relaxation training was generally more effective when patients had an adequate number of sessions, were trained in individual rather than group sessions, used audiotapes to supplement their training, and had enough time to gain a high level of skill with the techniques. In this analysis, progressive muscle relaxation seemed to work best with tension headache.

Other reviews (Blanchard & Andrasik, 1985; Lehrer, Carr, Sargunaraj, & Woolfolk, 1994; Syrjala & Chapman, 1984) have reached much the same conclusion; that is, the most successful use of relaxation training is in helping people cope with tension headache. In summary, these reviews suggest that relaxation training alone (1) significantly reduces a substantial number of chronic headaches, (2) is more effective than a placebo, and (3) is at least equal to biofeedback in decreasing tension headache pain.

However, progressive relaxation training is no panacea for pain reduction. Perhaps as many as 50% of tension headache patients do not experience significant relief through relaxation. For this reason, Edward Blanchard and Frank Andrasik (1985) viewed relaxation as a necessary first step in a pain management program, and one that may not be effective for all pain sufferers.

A second form of relaxation is meditation. Can meditative relaxation help people to cope with pain, stress, and anxiety? Jon Kabat-Zinn and his colleagues (Kabat-Zinn et al., 1985) studied the effectiveness of mindfulness meditation on chronic pain patients and found it to be more effective than a traditional intervention that included physical therapy, analgesics, and antidepressants. Patients trained to use mindfulness meditation reported a decrease in present pain, negative body image, depression, anxiety, and mood disturbance, and fewer psychological symptoms. Moreover, they decreased their use of pain medications, improved their activity levels, and increased their feelings of self-esteem. In another study (Kabat-Zinn et al., 1992), a meditation-based stress-reduction program for treating anxiety disorders was effective in over 90% of the participants with generalized anxiety disorder, panic disorder, or panic disorder with agoraphobia. Patients taught meditation techniques had significant reductions in anxiety and depression and maintained these gains at a 3-year follow-up (Miller, Fletcher, & Kabat-Zinn, 1995).

How does meditation compare with other behavioral treatments for treating stress and anxiety? The literature on progressive muscle relaxation, biofeedback, cognitive-behavioral strategies, and meditation includes few studies on meditation (Murphy, 1996). However, the studies that have evaluated meditation have found it was consistently more effective than any of the other approaches.

What is the effective ingredient in mindfulness meditation? Some evidence (Astin, 1997) suggests that meditation may be simply a powerful cognitive behavioral strategy for changing the way people respond to stressful life events. In any event, mindfulness meditation can be considered as an effective therapy for at least some stress-related disorders, and it may be at least as powerful as any other behavioral intervention.

Guided imagery is a third relaxation strategy for coping with pain, anxiety, and stress. However, the effectiveness of guided imagery is not yet well established because researchers have conducted only a relative few experimental studies on its efficacy. In a series of early studies, John Horan and his colleagues found that *in vivo* imagery reduced reported dental discomfort (Horan, Layng, & Pursell, 1976), childbirth anxiety and discomfort (Horan, 1973), and experimentally induced pain (Horan & Dellinger, 1974). Other studies found that guided imagery is more effective than either a therapist-attention group or a no-treatment control group in reducing anxiety and nausea both during and after chemotherapy (Lyles, Burish, Krozely, & Oldham, 1982); adds significantly to relaxation in helping severely burned patients cope with pain (Achterberg, Kenner, & Lawlis, 1988); is superior to biofeedback in treating migraine headache (Ilacqua, 1994); and is an effective technique for reducing postoperative pain and reducing duration of hospital stays in child surgical patients (Lambert, 1996).

Barb learned relaxation as part of her pain program and continues to practice relaxation for her chronic pain. She was amazed at how difficult it was to relax and how much practice it took to do so. She believes that relaxation helped her take control of her pain, and she is now committed to this method of pain control. Table 8.1 summarizes the effectiveness of relaxation techniques.

Hypnotic Treatment

Except for relaxation and acupuncture, hypnotic treatment is the oldest nonmedical treatment for pain. Early in the 19th century, physicians were using hypnotic processes as analgesia during surgery (Hilgard & Hilgard, 1994). The history of hypnosis, however, reveals a cycle of acceptance and rejection, and some controversy still surrounds its effectiveness as a treatment for pain (Hilgard & Hilgard, 1994).

Although trancelike conditions are as old as human history, modern hypnosis is usually thought to have had its beginnings in the last part of the 18th century, when Franz Anton Mesmer, an Austrian physician, conducted elaborate demonstrations in Paris. Mesmer's work was discredited by a committee of "scientific experts," but modifications of his technique, known as *mesmerism,* soon spread to other parts of the world. By the 1830s, mesmerism was being used by some surgeons as an anesthetic during major operations (Hilgard & Hilgard, 1994). With the discovery of chemical anesthetics, the popularity of hypnosis waned, but during the late 19th century, many European physicians, including Sigmund Freud, employed hypnotic procedures in the treatment of mental illness. Since the beginning of the 20th century, the popularity of hypnosis as a medical and psychological tool has continued to wax and wane. Its present position is still somewhat controversial, but a significant number of practitioners within medicine and psychology are taking advantage of the positive aspects of this procedure to treat health-related problems, especially the management of pain.

What Is Hypnotic Treatment?   Not only is the use of hypnotic processes still controversial, but the precise nature of hypnosis is also a debatable issue. Some authorities, such as Joseph Barber (1996) and Ernest Hilgard (1978) regard hypnosis as an altered *state* of consciousness in which the person's stream of consciousness is divided or dissociated. Joseph Barber believes that hypnotic analgesia works through a process of negative hallucination, or simply not perceiving something that one would ordinarily perceive. To Hilgard, the process of **induction**—that is, being placed into a hypnotic state—is central to the hypnotic process. After induction, the responsive person enters a state of divided or dissociated consciousness that is essentially different from the normal state. This altered state of consciousness allows people to respond to suggestion and to control physiological processes that they cannot control in the normal state of consciousness.

Table 8.1   Effectiveness of relaxation techniques

Problem	Findings	Studies
1. Tension headache	Relaxation is superior to placebo and equal to biofeedback.	Blanchard & Andrasik, 1985; Lehrer et al., 1994; Turner & Chapman, 1982a
2. Migraine headache in children	Relaxation added to biofeedback is more effective than placebos or drugs.	Hermann et al., 1995
3. Stress-related disorders	Progressive muscle relaxation helps in coping with headache, hypertension, and effects of chemotherapy in cancer patients.	Carlson & Hoyle, 1993
4. Anxiety disorders	Mindfulness meditation is better than physical therapy, analgesics, and antidepressants.	Kabat-Zinn et al., 1992; Miller et al., 1995
5. Worksite stress	Meditation techniques are consistently superior to other behavioral strategies.	Murphy, 1996
6. Dental discomfort and childbirth discomfort	Guided imagery is effective in coping with pain.	Horan et al., 1976; Horan, 1973
7. Unpleasant effects of chemotherapy	Guided imagery is more effective than placebos.	Lyles et al., 1982
8. Burn pain	Guided imagery adds to other relaxation strategies.	Achterberg at al., 1988
9. Migraine headache	Guided imagery is superior to biofeedback.	Ilacqua, 1994
10. Postoperative pain	Guided imagery reduces children's pain and shortens their hospital stay.	Lambert, 1996

In contrast, Theodore X. Barber (1982, 1984) views the hypnotic process as a more generalized *trait,* or a relatively permanent characteristic of people who respond well to suggestion. In addition, he rejects the notion that induction is necessary and holds that the suggestive procedures can be just as effective without the person's entering a trancelike state. Another view holds that hypnosis is a form of focused attention that makes it easier for people to relax and to learn to control their body functions (Olness, 1993). However, Joseph Barber (1996) insists that the hypnotic process involves something more than simple relaxation. Regardless of some of these technical differences, most current hypnotherapists believe that all hypnosis is self-hypnosis.

Although Joseph Barber contends that hypnotic induction is both more than and different from relaxation, a look at his technique reveals that relaxation training is a critical step in the process. Barber (1996) described six steps in his hypnotic technique, the first three of which closely resemble several relaxation training procedures discussed earlier. First, the hypnotherapist secures patients' attention by telling them that they have the capacity and imagination to retrain their own nervous system. This first step also includes the suggestion that patients should sit back in their chair, close their eyes, and relax. Second, the therapist narrows patients' range of attention by asking them to pay attention to the therapist's voice. Third, the therapist asks patients to further restrict their range of attention by directing it inward, concentrating, for example, on each breath. Barber's fourth step is to suggest dissociation; that is to suggest to patients that they become completely absorbed in the comfort of their own breathing. The therapist might also suggest that patients feel a tingling sensation in their finger tips, a sensation that will spread to the rest of their body. With a successful fourth step, induction is complete. Fifth, the therapist offers a therapeutic suggestion, telling patients that whatever is bothering them will soon disappear. In the final step, the therapist gives suggestions to end the induction, suggesting to patients that they will feel well and relaxed when they open their eyes. Although Barber's hypnotic treatment may be more than relaxation, it seems clear that relaxation training is an essential first component.

Despite the debate over the nature of the hypnotic state and the necessity of induction, most experimenters and clinicians agree that the hypnosuggestive technique is an important clinical tool, especially for the control of pain. However, not all patients profit equally from these procedures; some people are more suggestible than others, and these "good subjects" are better able to use hypnotic processes to cope with pain. What percentage of people are suggestible? Suggestibility seems to be widely distributed among the population, almost following a normal, bell-shaped curve. For this reason, clinicians need to determine the level of suggestibility of their patients before using hypnosis as an analgesic.

Does suggestion actually block pain or does it merely lower awareness of or reports of pain? Hilgard and Hilgard (1994) demonstrated that highly hypnotizable people given the suggestion that they feel no pain could still rate their pain as substantial if they were given instructions to report all their sensations. Even though they showed few behavioral signs of pain and verbalized little or no discomfort, these hypnotized people still rated their pain as substantial. People who have been hypnotized with a suggestion for no pain still show physiological reactions such as changes in

respiration, heart rate, and blood pressure that accompany increases in pain (Orne, 1980). Therefore, hypnosis probably does not lower pain but instead alters the awareness of pain.

How Effective Is Hypnotic Treatment?   Like other psychological inventions, hypnotherapy can be regarded as effective only if it proves more powerful than a placebo. Although the placebo effect depends on suggestion, research (Jacobs, Kurtz, & Strube, 1995) has shown an advantage for hypnotic suggestion over the placebo effect, at least for highly suggestible patients. Thus, for people who are easily hypnotized, hypnotherapy is more effective than a simple placebo. However, people who are low in hypnotizability tend to respond to hypnotic suggestions of analgesia at rates comparable to their response to placebos (Miller, Barabasz, & Barabasz, 1991). Nevertheless, the pain-controlling effects of hypnosis are real and do not depend on one's expectations. Individual differences in susceptibility may mitigate hypnotherapy as a pain reducer for some individuals, but other people can receive substantial analgesic benefits from this technique.

Thus, although authorities differ in their opinions concerning the nature of the mechanisms for hypnotic analgesia, few doubt that hypnosis works, at least with some patients. The list of pains that are responsive to hypnotic procedures is extensive, but headache, cancer pain, and burn pain have received the most attention. In addition, hypnotherapy has been used successfully for childbirth, dental treatment, low back pain, and pain associated with sickle cell disease.

Hypnotherapy can be useful in helping people cope with migraine, tension, and cluster headaches. For example, in one experimental study (ter-Kuile et al., 1994), chronic headache patients were randomly assigned to a therapy group or a waiting-list control group. People receiving hypnotherapy reported greater reduction in headache pain compared with those in the control group. Consistent with many other studies, this investigation found that highly hypnotizable participants reported less pain at posttreatment and follow-up than participants who were low in hypnotizability.

A diagnosis of cancer almost always produces anxiety, and the progress of cancer often produces pain. Hypnotherapeutic techniques have helped cancer patients cope with both anxiety and pain. A review of empirical studies (Genuis, 1995) on the efficacy of hypnotherapy with child and adolescent cancer patients showed that six of the seven studies on anxiety found a significant and positive effect for hypnosis, and all seven studies found that hypnotic procedures helped children and adolescents cope with pain. Incidentally, two other studies reported that hypnosis could help reduce vomiting resulting from chemotherapy. This review indicates that hypnotic techniques can help reduce anxiety, pain, and the unpleasant side effects of cancer treatment. A later study with pediatric cancer patients (Smith, Barabasz, & Barabasz, 1996) found that Hilgard's hypnotic treatment significantly lowered pain, anxiety, and distress in highly hypnotizable children, but that for low hypnotizable children, distraction was equal to the hypnotic treatment.

Hypnotherapy has also been used to treat burn pain. A review (Van der Does & Van Dyck, 1989) examined 28 studies that used hypnosis with burn patients and found consistent evidence that hypnotherapy is an effective analgesia for burn pain. However, this review found no evidence that hypnosis could speed the healing of burn wounds. An experimental study (Patterson, & Ptacek, 1997) investigated the efficacy of hypnotic procedures with burn patients. Severe burn patients were randomly assigned to either a hypnosis group or a control group that offered attention, information, and instructions on relaxation. When all patients were included in the analysis, pain scores of the two groups did not differ. However, when the researchers looked only at patients with very high pain reports at baseline, the hypnosis group reported less posttreatment pain than the control group.

In addition to easing headache, cancer pain, and burn pain, hypnotic treatments have been used successfully to control both pain and stress during childbirth and after delivery (Mairs, 1995); to reduce medication and lessen dental pain and anxiety in patients receiving dental surgery (Enqvist, & Fischer, 1997); to reduce pain and suffering in patients with low back pain (Burte, Burte, & Araoz, 1994); and to improve sleep, lessen medication, and alleviate pain in patients with sickle cell disease (Dinges, Whitehouse, et al., 1997)

Despite strong evidence that hypnosis can decrease acute pain and manage chronic pain, many health care providers have gross misunderstanding of this form of analgesia. A survey (Bryant, 1993) of a large number of burn therapists and rehabilitation therapists found that many of them were not aware of recent research on the efficacy of hypnotherapy and that some expressed many of the same misconceptions of hypnosis that nonprofessionals have. For example, some believed that hypnosis is an altered state of consciousness in which patients are not aware of their surroundings and possess an enhanced ability to recall past events. Such misconceptions discourage the use of hypnosis.

As Table 8.2 shows, the hypnotic process can be an effective tool for coping with pain. Nevertheless, more research is needed to identify those people who will respond favorably to hypnosis, under what conditions they will respond, and for what types of pain problems.

Biofeedback

Until the 1960s, most people in the Western world assumed that conscious control of such physiological processes as heart rate, the secretion of digestive juices, and the constriction of blood vessels was impossible. These biological functions do not require conscious attention for their regulation, and conscious attempts at regulation seem to have little effect on these functions controlled by the autonomic nervous system.

Then, during the late 1960s, a number of researchers began to explore the possibility of controlling biological processes traditionally believed to be beyond conscious control (Nigl, 1984). Their efforts culminated in the development of **biofeedback,**

Table 8.2   Effectiveness of hypnotic techniques

Problem	Findings	Studies
1. Headache	Hypnosis reduces pain, especially for highly hypnotizable patients.	ter-Kuile et al., 1994
2. Cancer pain in children	Hypnosis reduces pain and anxiety in pediatric cancer patients, especially for hypnotizable children.	Genuis, 1995; Smith et al., 1996
3. Burn pain	Hypnosis is better than placebo for severe pain, but does not speed healing.	Van der Dose & Van Dyck, 1989; Patterson & Ptacek, 1997
4. Childbirth discomfort	Hypnosis reduces pain and stress during childbirth and after delivery.	Mairs, 1995
5. Dental pain	Hypnosis reduces need for medication and lessens pain.	Enqvist & Fischer, 1997
6. Low back pain	Hypnosis lessens pain and suffering.	Burte et al., 1994
7. Pain from sickle cell disease	Hypnosis improves sleep, reduces medication, and lessens pain.	Dinges, Whitehouse, et al., 1997

the process of providing feedback information about the status of biological systems. Early experiments indicated that biofeedback made possible the control of some otherwise automatic functions. In 1969, Neal E. Miller reported a series of experiments in which he and his colleagues altered the levels of animals' visceral response through reinforcement. Some subjects received rewards for raising their heart rate and others for lowering it. Within a few hours, significant differences in heart rate appeared. Salivation, kidney function, intestinal contractions, and blood pressure also changed as a response to training. Miller, who used rats and dogs as subjects, expressed the belief that humans too could learn to control visceral responses.

Experiments by other investigators soon proved Miller correct. Joseph Kamiya (1969) and Barbara Brown (1970) both reported that humans are capable of learning to control their brain waves using electroencephalogram (EEG) biofeedback. A variety of biofeedback machines soon appeared on the market. Muscle tension, skin temperature, blood pressure, heart rate, gastric motility, skin conductance, and many other physiological measures can respond to biofeedback training.

What Is Biofeedback?   In biofeedback, biological responses are measured by electronic instruments, and the status of those responses is immediately available to the person being tested. In other words, a person gains information about changes in biological responses as they are taking place. This feedback allows the person to alter physiological responses that cannot be voluntarily controlled without the biofeedback information.

The type of biofeedback most commonly found in clinical use is **electromyograph (EMG) biofeedback.** EMG biofeedback reflects the activity of the skeletal muscles by measuring the electrical discharge in muscle fibers. The measurement is taken by attaching electrodes to the surface of the skin over the muscles to be monitored. The level of electrical activity reflects the degree of tension or relaxation of the muscles. The machine responds with a signal that varies in accordance to the electrical activity of the muscle. The electrodes may be placed over any muscle group; the choice of placement depends on the type of problem. Biofeedback can be used to increase muscle tension in rehabilitation or to decrease muscle tension in stress management. The most common use of EMG biofeedback is in the control of low back

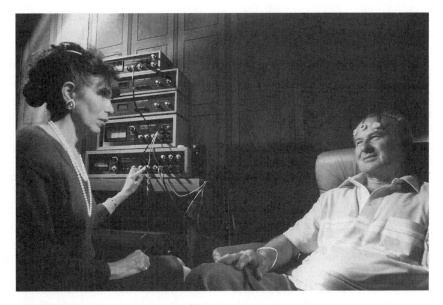

Electromyograph (EMG) biofeedback can help people lower muscle tension.

pain and headaches. Barb's pain program included a EMG biofeedback component, and she believes that monitoring her level of muscle tension helped her learn when she was tense and when she was more relaxed.

Thermal biofeedback, which is also frequently used to help people cope with stress and pain, is based on the principle that skin temperature varies in relation to levels of stress. High stress tends to constrict blood vessels whereas relaxation opens them. Therefore, cool surface skin temperature may indicate stress and tension; warm skin temperature suggests calm and relaxation.

Thermal biofeedback involves placing a **thermister**—a temperature-sensitive resistor—on the skin's surface. The thermister signals changes in skin temperature, thereby furnishing the information that allows control. The feedback signal, as with EMG biofeedback, may be auditory, visual, or both. The thermister is most often placed on fingers and less often on toes. These sites represent the most distal points in the circulatory system and are the most subject to temperature variations. However, temperature measurements taken from fingers or toes do not directly relate to any

pathological condition. Skin temperature may be an indirect measurement of tension and relaxation, or the fingers may represent vasoconstriction for the entire body. But in neither case can thermal biofeedback be seen as a direct intervention in the physiology that underlies any disorder.

The goal of thermal biofeedback is almost always to raise skin temperature. The vasodilation that causes warming accompanies relaxation. Migraine headache and **Raynaud's disease** are the disorders most commonly treated with thermal biofeedback. Raynaud's disease is a vasoconstrictive disorder in which the fingers (and less often the toes) suffer from restricted blood flow. Medical treatment involves surgery or drugs that dilate blood vessels, but both treatments have unwanted side effects. Biofeedback may offer an alternative treatment (Sedlacek & Taub, 1996).

How Effective Is Biofeedback? Biofeedback techniques are used for a wide range of disorders, including migraine and tension headaches, low back pain, and hypertension. To be a valuable coping technique, biofeedback must not only be superior to a placebo but should also produce better results than relaxation training, hypnosis, or any other behavioral intervention that does not require expensive technology.

Many programs for headache use thermal biofeedback; thermal biofeedback with relaxation can be effective for migraine and tension headaches (Blanchard at al., 1990b). This combination resulted in about a 50% reduction in pain—an improvement greater than that produced by a headache monitoring placebo but no more effective than a drug placebo. Similar results appeared in a meta-analysis of psychological interventions combining thermal biofeedback with relaxation training to produce a 43% reduction in headache activity (Holroyd & Penzien, 1990). A later summary of research (Compas, Haaga, Keefe, Leitenberg, & Williams, 1998) concluded that thermal biofeedback plus relaxation is more effective than a headache monitoring placebo, but no more effective than relaxation alone. EMG biofeedback is less frequently used to treat headache than thermal biofeedback. The findings regarding EMG biofeedback show it is effective, but no more so than thermal biofeedback plus relaxation training (Compas et al., 1998). Compared with an attention placebo, EMG and thermal biofeedback are generally more effective in controlling headache pain, but compared with relaxation and hypnosis, biofeedback offers no distinct advantage (Compas et al., 1998).

In spite of the prevalence of low back pain, biofeedback is not a common treatment for this pain syndrome. When used, it is rarely the only mode of treatment, which highlights a major problem in evaluating the effectiveness of biofeedback. Nearly all investigations have combined biofeedback with other treatment approaches. We discuss biofeedback combined with other techniques in the section on multimodal approaches.

Results from the few biofeedback studies on low back pain are somewhat mixed. One well-controlled study (Bush, Ditto, & Feuerstein, 1985) found a small gain for EMG biofeedback, but failed to find an advantage for the biofeedback group over either a placebo group or a no treat-ment group. In other words, even low back pain patients with no treatment tended to have less pain over time. However, a later study (Flor & Birbaumer, 1993) found some advantages when compared to cognitive-behavioral therapy and a conservative medical care control intervention. In this study, only the biofeedback group maintained significant reductions in pain after follow-up, suggesting that biofeedback may be of some use in alleviating low back pain.

Psychologists have also applied biofeedback techniques to the management of hypertension, or high blood pressure. In general, this approach to lowering blood pressure has had moderate success, but once again, the therapeutic ingredient might be relaxation. A study in Japan (Nakao et al., 1997) showed that biofeedback could decrease hypertension during laboratory mental stress experience. A study on biofeedback-assisted relaxation (Paran, Amir, & Yaniv, 1996) reported that patients with mild hypertension experienced a slight decrease in blood pressure and also a reduced need for hypertension drugs. A larger study (McGrady, 1994) showed some initial success for thermal biofeedback/relaxation training but no maintenance of this reduction in blood pressure 10 months later. These studies suggest some potential value for biofeedback in controlling hypertension, but they do not indicate that biofeedback alone is sufficient to manage blood pressure outside laboratory stress tests.

Because biofeedback requires a trained therapist and expensive equipment, it must provide effects that exceed those of relaxation, hypnosis, and other psychological interventions. The results of studies summarized in Table 8.3 suggest that it does not: Biofeedback alone is probably not a good choice for controlling headache pain, low back pain, or hypertension.

Behavior Modification

A fourth coping procedure health psychologists use is **behavior modification**, a process for changing behavior through the application of operant

Table 8.3 Effectiveness of biofeedback techniques

Problem	Findings	Studies
1. Migraine and tension headache	Thermal biofeedback plus relaxation produces a 45% to 50% reduction in headache activity.	Blanchard et al., 1990b; Holroyd & Penzien, 1990; Compas et al., 1998
2. Migraine headache	EMG biofeedback is more effective than a placebo and about as effective as thermal biofeedback.	Compas et al., 1998
3. Low back pain	EMG biofeedback has no immediate advantage over other interventions but may have a more lasting effect.	Bush et al., 1985; Flor & Birbaumer, 1993
4. Hypertension	Biofeedback-induced relaxation is moderately successful in temporarily controlling blood pressure.	Paran et al., 1996; McGrady, 1994; Nakao et al., 1997

conditioning principles. The goal of behavior modification is to shape *behavior,* not to alleviate *feelings* of stress or *sensations* of pain. Because stress is difficult to define in terms of specific behaviors, behavior modification is not often used for coping with stress. However, pain behaviors can be more clearly identified and thus lend themselves more easily to modification by operant conditioning techniques.

What Is Behavior Modification? People in pain usually communicate their discomfort to others. They complain, moan, sigh, limp, rub, grimace, miss work, or behave in a variety of other ways that indicate to other people that they are suffering. Many of these behaviors have been reinforced by the surroundings—that is, other people have in some manner rewarded these verbal and nonverbal expressions of pain.

Behavior modification strategies for coping with stress and pain are based on B. F. Skinner's (1987) notion that positive and negative reinforcers are central to operant conditioning. A **positive reinforcer** is any stimulus that, when added to a situation, increases the probability that the behavior it follows will recur. Positive reinforcers are also known as rewards. An example might be the attention and sympathy a person receives

from family and friends when exhibiting pain behaviors. A **negative reinforcer** is any aversive or painful stimulus that, when removed from a situation, increases the probability that the behavior it follows will recur. Examples are the relief from pain one experiences after taking pain medication and the avoidance of work or school responsibilities that can occur when a person shows pain.

Wilbert E. Fordyce (1974) was among the first to emphasize the role of operant conditioning in the perpetuation of pain behaviors. He recognized the *reward* value of increased attention and sympathy, financial compensation, relief from work and social obligations, and other positive reinforcers that frequently follow the various pain behaviors. Behavior modification techniques of pain management assume that pain behaviors are observable and can be reliably measured. Indeed, there is good evidence for these assumptions (Keefe & Block, 1982; McCracken, 1997). Once pain behaviors and their reinforcers have been identified, the process of behavior modification can begin. Nursing staff and patients' spouses can be trained to use praise and attention to reinforce more desirable behaviors and to withhold reinforcement when patients exhibit less desired pain behaviors. In other words, the inappropriate groans and complaints are now ignored while efforts toward greater physical activity and other positive behaviors are reinforced. Progress is noted by such criteria as amount of medication taken, absences from work, time in bed or off one's feet, number of pain complaints, physical activity, range of motion, and length of sitting tolerance.

How Effective Is Behavior Modification? Fordyce and his colleagues have successfully used behavior modification to improve mobility in pain patients. Using a single-subject design, Fordyce and his colleagues (Fordyce, Shelton, & Dundore, 1982) used behavior modification treatment for a young man suffering abdominal pain, dizziness, and disturbances in walking. As part of his therapy, the young man was given his choice of either walking the assigned distance at a predetermined speed or walking twice that distance at his own pace. The young man's mother was instructed to ignore him when he failed to walk and to encourage him when he showed progress in walking. The treatment intervention, which also included vocational counseling, was successful. At the end of treatment, the young man was walking more freely and complaining less of severe pain. Twenty-seven months later, the patient had maintained his gains despite no further treatment. Single-subject studies such as this show that behavior modification can work in individual cases, but they do not demonstrate the treatment's general efficacy.

The success of behavior modification in controlling pain is difficult to judge because many studies lacked adequate controls and, like biofeedback approaches, they employed multimodal treatment interventions. An early review (Turner & Chapman, 1982b) found some consistent trends for more than a dozen studies that used behavior modification to control a variety of pain syndromes (largely low back pain). One study (Nicholas, Wilson, & Goyen, 1991) found an initial advantage for behavior therapy in reducing medication and improving physical functioning of low back pain patients. However, another study (Turner & Clancy, 1988) suggested that this early advantage

for behavior modification may not continue after treatment.

How do behavior modification methods compare with traditional medical treatments for chronic low back pain? Fordyce and his associates (Fordyce, Brockway, Bergman, & Spengler, 1986) found some evidence to support the superiority of behavior methods over traditional medical treatment. Patients in the traditional management group received medication on an "as needed" basis and with the possibility of prescription renewal, while patients in the behavior therapy group were given medication on a time-contingent basis and with no renewal of the original prescription. In addition, the traditional treatment patients could stop their activity and exercises whenever they wished. For the behavior treatment patients, activity and exercises were completed on a predetermined basis. After 9 to 12 months, patients in the behavior management group were doing better than those treated with traditional procedures.

A later review of studies (Compas et al., 1998) confirmed the efficacy of behavior therapy, concluding that these techniques lead to improved psychological and physiological functioning for back pain patients. This research suggests that behavior-based programs of pain management are at least comparable in effectiveness to the more traditional physical therapy programs for managing back pain. Behavior modification programs are probably most effective in increasing levels of physical activity and decreasing use of medication—two important targets in any pain treatment regimen. Table 8.4 shows the effectiveness of behavior modification.

Cognitive Therapy

Cognitive therapy also uses reinforcement but places more emphasis on intrinsic or self-reinforcers than on reinforcers from therapists or other external sources. Cognitive therapy is based on the principle that people's beliefs, personal standards, and feelings of self-efficacy strongly affect their behavior (Bandura, 1977, 1986; Beck, 1976; Ellis, 1962)

Table 8.4   Effectiveness of behavior modification techniques

Problem	Findings	Studies
1. Low back pain and other pain syndromes	Behavior therapy improves physical activity and decreases medication.	Turner & Chapman, 1982b
2. Chronic low back pain	Behavior therapy may be better than traditional physical therapy methods.	Fordyce et al., 1986
3. Chronic low back pain	Behavior therapy is initially more effective than cognitive treatments, but this advantage is lost during follow-up.	Nicholas et al., 1991; Turner & Clancy, 1988

Cognitive therapies concentrate on techniques designed to change cognitions rather than on the immediate reinforcement of overt behavior.

Although he did not originally use the term *cognitive,* Albert Ellis (1962) evolved an approach called *rational emotive therapy* that became the precursor of modern cognitive therapies. According to Ellis, an analysis of a person's problem behavior reveals an underlying pattern of irrational or catastrophic thoughts. In other words, thoughts are the root of behavior problems. Once irrational cognitions have been identified, the therapist actively attacks these beliefs, with the goal of eliminating or changing them into more rational beliefs. Ellis believes that humans have the ability to use logic and to deal rationally with their problems. His therapy, then, is based on the assumption that people possess the ability to examine their belief systems logically, and to alter those systems when necessary.

Ellis contends that irrational beliefs form the basis for a variety of problems. All these problems are self-reinforced by an internal monologue in which people perpetuate their misery with continued self-statements of irrational beliefs and unreasonable expectations. Other people in similar situations may not "catastrophize" and thus may do better. The tendency to catastrophize was shown to be a mortality risk in a longitudinal study (Peterson, Seligman, Yurko, Martin, & Friedman, 1998). Expecting negative events to occur in many situations is hazardous to health, especially for men. These negative expectations may lead to poor problem solving and coping as well as social isolation and increased risks for violence. Therefore, a tendency to catastrophize can not only increase stress but also present health risks.

Ellis has proposed that the most effective way to alleviate stressful problems is to change the irrational beliefs. Escaping an unpleasant situation may not be possible, but learning to manage the situation with less stress is possible. The cognitive management occurs through the application of rational self-statements that lead to a realistic perception of the stressful situation and a more effective way to cope. An irrational, catastrophizing statement would be, "I didn't get the raise that I deserved, so everyone will be disappointed in me, and I'll never get the recognition that I deserve." The therapist would teach the person to substitute rational self-statements for irrational ones, decreasing the tendency to catastrophize. A rational statement might be "Even though I didn't get this raise, I can work to get others. If I am not as successful as I want to be in this job, I can succeed in other ways, and there are other jobs." Thus, the emotional element of the stress response is averted or minimized, and the person has a greater opportunity to cope rationally and positively with stress.

The experience of pain is one that can easily be turned into a catastrophe, and any exaggeration of feelings of pain can lead to maladaptive behaviors and further exacerbation of irrational beliefs. A study of dental patients (Chaves & Brown, 1987) found that some of them spontaneously used cognitive strategies to cope with pain and stress while others "catastrophized" their pain experiences. When the "copers" and the "catastrophizers" were compared, the researchers found that people who spontaneously coped with dental pain reported less stress but no less pain than did those who made a catastrophe of the situation. On the other hand, a later study (Keefe, Brown, Wallston, & Caldwell, 1989) showed that catastrophizing pain led to long-term exaggerations of pain. Rheumatoid arthritis pain sufferers who catastrophized their pain tended to report more intense pain, more functional impairments, and greater depression. This finding supports Ellis's contention that magnifying an event into a catastrophe will lead to increased emotional distress and elevated levels of pain.

What Is Cognitive Therapy?   Cognitive therapy rests on the assumption that a change in the interpretation of an event can change people's emotional and physiological reaction to that event. Although this approach typically uses operant conditioning techniques, it adds an emphasis on patients' ability to think about and evaluate their own behaviors. Because both behavior modification and cognitive therapy usually use multiple procedures, the two overlap a good bit, making accurate labeling of any multimodal package quite difficult.

As applied to pain management, cognitive therapy assumes that patients frequently exaggerate their pain-engendering thoughts, thus exacerbating their subjective feelings of pain and ultimately adding a psychological component to the physical experience of pain. Albert Bandura (1986) proposed that perceived self-efficacy can bring relief from pain by decreasing stress and bodily tension. For this reason, many cognitive therapists attempt in various ways to increase pain patients' feelings of self-efficacy—that is, their confidence that they can perform the behaviors necessary to produce desired outcomes.

Bandura hypothesized that cognitive therapy may block pain sensations at either the level of physiological transmission or the level of psychological awareness. He cited evidence suggesting that one's *belief* in the effectiveness of a placebo seems to release endorphins, the body's natural pain fighters (Bandura, 1986). These findings may explain why about one-third of all pain patients achieve relief from placebos. Because endorphins produce a biochemical reaction to placebos, at least some of the pain relief stemming from cognitive therapy techniques or any other type of psychological treatment is just as physically based as that attained through medication. Cognitive therapy also works to reduce pain on another level. Increased self-efficacy allows pain patients to return their attention to matters other than their pain. When people are confident that they can cope with impending increases in pain, they are less likely to dwell on the pain, thus decreasing their perceived suffering.

Psychologists have developed a variety of cognitive strategies for coping with pain and stress. Two of these are inoculation techniques and writing about strong negative emotions.

Inoculation Techniques   Dennis Turk, Donald Meichenbaum, and their associates (Meichenbaum & Turk, 1976; Turk, 1978; Turk & Rudy, 1992) have devised a cognitive program for pain management, and Meichenbaum and Roy Cameron (1983) have developed a parallel strategy for stress management. Both procedures rely on inoculation techniques; that is, they work in a manner analogous to vaccination. By introducing a weakened dose of a pathogen (in this case, the pathogen is a stressor) the therapist attempts to build some immunity against high levels of pain and stress.

Because pain is at least partially due to psychological factors, therapists who use inoculation techniques work first at getting patients to think differently about the source of their pain experience. During this *reconceptualization* stage, patients are encouraged to accept a psychological explanation for at least some of their pain. Once patients accept the potential effectiveness of psychologically based treatment, they are ready to enter the second stage—*acquisition and rehearsal of skills.* During this phase, patients learn relaxation and controlled breathing skills. Because relaxation is incompatible with tension and anxiety, learning to relax can be a valuable tool in managing pain. Patients also learn to direct their attention away from the pain experience by concentrating on a pleasant scene, such as a cool waterfall, or by focusing their attention outside themselves—for example, by counting spots on ceiling tiles or by thinking about a funny movie they have seen recently.

After patients have acquired and consolidated these skills, they are ready to enter the final, or *follow-through,* phase of treatment. During this stage, patients apply their coping skills to their natural environment. Physical activity and exercise are encouraged, to give patients a greater feeling of self-efficacy and a quantifiable means of evaluating their progress. Also during this stage, pain patients gradually increase the time between medication doses while decreasing their level of medication. During this follow-through stage, therapists give instructions to spouses and other family members in methods of ignoring patients' pain behaviors and of reinforcing such healthy behaviors as greater levels of physical activity, decreased use of medication, fewer visits to the pain clinic, or an increased number of days at work. Finally, with the help of their therapists, patients construct a posttreatment plan for coping with future pain. They must accept the reality that pain may return, sometimes more severe than ever, and that such a "relapse" is not a sign that the treatment was ineffective. Instead, the patients approach these pain episodes armed with a variety of self-help skills and with the confidence that they can cope with these experiences.

The **stress inoculation** program of Meichenbaum and Cameron (1983) is quite similar to Turk and Meichenbaum's method for coping with pain. Stress inoculation includes three stages: conceptu-alization, skills acquisition and rehearsal, and follow-through or application.

The *conceptualization* stage is a cognitive intervention in which the therapist works with clients to identify and clarify their problems. During this overtly educational stage, patients learn about stress inoculation and how this technique can reduce their stress. The *skills acquisition and rehearsal* stage involves both educational and behavioral components to enhance patients' repertoire of coping skills. At this time, patients learn and practice new ways of coping with stress. One of the goals of this stage is to improve self-instruction by changing cognitions, a process that includes monitoring one's internal monologue—that is, self-talk. During the *application and follow-through* stage, patients put into practice the cognitive changes they achieved in the two previous stages.

Inoculation training, either alone or in combination with other procedures, can be an effective intervention for pain and stress management for a variety of people in many painful and stressful situations. Research indicates that pain and stress inoculation can help athletes cope with painful injuries (Kerr & Goss, 1996; Ross & Berger, 1996); reduce depression, anxiety, and anger in high school students (Hains & Ellman, 1994); and decrease test anxiety among high school students (Sharma, Kumaraiah, & Mishra, 1996).

Expressing Emotions An additional cognitive strategy is the expression of strong, unpleasant emotions. James Pennebaker (1997a, 1997b) has studied the notion that talking or writing about negative events allows people to work toward a cognitive resolution of traumatic experiences. The therapeutic value of **catharsis**, or the venting of unpleasant emotions, goes back at least as far as Joseph Breuer and Sigmund Freud (1895/1955), but Pennebaker has recently been able to demonstrate the physical health benefits of talking or writing about traumatic events. In one study, (Pennebaker, Barger, & Tiebout, 1989) survivors of the Holocaust talked for 1 to 2 hours about their experiences during World War II while being measured for skin conductance level and heart rate.

Fourteen months later, the researchers collected data on health problems of the participants and found that the more survivors disclosed personally traumatic experiences, the better their subsequent health became.

Writing about negative experiences also seems to produce positive health results. Another study (Pennebaker, Colder, & Sharp, 1990) showed that students who ventilated feelings about entering college had fewer illnesses than those who merely wrote about superficial topics. A third study (Francis & Pennebaker, 1992) revealed that university employees age 22 to 70 who wrote about personal traumatic experiences had health advantages over those who wrote about nontraumatic experiences.

Pennebaker and his associates have examined several variables that may contribute to the health benefits of catharsis. They found that people who use negative emotion words improve more than those who use positive ones (Pennebaker, 1993); that nonverbal expression of traumatic experiences through art and music may be therapeutic (Berry & Pennebaker, 1993); and that writing about a particular topic (such as intimacy or school) helps people gain some cognitive resolution of that topic (Mancuso & Pennebaker, 1994). Pennebaker's research has added an effective and easily assessable tool to the arsenal of coping strategies. Expressing rather than denying negative experiences may benefit both psychological and physiological health.

How Effective Is Cognitive Therapy?   Evaluations of the effectiveness of cognitive therapy programs are difficult because widely diverse procedures have been placed under the rubric of cognitive therapy. As with behavioral therapies, cognitive programs often use a broad range of strategies, including relaxation training, biofeedback, behavior modification, systematic desensitization, and other techniques that are not strictly cognitive. Also, cognitive strategies themselves are not always used in the same way (Blanchard & Andrasik, 1985). Nevertheless, researchers have tested the effectiveness of cognitive therapy for a wide variety of stress and pain problems.

Cognitive therapy was as effective as relaxation training in relieving chronic low back pain (Turner & Jensen, 1993). Relaxation training, cognitive therapy, and a combination of the two techniques were all equally effective, and more effective than a waiting list control. A later review of research (Compas et al., 1998) reported that cognitive therapy for low back pain patients increased physical activity and improved psychological functioning. This review also suggested that cognitive behavioral group therapy may be able to reduce reliance on medication.

Combined cognitive and behavioral approaches have been shown to be effective with a variety of pain syndromes. A study with children suffering recurrent abdominal pain (Sanders, Shepherd, Cleghorn, & Woolford, 1994) compared a cognitive-behavioral approach with a standard pediatric care program and found that the cognitive-behavioral intervention was more effective in reducing pain, both at the end of treatment and after a 12-month follow-up. A review (Keefe & Van Horn, 1993) of studies dealing with rheumatoid arthritis pain found that cognitive-behavioral strategies were generally successful, at least for some arthritis patients.

In addition, research on the effectiveness of both stress inoculation training and emotional catharsis reveals that these forms of cognitive therapy show promise in helping people cope with pain and stress. A meta-analysis (Saunders, Driskell, Johnston, & Sales, 1996) of nearly 40 studies found that inoculation training was effective in decreasing anxiety and raising performance under stress. Also, Pennebaker (1997a, 1997b) provided evidence that personal self-disclosure not only improves emotional health but enhances physical health as well. Moreover, these positive effects of emotional catharsis extend to a variety of people, in myriad settings, across several Western cultures.

In summary, cognitively oriented treatment for stress and pain seems to be at least as effective as either relaxation training or biofeedback, but an important part of cognitive therapy programs may be the relaxation aspect. One possible advan-

Table 8.5 Effectiveness of cognitive therapy techniques

Problem	Findings	Studies
1. Chronic low back pain	Both cognitive therapy and a combination of cognitive therapy and relaxation diminish pain.	Turner & Jensen, 1993
2. Chronic low back pain	Cognitive therapy increases physical activity and improves psychological functioning.	Compas et al., 1998
3. Recurrent abdominal pain in children	Cognitive-behavioral therapy is more effective than a standard program.	Saunders et al., 1994
4. Rheumatoid arthritis	Cognitive-behavioral therapy can relieve at least some pain.	Keefe & Van Horn, 1993
5. Performance anxiety	Inoculation training reduces performance anxiety, state anxiety, and boosts performance under stress.	Saunders, et al., 1996
6. Physical and emotional distress	Emotional catharsis enhances both physical and emotional health.	Pennebaker, 1997a; 1997b

tage of cognitive approaches is their ability to change patients' self-perceived efficacy to cope with a range of stresses and pains and to reduce depression, emotionality, and irritability. Cognitive therapy appears to be an appropriate tool for many health-related behaviors. Its focus is broader than any of the other four psychological interventions we have discussed, all of which are primarily symptom oriented. Instead of concentrating on a specific behavior or behaviors, cognitive therapies take into account cognitive, affective, sensory, and behavioral components of a particular disorder. In other words, the goal of cognitive therapy is not limited to a specific target behavior such as stress reduction or pain management. Table 8.5 summarizes the effectiveness of cognitive therapy and the problems it can be used to treat.

Multimodal Approaches

Multimodal approaches to help people cope with pain and stress are interventions that include more than one and often several strategies. The pain program that Barb entered was a multimodal

program that included relaxation training, biofeedback, transcutaneous electrical nerve stimulation, and physical rehabilitation to control her low back pain. What are multimodal strategies and how effective are they?

What Are Multimodal Approaches? Multimodal approaches combine several effective techniques, such as relaxation training, hypnosis, biofeedback, behavior modification, cognitive therapies, and standard medical treatments. However, because the specific combination of techniques varies in different studies, a precise description of multimodal approaches is difficult. Moreover, evaluation of these approaches is complicated by their diversity of techniques.

How Effective Are Multimodal Approaches? Multimodal approaches should be at least as effective in reducing pain and stress as the most effective ingredient in the combined package. Research tends to support this supposition. For example, more than 70% of patients in a headache pain coping program experienced significant pain reduction and were able to reduce their medication by 50% or more (Scharff & Marcus, 1994). The program included education, information about medication management, physical therapy, and pain and stress management skills. This combination was significantly more effective than receiving no treatment.

Another study (Blanchard et al., 1990a) measured the effectiveness of cognitive therapy plus muscle relaxation compared to relaxation only for tension headache patients. Both treatments were more effective than no treatment or a sham treatment, but the addition of cognitive therapy did not increase effectiveness over relaxation alone. Also, a group of headache pain patients receiving a combination of thermal biofeedback, relaxation training, and cognitive therapy improved significantly more than a group that only monitored their headache pain, although the addition of cognitive therapy did not add to the effectiveness of biofeedback plus relaxation training (Blanchard et al., 1990b).

Another multimodal program combined relaxation training, cognitive therapy, and biofeedback for older chronic headache patients (Nicholson & Blanchard, 1993). The combined program allowed these patients to reduce their medication significantly after a 12-session treatment. At a 1-month follow-up, they were less depressed and less anxious than they were at the beginning of treatment.

An 11-year review of literature on worksite stress management (Murphy, 1996) revealed the effectiveness of multimodal programs. Individual studies in this review used a wide range of techniques, including progressive muscle relaxation, meditation, biofeedback, and cognitive-behavioral strategies. In addition, this review looked at studies that had used a combination of these procedures. As one would expect, the effectiveness of the single strategies varied greatly according to health outcome, existence of follow-up, and sample size. Of interest here was the finding that programs using a combination of approaches were generally more effective than programs using a single technique.

Thus, it seems that multimodal approaches are at least as effective as individual programs and possibly a little more so.

However, several problems exist in evaluating multimodal programs. First, although a combination of approaches usually results in lower levels of pain or stress, researchers and clinicians must consider whether the possible extra gain is worth the additional time and expense of a combination of strategies.

A second source of difficulty in evaluating all pain and stress coping programs is that more than one-third of patients involved in these programs also seek nontraditional therapies but do not disclose this fact to their physicians (Eisenberg et al., 1993). When participants in a study designed to test the efficacy of traditional pain reduction procedures are simultaneously seeking other treatments, no valid conclusions are possible concerning the effectiveness of the experimental treatment.

A third problem in evaluating the effectiveness of multimodal as well as other pain treatments is the placebo effect. Judith Turner and her associates (Turner et al., 1994) reviewed more than 200 studies on pain treatment to evaluate the importance of the placebo effect. They defined placebo as any nonspecific effect that results from patients' expectations and decreases their anxiety beyond that produced by traditional medical treatment. Turner et al. reported that traditional treatments such as surgery can produce strong placebo effects and that those effects are frequently much higher than the often-quoted 33% effectiveness.

Turner et al. (1994) suggested that pain patients usually improve for one or more of three reasons. First, pain is cyclical. People seek help and enroll in treatment studies when their pain is at its most intense. As the study continues, one would expect a reduction in pain even without treatment or without the placebo effect. For this reason, any treatment is likely to produce significant results because people simply return to their typical level of pain. Second, the intervention may actually help. Third, the program may produce nonspecific effects attributable to factors other than the specific treatment. Included in these nonspecific or "placebo effects" are the physician's attention, interest, concern, and expectations of positive results. Nonspecific effects also include the physician's reputation, the expense of the treatment, and the clinical setting. Turner et al. suggested that the placebo effect may explain nearly all of the benefits derived from a treatment.

Despite these difficulties, multimodal approaches to pain and stress management are generally effective. When used to control pain, they almost always result in reductions in pain medication, increases in patients' physical activity, and decreases in lost work time. Indeed, multimodal psychological treatments for pain are probably more effective than traditional medical treatments. Table 8.6 summarizes the effectiveness of some of the studies that used multimodal treatments.

In Summary

Among the techniques that health psychologists use to help people cope with stress and chronic pain are relaxation training, hypnotic procedures, biofeedback, behavior modification, and cognitive therapy. Four popular types of relaxation are: (1) progressive muscle relaxation, (2) meditative relaxation, (3) mindfulness meditation, and (4) guided imagery. All four approaches have demonstrated some success in helping patients cope with such stress-related problems as headache pain, anxiety disorder, dental pain, childbirth discomfort, worksite stress, and hypertension. Relaxation is generally more effective than a placebo and about as effective as biofeedback, which requires specialized machinery and therapists trained in its use.

Some debate still exists over the exact nature of hypnotic treatment, but there is little disagreement that hypnosis can be a powerful analgesic for managing pain. The benefits of hypnotherapy vary individually, but for suggestible people, hypnotic processes are an effective means of treating

headache, cancer pain, burn pain, hypertension, childbirth discomfort, dental pain, and the pain that accompanies sickle cell disease.

Biofeedback techniques provide immediate information to people concerning the status of their biological systems. Some evidence exists that biofeedback can be an effective procedure—either alone or in combination with other techniques—for lessening some kinds of pain. EMG and thermal biofeedback are effective in alleviating migraine and headache, reducing low back pain, and controlling hypertension.

Health psychologists also use behavior modification, a technique based on the principles of operant conditioning, to help people cope with pain. Behavior modification techniques are directed at altering pain behaviors, not lessening the sensations of pain. They are based on the assumption that withholding reinforcement for pain behaviors will decrease the likelihood that those behaviors will recur. When people are no longer rewarded for moaning, limping, missing work, or complaining, they tend to stop doing these things and begin to exhibit more nonpain behaviors. Behavior modification principles are most effective in reducing pain behaviors associated with low back pain and other muscular skeletal pains.

Cognitive therapy programs often rely on reinforcement techniques, but add a multitude of other strategies, including self-talk, self-efficacy, and self-evaluation of behavior. Because pain is at least partially due to psychological factors, cognitive therapists attempt to get patients to think differently about their pain experiences. One goal of cognitive treatment for pain is to increase patients' confidence that they can cope with increases in pain. This approach is effective for treating low back pain, rheumatoid arthritis, and performance anxiety. Cognitive therapists have developed a program for dealing with stress called stress inoculation, a procedure analogous to vaccination. Another successful procedure for coping with stress calls for patients to overtly express strong negative emotions through writing or talking.

Table 8.6 Effectiveness of multimodal techniques

Problem	Findings	Studies
1. Headache pain	Complex multimodal program reduced pain in more than 70% of patients, and patients decreased medication by 50%.	Scharff & Marcus, 1994
2. Chronic headache pain in elderly patients	Combined relaxation training, cognitive therapy, and biofeedback reduced pain medication, depression, and anxiety.	Nicholson & Blanchard, 1993
3. Worksite stress	Programs combining relaxation, meditation, biofeedback, and cognitive-behavioral therapy were more effective than single-technique programs.	Murphy, 1996
4. Headache pain	Multimodal programs were more effective than a placebo, but cognitive therapy added very little to relaxation.	Blanchard et al., 1990a
5. Headache pain	Thermal biofeedback with relaxation plus cognitive therapy was more effective than a headache monitoring program.	Blanchard et al., 1990b

Answers

This chapter addressed eight basic questions:

1. **How does social support influence coping?**

   Social support, defined as the emotional quality of one's social contacts, is inversely related to disease and death. Social support seems to influence coping in two ways. First, people with social support receive more encouragement and advice to seek medical care, and second, social support may provide a buffer against the physical effects of stress.

2. **How does personal control influence coping?**

   People with an internal locus of control believe that they control important events in their lives; these people generally cope better than people with an external locus of control. People's feelings that they are in control of the events of their life seem to have a positive im-

   pact on their health. Even small amounts of personal control can improve health and possibly extend life.

3. **How effective is relaxation training in coping with stress and pain?**

   Relaxation training can help people cope with a variety of stress and pain problems such as headache, chemotherapy side effects, anxiety, dental pain, and hypertension. Various relaxation training procedures are at least as effective as other psychological approaches to coping and more effective than a placebo.

4. **How effective is hypnotic treatment in coping with stress and pain?**

   For those who are suggestible, hypnotic processes are effective in treating headache, cancer pain, burn pain, childbirth discomfort, dental pain, and hypertension. People who are not suggestible would do better with another coping strategy.

5. **How effective is biofeedback in coping with stress and pain?**

   Biofeedback techniques are effective in alleviating migraine and tension headaches, anxiety, low back pain, and hypertension. However, biofeedback probably offers no advantage over relaxation and it has the disadvantage of requiring expensive equipment.

6. **How effective is behavior modification in coping with stress and pain?**

   Behavior modification involves withholding reinforcement for pain behaviors, which tends to eliminate those behaviors. This approach is especially effective for joint and low back pain.

7. **How effective is cognitive therapy in coping with stress and pain?**

   Cognitive therapy is hard to evaluate because it is often used in conjunction with other techniques. Two cognitively based approaches—stress inoculation and emotional expression—show some promise in helping people cope with stressful life experiences.

8. **How effective are multimodal approaches in coping with stress and pain?**

   In general terms, multimodal approaches are more effective than most types of placebo and probably at least as powerful as the most effective approach in the combination of techniques.

Glossary

behavior modification Shaping behavior by manipulating reinforcement in order to obtain a desired behavior.

catharsis The spoken or written expression of strong negative emotion, which may result in improvement in physiological or psychological health.

biofeedback The process of providing feedback information *about* the status of a biological system *to* that system.

electromyograph (EMG) biofeedback Feedback that reflects activity of the skeletal muscles.

induction The process of being placed into a hypnotic state.

negative reinforcer Any painful or aversive condition that, when removed from a situation, strengthens the behavior it follows.

positive reinforcer Any positively valued stimulus that, when added to a situation, strengthens the behavior it follows.

Raynaud's disease A vasoconstrictive disorder stemming from inadequate circulation in the extremities, especially the fingers or toes, and resulting in pain.

self-efficacy The belief that one is capable of performing the behaviors that will produce desired outcomes in any particular situation.

social contacts Number and kinds of people with whom one associates; members of one's social network.

social isolation The absence of specific role relationships.

social network Number and kinds of people with whom one associates; social contacts.

social support Both tangible and intangible support a person receives from other people.

stress inoculation A stress management technique in which patients are introduced to small amounts of stress and are given cognitive-behavioral strategies for dealing with those diminished levels of stress.

thermal biofeedback Feedback concerning changes in skin temperature.

thermister A temperature-sensitive resistor used in thermal biofeedback.

Suggested Readings

Fordyce, W. E. (1990). Contingency management. In J. J. Bonica (Ed.), *The management of pain* (2nd ed., pp. 1702–1710). Philadelphia: Lea & Febiger.

Wilbert Fordyce discusses terminology and principles of behavioral management of pain. Contingency management procedures typically target some combination of problem behaviors that include overmedication, reduced activity levels, excessive pain behaviors, deficits in well behavior, and inappropriate responses to pain behavior.

Hilgard, E. R., & Hilgard, J. R. (1994). *Hypnosis in the relief of pain (Rev. ed.). Los Altos, CA: Kaufmann. For those interested in hypnosis, this book offers a readable, comprehensive, and updated treatment of this means of pain control.*

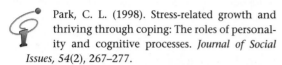 Park, C. L. (1998). Stress-related growth and thriving through coping: The roles of personality and cognitive processes. *Journal of Social Issues, 54*(2), 267–277.

Crystal Park takes an innovative approach by emphasizing the growth-enhancing potential of experiencing stress. She considers how personal characteristics influence positive consequences of stress, and reviews the role of appraisal and coping processes in stress-related growth. Available through InfoTrac College Edition by Wadsworth Publishing Company.

Pennebaker, J. W. (1997). Writing about emotional experiences as a therapeutic process. *Psychological Science, 8.* 162–168.

In this brief article, James Pennebaker discusses his technique of having patients write about their traumatic experiences, reports on the outcomes of this procedure, and reviews his and other people's research.

Schwarzer, R., & Leppin, A. (1992). Possible impact of social ties and support on morbidity and mortality. In H. O. E. Veiel & U. Baumann (Eds.), *The meaning and measurement of social support* (pp. 65–83). New York: Hemisphere.

Although this chapter is somewhat technical, it provides a solid background on the rationale for and research on social support and its relationship to morbidity and mortality.

Turner, J. A., Deyo, R. A., Loeser, J. D., Von Korff, M., & Fordyce, W. E. (1994). The importance of placebo effects in pain treatment and research. *Journal of the American Medical Association, 271,* 1609–1614.

An excellent review of the placebo in pain treatment, this article presents a broad definition of the placebo effect.

CHAPTER 9

Identifying Behavioral Factors in Cardiovascular Disease

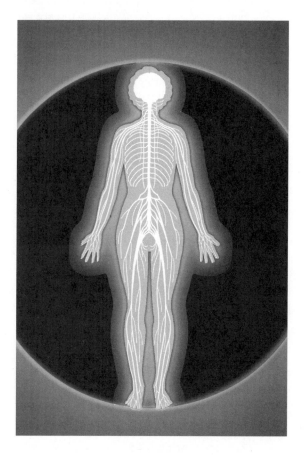

CASE STUDY
Jason: Building Cardiac Risk

CHAPTER OUTLINE

Questions

The Cardiovascular System

Measures of Cardiovascular Function

The Changing Rates of Cardiovascular Disease

Risk Factors in Cardiovascular Disease

Modifying Risk Factors for Cardiovascular Disease

Answers

Glossary

Suggested Readings

QUESTIONS

This chapter focuses on five basic questions:

1. What are the structures, functions, and disorders of the cardiovascular system?

2. What measurements of cardiovascular function can reveal damage?

3. How does lifestyle relate to cardiovascular health?

4. What are the risk factors for cardiovascular disease?

5. Can cardiovascular risk be lowered by modifying risk factors?

JASON: BUILDING CARDIAC RISK

Jason was determined that he would not undergo coronary bypass surgery, saying, "They're not going to take a vein out of my leg and put it in my heart. No way. I don't care if I die." Jason was not an immediate candidate for cardiac surgery who was refusing treatment but a 15-year-old adolescent whose father had undergone this procedure. The details of the surgery had made a dramatic impression on Jason, and he had become better acquainted with the risk factors for cardiovascular disease than most 15-year-olds.

Despite Jason's determination to avoid cardiovascular disease, he is at increased risk for several reasons. Jason's father developed heart disease in his early 40s, and this hereditary factor places Jason at increased risk. His African American ethnic background is another factor that increases his risk; African Americans experience cardiovascular disease and death at higher rates than European Americans (U.S. Bureau of the Census [USBC], 1998).

Although Jason knows that changing certain behaviors would lower his risk for heart disease, he refuses to consider such options. He says that he has no intention of restricting his diet by avoiding high-fat or salty foods. He plans to eat what he wants, and if he has a heart attack, then he has a heart attack. He is, however, strongly opposed to smoking, has felt no urge to experiment with cigarettes, and ridicules those who do. His attitudes about drinking are not as extreme, but he does not drink and feels that he will never be a smoker or a drinker.

Jason is competitive and impatient. His competitive attitude appears in his interactions with his peers and in his motivation for success. He is outgoing and likes to be the center of attention, and his wit allows him to achieve this goal often. However, he sometimes uses his wit to score points at others' expense. His motivation to succeed has not led to outstanding grades, but success in a career (which he has not yet chosen) is central to Jason. He believes that success, defined as making a lot of money, is very important. He cannot imagine being happy as an adult without career success and a comfortable life.

Jason's impatience extends to himself as well as to others. His impatience with himself occurs mostly when he cannot meet the high standards he has set for himself. Despite variable academic performance, Jason has a great deal of academic ability, and he judges his own performance critically. He is also critical of others who are less intellectually capable than he is and who cannot keep up with his verbal wit. The tendency to be openly critical of others and to use his wit to cut down others restricts his circle of friends to a few who enjoy his intelligence and sense of humor. However, Jason's parents are supportive and encouraging.

This chapter examines the behavioral risks for cardiovascular disease—the most frequent cause of death in the United States and other industrialized nations—and looks at Jason's risk from inherent and behavioral factors. But first it describes the cardiovascular system and methods of measuring cardiovascular function.

The Cardiovascular System

The cardiovascular system pumps blood throughout the body, providing a rapid-transport system for oxygen and nutrients and for the disposal of wastes. During normal functioning, the cardiovascular, respiratory, and digestive systems are integrated: The digestive system produces nutrients and the respiratory system furnishes oxygen, both of which circulate through the blood to various parts of the body. In addition, the endocrine system affects the cardiovascular system by stimulat-

ing or depressing the rate of cardiovascular activity. Although the cardiovascular system can be analyzed in isolation, it does not function that way.

This section briefly considers the functioning of the cardiovascular system, concentrating on the physiology underlying cardiovascular disease. The cardiovascular system consists of the heart and the blood vessels. By contracting and relaxing, the heart muscle pumps blood that circulates through the body. The circulation of blood allows the transport of oxygen to body cells and the removal

CHECK YOUR HEALTH RISKS

Check the items that apply to you.

- ❑ 1. Someone in my immediate family (a parent, sibling, aunt, uncle, or grandparent) died of heart disease before the age of 55.
- ❑ 2. I am diabetic.
- ❑ 3. I am male.
- ❑ 4. I am African American.
- ❑ 5. My blood pressure is at least 160 over 105.
- ❑ 6. My total cholesterol level is at least 240.
- ❑ 7. My HDL is less than 35.
- ❑ 8. The ratio of my total cholesterol to HDL is 6 to 1 or higher.
- ❑ 9. I am a current smoker.
- ❑ 10. I am a former smoker who has quit during the past 5 years.
- ❑ 11. I eat fruits and vegetables less than once a day.

- ❑ 12. My diet contains lots of red meat.
- ❑ 13. I almost never eat fish.
- ❑ 14. My diet is low in fiber.
- ❑ 15. I seem to be anxious most of the time.
- ❑ 16. I am an unmarried man.
- ❑ 17. I frequently get angry, and when I do I let everyone around me know about it.
- ❑ 18. I frequently get angry, and when I do I keep my anger to myself.

Each of these items represents a known risk factor for some type of cardiovascular disease. However, some items (such as Number 5) place you at a greater risk than others (such as Number 13). In general, however, the more of these items that apply to you, the greater your risk of heart disease or stroke.

---

of carbon dioxide and other wastes from cells. The entire circuit takes about 20 seconds when the body is at rest, but exertion speeds the process.

The blood's route through the body is pictured in Figure 9.1. Blood travels from the right ventricle of the heart to the lungs, where hemoglobin (one of the components of blood) becomes saturated with oxygen. From the lungs, oxygenated blood travels back to the left atrium of the heart, then to the left ventricle, and finally out to the rest of the body. The **arteries** that carry the oxygenated blood branch into vessels of smaller and smaller diameter, called **arterioles,** and finally terminate in tiny **capillaries** that connect arteries and **veins.** Oxygen diffuses out to body cells, and carbon dioxide and other chemical wastes pass into the blood so they may be disposed of. Blood that has been stripped of its oxygen returns to the heart by way of the system of veins, beginning with the tiny **venules** and ending with the two large veins that empty into the right atrium, the upper right chamber of the heart.

The Coronary Arteries

The blood supply to the heart muscle, the **myocardium,** is furnished by coronary arteries (see Figure 9.2). The two principal coronary arteries branch off from the aorta, the main artery that carries oxygenated blood from the heart. Left and right coronary arteries divide into smaller branches, providing the blood supply to the myocardium.

With each beat, the heart makes a slight twisting motion, which moves the coronary arteries. The coronary arteries, therefore, undergo a great deal of strain as part of their normal function. This movement of the heart has been hypothesized to almost inevitably cause injury to the coronary

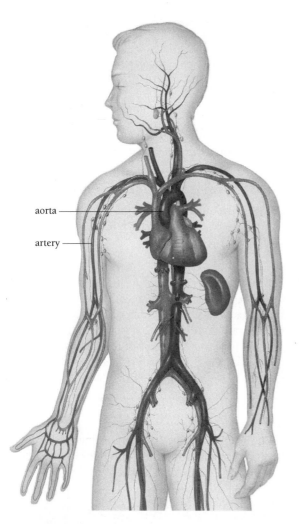

Figure 9.1 Cardiovascular circulation. *Source:* From *Introduction to Microbiology,* by J. Ingraham and C. Ingraham, p. 671. Copyright © 1995 Wadsworth Publishing Co. Used by permission.

arteries (Friedman & Rosenman, 1974). The damage can heal in two different ways. The preferable route involves the formation of small amounts of scar tissue and results in no serious problem. The second route involves the formation of **atheromatous plaques,** deposits composed of cholesterol and other lipids (fats), connective tissue, and muscle tissue. The plaques grow and calcify into a hard, bony substance that thickens the arterial

walls. The formation of plaques and the resulting occlusion of the arteries is called **atherosclerosis,** shown in Figure 9.3.

A related but different problem is **arteriosclerosis,** or the loss of elasticity of the arteries. The beating of the heart pushes blood through the arteries with great force, and arterial elasticity allows adaptation to this pressure. Loss of elasticity tends to make the cardiovascular system less capable of tolerating increases in cardiac blood volume. Hence, a potential danger exists during strenuous exercise for people with arteriosclerosis.

The formation of arterial plaques (atherosclerosis) and the "hardening" of the arteries (arteriosclerosis) often occur together. Both can affect any artery in the cardiovascular system, but when the coronary arteries are affected, the heart's oxygen supply may be threatened.

Coronary Artery Disease

Coronary artery disease (CAD) arises as a result of atherosclerosis and arteriosclerosis in the coronary arteries. No clearly visible, outward symptoms accompany the buildup of plaques in the coronary arteries; CAD can be developing while a person remains totally unaware of its progress. However, the plaques narrow the arteries and restrict the supply of blood to the myocardium. In addition, blood platelets tend to stick to and blood clots to form around the plaques. These blood clots can transform the partially obstructed artery into a completely closed one. Restriction of blood flow is called **ischemia.** If the coronary arteries do not allow enough blood to reach the heart muscle, the heart, like any other organ or tissue deprived of oxygen, will not function properly. When the heart is affected by CAD, **coronary heart disease (CHD)** has occurred.

One possible result of restriction of the blood supply to the myocardium is **angina pectoris,** a disorder with symptoms of crushing pain in the chest and difficulty in breathing. Angina is usually precipitated by exercise or stress because these conditions increase demand to the heart. With oxygen

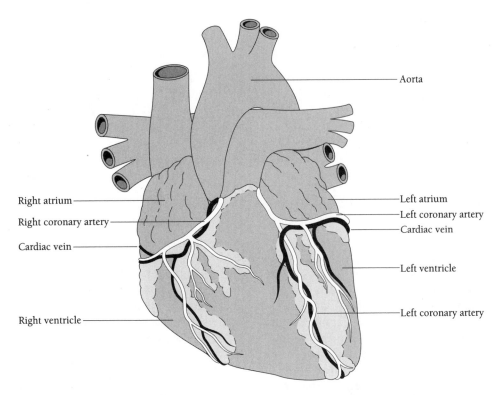

Aorta

Right atrium

Right coronary artery

Cardiac vein

Right ventricle

Left atrium

Left coronary artery

Cardiac vein

Left ventricle

Left coronary artery

Figure 9.2   Coronary arteries.

restriction, the reserve capacity of the cardiovascular system is reduced, and heart disease becomes evident. The uncomfortable symptoms of angina rarely last more than a few minutes, but angina is a sign of obstruction in the coronary arteries.

One approach to the treatment of CAD is surgery that replaces the blocked portion of the coronary artery (or arteries) with grafts of healthy veins, usually taken from the patient's leg. The surgeon attaches these grafts so that blood flows through the replacements, bypassing the blocked sections of the coronary arteries (see Figure 9.4). This treatment is the procedure that Jason refused to consider, but it is generally successful in relieving angina and improving the patient's quality of life, as it was for his father.

The number of bypass operations has increased to the hundreds of thousands in the United States

alone. Bypass surgery is expensive, carries some risk for death, and may not extend the patient's life significantly. The procedure does relieve angina and thus improves quality of life (Bypass Angioplasty Revascularization Investigation, 1997) The disease processes that led to blockage of the coronary arteries can also lead to obstruction of the replacement vessels. Therefore, people who have coronary bypass surgery may redevelop CAD; these patients must change their lifestyle if they are to prevent blockage of the replacement arteries.

Complete blockage of either coronary artery shuts off the blood flow and thus the oxygen supply to the myocardium. Like other tissue, the myocardium cannot survive without oxygen; therefore, coronary blockage results in the death of myocardial tissue, an infarction. **Myocardial infarction** is the medical term for the condition commonly

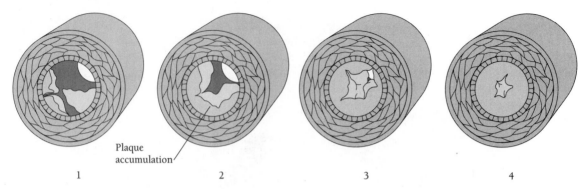

Plaque accumulation

1   2   3   4

Figure 9.3   Progressive atherosclerosis.

referred to as a heart attack. During myocardial infarction, the damage may be so extensive as to completely disrupt the heartbeat. In less severe cases, heart contractions may become less effective. The signals for a myocardial infarction include a feeling of weakness or dizziness combined with nausea, cold sweating, difficulty in breathing, and a sensation of crushing or squeezing pain in the chest, arms, shoulders, jaw, or back. Rapid loss of consciousness or death may occur, but the victim sometimes remains quite alert throughout the experience. The severity of symptoms depends on the extent of damage to the heart muscle.

Both angina pectoris and myocardial infarction are typically the result of atherosclerosis, which is most dangerous when it involves the coronary arteries. Continued thickening of the arterial walls restricts the flow of blood, causing angina. If the restriction is severe, heart tissue may die and the heart beat will be disrupted; that is, the person will experience a myocardial infarction.

In those people who survive a myocardial infarction (somewhat more than half do), the damaged portion of the myocardium will not regrow or repair itself. Instead, scar tissue forms at the infarcted area. Scar tissue does not have the elasticity and function of healthy tissue, so a heart attack lessens the capacity of the heart to pump blood efficiently. A myocardial infarction can limit the type and vigor of activities that a person can safely do, prompting some lifestyle changes. Frequently,

these changes result from cardiac patients' uncertainty about which activities are safe and from their fears about suffering another attack. Such fears have some basis. The coronary artery disease that caused a first attack can cause another, but future infarctions are not a certainty.

The process of cardiac rehabilitation often involves psychologists, who help cardiac patients adjust their lifestyle to minimize risk factors and lessen the chances of future attacks. Because heart disease is the most frequent cause of death in the United States, preventing heart attack and furnishing cardiac rehabilitation is a major task for the health care system. This chapter discusses the development and prevention of cardiovascular disease, and Chapter 11 discusses cardiac rehabilitation programs.

Stroke

Atherosclerosis and arteriosclerosis can also affect the arteries that serve the head and neck, thereby restricting the blood supply to the brain. Plaques may become detached from the artery wall, or one of the blood clots that tend to form on plaques may detach and flow through the circulatory system. Any obstruction in the arteries of the brain will restrict or completely stop the flow of blood to the area of the brain served by that portion of the system. A piece of material too small to obstruct an arteriole might completely block a capil-

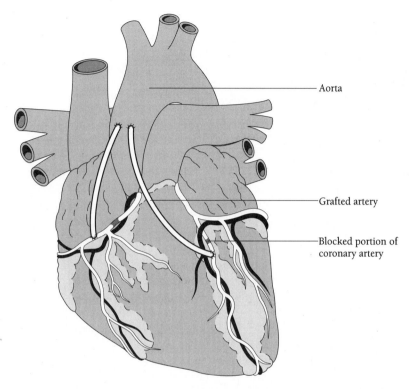

Aorta

Grafted artery

Blocked portion of
coronary artery

Figure 9.4   Coronary bypass.

lary. Oxygen deprivation causes the death of brain tissue within 3 to 5 minutes. This damage to the brain resulting from lack of oxygen is called a **stroke**, the third most frequent cause of death in the United States. But strokes have other causes as well—for example, a bubble of air (air embolism) or infection that impedes blood flow in the brain may also result in a stroke. In addition, the weakening of artery walls associated with arteriosclerosis may lead to an *aneurysm,* a sac formed by the ballooning of a weakened artery wall. Aneurysms may burst, causing a *hemorrhagic stroke* or death (see Figure 9.5).

A stroke damages neurons in the brain, and these neurons have no capacity to replace themselves. Therefore, death of any neuron results in the permanent loss of its function. The brain, however, contains billions of neurons. Rarely do people suffer from strokes that kill *all* neurons

controlling a particular function. More commonly, some of the neurons devoted to a particular function are lost, impairing brain function. Even though no neurons are replaced, the remaining healthy neural tissue compensates to some extent. For example, one specific area of the brain controls speech production. If this area is completely damaged by a stroke, the victim can no longer speak (but can still comprehend speech). A stroke that damages some of the neurons in this area results in partial loss of fluency and some difficulty in speaking. The extent of the loss is related to the amount of damage to the area; more extensive damage results in greater impairment. This same principle applies to other types of disabilities caused by stroke. Damage may be so extensive—or in such a critical area—as to bring about immediate death; or damage may be so slight as to go unnoticed.

Common stroke
is caused by a clot. Most often,
as in this illustration, the clot
forms where an artery has
been narrowed by
fatty deposits.

A hemorrhagic stroke
is caused by bleeding in
the brain due to a rupture
of a weakened artery.

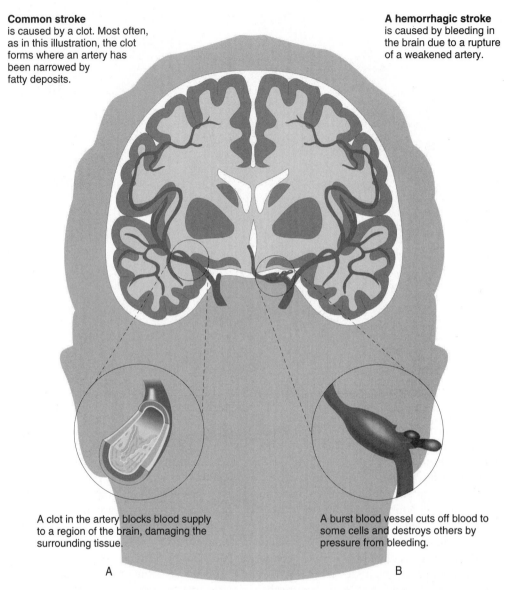

A clot in the artery blocks blood supply
to a region of the brain, damaging the
surrounding tissue.

A burst blood vessel cuts off blood to
some cells and destroys others by
pressure from bleeding.

A

B

Figure 9.5 **Two types of strokes. Common strokes are caused by blockage of an artery; hemorrhagic strokes are caused by the bursting of an artery in the brain.**   *Source:* From *An Invitation to
Health,* 7th ed. by Dianne Hales, p. 379. Copyright © 1997 by Brooks/Cole Publishing Co. Reprinted by permission
of Wadsworth Publishing Co.

Degenerative diseases of the cardiovascular
system, such as atherosclerosis and arteriosclerosis, are not the only cause of stroke. Blood clots
can form around internal wounds in the process
of healing and break away to float through the
circulatory system. However, the most common
cause of stroke is atherosclerosis. Blood clots can
form around atheromatous plaques, and a plaque

itself may detach from the artery wall, forming a floating hazard in the cardiovascular system that may result in a debilitating or deadly stroke.

Blood Pressure

When the heart pumps blood, the force must be substantial to power circulation for an entire cycle through the body and back to the heart. In a healthy cardiovascular system, the pressure in the arteries is not a problem because arteries are quite elastic. In a cardiovascular system diseased by atherosclerosis and arteriosclerosis, however, the pressure of the blood in the arteries can produce serious consequences. The narrowing of the arteries that occurs in atherosclerosis and the loss of elasticity that characterizes arteriosclerosis both tend to raise blood pressure and make the cardiovascular system less capable of adapting to the demands of heavy exercise and stress.

Blood pressure measurements are usually expressed by two numbers. The first number represents **systolic pressure**, the pressure generated by the heart's contraction. The second number represents **diastolic pressure**, or the pressure achieved between contractions, reflecting the elasticity of the vessel walls. Both numbers are measured by determining how high in millimeters (mm) a column of mercury (Hg) can be raised in a glass column.

Elevations of blood pressure can occur through several mechanisms. Some elevations in blood pressure are normal and even adaptive. Activation of the sympathetic nervous system, for example, increases heart rate and also causes constriction of the blood vessels, both of which raise blood pressure. The parasympathetic division blocks sympathetic action and returns blood pressure to its baseline rate, so sympathetic activation should not result in permanent increases in blood pressure. Other elevations in blood pressure, however, are neither normal nor adaptive; they are symptoms of cardiovascular disorder.

Millions of people in the United States have **hypertension**—that is, abnormally high blood pressure. This "silent" illness is the single best pre-

dictor of both heart attack and stroke, but it can also cause eye damage and kidney failure (see Figure 9.6). Hypertension is of two types—primary or essential hypertension and secondary hypertension. **Essential hypertension**, which accounts for 90% of the hypertension in the United States (Williams & Knight, 1994), refers to elevations of blood pressure that have no identified cause. It is positively related to such factors as age, African American ancestry, weight, sodium intake, tobacco use, and lack of exercise. **Secondary hypertension** is much less common than essential hypertension and stems from other diseases such as arteriosclerosis, kidney disorders, and some disorders of the endocrine system.

Table 9.1 shows the ranges for normal blood pressure, borderline hypertension, and hypertension. Despite beliefs to the contrary, people with hypertension are not able to diagnose their own blood pressure reliably (Meyer, Leventhal, & Gutman, 1985). Therefore, people can have dangerously elevated blood pressure and remain completely unaware of their vulnerability to heart attack and stroke.

Hypertension tends to progress from elevated systolic blood pressure coupled with normal or slightly elevated diastolic pressure to elevations of both systolic and diastolic blood pressure. Although systolic and diastolic hypertension may occur separately, people—especially older people—with hypertension typically experience elevations of both. Systolic pressure that exceeds 200 mm Hg presents a danger of rupture in the arterial walls (McClintic, 1978). A rupture of the aorta is usually fatal; a rupture of a cerebral artery results in a stroke that may be fatal. Diastolic hypertension tends to result in vascular damage that may injure organs served by the affected vessels, most commonly the kidneys, liver, pancreas, brain, and retina.

Because the underlying cause of essential hypertension is unknown, no treatment exists that will remedy its basic cause. Treatment tends to be oriented toward drugs or changes in behavior or lifestyle that can lower blood pressure. Because part of the treatment of hypertension involves

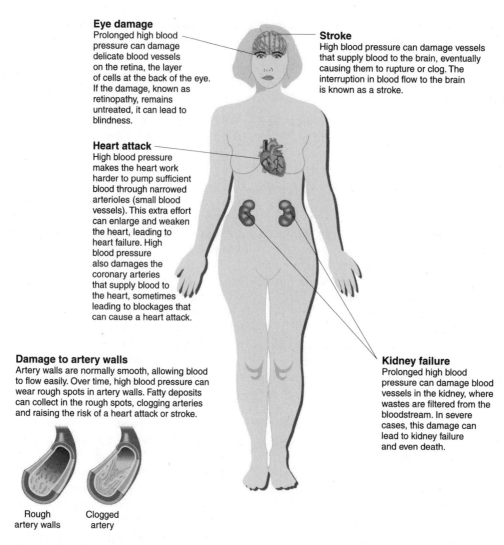

Eye damage
Prolonged high blood pressure can damage delicate blood vessels on the retina, the layer of cells at the back of the eye. If the damage, known as retinopathy, remains untreated, it can lead to blindness.

Stroke
High blood pressure can damage vessels that supply blood to the brain, eventually causing them to rupture or clog. The interruption in blood flow to the brain is known as a stroke.

Heart attack
High blood pressure makes the heart work harder to pump sufficient blood through narrowed arterioles (small blood vessels). This extra effort can enlarge and weaken the heart, leading to heart failure. High blood pressure also damages the coronary arteries that supply blood to the heart, sometimes leading to blockages that can cause a heart attack.

Damage to artery walls
Artery walls are normally smooth, allowing blood to flow easily. Over time, high blood pressure can wear rough spots in artery walls. Fatty deposits can collect in the rough spots, clogging arteries and raising the risk of a heart attack or stroke.

Rough
artery walls

Clogged
artery

Kidney failure
Prolonged high blood pressure can damage blood vessels in the kidney, where wastes are filtered from the bloodstream. In severe cases, this damage can lead to kidney failure and even death.

Figure 9.6   The consequences of high blood pressure.   *Source: An Invitation to Health,* 7th ed. by Dianne Hales, p. 379. Copyright © 1997 by Brooks/Cole Publishing Co. Reprinted by permission of Wadsworth Publishing Co.

behavioral changes, health psychologists have a role to play in encouraging such behaviors as controlling weight, maintaining a regular exercise program, and restricting sodium intake.

In Summary

The cardiovascular system consists of the heart and blood vessels. The heart pumps blood, which circulates throughout the body, supplying oxygen and removing waste products. The coronary arteries supply blood to the heart itself, and when atherosclerosis affects these arteries, coronary artery disease (CAD) occurs. In this disease process, plaques form within the arteries, restricting the blood supply to the heart muscle. The restriction can cause angina pectoris, with symptoms of chest pain and difficulty in breathing. Blocked

Table 9.1 Ranges of blood pressure (expressed in mm of Hg)

	Systolic	Diastolic
Normal	<140	<85
Borderline	140–159	85–104
Hypertensive	160 +	104 +

Source: Adapted from the *1984 Report of the Joint National Committee on Detection, Evaluation and Treatment of High Blood Pressure* (p. 8) by the U.S. Department of Health and Human Services (USDHHS), 1984, Washington, DC: U. S. Government Printing Office.

coronary arteries can also lead to a myocardial infarction (heart attack). When the oxygen supply to the brain is disrupted, stroke occurs. Stroke can affect any part of the brain and can vary in severity from minor to fatal. Hypertension—high blood pressure—is a predictor of both heart attack and stroke. Both behavioral and medical treatments can lower hypertension as well as other risk factors for cardiovascular disease.

Measures of Cardiovascular Function

For 55% of the people with coronary disease, a heart attack is the first symptom of a problem (Ellestad, 1996). Therefore, diagnosis of CAD is an urgent issue. Accurate diagnoses depend on reliable measures of both the functioning of the cardiovascular system and changes in that functioning.

The most common measurement of cardiovascular function is blood pressure. Blood pressure measurements suggest whether arteries have narrowed or lost elasticity or both. Because high blood pressure has many causes, hypertension does not always signal heart disease. Other techniques can assess cardiovascular function more precisely than the measurement of blood pressure, but none of these other assessments are as simple or as available

as blood pressure tests. Although there are no easy methods for the early diagnosis of CAD, several measures besides blood pressure are commonly used to detect potential cardiovascular problems.

Measurements of Electrical Activity in the Heart

An **electrocardiogram (ECG)** is a measurement of the electrical impulses produced by the heartbeat; this measurement is capable of revealing abnormalities in the resting heartbeat. People who show an abnormal ECG usually have some type of cardiovascular disorder. However, ECG readings cannot reveal the buildup of plaques in the coronary arteries. Consequently, dangerously advanced CAD may go undetected by an electrocardiogram.

A **stress test** measures the heart's electrical activity during exercise. Exercise increases oxygen demand by the heart muscle, so blockage of arteries is more easily detectable during exercise. Therefore, this measure is more sensitive and useful than an electrocardiogram in diagnosing heart problems. For example, an ECG cannot detect coronary artery blockage of less than 75%, even though such blockage is extensive. A stress test, however, can reveal blockage of around 50%. A 50% blockage in one coronary artery often fails to produce noticeable symptoms; thus stress testing is useful for discovering moderate yet significant levels of coronary artery blockage (Ellestad, 1996).

In a stress test, measuring electrodes are placed in a standard pattern on the torso, and then the person engages in progressively more strenuous exercise, typically either walking on a treadmill with an increasing slope or riding a stationary bicycle with increasing pedal resistance. As the exercise increases the body's demand for oxygen, the heart increases its action. If coronary arteries are partially blocked, the blood cannot be delivered fast enough to keep up with the increased demand. This restriction results in a pattern of electrical activity with a characteristic waveform that permits trained professionals to make a diagnosis of coronary heart disease.

Stress tests can provide additional diagnostic information about cardiovascular problems. People with angina pectoris may know that restriction of blood flow is the cause of their chest pains, but stress testing can inform them about the severity of the restriction. People with chest pains are sometimes given stress tests to determine whether their pains are a result of ischemia or some other cause. Stress tests are also recommended after myocardial infarction, as a way to measure damage to the heart, and after coronary bypass surgery, as a way to assess the effectiveness of the procedure (Ellestad, 1996). Stress tests are also recommended for previously sedentary people who decide to start an exercise program.

Angiography

The most definitive method of diagnosis for coronary artery disease is cardiac catheterization and **angiography.** Werner Forssmann was the first person to attempt cardiac angiography—on himself in 1929 (Ricciuti, 1997). The technique did not develop until the 1940s and 1950s, but it is now a routine diagnostic procedure. Angiography is used to determine the extent of coronary artery disease in cases of angina pectoris, after a positive result from a stress test, or after a myocardial infarction.

With cardiac angiography, the patient's heart is injected with a dye so that the coronary arteries are visible during X-ray. Injecting the dye involves inserting a catheter into a blood vessel in either the patient's arm or the groin and then threading it through the circulatory system to the heart. The heart pumps the released dye into the coronary arteries, allowing an X-ray to reveal the extent of the blockage as well as the areas where blood flow is reduced. For a complete diagnostic procedure, several catheterizations are necessary, and the procedure takes a total time of 1 to 2 hours. (Ricciuti, 1997).

Cardiac catheterization and angiography are invasive surgical procedures, but patients are awake and usually only lightly sedated. The procedure is uncomfortable and even painful, and patients are typically anxious about their health as well as the procedure itself. In addition, angiography carries some slight risk of injury or death. The chances of complications increase with patients who have more serious heart problems or diabetes (Ricciuti, 1997). Health psychologists can train patients in various techniques to relieve the stress and discomfort involved with this procedure (see Chapter 3).

Cardiac catheterization can be used in treatment as well as in diagnosis. Clot-dissolving drugs can be injected during a heart attack to dissolve the blood clot that precipitated the infarction, to minimize damage to the heart muscle. In addition, catheters with inflatable tips can reopen blocked arteries, preventing heart attacks.

Angioplasty is the procedure of inserting a balloon-tipped catheter into blocked arteries and inflating the tip to reduce artery blockage. First used successfully in 1977, angioplasty has now become routine (Ricciuti, 1997). Although angioplasty is an invasive surgical procedure, it is less risky than coronary bypass grafting. The success of angioplasty depends on the severity of the lesions, but the procedure is successful in at least 65% of cases. The main problem with angioplasty is the tendency for the blockage to reoccur in 25 to 35% of patients.

Catheterization can also be used to install a stent in an artery (Ricciuti, 1997). A stent is a metal device that can open a blocked artery and keep it open. Catheterization is also part of the process of removing artery blockages by breaking up the plaque or removing it. Catheterization is necessary for these treatment procedures, but diagnosis without surgical intervention is also a desirable goal. Several techniques allow diagnosis of various heart problems with less invasive technologies, but catheterization and angiography remain the best way to diagnose coronary artery blockage.

In Summary

Several techniques measure the functioning of the cardiovascular system. The simplest of these is a blood pressure reading, but this measurement cannot offer a complete diagnosis, because it does not reveal the cause of high blood pressure. The

ECG can determine cardiovascular abnormalities of a resting heartbeat. However, an exercise stress test is more valid and sensitive because it combines electrical measurement of the heart with the increased demands on the cardiovascular system that exercise produces. This technique can reveal blockage of the coronary arteries if substantial damage has occurred. Angiography, which involves X-raying the heart and coronary arteries, is currently considered the most precise diagnostic procedure. However, angiography requires placement of catheters in the heart, an invasive, uncomfortable, stressful procedure. All of these diagnostic procedures help health care professionals advise patients about the extent of damage and the possibility of surgery, angioplasty, and lifestyle changes.

The Changing Rates of Cardiovascular Disease

Throughout the 20th century, **cardiovascular disease (CVD)**, including various types of heart disease and stroke, was the leading cause of death for people in the United States, and the current rate of deaths from CVD is almost identical to the rate in 1920. However, the death rates between 1920 and 1995 changed dramatically. Figure 9.7 reveals a severe rise in CVD deaths from 1920 until the 1950s and 1960s. After 1960, the death rate dropped sharply until currently about less than 32% of all deaths in the United States are from heart disease and another 6.8% from stroke (USBC, 1998).

Reasons for the Decline in Death Rates

Is the decline in cardiac mortality a result mostly of changes in emergency coronary care or of changes to lifestyle? No definitive answer is currently possible. Beginning in the 1960s, many people in the United States began to change their lifestyle. They began to smoke less, be more aware of their blood pressure levels, control serum cholesterol levels, watch their weight, and follow a regular exercise program.

Many of these lifestyle changes were prompted by the publicity given to two monumental studies. The first was the Framingham Heart Study that began to issue reports during the 1960s implicating cigarette smoking, high cholesterol, hypertension, a sedentary lifestyle, and obesity as risk factors in cardiovascular disease (Voelker, 1998). The second study was the highly publicized 1964 Surgeon General's report (U.S. Public Health Service [USPHS], 1964), which found an unequivocal close association between cigarette smoking and heart disease. Many people became aware of these studies and began to alter their way of living.

Although these lifestyle changes closely parallel declining heart disease death rates, they offer no proof of a causal link between behavior changes and the drop in cardiovascular mortality. During this same period, medical care and technology continued to improve, and many cardiac patients who in earlier years would have died were saved by better and faster treatment. Although both factors—lifestyle changes and better medical care—have contributed to the declining death rate from heart disease, evidence began to emerge during the 1980s suggesting that changes in lifestyle may be at least as important as improved medical care in reducing deaths from myocardial infarction. One early study (Pell & Fayerweather, 1985) found a decline in the rate of *first* heart attack among men from the 1950s to the 1980s, signifying that changes in lifestyle may have prevented the onset of cardiovascular disease. More recently, investigators attempted to estimate the relative contributions of improved medical care and changes in lifestyle. One such study (Traven, Kuller, Ives, Rutan, & Perper, 1995) concluded that the 60% decline in coronary heart disease mortality for middle-aged European American men was due more to changes in lifestyle than to improvements in the treatment of heart disease. A report from the Framingham Heart Study (Sytkowski, D'Agostino, Belanger, & Kannel, 1996) also showed that more than one-half of the decline in cardiovascular disease mortality in women was attributable to changes in such lifestyle risk factors as obesity, cholesterol, blood pressure, and smoking. For

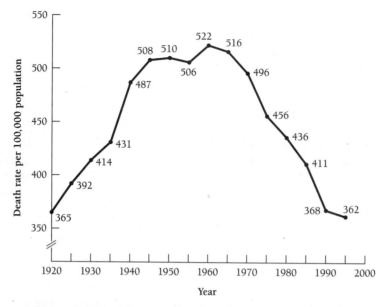

Figure 9.7   Death rates for major cardiovascular disease per 100,000 population, United States, 1920–1995.   *Source:* Data from *Historical Statistics of the United States: Colonial Times to 1970* (p. 58), by U.S. Bureau of the Census, 1975. Washington, DC: U.S. Government Printing Office; from *Statistical Abstracts of the United States: 1986* (p. 73), by U. S. Bureau of the Census, 1985, Washington, DC: U. S. Government Printing Office; and from *Statistical Abstracts of the United States, 1997* (117th edition, p. 94), by U. S. Bureau of the Census, 1997, Washington, DC: U. S. Government Printing Office.

men, about one-third to one-half of the decline was due to changes in these risk factors. Finally, a review of studies published in the United States (Hunink et al., 1997) found that more than 50% of the decline in coronary heart disease mortality was explained by behavior and lifestyle changes that protected people against both first and subsequent heart attacks and about 43% of CHD mortality decline was due to improvements in treatment. These studies suggest that the declining rates of death from heart disease may be about equally due to improved medical care and to changes in behavior and lifestyle.

Heart Disease Mortality throughout the World

The United States is only one of many industrialized Western countries that have seen lifestyle changes

and dramatic reductions in cardiovascular deaths among its population. One study from Finland (Jousilahti, Vartiainen, Toumilehto, Pekkanen, & Puska, 1995), for example, showed nearly a 50% reduction in coronary deaths of men and women during just the decade from 1972 to 1982. For this group, about one-half of the reduction in deaths was due to a healthier lifestyle, including reductions in total cholesterol, better control of blood pressure, and reductions in cigarette smoking. These changes are likely to continue to pay off in continued decreases in coronary mortality of 4% to 5% per year.

In New Zealand and Australia, nonfatal myocardial infarctions declined for both men and women by about 3% per year from the mid-1980s to the mid-1990s (Beaglehole et al., 1997). The rate of prehospitalized deaths declined more than deaths after hospitalization, which means that lifestyle changes rather than medical treatment have reduced the number of first heart attack deaths.

In Summary

Since the mid-1960s, deaths from coronary heart disease and stroke have steadily declined in the United States and most other industrialized nations. Although some of that decline is a result of better and faster coronary care, most authorities believe that lifestyle changes account for a significant amount of this decrease, perhaps as much as 50%. During the past 3 decades, millions of people in the United States quit smoking, became more aware of their blood pressure, watched their diet in order to control weight and cholesterol, and began an exercise program to lower their risk of heart disease.

Risk Factors in Cardiovascular Disease

Medical research has no exact answers as to what causes dangerous buildup of atheromatous plaques in the arteries of some people but not in others. However, research has linked several *risk factors* to cardiovascular disease. In Chapter 2, we defined a risk factor as any characteristic or condition that occurs with greater frequency in people with a disease than in people free from that disease. The risk factor approach does not reveal the underlying physiology in the development of the disorder; that is, it does not allow for the identification of a cause. Nor does it allow a precise prediction of who will be affected and who will remain healthy. The risk factor approach simply yields information concerning which conditions are associated—directly or indirectly—with a particular disease or disorder.

The risk factor approach to predicting heart disease began with the Framingham Heart Study in 1948, an investigation of more than 5,000 people in the town of Framingham, Massachusetts. The study was an epidemiological prospective de-

sign; thus all participants were free of heart disease at the beginning of the study. The original plan was to follow these people for 20 years to study heart disease and the factors related to its development. The results proved so valuable that the study has continued now for more than 50 years. In 1971, more than 5,000 children and their spouses were added to the study, and more recently, a third generation was included in order to follow the development of cardiovascular disease in the offspring of those original participants (Voelker, 1998).

During its early years, the Framingham study uncovered a number of risk factors for cardiovascular disease, including cigarette smoking, high cholesterol levels, elevated blood pressure, lack of physical activity, diet, and obesity. Other studies have found additional conditions that relate directly or indirectly to heart disease, and these include inherent risk factors such as diabetes, family history, gender, and ethnic background as well as psychosocial factors such as phobic anxiety, marital status, employment, hostility, and anger. Despite this impressive list, William Castelli, a long-time researcher with the Framingham study, believes that we currently know only about half the risk factors for heart disease (Voelker, 1998).

Inherent Risk Factors

Inherent risk factors result from genetic or physical conditions that cannot be modified through lifestyle changes. Because risk factors interact with one another so that a person with several risk factors is at greater risk than a person with only one, people with inherent risk factors have additional cause to reduce those risk factors that can be modified through lifestyle. For example, juvenile-onset diabetes is one inherent risk factor for CVD. People who have juvenile-onset diabetes are twice as likely to die of heart disease as those whose sugar metabolism is normal. Diabetics can decrease their risk by following a healthy lifestyle and by adhering to their medical regimen.

Age is the strongest inherent risk factor. Older people, of course, are more likely to die from all

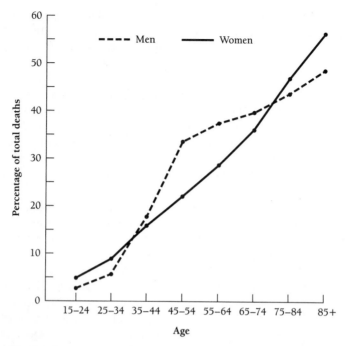

Figure 9.8 **The percentage of deaths from cardiovascular disease by age and gender, United States, 1991.**   *Source:* From *Statistical Abstracts of the United States, 1994* (114th ed., p. 94), by U.S. Department of Commerce, Bureau of the Census, 1994, Washington, DC: U. S. Government Printing Office.

causes than younger people. However, as people become older, the *ratio* of cardiovascular deaths to all-cause mortality increases. Figure 9.8 shows the rapid rise in the rate of cardiovascular mortality as people age. For young people 15 to 24 years of age, only about 2% of deaths are from cardiovascular disease, but for men and women 85 or older, at least half of deaths are due to heart disease and stroke. Figure 9.8 shows that for women below age 35 or above age 84, the percentage of deaths due to cardiovascular disease is higher than that of men even though men have a higher *rate* of cardiovascular death at all ages.

Family history is also an inherent risk factor for CVD. People with a history of cardiovascular disease in their family are more likely to die of heart disease than those with no such history; thus, Jason, our case study, is at risk because of his father's history of heart disease at an early age. Like other inherent risk factors, family history cannot be altered through lifestyle changes, but people with a family history of heart disease can lower their risk by changing those behaviors and lifestyles that can be altered.

Gender is another inherent risk factor. Heart disease is the leading cause of death in the United States for both women and men. However, men have a higher rate of death from CVD at every age, although the discrepancy is greatest for the middle-age years. Figure 9.9 shows that the rate of men's death from cardiovascular disease is about double that of women for ages 35 to 74. After that age, the percentage of women's deaths due to CVD increases sharply but still does not equal that of men.

What factors explain this gender gap? Hormones (Williams, 1989) and lifestyle (Matthews, 1989) have

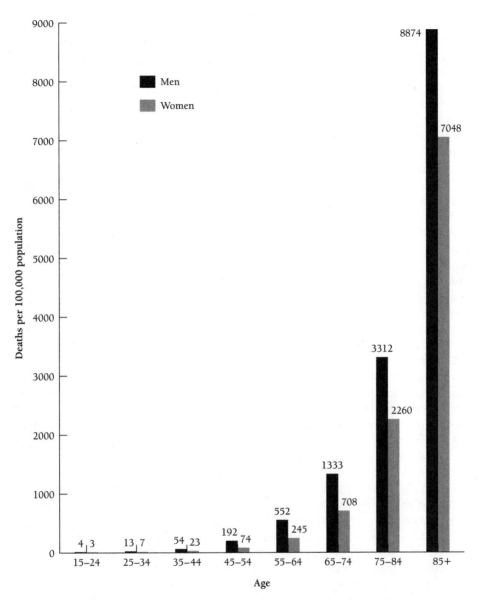

Figure 9.9 Cardiovascular disease mortality rates by age and gender, United States, 1993. *Source:* From *Statistical Abstracts of the United States, 1997* (117th ed., p. 97), by U.S. Department of Commerce, Bureau of the Census, 1997, Washington, DC: U.S. Government Printing Office.

both been hypothesized as factors, but lifestyle alone does not account for the gender gap. Statistically adjusting for lifestyle factors such as smoking, education, physical activity, cholesterol levels, and blood pressure did not change the risk for elderly men (Fried et al., 1998). Even with the same risk factors as women, men were still more than twice as likely to have died from coronary heart disease.

If gender is truly an inherent risk factor for CVD, then the differences between men and women should be similar throughout history, but the gender gap in heart disease was small until the 1920s (Nikiforov & Mamaev, 1998). Until that time, CVD deaths for men ages 25 to 74 years were only about 20% higher than women. From that time until the 1960s, the gap between men and women began to expand during middle age, as men's rates increased while women's rates declined. As a consequence, men now have twice the cardiovascular mortality as women during middle age. This historical perspective suggests that factors other than biology are at work in creating the gender gap, but it leaves the discrepancy unexplained.

Ethnic background is another risk for cardiovascular disease mortality. African Americans, compared with European Americans, have 40% higher coronary heart disease mortality and more than a twofold risk from ages 15 to 64 (Harry Rosenberg, Centers for Disease Control and Prevention, personal communication, September 23, 1998). Whether this increased risk for African Americans is inherent or related to social, economic, or behavioral factors remains in question.

African Americans tend to have the same risk factors for heart disease as do European Americans. However, the level of many of those risks is greater for African Americans, a discrepancy that exists even during childhood (Winkleby, Robinson, Sundquist, & Kraemer, 1999). The risks that are strongest for African Americans are high blood pressure, low income, and low educational level (Gillum, Mussolino, & Madans, 1998). The higher rates of cardiovascular death among African Americans may relate to their higher rate of hypertension, this risk may relate to greater cardiac reactivity (Light et al., 1993a). The tendency to react to stress by increased cardiac function may be a result of inherent factors, but some research has suggested that African Americans are particularly susceptible to increased blood pressure in reaction to racial discrimination. Nancy Krieger and her associates (Krieger & Sidney, 1996; Krieger, Sidney, &

Coakley, 1998) reported that part of the difference between African Americans and European Americans in blood pressure was due to experiences with racial discrimination. For low-income African American men, skin color related to both blood pressure and experiences with discrimination. However, for professional African American men and women skin color was unrelated to experiences of discrimination (Krieger et al., 1998). These studies suggest that reactions to racial discrimination may be partially responsible for the increased blood pressure levels among African Americans, but the issue is complicated by gender, skin color, and social class.

Some investigators (Rogers, 1992) have questioned whether African Americans would have any excess risk of cardiovascular disease if sociodemographic and economic factors such as marital status, family size, income, and educational level were controlled. However, socioeconomic status does not explain all the differences in cardiovascular risk factors for African American, Hispanic American, and European American women (Winkleby, Kraemer, Ahn, & Varady, 1998). Women with low socioeconomic status in all three groups had elevated risk factors compared with women with higher socioeconomic status, and African American and Hispanic American women had higher risk factors for CVD. However, after controlling for age and socioeconomic status (defined as education and family income), African American and Hispanic American women continued to have more risk factors than European American women. Therefore, high CVD risk factors are related to *both* socioeconomic level and ethnicity.

Although inherent risk factors cannot be changed, people with these risk factors are not necessarily destined to develop cardiovascular disease. Identifying people with inherent risk factors is important because such high-risk individuals can minimize their overall risk profile by changing the factors they can control through behavioral management and adjustments in lifestyle. For example, even with a family history of heart disease, people can control hypertension, quit

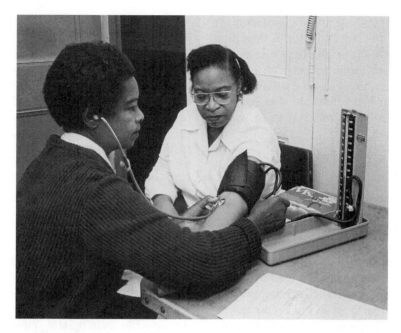

African Americans are more likely to have hypertension than European Americans.

smoking, and eat a healthy diet, thus lowering their *combined* risk factors.

Physiological Conditions

A second category of risk factors in cardiovascular disease includes the physiological conditions of hypertension and serum cholesterol level.

Hypertension   Hypertension is the single most important risk factor in cardiovascular disease, yet millions of people with high blood pressure are not aware of their vulnerability. Unlike most disorders, hypertension produces no overt symptoms, and dangerously elevated blood pressure levels commonly occur with no signals or symptoms. Most people believe that if their blood pressure were high they would be aware of the elevation (Meyer, Leventhal, & Gutman, 1985). Unfortunately, hypertension ordinarily has no discernible symptoms. At 15, Jason does not monitor his blood

pressure, and he takes a rather fatalistic attitude about developing hypertension.

Although the Framingham Heart Study was not the first to suggest that people with high blood pressure have more cardiovascular problems than those with normal blood pressure, it provided solid evidence of the importance of hypertension. The Framingham study (Dawber, 1980) divided blood pressure into three categories: normotensive (normal blood pressure), borderline, and hypertensive. Regardless of people's age or gender, their risk of cardiovascular disease increased with increases in blood pressure, clearly indicating that high blood pressure is a risk factor. Since that time, many other studies (e.g., Fried et al., 1998; Reed, MacLean, & Hayash, 1987) have confirmed the dose-response association between blood pressure and rate of cardiovascular disease.

If hypertension is a risk factor for heart disease and stroke, then factors related to hypertension should also relate to cardiovascular disease. One such factor is obesity, which the Framingham study found to be the best predictor of hypertension (Dawber, 1980). Although obesity itself does not always result in cardiovascular disease, one study (Manson et al., 1995) found that very heavy middle-age women had a fourfold risk. In summary, hypertension and factors related to hypertension are risks for CVD.

Serum Cholesterol Level   A second physiological condition related to cardiovascular disease is high serum cholesterol level. *Serum* or *blood cholesterol* is the level of cholesterol circulating through the blood stream; this level is related (but not perfectly related) to *dietary cholesterol,* or the amount of cholesterol in one's food. Cholesterol is a waxy, fat-like substance that is essential for human life as a component of cell membranes, insulation for neurons, and an ingredient in the production of certain hormones. The liver manufactures cholesterol, but cholesterol also comes from diet. Dietary cholesterol comes from animal fats and oils but not from vegetables or vegetable products. Although cholesterol is essential for life, too much may lead to cardiovascular disease.

After a person eats cholesterol, his or her bloodstream transports it as part of the process of digestion. A measurement of the amount of cholesterol carried in the serum (the liquid, cell-free part of the blood) is typically expressed in milligrams (mg) of cholesterol per deciliters (dl) of serum. This measurement is a ratio, but it is generally abbreviated to the cholesterol count. Thus, a cholesterol reading of 210 means 210 mg of cholesterol per deciliter of blood serum. But what does a cholesterol level of 210 mean? Is it good or bad?

Very high levels of cholesterol are dangerous. People with CHD tend to have high serum cholesterol levels, but how much cholesterol is too much? A long-term follow-up of young White men (Klag et al., 1993) found that cholesterol level at age 22 predicted incidence of cardiovascular disease, coronary heart disease, and cardiovascular deaths decades later. Men who had cholesterol levels of 209 to 315 were much more likely to develop coronary heart disease and die from cardiovascular disease than men who had total cholesterol levels of 118 to 172. An earlier report (Stamler, Wentworth, & Neaton, 1986) found not only elevated risk associated with high cholesterol but also a continuous relationship; that is, the higher the cholesterol level, the greater the risk. As cholesterol levels increased above 245, the risk for CVD increased from three to about four times that of men whose cholesterol level was below 180. The dose-response relationship between total cholesterol level and rate of death from coronary heart disease and stroke reveals only part of the story of cholesterol and cardiovascular disease.

Not all cholesterol is equally implicated in atherosclerosis (Gordon, Castelli, Hjortland, Kannel, & Dawber, 1977). Cholesterol circulates in the blood in several forms of **lipoproteins;** these lipoproteins can be distinguished by analyzing their density. The Framingham researchers found that **low-density lipoprotein (LDL)** was positively related to coronary heart disease, whereas **high-density lipoprotein (HDL)** was negatively related. Therefore, HDL seems to offer some protection against CVD, whereas LDL seems to promote atherosclerosis. Thus, LDL is sometimes referred to as "bad cholesterol" and HDL as "good cholesterol." Indeed, women's higher levels of HDL may be a partial explanation for the gender gap in heart disease (Davis et al., 1996).

During the past 20 years, much attention has centered on the ratio of total cholesterol to high-density lipoprotein. Total cholesterol is determined by adding the values for HDL, LDL, and 20% of very low-density lipoprotein (VLDL), also called **triglycerides.** A low ratio of total cholesterol to HDL is more desirable than a high ratio. Kenneth Cooper (1988) recommended ratios of less than 4.6 to 1.0 for men and less than 4.0 to 1.0 for women. That is, men should have HDL levels that are at least 22% of total cholesterol; women should have HDL levels that are at least 25% of total cholesterol. Most authorities now believe that a favorable balance of total cholesterol to HDL is more critical than total cholesterol in avoiding cardiovascular disease.

WOULD YOU BELIEVE...?

Cholesterol Level Is Related to Violent Death

Would you believe that lowering your cholesterol level may *increase* your chance of violent death, including suicide? Since the 1980s evidence has been accumulating that despite the positive relationship between cholesterol levels and incidence of coronary artery disease, low cholesterol does not lower all-cause mortality. Curiously, there seems to be a U-shaped relationship between total cholesterol and death from all causes, with both high and low levels of cholesterol associated with higher death rates. For example, a report from the Multiple Risk Factor Intervention Trial (Iso, Jacobs, Wentworth, Neaton, & Cohen, 1989) indicated the mortality rate for men with total cholesterol below 140 or above 300 was nearly twice as high as the mortality rate of men with cholesterol levels between 180 and 220.

Results of a review (Holme, 1990) confirmed the effectiveness of reducing total cholesterol on incidence of CHD, but the interventions to lower cholesterol *increased* total death rates. The possibility that violent deaths account for the difference was confirmed by two meta-analyses (Cumings & Psaty, 1994; Muldoon, Manuck, & Matthews, 1992), which revealed that men with low levels of cholesterol had significantly higher rates of deaths from violence or suicide. But why should low cholesterol be related to violent death? Researchers looking for the underlying connection discovered a link between low cholesterol and depression in men over 70 (Morgan, Palinkas, Barrett-Connor, & Wingard, 1993). Depression was about three times higher for men with cholesterol below 160 than for those with higher cholesterol.

Most of the earlier studies demonstrating a link between lower cholesterol and violent death involved cholesterol-reducing interventions and thus used participants who may have been experiencing the unpleasantness of a low-fat diet or the rigors of a tedious drug program. Could this deprivation have made them irritable and thus aggressive? More recent evidence does not support this hypothesis. A study of psychiatric patients (Mufti, Balon, & Arfken, 1998)

found that the strong relationship between low cholesterol levels and violent behavior could not be accounted for by cholesterol-lowering medication, alcohol use, or diet. However, research with animals by Jay Kaplan and his associates (Kaplan, Fontenot, Manuck & Muldoon, 1996; Kaplan et al., 1994) found that monkeys on a cholesterol-lowering diet behaved more aggressively than those on a high-fat diet, suggesting that a low-fat diet may be at least partially responsible for aggressive and violent behavior.

The frequently observed relationship between low cholesterol and violent death has led many authorities to rethink the standard recommendation to lower cholesterol. Gains from decreased CHD deaths are offset by increased deaths from other causes, including violent deaths. Researchers still have no satisfactory explanation for this intriguing finding, but David Jacobs and his associates (Jacobs, Muldoon, & Rästam, 1995) offered three possible explanations. First, certain diseases may cause lower cholesterol. This explanation may account for part of the relationship between low cholesterol and all-cause mortality. Low LDL was associated with cancer in one study (Fried et al., 1998), but this finding cannot explain the link between low cholesterol and non-illness mortality. The second explanation of Jacobs et al. is that some third factor, such as cigarette smoking, age, or socioeconomic status, may relate to both cholesterol and violent death. Although evidence from the Framingham study suggests that smoking may be implicated in excess deaths among people with total cholesterol below 160 (D'Agostino, Belanger, Kannel, & Higgins, 1995), these other factors are unlikely explanations because many of the studies have controlled for their potentially confounding factors. Third, there may be some overarching biological pathway by which serum cholesterol increases rate of violent death. To date, no such biological mechanism has been discovered, so in the meantime, the best advice may be to try to maintain a total cholesterol level that is neither too high nor too low.

Neither of these factors is as important in older people as they are in young and middle-aged people. Data from the Framingham study (Kronmal, Cain, Ye, & Omenn, 1993) revealed a significant positive relationship between total cholesterol levels and death from heart disease up to about age 60. From age 60 to 70, there was no significant relationship, and after age 80 total serum cholesterol levels may actually have a protective effect against death from cardiovascular disease. Therefore, cholesterol should be a concern through middle age, but older people can be less focused on attaining a low cholesterol level.

The findings on cholesterol and diet suggest several conclusions. First, cholesterol intake and blood cholesterol are related. Second, the relationship between dietary intake of cholesterol and blood cholesterol relates strongly to habitual diet—that is, eating habits maintained over many years. Lowering blood cholesterol level is possible, but the process is neither quick nor easy. Third, the guidelines that apply to young and middle-aged people do not apply to older people.

Behavioral Factors

A third category of risk factors includes all the behavioral correlates of cardiovascular disease, especially smoking and diet.

Smoking   Cigarette smoking is the leading behavioral risk factor for cardiovascular death in the United States, and more cigarette smokers die from cardiovascular disease than from all forms of cancer combined. Cigarette smokers are two to three times as likely to die from cardiovascular disease as nonsmokers, with at least 180,000 cardiovascular deaths a year due to smoking (USDHHS, 1995).

One recent study of lifestyle and biological risk factors for coronary heart disease (Twisk, Kemper, van Mechelen, & Post, 1997) looked at such factors as diet, physical activity, alcohol consumption, cholesterol levels, blood pressure, body fat, cardiopulmonary fitness, and smoking. Most life-style factors were relatively low risks, but cigarette smok-

ing was a strong risk for coronary heart disease. The link between smoking and heart disease has been well established for more than 30 years, and few studies are currently being conducted to confirm this association. Studies designed to discover a variety of cardiovascular risk factors (e.g., Fried et al., 1998) continue to find that high levels of cigarette smoking more than double one's chances of dying from cardiovascular disease. Passive smoking is not as dangerous, but exposure to environmental tobacco smoke raises the risk for cardiovascular disease by about 20% (Werner & Pearson, 1998).

Diet   Although obesity has long been suspected of being a risk factor for cardiovascular disease, evidence during the past 2 or 3 decades has suggested that *diet* contributes more to one's chances of developing heart disease than being overweight, which may not even be an independent risk factor for cardiovascular disease. Research during this period has suggested that diet may either increase or decrease one's chances of developing heart disease

The role of fat in the diet has received a great deal of attention; diets high in saturated fat increase one's risk for heart disease. Replacing saturated fat with other types of fat or oil is one strategy to reduce fat, but decreasing overall fat consumption is an even wiser choice (Trevisan et al., 1990).

Several different dietary components have been identified as protection against cardiovascular disease. For example, diets high in several vitamins reduce the risk. These vitamins are referred to as antioxidants because they seem to protect LDL from oxidation and thus from its potential damaging effects on the cardiovascular system. Included in this group are vitamin E, beta carotene, selenium, and riboflavin.

Consuming high levels of vitamin E lowered the CVD risk for female nurses (Stampfer et al., 1993) and male health care professionals (Rimm et al., 1993). The protective effects were not immediate, but after 2 years of taking vitamin E supplements, risks decreased. A measure of antioxidants in the blood, called serum carotenoids, also seems to protect against coronary disease

(Morris, Kritchevsky, & Davis, 1994). These studies suggest that regular consumption of vitamin E and beta carotene probably has some ability to protect against heart disease.

Fruits and vegetables, the main dietary sources of antioxidants, also provide fiber. A diet high in fiber is also related to decreases in coronary heart disease (Connor & Connor, 1997; Katan et al., 1997). In addition to fruits, vegetables, and grains, fish also seems to offer some protection against heart disease. The studies that have shown a benefit for fish consumption included only male participants, so the results are limited, but several studies (Albert et al., 1998; Daviglus et al., 1997) have shown that moderate fish consumption seems to protect men against myocardial infarction.

Psychosocial Factors

In addition to inherent factors, physiological conditions, and behaviors, researchers have identified a number of psychosocial factors that relate to heart disease. Included among these factors are anxiety level, education, income, marital status, and the Type A behavior pattern.

Anxiety For many years, people have suspected that high levels of anxiety may contribute to coronary death, but only relatively recently has evidence for this belief emerged. An 18- to 20-year follow-up of people with normal blood pressure at the beginning of the Framingham study (Markovitz, Matthews, Kannel, Cobb, & D'Agostino, 1993) revealed that men who had heightened anxiety were more than twice as likely as men with lower anxiety levels to develop hypertension during middle age. This relationship did not hold for older men or for women. A prospective study (Kawachi et al., 1994) showed that men who experienced phobic anxiety were three times more likely to suffer sudden death from heart disease than men who were lower in anxiety. A 32-year case-control follow-up study (Kawachi, Sparrow, Vokonas, & Weiss, 1994) found a similarly elevated risk of sudden death from heart disease but

showed that anxiety was unrelated to the risk for nonfatal myocardial infarction or angina, suggesting that anxiety contributes to the deadliness of the disease.

Educational Level and Income Low educational level and low income are two additional risk factors for heart disease. A prospective study (Eaker, Pinsky, & Castelli, 1992) found that employed women and homemakers with little education were at increased risk of myocardial infarction. Other studies (e.g., Fried et al., 1998) reported that both women and men with less than a high school education had nearly twice the rate of cardiovascular mortality as men and women with higher levels of education. Also, the National Health and Nutrition Examination Survey (Gillum et al., 1998) found that both African American and European American men and women with fewer than 12 years of school were at an increased risk for coronary heart disease, but the risk was greatest for African American men. For this group, low education was an even higher risk than elevated blood pressure.

Income level is another risk factor for coronary heart disease; people with lower incomes have higher rates of heart disease than people in the higher income brackets. Redford Williams and his associates (1992) looked at the survival rates of male and female patients with coronary artery disease and found that those with incomes of $40,000 or more had nearly double the survival rate of those with incomes of $10,000 or less. Similarly, Linda Fried and her associates (1998) reported that older people with incomes of less than $50,000 a year were nearly twice as likely to die of cardiovascular disease as those with incomes of $50,000 or more. These findings suggest that people who lack financial or educational resources are probably less able or less likely to seek medical care—conditions that place them at a greater risk for a variety of disorders, including heart disease.

Marriage and Social Support Being single and lacking social support are also coronary risk factors, at least for some people. Unmarried people who lack someone in whom they can confide are much more likely to die of coronary artery disease than people who have a spouse, a confidant, or both (Williams et al., 1992). For people who have already had a heart attack, living alone can be an independent risk for additional heart problems. One study (Case, Moss, Case, McDermott, & Eberly, 1992) found that 6 months after having a heart attack, patients who lived alone were nearly twice as likely as those who lived with another person to have had a recurrent cardiac event.

These studies confirm results from other research on social support discussed in Chapter 8, which indicated that people who have a wide circle of friends or who feel they can confide in another person are less likely to die of stress-related diseases. Social support may reduce risk of cardiovascular mortality when a spouse or friend encourages a patient to maintain a healthy lifestyle, to seek medical attention, and to comply with medical advice.

The Type A Behavior Pattern   Another behavioral factor that has received a plethora of research attention is the Type A behavior pattern. However, most researchers now believe that the Type A concept is too general and that only one of its components—overt expressions of hostility—contributes to coronary heart disease.

The Type A behavior pattern is a concept originated by two cardiologists, Meyer Friedman and Ray Rosenman (Friedman & Rosenman, 1974; Rosenman et al., 1975). Friedman and Rosenman hypothesized that people can be divided into two categories, Type A and Type B. People with the Type A behavioral pattern are hostile, competitive, concerned with numbers and the acquisition of objects, and possessed of an exaggerated sense of time urgency. The Type B behavior pattern is characterized by a lack of time urgency, competitiveness, and hostility.

Friedman and Rosenman originated the Type A behavior pattern as a result of their observations during the 1960s that most of their coronary patients exhibited these behaviors. An early prospective study—the Western Collaborative Group Study (Rosenman et al., 1975)—showed that Type A men were about twice as likely as Type B men to experience coronary heart disease. However, other research has failed to find strong support for the relationship between the Type A behavior pattern and development of CHD (Ragland & Brand, 1988).

The inability of a global Type A behavior pattern to consistently predict heart disease has led investigators to analyze the component behaviors in the Type A pattern to determine whether some one behavior or some constellation of behaviors might yield a more valid predictor. Researchers became increasingly convinced that the global Type A behavior pattern, as defined by extreme ambition, competitiveness, impatience, hostility, and time urgency, is *not* a risk factor for coronary artery disease (Siegman, Anderson, Herbst, Boyle, & Wilkinson, 1992). Instead, they began to focus on one possible toxic component of the Type A behavior pattern—namely *hostility.*

Hostility   Beginning in the 1980s, a large body of research emerged that demonstrated a link between hostility and heart disease (Dembroski & MacDougall, 1985; Dembroski, MacDougall, Williams, Haney, & Blumenthal, 1985). Indeed, hostility is a better predictor of coronary artery blockage than Type A behavior (Williams et al., 1980), and hostility is associated with increased coronary and all-cause mortality for both women and men (Barefoot, Larsen, von der Lieth, & Schroll, 1995). Redford Williams (1989) presented evidence that one type of hostility—cynical hostility—is especially harmful. Williams contended that people who mistrust others, think the worst of humanity, and interact with others with cynical hostility are harming themselves and their hearts. Furthermore, he suggested that people who use *anger* as a response to interpersonal problems have an elevated risk for heart disease.

To investigate the relationship between hostility and heart disease, researchers have used several measures of hostility, particularly the Cook-Medley

Hostility (Ho) Index (Cook & Medley, 1954). The Cook-Medley consists of 50 items taken from the original Minnesota Multiphasic Personality Inventory (MMPI) and therefore offers the advantage of being part of a widely administered psychological test. The Ho scale of the Cook-Medley measures suspiciousness, resentment, frequent anger, and cynical mistrust of others more than it measures the tendency to behave violently. Recently, Erika Rosenberg and her associates (Rosenberg, Ekman, & Blumenthal, 1998) measured the affective component of Ho and found that facial expressions of contempt in coronary heart disease patients were accurate reflections of hostility.

Although hostility is related to coronary mortality (Ranchor, Sanderman, Bouma, Buunk, & van den Heuvel, 1997), it is also related to other causes of death. Thus, hostility is not a risk specific to cardiovascular disease. In addition, hostility is not an independent predictor of heart disease; it is related to other behaviors that relate to heart disease. These include higher body weight and blood pressure (Siegler, Peterson, Barefoot, & Williams, 1992), alcohol consumption and smoking (Everson et al., 1997), and negative life events and low social support (Scherwitz, Perkins, Chesney, & Hughes, 1991). Controlling for alcohol consumption, smoking, and body weight caused the relationship between hostility and coronary heart disease to disappear (Everson et al., 1997), demonstrating that hostility is not an independent risk factor for CHD.

Research on the relationship between hostility and cardiovascular disease continues, and hostility as a factor in disease remains an active question in health psychology. However, many researchers interested in psychosocial factors in cardiovascular disease have narrowed their investigations to specific components of hostility, just as a decade earlier other researchers sought to discover the specific toxic components of the Type A behavior pattern. Those efforts have focused on anger.

Anger   Hostility and anger are related, but anger can be defined as an unpleasant *emotion* accompanied by physiological arousal and usually lasting for a relatively short duration (Smith, 1994). On the other hand, hostility involves a negative *attitude* toward others and may be of long duration. The *experience* of anger probably does not threaten cardiovascular functioning, but the *expression* of anger may well be a risk factor for coronary artery disease (Siegman, Dembroski, & Ringel, 1987). The *expression* of anger-hostility was positively related to the severity of coronary artery disease (CAD) in angiographic patients. Examples of behaviors that related to severity of coronary artery disease were those that involved yelling back when someone yells at you, raising your voice when arguing, and throwing temper tantrums. This relationship between expression of anger and CAD was independent of traditional risk factors such as cholesterol level and blood pressure (except for patients 65 or older). The significance of this research is that the mere experience of anger did not relate positively to severity of coronary artery disease, but the outward expression of anger did.

Anger and Cardiovascular Reactivity   Why should the expression of anger relate to coronary artery disease? Aron Siegman and his colleagues demonstrated that provoked anger in a laboratory setting increases some measures of cardiovascular reactivity (CVR), specifically increases in systolic and diastolic blood pressure. If increased cardiovascular reactivity generally accompanies expressions of anger, perhaps the continual physical or verbal expression of anger over many years may increase one's risk of cardiovascular disease.

In one study of male undergraduates, Siegman and his associates (Siegman, Anderson, Herbst, Boyle, & Wilkinson, 1992) measured cardiovascular reactivity in a situation that involved a stressful laboratory situation. They found that participants' heart rate and diastolic and systolic blood pressure increased and that participants generally felt a great deal of anger after being provoked. However, their *experience* of anger-hostility was unrelated to their level of reactivity. In contrast, their *expression* of anger-hostility was significantly related to both systolic and diastolic blood

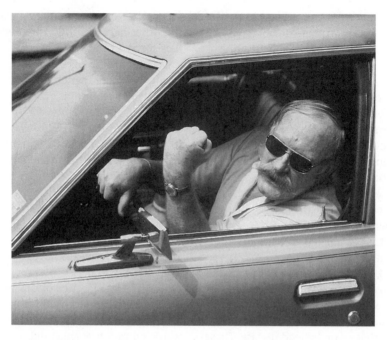

Hostility and expressed anger are risk factors for cardiovascular disease.

pressure but not to heart rate. These results suggest that men, when provoked, show increased levels of cardiovascular reactivity.

Women may not experience comparable reactivity when provoked. Provoked men, but not women, showed increased cardiovascular reactivity as they increased their outward expression of anger (Burns & Katkin, 1993). Similarly, husbands experienced increases in heart rate and systolic blood pressure while attempting to control their wives, but the wives experienced no comparable reactivity while trying to control their husbands (Smith & Brown, 1991). Interestingly, the wives experienced an increase in systolic blood pressure only at the times their husbands were expressing cynical hostility.

This research suggests that provoked anger increases CVR in cynically hostile men but not in women. If psychophysical factors can cause heart disease, these findings may partially explain the different rates of early CHD for men and women. The findings concerning the risks of expressing anger raise the question, Is it healthier to suppress anger?

Suppressed Anger Ted Dembroski and his colleagues reported on two studies suggesting that suppressed anger, or Anger-In, was a toxic element in heart disease. In the first study, Dembroski et al. (1985) found that Potential for Hostility and Anger-In were consistent predictors of severity of coronary artery disease (CAD) for both women and men. The second study (MacDougall, Dembroski, Dimsdale, & Hackett, 1985) found a significant relationship between Anger-In scores and CAD for a group of male patients who had received cardiac catheterization. Once again, these researchers found no value in the global Type A behavior pattern as a predictor of coronary artery disease.

Although results from these studies seem to indicate that suppressed anger may be harmful, it is possible that patients' suppression of anger may be a *result* of heart disease rather than a contributor to it. Also, the relationship between Anger-In (or the suppression of anger) may result from doctors telling heart patients to avoid situations in which they may be provoked to anger and to keep their angry feelings to themselves (Mendes de Leon, 1992). This advice has some validity in light of the findings that an outward expression of anger is predictive of coronary artery disease. But this recommendation should be given to people (especially men) *before* they develop heart disease. Once people are diagnosed with heart disease, anger, whether expressed or suppressed, seems to exacerbate their condition.

Figure 9.10 shows the evolution of the Type A behavior pattern to hostility, to anger, and finally to expressed anger. Although research evidence to date is not unanimous, it does suggest that physical and/or verbal expression of anger may be a behavioral risk factor for the development of cardiovascular disease.

Although the belief that hostility and anger somehow cause heart disease is centuries old (Williams, 1993), psychophysiological research has only recently begun to confirm this notion. Still, evidence is lacking that any component of the Type A behavior pattern, including hostility and anger, is a strong independent risk for cardiovascular disease in people generally. Presently, personality factors do not appear to put people (men and women, Black and White, young and old) at the same elevated risk for heart disease as do traditional risk factors, such as cigarette smoking, hypertension, or high cholesterol levels. However, evidence suggests that hostility/anger interacts with these latter two risks to increase a person's risk for heart disease.

In Summary

Although the exact causes of coronary artery disease are not fully understood, an accumulating body of evidence points to certain risk factors. These factors include such inherent risks as family history of heart disease, gender, age, and ethnic background. Although none of these factors can be

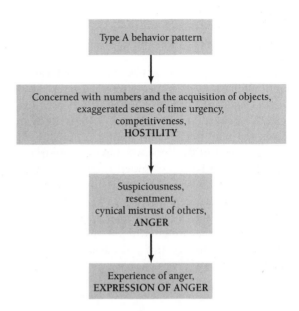

Note: **BOLDFACE** denotes components suggested by research to be the best link to heart disease.

Figure 9.10   The evolution of expressed anger from the Type A behavior pattern.

changed, people who are inherently at risk can modify other risks and thus lower their chances of developing heart disease. Other risk factors include physiological conditions such as hypertension and high serum cholesterol levels. Hypertension is the best predictor of coronary artery disease, and a dose-response relationship exists between blood pressure level and risk for heart disease. Total cholesterol level is also related to coronary artery disease, but the *ratio* of total cholesterol to high-density lipoprotein (HDL) is a more critical risk factor.

Behavioral conditions such as smoking and imprudent eating also relate to heart disease. Cigarette smokers have a two- to threefold risk of developing heart disease, but nonsmokers exposed to tobacco probably have only a very slight risk. Eating foods high in saturated fat and consuming low levels of fiber and antioxidants (vitamin E and beta carotene) add to one's risk of heart disease.

Psychosocial risk factors related to coronary artery disease include anxiety, education and income, marriage and social support, and the hostility/anger component of the Type A behavior pattern. People with persistent anxiety have elevated risks for CAD, as do people with low levels of education and income. However, being married and/or having a confidant can lower one's risk for heart disease. The global Type A behavior pattern does not seem to be an independent risk factor. Hostility is a component of the Type A behavior pattern, but hostility itself is not an independent risk factor. One of its dimensions—anger—has potentially lethal consequences. However, the mere experience of anger seems to have no detrimental effect on cardiovascular functioning. Rather, the *expression* of anger may be the toxic agent underlying some CAD disease.

Modifying Risk Factors for Cardiovascular Disease

Psychology's main contribution to cardiovascular health has focused on changing behaviors related to heart disease and stroke. Psychologists also participate in cardiac rehabilitation by helping patients change their behaviors so they will lower their risk of having another heart attack. The role of psychologists in cardiac rehabilitation and other chronic illnesses is discussed in Chapter 11.

Coronary heart disease and stroke are closely associated with several unhealthy behaviors and living habits, presenting the rationale for the involvement of health psychologists in modifying risk factors for cardiovascular disease. Most of these behaviors are acquired over many years, beginning in childhood, and most are resistant to change. Children at high risk for cardiovascular disease because of elevated cholesterol levels, above ideal weight, and high blood pressure tended to remain at high risk when they became young adults (Myers, Coughlin, Webber, Srinivasan, & Berenson, 1995); that is, cardiovascular risk factors begin during childhood and persist into adulthood. Long-standing habits make advice to go on a diet or to stop smoking ineffective in altering these behaviors. People who enjoy eating eggs and red meats

(and who have done so since they were children) often have quite a bit of trouble changing their eating patterns. People who have smoked two or three packs of cigarettes a day for 10 or 15 years may not find it easy to quit. But psychologists have traditionally been concerned with changing behavior, and many of their techniques can be used to modify behaviors that place people at risk for developing cardiovascular disease.

Before people will cooperate with programs to change their behavior, they must perceive that these behaviors are risk factors that place them in jeopardy. People's perceptions can be colored by potentially deadly biases that decrease their perceptions of risk (Avis, Smith, & McKinlay, 1989). People recognize established risk factors in calculating their personal risk, but they display what Neil Weinstein (1984) called *optimistic bias* in assessing their risk. That is, people tend to believe that these risk factors increase others' risk but not their own. This tendency to exempt oneself from risks, especially behavioral risks, is a strong influence on the perception of personal risk, and that perception can affect a person's willingness to change his or her behavior. Accurate feedback about one's risk status can decrease optimistic bias (Avis et al., 1989; Weinstein, 1983). People with an accurate perception of risk are more likely to do something about changing their risk factors for coronary heart disease.

The most serious behavioral risk factor in cardiovascular disease is cigarette smoking, a behavior also implicated in a variety of other disorders, especially lung cancer. For this reason, all of Chapter 13 is devoted to a discussion of tobacco use. Although hypertension and serum cholesterol are not behaviors and thus cannot be directly modified through psychological interventions, both can be affected indirectly through changes in behavior.

Reducing Hypertension

Lowering high blood pressure into the normal range is difficult, because a number of physiological mechanisms act to keep blood pressure at a set point (Linden, 1988). At least eight different feed-

BECOMING HEALTHIER

1. Know about your family risk for heart disease. Although you cannot change this risk factor, knowing that you are at high risk can motivate you to change some of your modifiable risk factors.

2. Have your blood pressure checked. If it's in the normal range, you can keep it that way by exercising, controlling your weight, and moderating alcohol consumption. Also, try some of the relaxation techniques we discussed in Chapter 8. If your blood pressure is in the hypertensive range, consult a physician.

3. Know your cholesterol level, but be sure to ask for a complete profile, one that includes measures of both HDL and LDL as well as the ratio of total cholesterol to HDL.

4. If you are a smoker who has tried to quit but failed, keep trying. Many ex-smokers made multiple attempts before successfully quitting.

5. Keep a food diary for at least 1 week. Note the amount of saturated fat you ate, the approximate number of calories consumed per day, and the amount of fruits and vegetables you ate. A heart-healthy diet includes five servings of fruits and vegetables per day.

6. If you are persistently angry and react to anger-arousing events with loud, sudden explosions of anger, try to change your reactions by expressing your frustrations in a soft, quite voice.

---

back systems either raise or lower blood pressure when the body senses that blood pressure is out of the critical zone. The body may perpetuate hypertension by means of these feedback mechanisms, regulating blood pressure to the hypertensive level instead of regulating it into the normal range (Linden, 1988). Because complex feedback systems work against rather than for the maintenance of appropriate blood pressure, hypertension tends to be difficult to control.

Interventions aimed toward hypertension usually try to control blood pressure through antihypertensive drug therapy, and four different types of drugs help to control blood pressure through different physical mechanisms. These drugs vary in expense and potential for side effects, and recommendations include prescribing those with the least risk for side effects first (Siegel & Lopez, 1997). All require a physician's prescription, and patients should be periodically monitored while taking them to achieve the best control of blood pressure with the fewest side effects. Because hypertension presents no unpleasant symptoms, many patients are reluctant to continue with a daily medication that may cause unpleasant side effects. (The factors affecting adherence with this and other medical regimens were discussed in Chapter 4.)

Several behaviors relate to both the development and the treatment of hypertension. Obesity is correlated with hypertension, and many obese people who lose weight lower their blood pressure into the normal range. Regular exercise has also been found effective in controlling hypertension (exercise is discussed in Chapter 16). Sodium intake relates to hypertension, and hypertensive patients have been advised to eat less salt. Recent research (Alderman, Cohen, & Madhavan, 1998) has questioned the wisdom of recommending sodium restriction as a prevention for hypertension. However, some people with hypertension can lower their blood pressure by restricting their sodium intake.

Drugs may be the most common strategy for controlling hypertension, but there are also non-pharmacological, behavioral treatments, including stress management (as discussed in Chapter 8.) Other behavioral programs include weight loss, sodium restriction, and alcohol restriction. These changes in behavior can make a difference for people with hypertension. One study (Langford et al., 1985) examined nearly 500 hypertensive individuals who had been on medication for 5 years and whose blood pressure had been reduced to the normal range with medication. After discontinuing their medication, participants were assigned to one of three conditions: a sodium-restricted diet, a weight-loss diet, or a control group. Success with either the weight-loss or the sodium-restricted diet was likely to keep a participant in the normal range without medication. In all, 78% of those who restricted their sodium intake and 72% of those who reduced their weight were successful at maintaining normal blood pressure without medication.

Relaxation training may also be an effective tool for lowering blood pressure. Borderline hypertensive men were able to reduce their blood pressure to a normal range through relaxation therapy (Davison, Williams, Nezami, Bice, & DeQuattro, 1991). These findings strongly suggest that hypertension can be modified through behavioral intervention and that continued medication may not be necessary for many hypertensives who reduce weight, control their diet, and learn relaxation techniques.

Lowering Serum Cholesterol

Interventions aimed at lowering cholesterol levels can include drugs, dietary changes, or both. Cholesterol-lowering drugs such as the *statin* drugs are frequently prescribed for patients with high total cholesterol levels. These drugs act by blocking an enzyme that the liver needs to manufacture cholesterol, and they lower LDL and raise HDL. Other drugs lower cholesterol through different biological actions, but all tend to have the beneficial effects of lowering overall cholesterol levels, lowering LDL, and raising HDL. These drugs are effective (Hebert, Gaziano, Chan, & Hennekens, 1997), but all are prescription medications that cost money and have side effects.

For postmenopausal women, estrogen replacement therapy is also a strategy for lowering cho-

lesterol. The difference in cardiovascular disease in women before and after menopause has led to the belief that estrogen can lower CVD risks. Many observational studies have shown such benefits, but an experimental study (Hulley et al., 1998) showed that although estrogen-replacement therapy lowered cholesterol, it provided no survival advantage for women who had already developed cardiovascular disease. Indeed, women who began this therapy had elevated risks for other diseases, making estrogen replacement a bad choice for postmenopausal women with coronary disease.

For those with very high cholesterol levels, cholesterol-lowering drugs are probably the best choice, but dietary modification may be a more appropriate approach to lowering cholesterol levels for the majority of the population (Wilson, Christiansen, Anderson, & Kannel, 1989). Can people learn to adjust their eating habits sufficiently to affect serum cholesterol levels? Evidence from a meta-analysis of dietary interventions (Brunner et al., 1997) indicated that dietary changes can be effective in improving cardiovascular risk factors. The changes in serum cholesterol levels tended to be modest. Even diets with severe fat restrictions usually do not allow a reduction of high cholesterol levels without some other intervention (Knopp et al., 1997). Therefore, dietary changes alone are not likely to be sufficient to lower dangerously high cholesterol.

Does lowering cholesterol result in decreased deaths from coronary heart disease? Although reductions in total cholesterol do not produce comparable reductions in all-cause mortality (Katerndahl & Lawler, 1999) they do bring about decreases in deaths from heart disease—at least in men (Jacobs et al., 1992). Little research has concentrated on women, and many cholesterol-lowering trials have excluded female participants, resulting in scant and sometimes inconsistent findings. One review (Walsh & Grady, 1995) concluded that healthy women showed no benefit from cholesterol lowering, but another study (Verschuren & Kromhout, 1995) showed a strong relationship between cholesterol level and CHD mortality.

The recommendations for cholesterol lowering, therefore, are complex. For men, lowering total cholesterol by at least 8% to 9% will probably result in a 15% to 20% reduction in CHD, but unless total cholesterol is over 240, the reduction of heart disease may be offset by mortality from other causes. For women, lowering cholesterol will not produce the same benefits or risks as for men, but women with existing coronary artery disease may benefit.

Modifying Psychosocial Risk Factors

Earlier, we discussed research strongly suggestive that hostility and its anger component are the toxic elements in the Type A behavior pattern. If this is so, then a reduction in hostility and anger should prove therapeutic. Redford Williams (1989) has suggested that becoming more trusting is the antidote to cynical hostility. He outlined a 12-step program through which people can decrease their cynicism and hostility and thus lower their risk of heart disease. The steps constitute a type of cognitive therapy in which people become aware of their attitudes, stop cynical thoughts, reason with themselves, and practice trust and relaxation.

Anger, too, can be dealt with in a therapeutic manner, and clinical health psychologists have recommended a variety of strategies for coping with anger. The goal of intervention strategies is not to eliminate anger but to cope with it. Aron Siegman and Selena Cappell Snow (1997) asked college students to participate in three experimental conditions (1) Anger-Out, in which anger-arousing events were expressed loudly and quickly; (2) Anger-In, in which students relived their anger inwardly, that is in their imagination; and (3) Mood-incongruent speech, in which students expressed their anger softly and slowly—that is, in a manner incongruent with their strong emotion. As Siegman and Snow hypothesized, only participants who expressed anger openly and loudly experienced significant cardiovascular reactivity, as measured by blood pressure readings and heart rate. Participants who relived their anger-arousing

experience in imagination or who expressed it in a soft, slow manner had almost no increase in reactivity. These results suggest that people may buffer any toxic elements of anger by reliving the event in imagination or by speaking softly and slowly about the event.

Research has shown that several techniques for managing anger can be successful (Deffenbacher, 1994). One such strategy is relaxation training, which we discussed in Chapter 8. Another approach involves learning new social and communication skills. Perpetually angry people can learn to negotiate with others, to be more assertive, and to become aware of cues others give that typically provoke angry responses. In addition, people can remove themselves from provocative situations before they become angry, or they can do something else. In interpersonal encounters, people can call "time out," count backward from 10, or use self-talk as a reminder that the situation won't last forever. Humor is another potentially effective means of coping with anger, but one must be careful with its use. Sarcastic or hostile humor can incite additional anger, but silliness or mock exaggerations often defuse potentially volatile situations.

Also, Deffenbacher and Robert Stark (1992) presented evidence that relaxation coping skills are effective means of dealing with anger. They used a combination of progressive relaxation, deep breathing exercises, tension-reduction training, relaxing to the slow repetition of the word "relax," and relaxation imagery, in which the person imagines a peaceful scene. People who learned these skills experienced significant reductions in anger compared with people in a no-treatment control group. Moreover, the relaxation group maintained its ability to cope with anger after 1 year.

In Summary

Some cardiovascular risk factors can be changed through psychological interventions. Hypertension is subject to some modification, and behavioral interventions have been moderately successful in lowering high blood pressure. Diets that are low in fatty foods help maintain healthy cholesterol levels, but once elevated, total cholesterol levels are resistant to change through behavioral means. However, research suggests that long-term changes in diet can lower total cholesterol as much as 7% to 10%, perhaps without reducing HDL.

The anger component of hostility can also be modified through practice and training. People can learn to recognize their anger and to express it verbally in a soft, slow voice or to cope with it by a variety of other strategies designed to prevent the anger from turning to rage or fury. Because anger has some association with heart disease, people at risk for cardiovascular disease who also have problems with anger control can reduce that risk through these various coping and relaxation strategies.

Answers

This chapter addressed five basic questions:

1. **What are the structures, functions, and disorders of the cardiovascular system?**

   The cardiovascular system includes the heart and blood vessels (veins, venules, arteries, arterioles, and capillaries). The heart pumps blood throughout the body, delivering oxygen and removing wastes from body cells. Disorders of the cardiovascular system include (1) coronary artery disease (CAD), which occurs when the arteries that supply blood to the heart become clogged with plaque, restricting the blood supply to the heart muscle; (2) angina pectoris, a nonfatal disorder with symptoms of chest pain and difficulty in breathing; (3) myocardial infarction (heart attack), caused by blockage of coronary arteries; (4) stroke, which occurs when the oxygen supply to the brain is disrupted; and (5) hypertension (high blood pressure), a silent disorder but a good predictor of both heart attack and stroke. Heart attack and stroke account for over 30% of deaths in the United States.

2. **What measurements of cardiovascular function can reveal damage?**

   Two measurements that can reveal cardiovascular damage are blood pressure assessment and the electrocardiogram. However, neither can reveal blockage to the coronary arteries. An exercise electrocardiogram (stress test) can reveal coronary artery blockage for severe damage. The most accurate test for coronary artery blockage is angiography, imaging of the coronary arteries. This procedure has the disadvantage of requiring an invasive procedure, namely cardiac catheterization.

3. **How does lifestyle relate to cardiovascular health?**

   Lifestyle factors such as cigarette smoking, diet, and regular physical activity all relate to cardiovascular health. During the past 3 decades, deaths from heart disease steadily decreased in the United States, with perhaps as much as 50% of that drop a result of changes in behavior and lifestyle. During this same time period, millions of people quit smoking, altered their diet to control weight and cholesterol, and began an exercise program.

4. **What are the risk factors for cardiovascular disease?**

   Beginning with the Framingham study, researchers have discovered a number of cardiovascular risk factors. These include (1) inherent risk, (2) physiological risks, (3) behavioral and lifestyle risks, and (4) psychosocial risks. Inherent risk factors, such as family history, age, gender, and ethnicity, cannot be changed, but people with inherent risk can alter their other risks to lower their chances of developing heart disease. The two primary physiological risk factors are hypertension and high cholesterol, and diet can play a role in controlling each of these. Behavioral factors in CVD include smoking and a diet high in saturated fat and low in fiber and antioxidant vitamins. Psychosocial risks include persistently high levels of anxiety, low educational levels, low income, lack of social support, and loud, violent expressions of anger.

5. **Can cardiovascular risk be lowered by modifying risk factors?**

Hypertension can be controlled by drugs, sodium restriction, and relaxation techniques. Cholesterol levels can be lowered through drugs and, to some extent, through diet. Lowering the ratio of total cholesterol to HDL is probably a better idea. Both regular exercise and moderate consumption of alcohol can improve this ratio. Also, people can learn to modify loud, quick outbursts of anger by expressing their frustrations in a soft, slow manner or by using various relaxation techniques.

Glossary

angina pectoris A disorder involving a restricted blood supply to the myocardium, which results in chest pain and restricted breathing.

angiography A method of viewing cardiovascular damage through the use of X-ray pictures and the injection of dye into the circulatory system.

angioplasty Medical intervention in which a catheter with an inflatable tip is passed into an obstructed artery in order to flatten atherosclerotic deposits of plaque.

arteries Vessels carrying blood away from the heart.

arterioles Small branches of an artery.

arteriosclerosis A condition marked by loss of elasticity and hardening of arteries.

atheromatous plaques Deposits of cholesterol and other lipids, connective tissue, and muscle tissue.

atherosclerosis The formation of plaque within the arteries.

capillaries Very small vessels that connect arteries and veins.

cardiovascular disease Disorders of the circulatory system, including coronary heart disease and stroke.

coronary artery disease (CAD) A disorder of the myocardium arising from atherosclerosis and/or arteriosclerosis.

coronary heart disease (CHD) A disorder in which blockage of the coronary arteries affects the functioning of the heart.

diastolic pressure A measure of blood pressure between contractions of the heart.

electrocardiogram (ECG) A measure of the heart's electrical signals.

essential hypertension Elevations of blood pressure that have no known cause.

high-density lipoprotein (HDL) A form of lipoprotein that confers some protection against coronary heart disease.

hypertension Abnormally high blood pressure, with either a systolic reading in excess of 160 or a diastolic reading in excess of 105.

ischemia Restriction of blood flow to tissue or organs; often used with reference to the heart.

lipoproteins Substances in the blood consisting of lipid and protein.

low-density lipoprotein (LDL) A form of lipoprotein found to be positively related to coronary heart disease.

myocardial infarction Heart attack.

myocardium The heart muscle.

secondary hypertension Elevations in blood pressure that are triggered by other diseases.

stress test An exercise test to diagnose coronary heart disease.

stroke Damage to the brain resulting from lack of oxygen; typically the result of cardiovascular disease.

systolic pressure A measure of blood pressure generated by the heart's contraction.

triglycerides A group of molecules consisting of glycerol and three fatty acids; one of the components of serum lipids that has been implicated in the formation of atherosclerotic plaque.

veins Vessels that carry blood to the heart.

venules The smallest veins.

Suggested Readings

Cooper, K. H. (1994). *Dr. Kenneth H. Cooper's antioxidant revolution.* Nashville, TN: Nelson.

In this very readable book, Kenneth Cooper, one of the early promoters of aerobic exercise for a healthy heart, discusses the value of antioxidants, including vitamin E.

Dolnick, E. (1995). Hot heads and heart attacks. *Health, 9*(4), 58–64.

This readable article traces the evolution of the Type A behavior pattern to anger as the underlying risk for heart disease. Dolnick points out the importance of behavioral factors in cardiovascular disease and suggests ways to manage anger to lower risk. Available through InfoTrac College Edition by Wadsworth Publishing Company.

Siegman, A. W. (1994). From Type A to hostility to anger: Reflections on the history of coronary-prone behavior. In A. W. Siegman & T. W. Smith (Eds.), *Anger, hostility, and the heart* (pp. 1–21). Hillsdale, NJ: Erlbaum.

One of the leading advocates of the notion that anger is the toxic component of the Type A behavior pattern discusses the evolution of Type A to hostility to anger.

Voelker, R. (1998). A "family heirloom" turns 50. *Journal of the American Medical Association, 179*, 1241–1245.

Rebecca Voelker's interview with William Castelli, who directed the famous Framingham Heart Study from 1965 to 1995, reveals an interesting history of this study. Castelli contends that epidemiologists still know only about one half of the risk factors for heart disease.

CHAPTER 10

Identifying Behavioral Factors in Cancer

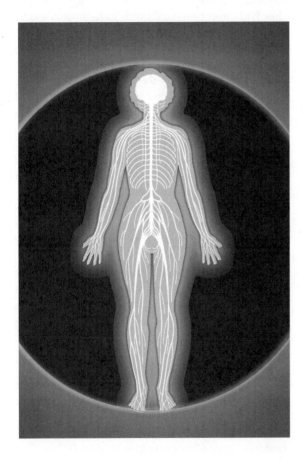

QUESTIONS

This chapter focuses on six basic questions:

1. What is cancer?

2. How deadly is cancer?

3. What are the behavioral risk factors for cancer?

4. What are the uncontrollable risk factors for cancer?

5. What are the psychological risk factors for cancer?

6. What psychosocial factors relate to cancer survival?

VICTORIA: A LIFE-THREATENING DISEASE AT 16

Victoria was a 16-year-old high school junior when she was diagnosed with **non-Hodgkin's lymphoma,** cancer of the lymphatic system. She had noticed a lump on her head and knew of no reason for it. Her mother took Victoria to her pediatrician, who referred her to several specialists. One of these specialists was a dermatologist who took a **biopsy** and diagnosed lymphoma.

The dermatologist did not explain his reasoning or the procedures. Even when he told Victoria and her mother that the lump was lymphoma, he didn't really explain what it was or what she should expect. He did, however, refer her to an **oncologist,** a physician who specializes in the treatment of cancer. The oncologist conducted further tests and confirmed the diagnosis.

Victoria's parents were not pleased with her medical care and took her to a large research hospital that specializes in children's cancer. The hospital physicians repeated some of the testing and rapidly confirmed the diagnosis of lymphoma. The treatment she received there was different—the staff was always completely honest and ready to explain any facet of the diagnosis and treatment. They were also prepared to deal with her reaction to her diagnosis, the first of which was anger. She was angry with everyone for a while.

Her doctors' understanding helped her assimilate her diagnosis and accept the treatment, which consisted of a 3-month regimen of intensive chemotherapy followed by 6 months of less intensive treatment. Her experience during the 3 months of intensive chemotherapy was terrible. She lost 30 pounds, she experienced muscle atrophy and coordination problems, and her hair fell out. But the treatment worked: The tumor started to shrink from the first treatment.

Victoria's life was disrupted by her illness as well as by the treatment. In addition to the difficulties of traveling to the hospital to receive treatment and coping with its side effects, she was faced with changes in her life due to her illness. Her friends treated her differently, becoming awkward around her and not knowing what to say. Victoria knew that they had never been faced with a life-threatening illness in someone their own age. "I didn't think it could happen to anyone I knew," she said. She had been dating a young man for about 3 months when she was diagnosed, and she thought that her illness would end their relationship. She told him that if he couldn't handle it, she would understand. He said that he thought he could, and he did.

Victoria could not attend school during her treatment but received home schooling and graduated from high school with her class. She remembers that keeping up with the school work was not difficult, but being alone was. Rather than going to school and being with her friends, she had to study at home by herself. She believes that the experience changed her, making her less sociable and less outgoing.

Victoria's lymphoma went into remission and has remained so. Although her diagnosis and treatment were difficult and painful, she said that she always thought, "It could have been worse." She never believed she was going to die and never tried to live each day as though it was her last. She did, however, lose her feeling of invincibility.

In this chapter, we examine cancer, the second most frequent cause of death in the United States and many other industrialized countries. We look at the demographics and risk factors for cancer and discuss behavioral changes that can help to alter risk factors. First, however, we define cancer and describe its biology.

Cancer and Its Changing Mortality Rates

The first medical document to describe cancer was the *Ebers Papyrus,* written around 1,500 B.C.E. That document did not give a detailed description of cancer, only a description of the swellings that accompany some tumors. Hippocrates gave the disorder the name *cancer,* and the Roman physician, Galen, first used the word *tumor.* These ancient physicians did not know much about

✓ CHECK YOUR HEALTH RISKS

Check the items that apply to you.

❑ 1. Someone in my immediate family (a parent, sibling, aunt, uncle, grandparent) developed cancer before age 50.

❑ 2. I am African American.

❑ 3. I have or have had a job where I was regularly exposed to radiation or hazardous chemicals.

❑ 4. I am a current smoker.

❑ 5. I am a former smoker who quit during the past 15 years.

❑ 6. I have used tobacco products other than cigarettes (such as chewing tobacco, a pipe, or cigars).

❑ 7. My diet is high in fat.

❑ 8. My diet includes lots of smoked, salt-cured, or pickled foods.

❑ 9. I rarely eat fruits or vegetables.

❑ 10. My diet is low in fiber.

❑ 11. I have light-colored skin, but I like to get at least one nice tan every year.

❑ 12. I have had more than 15 sexual partners during my life.

❑ 13. I have had unprotected sex with a partner who was at high risk for HIV infection.

❑ 14. I am a woman over age 30 who has not given birth to a child.

❑ 15. I have at least two alcoholic drinks every day.

❑ 16. I do not engage in any kind of exercise on a regular basis.

Each of these items represents a known risk factor for some type of cancer. However, the behaviors related to smoking and diet (Items 4–10) place you at a greater risk than other behaviors, such as Item 15 (alcohol) or Item 16 (exercise). In general, however, the more of these items that apply to you, the greater your risk of cancer.

---

cancer, however, because they did not have microscopes or use dissection, two procedures that greatly facilitated an understanding of cancer (Braun, 1977).

What Is Cancer?

Cancer is a group of diseases characterized by the presence of new cells that grow and spread beyond control. During the 19th century, the great physiologist, Johannes Muller, discovered that tumors, like other tissues, consisted of cells and were not formless collections of material. However, their growth seemed unrestrained by the mechanisms that control other body cells.

The finding that tumors consist of cells did not shed light on what causes their growth. During the 19th century, the leading theory of cancer was that a parasite or infectious agent caused the disorder, but researchers could find no such agent. Because of this failure, a mutation theory arose holding that cancer originates because of a change in the cell, a mutation. The cell continues to grow and reproduce in its mutated form, and the result is a tumor.

Research during the late 19th and early 20th centuries found that a large number of agents—chemical, physical, and biological—cause cancers (Braun, 1977). Interestingly, each of these different agents can cause identical tumors. For example, a chemical such as benzene and a physical agent such as X-rays can precipitate the same tumor at the same site. Cancers can even develop in laboratory cell cultures, apparently spontaneously.

This diversity of origin complicates the search for the cause of cancer because cancer does not have a single cause.

Nor are cancers unique to humans. All animals get cancers, as do plants. Indeed, any cell that is capable of division can be transformed into a cancer cell. In addition to the diverse causes of cancer, many different types exist. However, different cancers share certain characteristics, the most common of which is the presence of **neoplastic** tissue cells. Neoplastic cells are characterized by new and nearly unlimited growth that robs the host of nutrients and that yields no compensatory beneficial effects. All true cancers share this characteristic of neoplastic growth.

Neoplastic cells may be **benign** or **malignant**, although this distinction is not always easy to determine (Levy, 1985). Both types consist of altered cells that reproduce true to their altered type. However, benign and malignant neoplasms have some differences: Benign growths tend to remain localized, whereas malignant tumors tend to spread and establish secondary colonies. The tendency for benign tumors to remain localized usually makes them less threatening than malignant tumors, but not all benign tumors are harmless. Malignant tumors are much more dangerous, because they invade and destroy surrounding tissue and may also move or **metastasize** through blood or lymph and thus spread to other sites in the body.

The most dangerous characteristic of tumor cells is their autonomy—that is, their ability to grow without regard to the needs of other body cells and without being subject to the restraints of growth that govern other cells. This unrestrained tumor growth makes cancer capable of overwhelming its host, damaging other organs or physiological processes, or using nutrients necessary for body functions. The tumor takes priority, becoming like a parasite on its host.

Malignant growths can be divided into four main groups—**carcinomas, sarcomas, leukemias,** and **lymphomas.** Carcinomas are cancers of the epithelial tissue, cells that line the outer and inner surfaces of the body, such as skin, stomach lining, and mucous membranes. Sarcomas are cancers that arise from cells in connective tissue, such as bone, muscles, and cartilage. Leukemias are cancers that originate in the blood or blood-forming cells, such as stem cells in the bone marrow. Three types of cancers—carcinomas, sarcomas, and leukemias—account for over 95% of malignancies (Braun, 1977). Victoria's cancer, lymphoma, a cancer of the lymphatic system, was one of the rarer types of cancer.

Humans have about five times more connective tissue than epithelial tissue; yet carcinomas account for about 85% of all cancers in adults (Braun, 1977), and sarcomas account for only 2%. The rate of sarcoma development stays constant regardless of a person's age, but the rate of carcinoma increases markedly with age. The reason for the increased frequency of carcinoma has to do with its exposure to substances that promote cancer. Environmental **carcinogens** would be much more likely to come into contact with the epithelial tissue that covers the body (inside and out) than the connective tissue inside the body.

Although some people may have a genetic predisposition to cancer, the disease itself is almost never inherited. Behavior and lifestyle are the primary contributors to cancer, and our concern is with those behaviors and lifestyles that have been identified as risk factors in the development of cancer.

The Changing Mortality Rates from Cancer

During the 20th century, the overall mortality rates from cancer in the United States showed a steady increase. Death rates in 1993 were more than three times higher than in 1900. However, after 1993, and for the first time since records have been kept, the death rates from cancer began to decline. Figure 10.1 shows the total cancer death rates in the United States from 1900 to 1996.

Does the slight drop from 1993 to 1996 represent a statistical anomaly or does it signal the beginning of a long-term downward trend in cancer deaths in the United States? If present trends con-

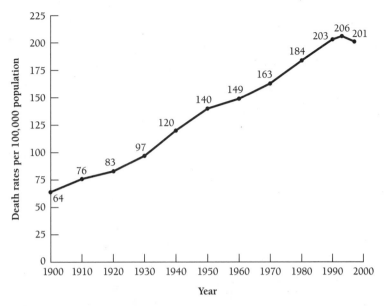

Figure 10.1 Death rates from cancer per 100,000 population, United States, 1900 to 1997. *Sources:* Data from *Historical Statistics of the United States: Colonial Times to 1970, Part 1* (p. 68), by U. S. Bureau of the Census, 1975, Washington, DC: U. S. Government Printing Office; *Health, United States, 1998* (p. 231), Washington, DC. U.S. Government Printing Office; and "Births and Deaths: Preliminary Data for 1997" (p. 7) by S. J. Ventura, R. N. Anderson, J. A. Martin, & B. L. Smith, 1998, *National Vital Statistics Report, 47*(4).

tinue, death rates for three of the four most deadly cancers (breast, prostate, and colon-rectum) will decrease. The most lethal of all cancers—lung cancer—is decreasing for men but still increasing for women. Prediction of long-term trends in lung cancer mortality depends on future trends in tobacco consumption. If women continue their gradual decrease in cigarette smoking, then lung cancer deaths among women should begin to level off and then decrease in the next 10 to 15 years. But if the use of cigarettes continues to increase among teenagers, then lung cancer rates for both women and men may once again begin to rise.

Predicting cancer death rates is also complicated by the shifting mortality rates from other diseases, particularly cardiovascular disease. Cancer and cardiovascular disease are likely to remain the two leading causes of death in the United States for a number of years. Thus, as deaths from cancer decrease, people live long enough to develop cardiovascular disease, just as any drop in cardiovascular deaths might add to cancer mortality. Two other factors contributing to cancer death rates are the more sophisticated techniques for diagnosing cancer and the rise of AIDS-related cancer deaths, especially non-Hodgkin's lymphoma, invasive cervical cancer, and **Kaposi's sarcoma.**

Rather than considering total cancer mortality rates, it may be productive to look at trends in death rates for people under age 55. As seen in Figure 10.2, death rates for young and middle-aged women have been declining since 1950. For men age 45 to 54, the drop in cancer mortality has been sharp, but it did not begin until 1980. For younger men, the gradual decline in cancer death rates began around 1970 (see Figure 10.3). Thus, the decrease in cancer mortality among young and middle-aged women and men is not new, although the drop in total cancer deaths is.

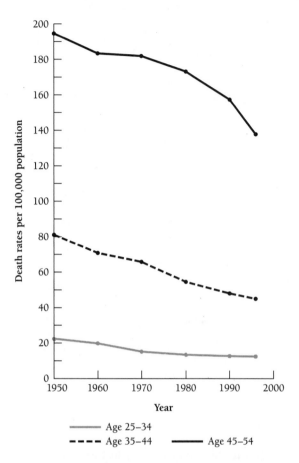

Figure 10.2 Cancer death rates by age, women, United States, 1950 to 1996.   *Sources:* Data from *Statistical Abstracts of the United States, 1994* (p. 99), by U.S. Bureau of the Census, 1994, Washington, DC.: U.S. Government Printing Office and the National Vital Statistics Systems; and Health, *United States, 1998* (p. 231), by USDHHS U.S. Department of Health and Human Services, 1998, Washington, DC.: U.S. Government Printing Office.

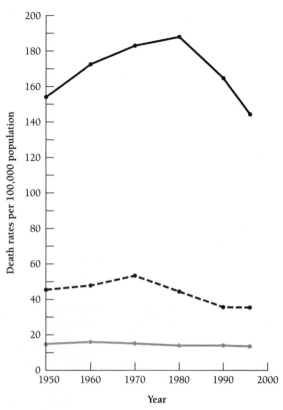

Figure 10.3 Cancer death rates by age, men, United States, 1950 to 1996.   *Sources:* Data from *Statistical Abstracts of the United States, 1994* (p. 99) by U.S. Bureau of the Census, 1994, Washington, DC.: U.S. Government Printing Office and the National Vital Statistics Systems; *Health, United States, 1998* (p. 231), by USDHHS U.S. Department of Health and Human Services, 1998, Washington, DC.: U.S. Government Printing Office.

Is this recent drop in overall cancer mortality due to better treatment or to more effective preventive measures? Current evidence indicates that both improved treatment and a reduction in risk factors have contributed to the decrease in cancer deaths. The 5-year survival rates—especially for breast cancer—have increased in recent years, suggesting improved treatment measures. At the same time, the incidence of *new* cases has generally declined, suggesting more effective prevention (American Cancer Society, 1996).

Although cancer incidence and mortality have both begun to decline, not all cancer sites have been equally affected. When cancer mortality rates for selected body sites are examined, an interesting picture emerges. For men, the four leading sites are lung, prostate, colon and rectum, and pancreas, with lung cancer deaths far exceeding the sum of the other three leading sites (American Cancer Society, 1998a). Figure 10.4 shows the

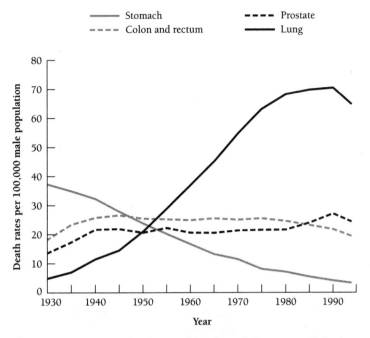

——— Stomach   ╍╍╍╍ Prostate
╌╌╌╌ Colon and rectum   ——— Lung

Figure 10.4   Cancer death rates for selected sites, men, United States, 1930 to 1994.   *Source:* Data from *Cancer Facts & Figures—1998* (p. 2), American Cancer Society.

changing patterns of cancer deaths for men in the United States. Note the decline in lung cancer deaths for men from 1990 to 1994. This decline follows a drop in men's cigarette smoking by about 30 years.

For women, the four cancer sites leading to the largest number of deaths are lung, breast, colon and rectum, and pancreas. Stomach cancer death rates for women, like those for men, have shown a consistent decline during the past 70 years. Unfortunately, death rates from lung cancer among women have shown a sharp rise since about 1965, but they still remain lower for women than for men. Figure 10.5 reveals the changing patterns of cancer deaths for women in the United States. Note the possible beginning of a leveling trend in lung cancer deaths for women. If more women quit smoking or never begin, lung cancer mortality rates will probably begin to decline during the next decade. Note also that breast cancer death rates have declined only slightly since

1990, despite a growing percentage of women who have survived breast cancer for at least 5 years. This reflects an increased incidence of new cases throughout the 1980s and early 1990s. In recent years, however, the incidence rates for breast cancer have leveled off, a situation that forecasts a steady decline in breast cancer mortality. Finally, compare the colon and rectum cancer death rates for men and women. For reasons not yet fully understood, the rates for women have decreased steadily since about 1945, while those for men have been more resistant to decline.

In Summary

Cancer is a group of diseases characterized by the presence of neoplastic cells that grow and spread without control. These new cells may form *benign* tumors, which tend to remain localized, or *malignant* tumors, which tend to spread to other tissues and may *metasasize* and spread to other organs.

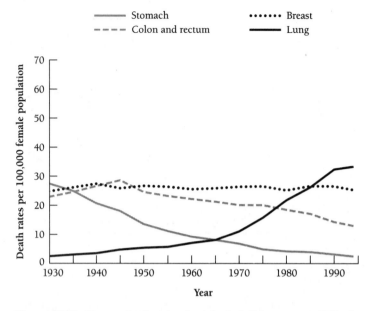

Figure 10.5   Cancer death rates for selected sites, women, United States, 1930 to 1994.   *Source:* Data from *Cancer Facts & Figures—1998* (p. 3), American Cancer Society.

Death rates from cancer increased more than threefold during the first 9½ decades of the 20th century, but they began to decline during the mid-1990s. Some of that threefold increase was due to (1) more accurate techniques for diagnosing cancer; (2) a decline in cardiovascular death rates, which means that people would live long enough to die of cancer; (3) the rapid rise of AIDS-related cancer deaths; and (4) a sharp increase in lung cancer, which is closely tied to cigarette smoking. In more recent years, cancer death rates for nearly all sites have begun to decline. The most important exception is lung cancer mortality for women, and that rate may be beginning to level off, a trend that would follow lung cancer deaths among men.

Behavioral Risk Factors for Cancer

Cancer results from an interaction of genetic, behavioral, and environmental conditions, most of which are still not clearly understood. As with car-

diovascular diseases, however, a number of cancer risk factors have been identified. Recall that risk factors do not necessarily *cause* a disease, but they do predict the likelihood of a person developing or dying from that disease.

Most risk factors for cancer involve personal behavior and lifestyle, especially smoking and diet. About two-thirds of all cancer deaths in the United States are associated with either smoking cigarettes or eating unwisely (Doll & Peto, 1981). Cigarettes and diet are not the only known behavioral risk factors; alcohol, physical inactivity, exposure to ultraviolet light, and sexual behavior are also associated with cancer.

Smoking

Cigarette smoking is the primary cause of preventable deaths in the United States, accounting for about 400,000 deaths per year (USDHHS, 1998a). Although tobacco use contributes to more deaths from cardiovascular disease than from cancer, it is the leading cause of cancer deaths.

About 90% of lung cancer deaths in men and 80% in women are attributed to cigarette smoking (Heusinkveld, 1997). Although the vast majority of smoking-related cancer deaths are from lung cancer, smoking is also implicated in deaths for several other cancers, including leukemia and cancers of the lip, oral cavity, pharynx, esophagus, pancreas, larynx, trachea, urinary bladder, and kidney.

What Is the Risk?   Epidemiologists generally agree that sufficient research evidence exists for a causal relationship between cigarette smoking and lung cancer. Chapter 2 included a review of that evidence and also explained how epidemiologists can infer causation from nonexperimental studies. A strong case for a causal relationship between smoking and lung cancer can be seen by observing the way lung cancer rates track smoking rates. About 15 to 20 years after smoking rates began to increase for men, lung cancer rates started a steep rise; about 15 to 20 years after smoking rates increased for women, lung cancer rates began to rise. During the time that lung cancer rates were going up for both men and women smokers, rates for nonsmokers remained stable (Thun, Day-Lally, Calle, Flanders, & Heath, 1995). About 25 years after cigarette consumption decreased for men, lung cancer death rates for men began to drop; the decline in smoking among women has been more gradual than among men, and their lung cancer mortality rates have also been slower to show a decline. Low-income men smoke more than high-income men, and they have a higher lung cancer mortality rate; low-income women smoke a little less than high-income women, and they have a slightly lower rate of lung cancer mortality (USD-HHS, 1998a). The dose-response relationship between cigarette smoking and lung cancer and the close tracking of smoking rates and lung cancer rates provides compelling evidence for a causal relationship between smoking behavior and the development of lung cancer.

How high is the risk for lung cancer among cigarette smokers? A conservative estimate (Lubin, Richter, & Blot, 1984) placed the relative risk at 9.0, meaning that lung cancer was nine times higher among smokers than among nonsmokers. The risk that cigarette smokers have of dying of lung cancer is the strongest link between any behavior and a major cause of death. In Chapter 2 we saw that a relative risk of 1.3 can suggest causality and that a relative risk of 2.0 or greater is considered strong. Thus, cigarette smokers' relative risk in the vicinity of 9.0 for lung cancer clearly establishes smoking as a primary contributor to death from lung cancer—the leading cancer-related death for both men and women. This link is so well established that epidemiologists now have moved beyond conducting research in this area. Instead, they are more concerned with the risk to passive smokers—that is, people exposed to the smoke of others. (See Chapter 13 for a review of this research.)

Cigarette smoking also contributes to breast cancer. Women who smoke and women who live with a smoker have an elevated risk for both breast cancer incidence and breast cancer mortality, and the risk is dose-related. One study (Calle, Miracle-McMahill, Thun, & Heath, 1994) found that women who smoked 40 or more cigarettes daily had a 75% increase in breast cancer, whereas those who smoked 10 to 19 cigarettes a day had only a 20% increase. Also, the number of years of smoking history was directly related to risk of breast cancer, as was early initiation of smoking. Because of the dose-response relationship in terms of number of cigarettes smoked daily, number of years smoked, and age of initiation, this study presents powerful evidence that smoking increases a woman's chances of dying of breast cancer.

These studies leave no doubt that cigarette smoking is a primary factor in the incidence of cancer, especially lung cancer. Research reports vary somewhat with regard to the level of risk of lung and other cancers for cigarette smokers, but such fluctuations are partially explained by the fact that cancers are multidetermined. Besides smoking, such factors as polluted air, socioeconomic level, occupation, ethnic background, and building material in one's house have all been linked to lung cancer. Each of these has an additive or possibly a *synergistic effect* with smoking

(Millar, 1983), so studies of different populations may yield quite different risk factor rates. In addition, the number of cigarettes consumed is directly related to risk factor rates for lung cancer, and this dose-response relationship is perhaps the clearest evidence implicating cigarette smoking and lung cancer.

What Is the Perceived Risk?   Despite their heightened vulnerability to cancer, many smokers do not perceive that their behavior puts them at risk. They show what Neil Weinstein (1984) referred to as an *optimistic bias* concerning their chances of dying from cigarette-related causes. One study of high school students (Reppucci, Revenson, Aber, & Reppucci, 1991) found that both smokers and nonsmokers recognized a significant relationship between smoking and lung cancer. However, the smokers judged their chances of developing lung cancer as average despite evidence suggesting that they have nearly a tenfold chance compared with nonsmokers of dying of this disease. Adult smokers, too, have an optimistic bias concerning their personal risks from smoking. Michael Schoenbaum (1997) asked middle-aged (1) lifelong nonsmokers, (2) former smokers, (2) current light smokers, and (4) current heavy smokers to estimate their chances of living to age 75. The first three categories made fairly accurate guesses, but heavy smokers greatly overestimated their chances of living to age 75. Another study (Brownson et al., 1992) found that both current and former smokers were less likely to believe that cigarette smoking caused lung cancer, and current smokers were less likely than ex-smokers to endorse this belief. Also, smokers were more likely than nonsmokers to say that smoking tastes good, smells good, is sociable, or is good for one's nerves (van Assema, Pieterse, Kok, Eriksen, & de Vries, 1993).

Is Smoking Ever Safe?   Is smoking ever safe? As cigarette smoking rates declined, cigar smoking increased 45% during the period from 1993 to 1996 (American Cancer Society, 1998). Many people have taken up cigars and pipes in the belief that they are less hazardous than cigarettes. Is this belief justified? Evidence suggests that cigars and pipes are safer than cigarettes, but each has a relatively high risk for lung cancer. One study (Lubin et al., 1984) found that the relative risk for cigarette-only smokers was 9.0 whereas the risks for cigar-only and pipe-only smokers were 2.9, and 2.5, respectively. Interestingly, when cigars or pipes were combined with cigarettes, the relative risk for lung cancer increased dramatically. Cigars and cigarettes combined yielded a 6.9 risk, whereas pipes and cigarettes raised the relative risk to 8.1, or nearly as high as cigarettes alone. Results from this research are clear; *smoking any tobacco product is never safe.*

Diet

Another risk factor for cancer is an unhealthy diet. The American Cancer Society (1998) estimated that one-third of all cancer deaths in the United States are a result of dietary choices, but other estimates (Simone, 1983) yield rates as high as 50%. Poor dietary practices are associated with cancers of the breast, stomach, uterus, endometrium, rectum, colon, kidneys, small intestine, pancreas, liver, ovary, bladder, prostate, mouth, pharynx, thyroid, and esophagus.

Foods That May Cause Cancer   Unwise eating includes selecting foods high in carcinogens, either as natural components or as food additives. "Natural" foods—those without added chemicals or preservatives—are not necessarily safer than those containing preservatives, and some may be less so. Also, the lack of preservatives can result in high levels of bacteria and fungi. Spoiled food is a risk factor in stomach cancer, and the sharp decline in this cancer (see Figures 10.4 and 10.5) is due in part to increased refrigeration during the last 70 years and to lower consumption of salt-cured foods, smoked foods, and foods stored at room temperature.

Dietary fat contributes to high cholesterol—an established risk for cardiovascular disease—but is such a diet also a risk for cancer? A number of studies have investigated this question, especially as it relates to breast cancer. In general, the evidence for a direct relationship between fat consumption and breast cancer is somewhat complex.

Researchers with the Nurses' Health Study (Holmes et al., 1999; Willett et al., 1992) found that eating a high-fat diet did not increase women's chances of breast cancer. Another report from the Nurses' study (Huang et al., 1997) showed that a history of being overweight was not a risk for breast cancer and was actually associated with a lower incidence of breast cancer before menopause. However, weight *gain* after age 18 was positively associated with breast cancer after menopause, especially in women who never used hormone replacement therapy.

Women in the Nurses' study may not be typical of all women in the United States, because even those in the upper 20% of fat intake may be eating only slightly more fat than those in the bottom group. Italian women have a greater variation in fat intake, and an investigation of the link (Toniolo, Riboli, Protta, Charrel, & Coppa, 1989) showed that cancer patients had a slightly higher consumption of protein and nonvegetable fats compared to healthy women. The breast cancer patients' slightly elevated consumption of fat was due almost entirely to their very high consumption of milk, high-fat cheese, and butter. Women who consumed half their calories as fat had breast cancer rates that were three times higher than average. In addition, both saturated fats and animal protein were implicated in increased breast cancer rates.

Diet may also be related to lung cancer. Researchers with the Western Electric study (Shekelle, Rossof, & Stamler, 1991) followed a large group of men for 24 years and found that increases in dietary cholesterol were directly related to their chances of developing lung cancer. Men who consumed high levels of cholesterol had nearly twice the rate of lung cancer as men who were low consumers of cholesterol, and men who consumed an intermediate level had an intermediate risk. How-ever, the increased risk seemed to be limited to dietary cholesterol from eggs.

Colon cancer may be related to diet. A diet high in red meat, processed meat, fast foods, refined grains, sugar-laden foods, and few fruits and vegetables was found to be positively related to colon cancer (Slattery, Boucher, Caan, Potter, & Ma, 1998). This pattern is typical of many people in the United States, placing large parts of the population at increased risk. In contrast, a diet high in fruit, vegetables, fish, and poultry but low in red and processed meat was protective against colon cancer. No one food was associated with the development of colon cancer, but patterns of eating were. In addition, the diet pattern associated with colon cancer was also linked to low levels of physical activity and heavier weight, both of which are risk factors for other diseases.

Foods That May Protect against Cancer   If certain eating practices increase the risk for cancer, do other dietary measures protect against this disease? Which foods should people consume to reduce their risk for cancer? Research in this area has focused both on types of foods that relate to lowered risks for cancer of different sites and on nutrients that may protect against the development or proliferation of cancer (see the Would You Believe . . . ? box).

Deficiencies in vitamin A result in deterioration of the stomach's protective lining; this situation has prompted several investigators to look for a possible association between cancer and low intake of vitamin A and **beta-carotene,** a form of vitamin A found in plentiful supply in vegetables such as carrots and sweet potatoes. A review of many of these early studies (Peto, Doll, Buckley, & Spron, 1981) concluded that there is a weak connection between beta-carotene intake and cancer, and later studies (Hunter et al., 1993; Yong et al., 1997) have tended to support the hypothesis that moderate amounts of dietary vitamin A probably provide some protection against lung and stomach cancer.

Twenty years ago, Linus Pauling (1980) created much interest and some controversy with his

WOULD YOU BELIEVE...?

Pizza May Prevent Cancer

Would you believe that pizza may prevent cancer? A growing body of evidence indicates that pizza contains a specific nutrient that has some ability to prevent malignancies from forming and proliferating. A great deal of research has gone into identifying the dietary risks for cancer, and this research has led to general recommendations to eat a diet high in fruits and vegetables and to avoid diets with a lot of fat, meat (especially well-done meat), and alcohol (Cummings & Bingham, 1998).

However, research is also beginning to find that a number of specific nutrients have the ability to influence cancer in a number of ways. For example, pizza includes tomato sauce, which contains lycopene, a type of chemical that is inversely related to the development of cancer (Giovannucci, 1999). That is, people who eat more tomatoes are less likely to get cancer, and cooked tomato products, like the sauce on pizza, seem to be especially effective. Tomato products are not the only foods that may lower cancer risk.

At the earliest stage of prevention, antioxidants can counteract carcinogens before they damage cells; the polyphenols in green tea as well as the lycopene in cooked tomatoes seem to work in this way (Cowley, 1998). After entering the body, carcinogens are converted from precursors into agents that damage DNA and produce malignancies. You can slow this process, however, by eating lots of vegetables, including tomato paste and garlic.

Another possibility for the preventive power of nutrients comes from the body's ability to destroy damaged or mutated cells; the omega-3 fatty acids found in flaxseed and fatty fish may have the ability to hinder tumor growth. Not all fats are protective, however; the fat in corn and safflower oils are believed to promote tumor growth (Cowley, 1998). Therefore, a low-fat diet is a good general dietary strategy for lowering cancer risk. More specifically, eating fish and flaxseed may help protect against cancer.

Tissues of reproductive organs are especially vulnerable to malignancies, and estrogen is a culprit for breast cancer in women. Soy products can diminish the estrogen risk, because soy contains a chemical that binds to estrogen receptors but is much weaker than estrogen, diminishing the effect. This substitution can be an advantage in slowing cell division and thus tumor growth. Countries in which soy is an important part of the diet have lower rates of both breast and prostate cancer than the United States (Cowley, 1998).

Another possible route for protection comes from nutrients that suppress tumor growth. Like other growing cells, malignancies depend on growth factors to establish and promote growth, and suppression of these factors can thwart cancer proliferation. A chemical in red grapes, carrots, rosemary, and turmeric has the ability to block blood vessel formation, thus preventing a tumor from establishing itself (Cowley, 1998). Eating these foods will not cure cancer, and most of the research on the preventive powers of nutrients have been carried out on rats. However, diet is a factor in the establishment and spread of cancer, so a cancer-healthy diet exists. This diet includes foods with specific nutrients that seem to offer protection against particular types of cancer—so have a slice of pizza.

---

claim that taking large doses of vitamin C (ascorbic acid) was an effective protector against cancer. Ascorbic acid acts as a nitrite scavenger and antioxidant, thus inhibiting the formation of **nitrosamine** carcinogens. For this reason, vitamin C does appear to have some *potential* to protect against cancer. Epidemiological evidence suggests that diets high in vitamin C provide moderate protection against lung cancer. For example, the First National Health and Nutrition Examination

Survey (NHANES I) (Yong et al., 1997) found that adults in the top level of vitamin C consumption, compared with those in the bottom level, had only two-thirds the incidence of lung cancer.

Selenium is an important trace element found in grain products and in meat from grain-fed animals. It enters the food chain through the soil, but not all soils throughout the world contain equal amounts of selenium. In excess, selenium is toxic, but in moderate amounts, it may provide some protection against cancer. Selenium deficiency is related to cancer in animals (Newberne & Suphakarn, 1983) and possibly in humans (Salonen, Alfthan, Huttunen, & Puska, 1984). These findings suggest that moderate levels of selenium provide some protection against cancer, but offer no evidence that added amounts of this nutrient are protective.

Indeed, little evidence suggests that adding vitamin supplements is an effective approach to further lowering of one's risk of cancer. For example, the NHANES I study (Yong, et al., 1997) found that dietary consumption of vitamin E, vitamin C, and vitamin A all had some ability to reduce lung cancer in some people but found no added benefit in supplementing these vitamins. Moreover, one randomized, double-blind, placebo-controlled study (Omenn et al., 1996) found that a combination of beta-carotene and vitamin A seemed to *promote* lung cancer. In contrast, a study of male physicians (Hennekens et al., 1996) used only beta-carotene supplements and found neither harm nor benefit; that is beta-carotene supplements—not combined with vitamin A— neither raised nor lowered these men's incidence of cancer or cardiovascular disease.

Researchers have also looked at dietary flavonoids as a possible buffer against lung and other cancers. Flavonoids, which are products of plant metabolism, are effective antioxidants and thus have some potential to protect against cancer. Apples are an excellent source of flavonoids, but other good sources include onions, garlic, scallions, and leeks. High levels of dietary flavonoids are moderately associated with low levels of lung cancer and other cancers in men and women

(Knekt et al., 1997). The association was due mainly to the strong inverse relationship between dietary intake of flavonoids and rate of lung cancer. The protective effect of flavonoids was independent of vitamin E, vitamin C, and beta-carotene and was strongest for nonsmokers.

Evidence that high-fiber diets provide protection against colon and rectum cancers is not yet clear. Some studies (Steinmetz, Kushi, Bostick, Folsom, & Potter, 1994) have found that fruits and vegetables (except for garlic) offer little protection against colon cancer. However, a later study (Slattery et al., 1998) found that a "prudent" pattern of eating helps reduce one's risk of colon cancer. A "prudent" diet consists of all types of fruits and vegetables, some fish and poultry, but very little red meat, processed meat, or sugar-laden foods. This is the same study that found that a "Western" eating pattern—lots of red meat, processed meat, fast foods, refined grains, and sugar—was positively related to colon cancer.

In summary, current knowledge suggests that some dietary components are related to reduced cancer risk. The specific components have not been identified, making supplementation a poor strategy. Instead, results of many studies suggest that a diet high in fruits, vegetables, and grains is cancer-healthy as well as heart-healthy (see Chapter 9). Conversely, diets high in animal fat have been found to be related to both diseases. The specific source of cancer protective effects is the topic of a growing body of research that may yield more certain dietary recommendations. Table 10.1 summarizes some of the research on diet and cancer.

Alcohol

For cancers of all sites, alcohol is not as strong a risk factor as either smoking or imprudent diet. Nevertheless, alcohol has been implicated in cancers of the tongue, tonsils, esophagus, pancreas, breast, and liver. Pancreatic cancer has a special affinity to alcohol consumption, and some evidence ties alcohol consumption to liver cancer. The liver has primary responsibility for detoxifying alcohol. Therefore, persistent and excessive

Table 10.1   Diet and its effects on cancer

Type of Food	Findings	Studies
1. High-fat diet	No effect on breast cancer	Huang et al., 1997; Willett et al., 1992
	Increased risk of colon cancer	Slattery et al., 1998
2. Very high consumption of milk, cheese, & butter	Triples chance of breast cancer	Toniolo et al., 1989
3. High cholesterol diet	Increases chance of lung cancer	Shekelle et al., 1991
4. Dietary vitamin A	Some protection against lung & stomach cancer	Hunter et al., 1993; Yong et al., 1997
5. Dietary vitamin C	Reduces lung cancer by one-third	Yong et al., 1997
6. Moderate levels of sodium	Offers some protection against cancer for some people	Salonen et al., 1984
7. Vitamin E & C supplements	No added benefit in protecting against lung cancer	Yong et al., 1997
8. Combination of vitamin A & beta-carotene	May promote lung cancer	Omenn et al., 1996
9. Beta-carotene	No harm, no benefit for supplements alone	Hennekens et al., 1996
10. Dietary flavonoids (apples, onions, etc.)	Reduce all cancer, but especially lung cancer	Knekt et al., 1997
11. High-fiber diet	Mixed evidence as a protector against colon cancer	Slattery et al., 1998; Steinmetz et al., 1994

drinking often leads to cirrhosis of the liver, a degenerative disease that curtails the organ's effectiveness. Cancer is more likely to occur in cirrhotic livers than in healthy ones (Leevy, Gellene, & Ning, 1964), but liver cancer is not common, and alcohol abusers are likely to die of a variety of other causes (Monson & Lyon, 1975). Alcohol-related liver cancer is responsible for relatively few deaths in the United States (USDHHS, 1993).

Alcohol may have some association with breast cancer, but the evidence is not overwhelming. A study by the American Health Foundation (Harris & Wynder, 1988) compared women with breast cancer with female hospital patients who were free of breast cancer. These researchers found no relationship between alcohol and the development of breast cancer—except for thinner women for whom the association was quite weak. A later

study (Vaeth & Satariano, 1998) found that newly diagnosed breast cancer patients were somewhat more likely to have been frequent drinkers as opposed to being either infrequent drinkers or abstainers during the year prior to diagnosis. Results from these studies support the notion that, although alcohol may increase the risk of breast cancer in some women, it is not a large risk for women as a group.

Alcohol also has a synergistic effect with smoking, so people who both smoke and drink heavily have a relative risk for certain cancers exceeding that of the two independent risk factors added together. For example, a review of earlier studies (Flanders & Rothman, 1982) found a synergistic effect of alcohol and tobacco on cancer of the larynx. Exposure to both substances increases the risk for laryngeal cancer by about 50% more than would be expected if the effect were merely additive. These data suggest that people who both drink excessively and smoke heavily could substantially reduce their chances of developing laryngeal cancer by giving up one or the other unhealthy practice. Quitting both, of course, would reduce the risk still more.

Physical Activity

Can exercise cause cancer, or does it have a protective effect? Some evidence suggests that both alternatives may be possible, although much more research is needed before the answer is clear. Several studies have reported on the relationship between physical activity and breast cancer. Although some early studies (Paffenbarger, Hyde, & Wing, 1987) found no association between breast cancer and physical activity, later research is beginning to demonstrate consistent evidence that a regular routine of physical activity is one way in which women can help protect themselves against breast cancer. One study (Bernstein, Henderson, Hanisch, Sullivan-Halley, & Ross, 1994) reported that women who began a physical activity program when they were young cut their risk for breast cancer in half, provided they exercised at least 4 hours a week. A second study (Thune, Brenn, Lund, & Gaard, 1997) found much the same results. This study showed that women whose exercise programs included at least 4 hours a week of activity greatly reduced their risk of breast cancer. The gains were larger for premenopausal women. These studies suggest that young women who adopt a regular exercise program can reduce their chances of breast cancer.

Evidence for a relationship between physical activity and prostate cancer is also mixed, with some studies showing a positive association and others a negative relationship. A case-control study (Le Marchand, Kolonel, & Yoshizawa, 1991) compared men with prostate cancer with a group of controls and found that older men who had spent most of their lives in sedentary or low-activity jobs had lower rates of prostate cancer than men who

had worked on more active jobs. For younger men, however, no relationship emerged between work at physically active jobs and incidence of prostate cancer. One weakness of this study was the lack of assessment of leisure-time activity, which may affect overall activity levels. In contrast, Ralph Paffenbarger and his colleagues (Lee, Paffenbarger, & Hsieh, 1992) measured all types of activity and found that physically active men had a much reduced rate of prostate cancer compared with men who exercised infrequently or not at all. These researchers hypothesized that physical activity may protect against prostate cancer because it moderates the production of testosterone, a hormone that seems to increase the risk of prostate cancer.

As for colon cancer, physical activity seems to offer some protection to both men and women. Martha Slattery and her group (Slattery, Schumacher, Smith, West, & Abd-Elghany, 1990) found that regular exercise helped protect against colon cancer and concluded that physical activity may buffer some of the harmful effects of a high-fat, high-protein diet. From these studies, we can conclude that regular leisure-time physical activity probably does not contribute to the development of cancer. The potential risks and benefits of physical activity are discussed more fully in Chapter 16.

Ultraviolet Light

Exposure to ultraviolet light, particularly from the sun, has long been recognized as a cause of skin cancer, especially for light-skinned people (Levy, 1985). Yet 25% of White adults in the United States sunbathe frequently and one-fourth of those do not use sunscreens at the recommended levels (Koh et al., 1997). Both cumulative exposure and occasional severe sunburn seem to relate to subsequent risk of skin cancer. Since the mid-1970s, the incidence of skin cancer has risen dramatically, but because this form of cancer has a low mortality rate, it has only slightly affected total cancer mortality statistics. Not all skin cancers,

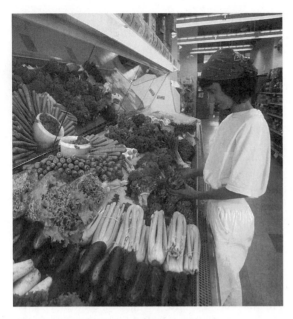

A diet high in fruits and vegetables offers protection against both cancer and cardiovascular disease.

however, are innocuous. One form, malignant melanoma, can be deadly. Malignant melanoma is especially prevalent among light-skinned people exposed to the sun.

Although skin cancer is associated with a behavioral risk (voluntary exposure to the sun over a long period of time), it also has a strong genetic component. Light-skinned, fair-haired, blue-eyed individuals, compared with dark-skinned people, are more likely to develop skin cancer, and much of their damage occurs with sun exposure during childhood. From the 1950s to the present, the death rate from malignant melanoma increased progressively. However, the rate of that progression has begun to decline, and at least one expert (Lee, 1997) projects that malignant melanoma mortality rates will soon stabilize.

In the United States 50 years ago, a clear pattern existed between residence in southern states and high deaths rates from melanoma among light-skinned people. During the past 45 years, this relationship between melanoma mortality

rates and geographic latitude has gradually decreased. Geography is no longer a risk factor for women and is a decreasing risk factor for men. Indeed, by the year 2010, this risk may vanish entirely (Lee, 1997).

Even if geography ceases to be a risk for malignant melanoma, fair-skin people will remain vulnerable to this disease. These people should avoid prolonged and frequent exposure to the sun by taking protective measures, including using sunscreen lotions and wearing protective clothing while exposed to the sun. Presently, the group *least* likely to protect themselves against the harmful effects of the sun are young White men who have no history of skin cancer (Hall, May, Lew, Koh, & Nadel, 1997).

Sexual Behavior

Some sexual behaviors also contribute to cancer deaths, especially cancers resulting from acquired immune deficiency syndrome (AIDS). Two common forms of AIDS-related cancers are Kaposi's sarcoma and non-Hodgkin's lymphoma. Kaposi's sarcoma is a malignancy characterized by soft, dark blue or purple nodules on the skin, often with large lesions. The lesions can be so small as to look like a rash but can grow to be large and disfiguring. Besides covering the skin, these lesions can spread to the lung, spleen, bladder, lymph nodes, mouth, and adrenal glands. Until the 1980s, this type of cancer was quite rare and was limited mostly to older men with a Mediterranean or Jewish background. However, AIDS-related Kaposi's sarcoma occurs in every age group and in both men and women. But not all people with AIDS are equally susceptible to this disease; gay men with AIDS are much more likely to develop Kaposi's sarcoma than people who developed AIDS due to injection drug use or to heterosexual contact (Schulz, Boshoff, & Weiss, 1996). For reasons scientists do not yet understand, incidence of Kaposi's sarcoma is decreasing, but the proportion of AIDS patients who have died of this cancer has remained about the same.

Non-Hodgkin's lymphoma is characterized by rapidly growing tumors that are spread through the circulatory or lymphatic systems. Most people with non-Hodgkin's lymphoma, like Victoria, do *not* have AIDS, but a positive human immunodeficiency virus (HIV) test combined with aggressive non-Hodgkin's lymphoma is sufficient to establish an AIDS diagnosis. Like Kaposi's sarcoma, non-Hodgkin's lymphoma can occur in AIDS patients of all ages and both genders. The greatest risk for AIDS-related cancers continues to be unprotected sex with an HIV-positive partner.

The presence of invasive cervical cancer has also become a basis for diagnosing AIDS (CDC, 1992), but the majority of cases of cervical cancer are unrelated to HIV infection. Cancer of the cervix accounts for only a small number of all cancer deaths among women in the United States, but some women are at greater risk than others. Women in low socioeconomic groups, those who have had many sex partners, those whose first sexual intercourse experience occurred early in life, and those who have had early pregnancies are most vulnerable to cervical cancer.

Cervical cancer is related not only to the sexual behavior of women but also to the sex practices of their male partners. When men have multiple sex partners, specifically with women who have had many sex partners and also at an early age, their female sex partners are at an increased risk of cervical cancer. Poor sexual hygiene is also implicated in this disease, and evidence suggests that the use of barrier forms of contraception, including diaphragms and condoms, lowers the risk for cervical cancer (Levy, 1985).

Other sexual practices put both women and men at risk for cancer. For women, early age at first intercourse and a large number of sex partners are both strongly implicated in the development of cancer of the cervix, vagina, and ovary. However, some of the danger is offset by physiological changes in women's bodies resulting from pregnancy and childbirth that seem to protect against breast, ovarian, and endometrial cancers. These cancers are less common in women who have had children early in life compared with those who have had children later in life or who have no children; that is, a strong inverse relationship exists between development of breast cancer and age of first childbearing (Levy, 1985). Having a first child later in the childbearing years does not confer the same protection as it does during early years.

In Summary

Approximately two-thirds of cancer deaths in the United States are associated with lifestyle and personal behavior, with cigarette smoking and imprudent eating being the two leading behavioral risk factors. In addition, research has related alcohol, ultraviolet light, and sexual behavior to cancer.

Cigarette smoking is the leading risk factor for lung cancer. Although not all cigarette smokers die of lung cancer and some nonsmokers develop this disease, clear evidence exists that smokers have a greatly increased chance of developing some form of cancer, particularly lung cancer. The more cigarettes per day people smoke and the more years they continue this practice, the more they are at risk. Cigars and pipes are safer than cigarettes, but they carry a substantial risk for several types of cancer, particularly lung cancer. Cancers of the mouth, pharynx, and esophagus have also been associated with cigars, pipes, snuff, and chewing tobacco as well as with cigarettes.

Poor dietary habits, especially high-fat diets, are related to cancers of the digestive and excretory systems, breasts, and lungs. Women who consume half their calories in fat have an elevated chance of developing breast cancer, but the relationship between specific diets and various cancers is quite complex. Currently, no convincing evidence exists that proper diet is a cure for cancer, but several studies suggest a preventive effect for diets high in vitamin A, beta-carotene, vitamin C, selenium, and flavonoids.

Alcohol is probably only a weak risk factor for cancer. Nevertheless, it has a synergistic effect with cigarette smoking; when the two are combined,

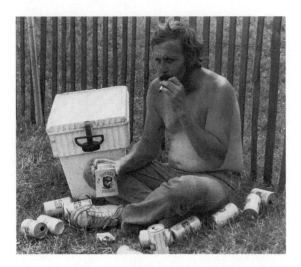

Risks from smoking, drinking, and sun exposure can have a synergistic effect, multiplying the chances of developing cancer.

the total relative risk is much greater than the two factors added together. Lack of physical activity and exposure to ultraviolet light are additional risk factors for cancer. Also, certain sexual behaviors relate to cervical cancer as well as to cancers associated with AIDS—Kaposi's sarcoma and non-Hodgkin's lymphoma.

Risk Factors beyond Personal Control

Most risk factors for cancer result from personal behavior, especially diet and smoking. However, some risks are largely beyond personal control, and these include both environmental and inherent risks.

Environmental Risk Factors

Environmental cancer risk factors include such conditions as exposure to radiation, asbestos, pesticides and other chemicals, and may also include living near a nuclear facility. In addition, arsenic, benzene, chromium, nickel, vinyl chloride, and various petroleum products are possible suspects in a number of cancers (Shaw, 1981).

Long-time exposure to radiation produces a slight risk for cancers of all kinds. A study in Canada (Ashmore et al., 1998) looked at more than 200,000 workers who had been exposed to occupational radiation between 1951 and 1983 to determine if such exposure increased their risks of cancer deaths. The investigators measured radiation exposure in dental, medical, industrial, and nuclear power workers and later compared their death rates to expected death rates. Three interesting findings emerged from this study: First, of these four occupational groups, only people who worked in a nuclear power plant had a significant lifetime accumulation of radiation; second, for men (but not women) cancer death rates increased with cumulative radiation exposure; and third, death rates from cardiovascular disease (for both men and women) and death rates from accidents (for men only) also increased with cumulative exposure to radiation. The authors had no explanation for the association between cardiovascular disease death rates and radiation exposure. These results suggest that long-time occupational exposure to high levels of radiation increases the risk of death from some cancers and for some people, but it also increases the risk of death from cardiovascular disease and contributes to all-cause mortality.

Does living near a nuclear plant increase the chances of dying of cancer? Presently, scientists have found no evidence that simply residing near a nuclear power plant causes cancer or elevates one's risk for cancer. A study (Jablon, Hrubec, & Boise, 1991) that investigated this question compared cancer mortality rates of people living in U.S. counties where nuclear facilities were located with the rates of people living in counties without such facilities. This large-scale study, which included more than 40 million people covering a 35-year period, found *no* increased cancer mortality for people living near nuclear electrical generating plants.

Does working with utility lines or living near electric power lines present a risk for cancer? Although many people who work with or live near electro-magnetic fields believe that they have an elevated risk of cancer, scientific research does not confirm these beliefs. A study in Denmark (Johansen & Olsen, 1998) found no support for the belief that occupational exposure to magnetic fields is associated with an increased cancer risk. Another investigation of occupational risk for leukemia in Los Angeles County (Kheifets, London, & Peters, 1997) reported that power line workers have no increased risk for that disease. As for any danger from living near power lines, Edward Campion (1997) looked at 18 years of research on all cancer as well as specific cancers and concluded that no convincing evidence exists that power lines can cause cancer or any other health hazard. Campion noted that small, poorly controlled early studies suggesting a link between cancer and living near power lines generated stories in the popular media, causing many people to be concerned without reason.

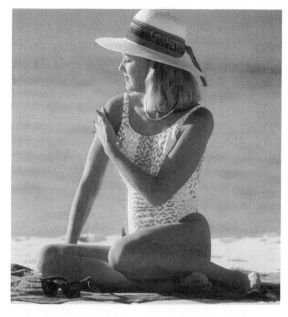

Protective clothing and sunscreen can decrease the risks associated with exposure to ultraviolet light.

Inherent Risk Factors for Cancer

Inherent risks for cancer include such factors as family history, ethnic background, and age. Although these risks are beyond personal control, people with inherent risk factors for cancer can reduce their risk by modifying their behavioral and psychological risk factors.

Only about 1% to 2% of cancers are inherited (Ellenhorst-Ryan, 1997), but genetic predisposition can interact with other risk factors to increase a person's risk for cancer. For example, people with light-colored skin who accumulate many hours of sunlight increase their chances of developing skin cancer.

Family History Genetic *predisposition* may play a role in a large number of cancers, but most research on family history has centered on breast cancer. Having a mother or sister with early breast cancer doubles or triples a woman's risk for this disease. The Nurses' Health Study (Colditz et al., 1993) observed women whose mothers had been diagnosed with breast cancer and compared their cancer rates to those of women whose mothers had no history of breast cancer. Women whose mothers had been diagnosed with breast cancer before age 40 were more than twice as likely to have breast cancer. Those who had a sister with breast cancer also had a twofold chance of developing this same disease, and having both a sister and a mother with breast cancer increased a woman's risk by about two and a half times. Similarly, a study of Mormon women in Utah (Slattery & Kerber, 1993) found that women with the strongest family history of cancer had three times the risk of breast cancer compared to those with the lowest risk. Looking at this issue from a different view, approximately one-third of all women with breast cancer have a family history of the disease (Esplen et al., 1998).

Ethnic Background Compared with European Americans, African Americans have about a 40% to 50% greater incidence of and mortality from cancer. However, Hispanic Americans, Asian Americans, and Native Americans have lower rates than either African Americans or European Americans (USD-HHS, 1998b). Reasons for these discrepancies appear to be due more to behavioral and psychosocial factors than to biology. For example, although Asian Americans generally have lower total cancer death rates than European Americans, they have a much higher mortality rate for stomach cancer, which is strongly influenced by diet (Miller et al., 1996).

Minority status plays a greater role in survival of cancer than it does in incidence of this disease. For cancer sites with a high rate of 5-year survival, the discrepancy between incidence and mortality widens with ethnic background. With breast cancer, for example, Non-Hispanic White women have a higher incidence rate than African American women, but African American women have a higher mortality rate from cancer (Miller et al., 1996).

How does minority status contribute to cancer outcomes—that is, length of survival and quality of life? A comprehensive review of research on this question (Meyerowitz, Richardson, Hudson, & Leedham, 1998) showed that several variables contribute to different cancer outcomes among ethnic groups. These variables include socioeconomic status, knowledge about cancer and its treatment, and attitudes toward the disease. These factors can affect access to medical care as well as adherence to medical advice. Access and adherence, in turn, influence both survival time and quality of life. No direct link exists between ethnicity itself and cancer outcome; the association between ethnic background and cancer mortality stems from differences in access, adherence, knowledge and attitudes, and socioeconomic status.

Age The strongest risk factor for cancer is advancing age; the older people become, the greater their chances of developing and dying of cancer. Figure 10.6 shows a steep increase in cancer mortality by age for both men and women, but especially for men. (However, the disparity in rates for

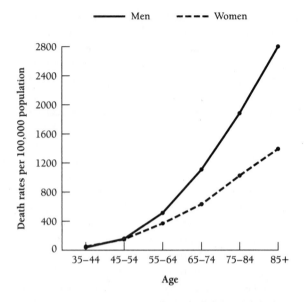

Figure 10.6 Cancer death rates by age and gender, per 100,000 of U.S. population, 1996. *Source:* Data from *Health, United States, 1998* (p. 231), U.S. Department of Health and Human Services, 1998, Washington, DC.: U.S. Government Printing Office.

men and women has diminished slightly since 1992.)

Age, of course, is an increasing risk for many other illnesses, including cardiovascular disease. Indeed, cancer mortality does not increase as rapidly with age as does cardiovascular mortality. Yet, advancing age remains the single most powerful inherent risk factor for cancer.

In Summary

Inherent risks for cancer include family history, ethnic background, and age. Cancer is almost never inherited, but family history and a genetic predisposition play a major a role in its development. A woman who has a mother or sister with breast cancer has a two- to threefold chance of developing that disease. About one-third of all women with breast cancer have a family history of the disease.

African Americans have a higher cancer incidence and death rates than European Americans, but people from other ethnic backgrounds have a lower incidence. These differences are not due to biology but to differences in socioeconomic status, knowledge about cancer, and attitudes toward the disease. Each of these is related to both the incidence of cancer and to 5-year survival with the disease.

The strongest risk factor for cancer is advancing age. The older one becomes, the greater that person's risk for cancer. Both men and women increase their risk for cancer as they get older, but men have an even greater increase than women.

Psychological Risk Factors for Cancer

Psychological factors can also place some people at risk for cancer. In general, psychological factors are not strong risk factors, but they can interact with inherent and behavioral risks to increase ones' chances for cancer. The two psychological factors that have produced the most research interest are suppression of emotion and depression.

Suppression of Emotion

Since the days of the Greek physician Galen (131–201 C.E.), people have theorized about the relationship between personality traits and certain diseases, including cancer. Some investigators have advanced the notion of a cancer-prone personality, or a Type C (for cancer) behavior pattern (Soloman, 1987). However, careful reviews (Spiegel & Kato, 1996; Watson & Greer, 1998) have uncovered no substantive evidence for the existence of such a global personality trait.

Nevertheless, specific personal characteristics such as the denial of unpleasant experiences and an inability to express emotion are risks for the development of cancer. During the 1970s, evidence began to emerge showing that the suppression of emotion was positively related to incidence of cancer. One of these early studies by Steven Greer and Thomas Morris (1978) investigated the relationship between suppression of emotion and cancer. In this prospective study, women admitted to a hospital for biopsy of a lump in the breast all had reasons to be anxious while waiting for their test results. Greer and Morris placed the women into one of three groups: (1) those who suppressed emotion, (2) those who were extreme in their expression of feelings, and (3) those who were apparently normal in their emotional response. A 5-year follow-up revealed that the suppression or denial of anger was significantly related to increased chances of a later diagnosis of breast cancer. These findings led many other researchers to study the relationship between suppression of emotion and incidence of cancer.

A study with male patients at a Veterans Administration hospital (Dattore, Shontz, & Coyne, 1980) also found that suppression of emotion was related to later development of cancer. Ten years prior to diagnosis, these veterans had filled out the Minnesota Multiphasic Personality Inventory (MMPI), giving the researchers early information on their tendencies to suppress emotion. Men later diagnosed with cancer were more likely than other participants to have suppressed emotion during a period of years prior to the onset of cancer.

A 30-year follow-up of medical school students (Shaffer, Graves, Swank, & Pearson, 1987) demonstrated the relationship between repression of emotion and cancer. These medical students had taken a series of psychological tests and questionnaires, which allowed researchers to assign students to groups based on their scores. Only 1% of physicians in the group characterized by "acting out" behaviors and by overt expression of emotion had developed cancer 30 years later. However, physicians who suppressed their emotions and who were characterized as loners were 16 times more likely to have developed cancer than physicians in the acting-out group.

Again, these results suggest that suppression of emotion may relate to subsequent development of cancer. However, a thorough literature review by David Spiegel and Pamela Kato (1996) revealed that suppression of emotion is the only personality trait to show any consistent relationship with cancer incidence. Later, we examine the effects of emotional suppression on survival of cancer patients. First, however, we look at the relationship between depression and cancer.

Depression

Several studies have examined the relationship between clinical depression and the subsequent development of cancer, but these studies have failed to yield a clear picture of any relationship. An early study (Dattore et al., 1980) showed that cancer patients not only were more likely to suppress emotion but also to score high on the Depression scale of the MMPI years before they developed cancer. Another study (Shekelle et al., 1981) showed that men assessed as depressed were at elevated risk for cancer 17 years later. A follow-up report on this study (Persky, Kempthrone-Rawson, & Shekelle, 1987) showed somewhat different results: Depression was a risk factor for dying of cancer but not for developing it. That is, this follow-up investigation found an increased rate of cancer *deaths* for men who were significantly depressed 20 years earlier but not a higher *incidence* of cancer. These results suggest that depression may promote established cancers, but it probably does not initiate them. However, a later study by (Zonderman, Costa, & McCrae, 1989) showed no significant relationship between depression and either cancer morbidity or mortality. This investigation followed participants in the National Health and Nutrition Examination Survey for 10 and 15 years and found no difference in cancer incidence or cancer deaths between cheerful people and depressed people.

Taken together, this body of research does not leave a clear picture of the relationship between depression and cancer. After reviewing this research, Spiegel and Kato (1996) concluded that

there is little support for any relationship between depression and incidence of cancer and no evidence of a *causal* association.

In Summary

Psychological risk factors for developing cancer generally are not as powerful as psychological factors for increasing survival time of cancer patients. In addition, a causal link between psychological risk factors and the development of cancer has not yet been established. Nevertheless, research has shown that certain psychological factors may be related to incidence as well as the mortality of cancer. Strongest of these psychological risk factors is a pattern of suppressing emotion. People who suppress their feelings, particularly anger and hostility, have an increased risk for cancer. Less evidence exists for a consistent relationship between depression and cancer.

Psychosocial Factors and Survival of Cancer Patients

Once people develop cancer, can they improve their chances of survival through nonmedical means? More precisely, do psychosocial factors such as social support, a "fighting spirit," or marital status play a role in length of survival of cancer patients? Are nonmedical interventions successful in prolonging the lives of cancer patients? Can psychotherapy be an effective tool in changing behaviors associated with the cancer-prone personality?

Despite some negative findings, a growing body of research indicates that psychosocial factors are important in cancer survival. Early studies (Pettingale, Morris, Greer, & Haybittle, 1985) found that patients who fight angrily against the diagnosis of cancer tend to live longer than those who calmly accept their fate. Interestingly, those cancer patients who were poorly adjusted to their illness outlived those who were more psycho-

BECOMING HEALTHIER

1. Know your family history for cancer. Although you cannot alter this risk factor, you can change modifiable behaviors that relate to cancer.

2. If you smoke, try to quit and keep trying. Most ex-smokers tried more than once to quit before they were successful. Also, don't switch to cigars or pipes. Remember, too, that smoking interacts with alcohol to create an even higher risk for cancer.

3. Keep a food diary for at least one week, (We also recommended this for Chapter 9). Note the amount of fat and the number of servings of fruits and vegetables. Imprudent eating relates to a number of cancers, including lung cancer.

4. If you are currently sedentary, take up some type of exercise program. Begin slowly at first and try to make it fun. (We have more recommendations for this at the end of Chapter 16.)

5. Practice expressing your emotions, especially anger and hostility, in a quiet, soft, and slow manner. Don't suppress your feelings; recognize them, but don't traumatize other people with a violent expression, although if you have been diagnosed with cancer, go ahead and vent your feelings.

6. If you are frequently depressed or if you have a hopeless/helpless attitude toward life, seek professional help. Qualified psychologists and counselors may be able to help you change your behavior and way of looking at things.

logically adjusted and more accepting of their cancer diagnosis. Specifically, the long-term survivors had higher levels of anxiety, depression, and guilt as well as stronger feelings of alienation. Patients who did not survive the first year were less hostile, better adjusted to their illness, and showed less anger and fewer feelings of discontentment. A review of later studies by Spiegel and Kato (1996) concluded that a "fighting spirit" tends to help cancer patients prolong their life, whereas a hopeless/helpless attitude and difficulty in expressing distress are related to a shorter survival time.

Another psychosocial factor that relates to length of survival is social support. Such social support can come from at least two sources—marital status and supportive psychotherapy. Married people seem to be able to survive cancer better than unmarried persons. Married patients are more likely to be diagnosed earlier than unmarried persons and they are more likely to receive early treatment (Goodwin, Hunt, Key, & Samet, 1987).

But even after controlling for early diagnosis and treatment, married persons still have better survival rates.

Why do married people survive cancer longer than unmarried people? A later study (Reynolds & Kaplan, 1990) provided at least a partial answer to this question: Married people enjoy more social support. Subsequent research has shown that strong social support and an extensive social network are positively related to length of survival of cancer patients, whereas social isolation is negatively related to survival time (Helgeson, Cohen, & Fritz, 1998; Spiegel & Kato, 1996). Social support and social networks can help cancer patients directly by increasing access to information, strengthening a sense of personal control, fostering self-esteem, and boosting feelings of optimism (Helgeson et al., 1998); and indirectly by providing a buffer against stress (Spiegel & Kato, 1996). After a review of the research, Vicki Helgeson and her colleagues found evidence that social networks may lessen a cancer patient's risk for death or recurrence, but that the evidence is much stronger for the notion that social ties can lengthen time of survival. As for the buffering hypothesis, Spiegel and Kato found little evidence for its underlying assumption, namely that stress can shorten survival time of cancer patients. Therefore, little or no evidence exists that social support can buffer the negative effects of stress on cancer and contribute to patients' survival time. Nevertheless, research suggests that adequate social support seems to prolong the life of cancer patients and, in some cases, lower their risk of dying of cancer.

In addition to a fighting spirit and marital status, certain types of psychotherapy may relate to survival time of cancer patients. The benefits of psychotherapy and counseling to alleviate stress and improve patients' emotional well-being are well established (Jacobsen & Hann, 1998), but the ability of psychological interventions to extend the life of cancer patients is less firmly established. Perhaps the most dramatic study to show the efficacy of a psychological intervention to prolong the life of cancer patients was conducted by David Spiegel and his colleagues (Spiegel, Kraemer, Bloom, & Gottheil, 1989). Spiegel et al. randomly assigned women with metastatic breast cancer to either regular treatment or regular treatment plus participation in a support group. The support groups consisted of weekly 90-minute meetings in which the women were free to express fears and other negative emotions. Spiegel (1993) reported that he had expected the groups to benefit the women emotionally, but he had not expected the experience to lengthen their lives. However, the women who participated in the group therapy lived an average of 18 months longer than comparable women who received only medical treatment.

A later review of studies by Spiegel and his associates (Classen, Sephton, Diamond & Spiegel, 1998) reported less dramatic findings. Studies in this review yielded mixed results, but those that did find some benefit for psychological interventions tended to have some common elements— namely, strong social support, group therapy with

patients of similar cancer conditions, an educational component, and information on coping strategies.

In Summary

Once people have been diagnosed with cancer, they can affect their survival time by adopting a "fighting spirit," having strong emotional and social support, joining support groups, or attending group psychotherapy sessions. Poor adjustment and a nonacceptance of the cancer diagnosis are *positive* traits for cancer patients and tend to prolong their lives. For several reasons, cancer patients who are married tend to live longer than those who are not. Supportive therapy that allows the expression of negative emotions increases survival time and demonstrates the power of psychosocial factors in cancer survival. Psychotherapeutic interventions that provide the best chance of extending the life of cancer patients are those that include a supportive environment, group therapy, education, and training in coping techniques.

Answers

This chapter addressed six basic questions:

1. **What is cancer?**

   Cancer is a group of diseases characterized by the presence of new (neoplastic) cells that grow and spread beyond control. These cells may be either benign or malignant, and both types of neoplastic cells can be dangerous. Malignant cells sometimes metastasize and spread through the blood or lymph to other organs of the body; thus, malignancies are life threatening.

2. **How deadly is cancer?**

   Cancer is the second leading cause of death in the United States, accounting for about 20% of deaths. During the first 9½ decades of the

20th century, cancer rates in the United States rose threefold, but since the mid-1990s, the death rates have begun to decline. One important exception is the rise in lung cancer mortality among women; lung cancer deaths have decreased among men but remain the most deadly form of cancer for both men and women.

3. What are the behavioral risk factors for cancer?

As many as two-thirds of all cancer deaths in the United States have been attributed to either smoking or unwise dietary choices. Smoking cigarettes raises the risk of lung cancer by nearly 10 times, but smoking also accounts for other cancer deaths. Cigars and pipes are less dangerous than cigarettes, but they each present a very high risk for cancer.

High-fat diets are related to cancer of several sites, whereas diets that include lots of fruits, vegetables, and grains seem to offer some protection against cancer. Alcohol is not as strong a risk for cancer as diet but, when combined with smoking, increases risk sharply. A sedentary lifestyle also presents a risk, especially for breast cancer, and exposure to ultraviolet light and sexual behaviors can increase the risks for various cancers.

4. What are the uncontrollable risk factors for cancer?

The uncontrollable risk factors for cancer include family history, ethnic background, and age. Family history is a factor in many types of cancer, and women whose mothers or sisters had breast cancer have a two- to threefold risk for breast cancer. Ethnic background is also a factor; compared with European Americans, African Americans have a significantly higher rate of mortality from cancer, but other ethnic groups have a lower rate. Advancing age is the single most powerful mortality risk for cancer, but age is an even greater risk for death from cardiovascular diseases.

5. What are the psychological risk factors for cancer?

Psychological risk factors for cancer are not as powerful as behavioral risks. Research has shown that the suppression of emotion, especially anger and hostility, can increase cancer risk. The link between depression and cancer is weaker.

6. What psychosocial factors relate to cancer survival?

The same psychological traits that increase the risk for developing cancer—suppression of emotion and depression—are even more closely related to the survival of cancer patients. People with cancer improve their chances of survival if they actively fight against their disease, rather than passively accepting it, and learn how to express negative emotions rather than suppressing them.

Glossary

benign Limited in cell growth to a single tumor.

beta-carotene A form of vitamin A found in abundance in vegetables such as carrots and sweet potatoes.

biopsy A diagnostic procedure in which living tissue is removed from the body and examined for possible disease.

cancer A group of diseases characterized by the presence of new cells that grow and spread beyond control.

carcinogen A substance that induces cancer.

carcinoma Cancer of the epithelial tissues.

Kaposi's sarcoma A malignancy characterized by multiple soft, dark blue or purple nodules on the skin, with hemorrhages.

leukemia Cancer originating in blood or blood-producing cells.

lymphoma Cancer of the lymphoid tissues, including lymph nodes.

malignant Having the ability not only to grow but also to spread to other parts of the body.

metastasize To undergo metastasis, the spread of malignancy from one part of the body to another by way of the blood or lymph systems.

neoplastic Characterized by new, abnormal growth of cells.

nitrosamines Powerful carcinogens that may be produced by nitrites.

non-Hodgkin's lymphoma A malignancy characterized by rapidly growing tumors that are spread through the circulatory or lymphatic systems.

oncologist A physician who specializes in the treatment of cancer.

sarcoma Cancer of the connective tissues.

Suggested Readings

Dollinger, M., Rosenbaum, E. H., & Cable, G. (1991). *Everyone's guide to cancer therapy.* Kansas City: Somerville.

For anyone with cancer or who has a loved one or family member with cancer, this very readable book contains answers to frequently asked questions.

Fife, B. L. (1994). The conceptualization of meaning in illness. *Social Science in Medicine, 38,* 309–316.

Betsy Fife examines patients' search for meaning in their illness. She studied cancer patients, asking them about the social circumstances of their illness and how they came to understand it and their lives.

Ott, P. J., & Levy, S. M. (1994). Cancer in women. In V. J. Adesso, D. M. Reddy, & R. Fleming (Eds.), *Psychological perspectives on women's health* (pp. 83–98). Washington, DC: Taylor & Francis.

Peggy Ott and Sandra Levy discuss psychological aspects of cancer in women, with emphasis on breast and gynecological cancers. Pertinent topics include prevention, psychological adjustment to cancer, and psychological factors in survival rates.

Perera, F. P. (1997). Environment and cancer: Who are susceptible? *Science, 278,* 1068–1073.

This article reviews the evidence linking environmental factors such as smoking, diet, and pollutants with cancer, and the interaction of these environmental factors with individual differences arising from genetic factors, ethnic background, and gender. Thus, the article explores complex relationships that produce cancer. Available through InfoTrac College Edition by Wadsworth Publishing Company.

CHAPTER 11

Living with Chronic Illness

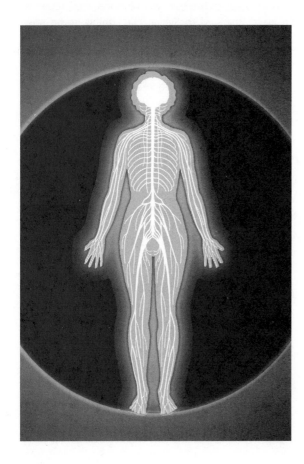

QUESTIONS

This chapter focuses on six basic questions:

1. What is the impact of chronic illness?

2. What is involved in cardiac rehabilitation programs?

3. How can patients be helped in coping with cancer?

4. What is involved in adjusting to diabetes?

5. How can HIV infection be managed?

6. What is the impact of Alzheimer's disease on patients and their families?

BRENDA'S MOTHER, SYLVIA

Brenda was concerned about her mother, Sylvia, who seemed to be more and more forgetful. At first, Brenda attributed the lapses in Sylvia's memory to her age. She was 81 and entitled to be forgetful at times, but the times were becoming progressively more frequent and disturbing. One day when she was visiting her mother, Brenda noticed that the electric stove in the kitchen was still turned on to the highest setting. She turned it off without saying anything to Sylvia. Later that afternoon, Brenda asked her mother what she had fixed for dinner and was quite surprised when Sylvia replied that she had forgotten to eat. Could it be that Sylvia had turned on the stove and then forgotten to cook anything? The question bothered Brenda.

Several months later when Brenda was visiting her mother, Sylvia suddenly became angry and accused her daughter of throwing away her reading glasses. "You threw out my glasses," Sylvia shouted. "You don't want me to read the newspaper. What are you trying to do to me?" Brenda tried to assure her mother that she had not thrown out her glasses and that she wasn't trying to do anything to her, but Sylvia remained unconvinced.

As time passed, Sylvia's failing memory became even more disconcerting to Brenda. Sylvia often forgot to eat, to bathe, to comb her hair, or to feed her cat. Moreover, she repeatedly confused the names of her children, lost interest in reading and watching television, failed to understand directions, and had difficulty making herself understood.

Sylvia was aware of her loss of memory and would become angry at herself when she could not think of names for simple objects like the chair, the table, or the radio. Her memory for past events seemed to be largely unaffected. She frequently showed old photo albums to Brenda and told stories about the people in the pictures. However, she had little memory for what happened the day before or even the minute before. One day when Brenda was preparing to leave, she said to Sylvia, "I'm going home now, Mother. Do you understand?" Sylvia replied that she did, but when Brenda started for the door, Sylvia asked, "Where are you going?"

Brenda had two brothers and an older sister, but they lived in other cities, and the closest was more than 200 miles away. Brenda knew that she would be the one primarily responsible for her mother. She wondered whether her mother might have Alzheimer's disease, so she sought the opinion of Sylvia's physician. The doctor was unable to confirm a diagnosis and pointed out that no absolute diagnosis of Alzheimer's disease is possible while the patient is still living. Only by eliminating other possible causes of Sylvia's dementia, the doctor told Brenda, could he determine that Sylvia was likely to have Alzheimer's disease.

This chapter looks at the consequences of living with chronic illnesses, such as Alzheimer's disease, cancer, cardiovascular disease, diabetes, and AIDS, but other chronic illnesses share many elements with these. The physiology of the diseases varies, but the emotional and physical adjustments, the disruption of family dynamics, the need for continued medical care, and the necessity for self-management also apply to such chronic diseases as asthma, arthritis, kidney disease, head injury, and spinal cord injury.

The Impact of Chronic Illness

Long-lasting, chronic diseases are now far more common in the United States than short-term, acute ones. At any point in time, half the U.S. population is affected by chronic disease, and virtually everyone will eventually develop some type of chronic condition (Taylor & Aspinwall, 1993). Most of these conditions are not severe or life-threatening, but the number of people affected presents a major problem for the medical profession and for health psychology, because such conditions affect not only the person with the disease but friends and family members as well. As Chapter 1 explained, the patterns of death and disease in the United States have changed during the past 100 years. Acute diseases such as pneumonia and influenza were once among the leading causes of death, but today such chronic diseases as heart disease and cancer have replaced them as the leading causes. Acute diseases do not last long; people are either cured relatively quickly or die rapidly. Chronic diseases, on the other hand, are lingering and if fatal, they cause death only after a lengthy period of illness. During this period, symptoms are not necessarily constant. People with chronic diseases may feel relatively well at times and very sick at other times, but they are never completely healthy.

According to Howard Leventhal and his colleagues (Leventhal, Nerenz, & Steele, 1984; Meyer, Leventhal, & Gutman, 1985), people tend to conceptualize diseases as acute rather than chronic. These researchers have found that people with a chronic disease (namely, hypertension) thought about this disorder as though it were acute, believing that they would not be in treatment for the rest of their lives and that they would eventually recover. These beliefs would be correct about an acute disease, but they represent a distorted view of a chronic disease like hypertension. The research of Leventhal and his colleagues suggests that people have trouble understanding that chronic diseases will continue indefinitely; instead, they tend to apply their knowledge of acute disease to any disorder they develop.

Serious chronic illness presents a crisis in people's lives that frequently goes beyond adjusting to the disease itself. For instance, chronic illness may produce financial hardships, change the way patients see themselves, and severely affect relationships with family members and friends.

Chronic illness can be analyzed in terms of crisis theory (Moos & Schaefer, 1984). *Crisis theory* deals with the impact of disruptions on established patterns of personal and social functioning. This theory holds that individuals need to operate in a state of equilibrium. When that state is disrupted for any reason, including illness, people rely on previously successful ways of responding in an effort to restore balance. A crisis exists when events are so unusual or major that habitual patterns of coping are inadequate. People then experience heightened feelings of anxiety, fear, and stress. Because people cannot tolerate a crisis state for very long, they adopt new ways of responding. Some of these new patterns of coping may lead to healthy adaptation, but others result in unhealthy adjustment and psychological deterioration. The crisis itself is neither healthy nor pathological. Rather, it is a turning point in a person's life, resulting in either a healthy adjustment to the precipitating event or a psychologically unhealthy adaptation. Crisis theory suggests that chronic illness would not inevitably bring about psychological distress. A person might react to the illness in either a positive or a negative manner.

Impact on the Patient

In one way or another, all patients must cope with their illness, but this task is not easy. Patients must deal with the symptoms of the disease along with the stresses of the treatment. As Chapter 3 explained, interactions with the health care system tend to deprive people not only of their sense of competence and mastery but also of their rights and privileges; that is, health care tends to result in the "nonperson" treatment for sick people. Loss of personal control and threats to self-esteem are two of the changes that patients with chronic illnesses must face (Fife, 1994). Being ill leads to feelings of vulnerability and loss of control over the future as well as changes in how others think of patients and how patients think of themselves. Because of the time course of chronic diseases, patients with these conditions face problems beyond those that patients with an acute disease must manage.

Several studies have explored the impact of chronic illness on the lives of patients. Research that evaluated the functioning of a large group of patients with a variety of chronic illnesses (Stewart et al., 1989) found that patients with chronic illnesses showed worse social and physical functioning, poorer mental health, and greater pain than patients without chronic illnesses. Hypertension produced the lowest impact on functioning, and gastrointestinal disorders and heart disease the highest. Patients with more than one chronic condition showed greater decrements in functioning than patients with only one chronic disease. The degree of intrusiveness of symptoms correlated with the time required for treatment of the condition, the symptoms, the amount of fatigue, and the degree to which the illness interfered with daily activities (Devins et al., 1990). Thus, chronic illnesses differ in their impact, not only in severity but also in how much they disrupt patients' lives. Even serious diseases that have few symptoms and allow patients to function at near normal levels do not produce the adjustment problems caused by less serious but more intrusive diseases.

A major impact of chronic illness involves the changes that occur in how people think of themselves; that is, the diagnosis of a chronic disease changes self-perception. Diagnosis of a disease such as cancer changes people's lives, and they go through a process of understanding the meaning of their illness and integrating it into their lives and their perceptions of themselves. Developing such an understanding was an important part of coping for the cancer patients in one study (Fife, 1994). The patients' illness and treatment forced many of them to reevaluate their lives, relationships, and body image. Some found positive as well as negative aspects to the experience. None of them, however, remained as they were before their diagnosis, and none imagined that their lives would ever be the same.

People with chronic diseases tend to adopt a number of coping strategies to deal with their illness, including attempts to focus on the positive aspect of the disease (Dunkel-Schetter, Feinstein, Taylor, & Falke, 1992). Besides focusing on the positive, the patients who experienced the least emotional distress tended to seek social support and to try to distance themselves emotionally from their illness. Those who experienced more emotional distress tended to cope by using strategies of cognitive or behavioral avoidance, such as wishing that the situation would go away or avoiding the situation by misusing drugs, alco-

hol, or food. In summary, people with chronic illnesses—like other stressed people—use a variety of coping strategies, but some strategies are more effective than others.

Like patients with acute diseases, those with chronic conditions must develop and maintain relationships with health care providers (Moos & Schaefer, 1984), but the characteristics of these relationships differ. People with an acute illness usually believe in the power of modern medicine and are optimistic about cures. This attitude is shared by health care workers, creating a positive climate of trust and optimism. Conversely, people with a chronic illness may have a somewhat hopeless attitude toward their condition, an attitude often reflected in their relationship with their physician. Health care providers too may feel less positive about those with chronic conditions. These feelings can create a difficult climate for treatment, with patients questioning and resisting health care providers, and providers feeling frustrated and annoyed with patients who fail to follow treatment regimens and who do not get better.

Negative emotions are common among the chronically ill due to the uncertain course of chronic disease, and physicians often feel less than adequately prepared to help patients deal with these emotional reactions (Moos & Schaefer, 1984). Such deficits have led to two types of supplements: psychological interventions and support groups. For many chronic illnesses, health psychologists have created interventions that emphasize the management of emotions. Support groups have also addressed this need by providing emotional support to patients or family members who must confront an illness with little chance of a cure. These services supplement traditional health care and help chronically ill patients to maintain compliance with the prescribed regimen and sustain a working relationship with health care providers. A meta-analysis of studies dealing with the effectiveness of psychosocial interventions with cancer patients (Meyer & Mark, 1995) showed that a variety of behavioral, informational, and ed-

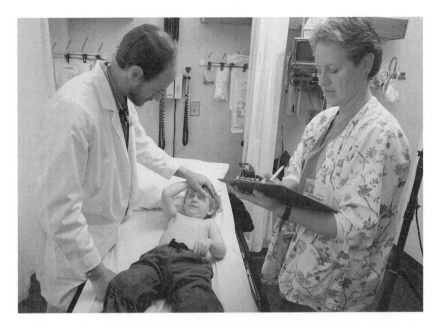

A chronically ill child can create financial and emotional problems within the family.

ucational methods helped patients adjust emotionally and functionally to their symptoms and their treatment.

Sustaining personal relationships is another challenge for those who are ill (Moos & Schaefer, 1984). When people become ill, their behavior often changes, and the relationships and the expectations of their friends and family members undergo significant shifts, even though social support is an important factor in maintaining health (Berkman & Syme, 1979; Wiley & Camacho, 1980). These changes are partly due to their role as sick people. However, people who are chronically ill do not fit the sick role as well as those who are acutely ill. Therefore, chronic illness can have a great impact on the families of the chronically ill.

Impact on the Family

Illness is a crisis not only for people who are ill but also for their families. As Sylvia's illness progressed, she became unable to live alone. She sometimes wandered about her neighborhood in the middle of the night, forgot to eat, set fires in her house to burn old letters, and behaved in other dangerous ways that made living alone an impossibility. Brenda realized that her mother needed constant care and vigilance, so she and her husband, Bob, decided to move Sylvia into their home. Sylvia resented this notion, claiming that nothing was wrong with her and that Brenda was trying to steal her money. With much rancor and bitterness all around, the move was made. Although Sylvia had previously spent a great deal of time in her daughter's house, this move confused and disoriented her. She couldn't find her personal belongings and had trouble understanding how to move from one room to another. She became increasingly angry at Brenda, her primary caregiver, and complained to Bob that "that woman (meaning Brenda) is mean to me." Paradoxically, Sylvia directed her fury almost exclusively at Brenda, the one person who spent so much time and effort caring for her. Brenda was unable to continue her law practice and care for her mother, so she gave up her practice to be with Sylvia 24 hours a day. Bob tried to relieve his wife whenever possible, but he too was a lawyer, and his income was important, so he worked longer hours to help make up for Brenda's loss of income. During the 3 years that Sylvia lived with Brenda and Bob, Brenda felt stressed and confined. Often she wondered who was the real victim of her mother's disease.

In adults like Sylvia, chronic illness may cause a redefinition of identity (Fife, 1994; Moos, 1984) and a change in relationships with others. Chronic illness in children also changes the lives not only of the patients but of the entire family, as parents and siblings try to maintain a family life while coping with therapy for the sick child.

The relationship between married partners often undergoes changes when one of them develops a chronic illness. An analysis of coping responses in married couples with one partner undergoing kidney dialysis for renal failure (Palmer, Canzona, & Wai, 1984) showed that couples with flexible roles adapted better than those couples with fixed, inflexible roles. The treatment was not the major source of problems; rather, difficulties arose from a discrepancy between the patients' view of their problems and the partners' view of the patients' problems. These differing views contributed to feelings of being misunderstood and abandoned. Many couples became closer but not more satisfied with their relationship, because the closeness was a result of dependency and came at the price of sacrificing one partner for the other's needs. Other research (Helgeson, 1993) confirmed the changes in couples' relationships as a result of chronic illness as well as a tendency for partners to believe that their relationships had returned to "normal" when they had not.

Chronically ill parents can also experience changes that produce problems in their relationships with their children; these changes are most pronounced for children with a terminally ill parent (Christ et al., 1993). As part of the sick role, a parent may lose the authority to discipline a child, or a sick parent may be protected from children's misbehavior because of the illness. Children may avoid consulting a sick parent so as not to further burden the parent, leading to decreased closeness. Children may be even less comfortable than adults with sick people and may change their behavior toward their sick parent as a result. Children may fear or experience changes in family life, and their role in the family may change as a result of a parent's illness. Young children may even feel guilt for their parent's illness because they do not understand that their misbehavior played no role in the development of the illness, and they may fear that their other parent will also get sick.

For adults, the changes that come with illness can alter their relationships and redefine their identity, but for children who are sick, illness can be an important factor in their identity formation. Although the rates of childhood diseases have fallen dramatically in the 20th century, a significant number of children still experience chronic diseases (Newacheck & Taylor, 1992). The majority of these illnesses are relatively minor, but many children experience severe chronic conditions such as cancer, asthma, rheumatoid arthritis, and diabetes, conditions that limit mobility and activity. For some children, these restrictions are very difficult, leading to isolation, depression, and distress, whereas other children cope more effectively (Brunnquell & Hall, 1984). Children who tend to be physically active and who have formed friendships based on activity find restrictions difficult. Health care providers and parents can help these children make adjustments by offering alternative or modified activities.

Families of sick children tend to be emotionally and physically fatigued (Garrison & McQuiston, 1989). A child who is ill requires a great deal of emotional support, most of which is supplied by mothers. These efforts can leave mothers so drained that they have little emotional energy left for their husbands, which can leave husbands feeling abandoned, angry and finally, guilty over these feelings. Added to these negative feelings are concerns over the financial demands of the illness and continuing concern for the sick child. Furthermore, a child's chronic illness can lead to sibling jealousy. Dependence in sick children can easily lead to overdependence, and they can learn to manipulate the family by becoming angry or depressed when they do not get their way. A child's illness, then, can disrupt family functioning at all levels, stressing each member's ability to cope.

Recommendations for families include trying to find some positive aspect of their child's illness (Moos, 1984). One example of this would be to look for ways in which the crisis might bring the family closer together and make family members feel less reluctant to express their feelings. Families should also find ways to express their negative emotions, such as anger and frustration over their situation. Families with sick children should also set aside time for themselves and not spend all their energy caring for the sick child. As a result of their own unmet emotional needs, many parents have joined support groups for families of children with chronic illnesses. These support groups can help families manage their emotions as well as receive information about their child's condition.

In Summary

Chronic illness affects not only the afflicted person but friends and family members as well. Unlike infectious diseases that last for a relatively short time, chronic illnesses such as heart disease, cancer, diabetes, AIDS, and Alzheimer's disease may persist for years.

Long-term chronic illnesses frequently bring about a crisis in people's lives, change the way patients see themselves, produce financial hardship, and disrupt family dynamics. Chronically ill patients have physiological, social, and emotional needs that are different from those of healthy people, and finding ways to satisfy these needs is part of the coping process. The social and emotional needs may be neglected by health care professionals who attend to the patient's physical needs. Health psychologists and support groups help provide for the emotional needs associated with chronic illness. Although some elements are common to all chronic diseases, special problems exist for people living with cardiovascular disease, cancer, diabetes, AIDS, and Alzheimer's disease.

Following a Cardiac Rehabilitation Program

Charlie had been retired from his job at a chemical plant less than 2 years when he began to experience signs of heart disease. For almost 15 years his jobs had included a lot of physical activity, but his last job in industrial relations was both stressful and sedentary. During this time, he developed hypertension and started taking medication. Also, he first began to have trouble with his weight and to feel more quickly out of breath when he changed from an active job to a sedentary one. After his retirement, his exercise was limited to fishing and hunting, and he continued to smoke and enjoy eating. One day he felt a deep, severe pain in his chest, shoulders, and arms. He immediately interpreted this pain as a heart attack, called for help, and was taken to a hospital.

An angiogram revealed that Charlie had 100%, 99%, and 95% blockage of three coronary arteries. The physicians who treated him decided that he was not a good candidate for angioplasty and that he should have coronary bypass surgery. Charlie thought, "Let's get this thing over with so I can start recuperating," and the arrangements were made for triple bypass surgery.

In the intensive coronary care unit (ICCU), Charlie developed a respiratory complication that prolonged the normally painful and stressful stay in ICCU. Charlie started to wonder if he would survive, and at one point, he became convinced that the hospital staff was going to leave and abandon the care of all the patients in ICCU. When the shift changed Charlie decided to leave rather than stay in the hospital, and, in his attempt to leave the hospital, he disconnected the intravenous lines and electrode leads to the monitoring machinery. He stayed only because he was restrained.

Despite the complications and the bypass surgery, Charlie recovered from his heart attack and cardiac surgery with no serious damage to his heart. As part of his rehabilitation program, he was advised to quit smoking, lose weight, and begin regular exercise. Charlie quit smoking immediately but found losing weight difficult. At first he lost some weight but then regained it. Charlie's exercise program consisted of walking a quarter of a mile for one week and then increasing the distance by one quarter mile per week until he could walk two miles in 30 minutes. Charlie now finds the distance no problem but has difficulty walking at the recommended pace. However, he feels better when he sticks to his exercise schedule, so he tries to exercise at least every other day.

In addition to changing his lifestyle, Charlie takes several medications for his heart and blood pressure. Once a year he undergoes a complete medical examination that includes an exercise stress test. Although he experienced depression that lasted for over a year after his cardiac surgery, Charlie says that he feels fine now, 3 years after his heart attack. His wife and family are pleased at his recovery, but they want him to be even more concerned about losing weight and sticking to his regimen for rehabilitation.

Cardiac rehabilitation programs can encompass a number of conditions and include a variety of activities, as Charlie's did. People who have experienced a heart attack participate in cardiac rehabilitation programs to restore their physical, social, and economic usefulness. Most programs of cardiac rehabilitation are similar to the one that Charlie followed. They include adherence to a regimen of medication, smoking cessation, a gradual increase in exercise, dietary changes to lower fat intake, and possibly psychological interventions to alleviate depression and change hostility. The exercise components vary according to the extent of damage to the heart and may include attendance at exercise classes supervised by health care personnel who can provide emergency care for cardiac complications.

Health psychologists have designed and implemented programs that supplement the standard cardiac rehabilitation programs. In addition to researching the problems with implementing general lifestyle change programs, health psychologists have researched and designed interventions for the particular adjustment problems of heart disease patients and their families.

Are rehabilitation programs effective in increasing the life expectancy of those who have experienced a heart attack? Evaluations of cardiac rehabilitation programs (Linden, Stossel, & Maurice, 1996; Oldridge, Guyatt, Fischer, & Rimm, 1988) indicate that they are. Individuals who participated in a cardiac rehabilitation program had lower death rates from cardiovascular disease. In addition, a meta-analysis evaluating the addition of psychosocial treatment to cardiac rehabilitation (Linden et al., 1996) showed that these components were effective in reducing mortality and morbidity as well as in reducing psychological distress.

Lifestyle Changes

Programs for cardiac rehabilitation emphasize lifestyle changes and, in that respect, are similar to the programs designed to lower risk factors for cardiovascular disease. However, cardiac rehabilitation patients have already experienced dramatic signs of the disease and thus may be more highly motivated to change their behavior than people trying to prevent the disease. Their behavior, then, may differ from those at risk for heart disease, and so we can consider research in the context of cardiac rehabilitation.

One approach that has been successful with people who have experienced heart disease is a program originated by Dean Ornish and his colleagues (Ornish et al., 1990, 1998). This program tested the possibility of reversing coronary artery damage by introducing substantial changes in lifestyle. Although similar to the interventions that attempt to alter risk factors, this program was more comprehensive and imposed more stringent modifications. Diet, an important part of the program, was much more restricted in its allowance of fat than most cardiac rehabilitation or cholesterol-lowering diets. The American Heart Association's guidelines recommend that no more than 30% of calories come from fat. In the Ornish program, participants were allowed only 10% of calories from fat, necessitating a vegetarian diet with no added fats from oils, eggs, butter, or nuts. Ornish (1995) contends that a diet in which 30% of calories come from fat is not sufficient to *reverse* coronary artery disease (CAD), although such a diet may be sufficient to *prevent* the development of CAD. In addition to the dietary restrictions, participants received stress management training and were encouraged to stop smoking, moderate their alcohol intake, and start exercising. A control group in this study followed a typical program intended to lower risk factors for people with coronary heart disease, including eating a low-fat diet, quitting smoking, and increasing physical activity.

After 1 year of the program, Ornish and his colleagues (1990) found that 82% of their patients in the treatment group showed a regression of plaques in the coronary arteries, a truly difficult achievement. Compared with the control group, patients in the treatment group had significantly less blockage of their coronary arteries, and those who most faithfully followed the program showed the most dramatic changes. This program also showed improvements in blood flow (Gould et al., 1995) and in artery blockage and number of coronary events (Ornish et al., 1998) after 5 years on the program, which compares favorably with standard risk modification. These studies demonstrated that a change in the coronary arteries can occur without the use of drugs that alter cholesterol levels and without coronary bypass surgery.

Programs that attempt to lower risk factors for cardiovascular disease share many goals with the programs that assist in cardiac rehabilitation. Both types of programs aim to increase physical activity, decrease smoking, lower dietary fat, and moderate alcohol intake. However, the psychological impact of heart surgery or heart attack differs from the impact of simply being at risk for heart disease. Cardiac patients have reported a variety of psychological reactions after developing heart disease.

Psychological Reactions after Heart Disease

Patients recovering from heart disease, as well as their spouses, often experience a variety of psychological reactions that include depression, anxiety, anger, fear, guilt, and interpersonal conflict. In addition, up to 50% of patients suffer serious psychiatric disturbances such as delusions and paranoia, called *postoperative delirium* (Sotile, 1996). These symptoms rarely last longer than 2 or 3 days. Charlie's delusion that the hospital staff would abandon him and the other ICCU patients is typical of the type of disturbance common among cardiac surgery patients, but his disturbance lasted only a few hours rather than a few days.

Depression is the most common and persistent problem for survivors of a heart attack; cardiac patients reported more serious depression after 1 year than healthy people (Holahan, Moos, Holahan, & Brennan, 1995). Women with cardiac problems were especially vulnerable to depression, but both women and men benefited from social support and active coping efforts, making these components good candidates for inclusion in cardiac rehabilitation programs. In addition, depressed survivors of heart attack were more likely than nondepressed survivors to suffer additional cardiac problems during the year following their heart attack (Frasure-Smith, Lespérance, & Talajic, 1995). Depression is not limited to the person who experiences the heart attack: Wives whose husbands have had a heart attack also reported depression (Michela, 1987).

The emotional support provided by spouses can be important in recovery from heart disease, and married people tend to receive more emotional support than their unmarried counterparts (Kulik & Mahler, 1993). This emotional support is related to emotional adjustment, quality of life, and compliance with lifestyle changes such as exercise and smoking cessation. Developing emotional support is one psychological strategy to help cardiac patients improve (Sotile, 1996).

The belief that sexual activity increases the chances of subsequent heart attack can affect both husbands and wives after a heart attack. This belief, however, is a myth—a myth that probably has its basis in the elevation of heart rate during sex, especially during orgasm. Heart rate does not rise to a dangerous level during sex, so sexual activity poses little threat to those who have experienced a heart attack. Despite these reassurances, couples may be uncomfortable concerning sex and may return to sexual activity only gradually (Michela, 1987).

Many people attach special significance to the heart, and therefore cardiac surgery can be a psychologically meaningful and fearful experience. The fear of death from heart surgery is based on real risk, but cardiac patients tend to perceive the risk of death as 50–50, even when their surgeons have repeatedly presented risk figures that were more accurate and more optimistic (Goldman & Kimball, 1985). Charlie's feelings were not consistent with these results; he never felt that he was in danger of dying from the surgery, and he felt eager to proceed with his recovery. Such optimism is beneficial in recovery from cardiac bypass surgery (Scheier et al., 1989), but the beneficial element in optimism may be the feeling of control that accompanies optimism (Fitzgerald, Tennen, Afflect, & Pransky, 1993).

Although most patients report improvements attributable to their cardiac surgery (Goldman & Kimball, 1985), not all do. Psychological problems cause difficulties in those who do not report improvement. Charlie is one of the majority of patients who feel benefited by surgery. His depres-sion decreased after a year, and he now feels neither physical nor psychological problems due to his heart disease and surgery.

Psychological Interventions in Cardiac Rehabilitation

Psychological interventions with cardiac patients usually begin while patients are still in the hospital (Sotile, 1996). Although many cardiac patients see no need for psychological assistance and may even be upset if someone else requests psychological attention for them, psychological counseling can ameliorate the experience of hospitalization, counteract some of the anxiety of being monitored while in intensive care, and increase the patient's confidence in the hospital's equipment and personnel. Families, too, need to understand the ramifications of the patient's heart disease, and most cardiac care programs include information to refute the common misconceptions about recovery from heart disease.

Psychological interventions can be effective in dealing with anxiety and depression, the most common psychological problems in heart patients. A program of in-hospital counseling tested the effectiveness of counseling for heart attack survivors and spouses (Thompson & Meddis, 1990a, 1990b). The program consisted of four 30-minute counseling sessions that took place while the patients were still in the hospital. The patients and their spouses reported significantly less depression and anxiety; these differences persisted in a 6-month follow-up. This program demonstrates that a simple psychological intervention can be effective for cardiac patients and their families.

Another research project (Fontana, Kerns, Rosenberg, & Colonese, 1989) evaluated the effect of social support on recovery after hospitalization for heart disease. These researchers found social support lessens the experience of both stress and distress and that social support was more important in the first 6 months after hospitalization than in the next 6 months. These results suggest the value of both psychological interventions for the patients and support groups for the families. Families that understand cardiac rehabilitation can help the patients by improving the critical factor of social support.

In Summary

Both heart attack and cardiac surgery can cause psychological problems for patients and their families. Depression is the most common and persistent psychological problem for those who have undergone cardiac surgery. Not only do patients experience depression, but the wives of men who have had heart attacks also feel depressed. Fear and anxiety are also frequent emotions and can introduce conflict into families that changes the nature of marital relationships. Some patients experience symptoms of severe psychological problems within several days after surgery, but these symptoms persist for only a few days.

Cardiac rehabilitation programs attempt to help heart patients increase their level of physical, social, and psychological functioning. These programs typically include regimens for lifestyle changes as well as interventions aimed at reducing the harmful psychological effects of coronary heart disease on patients and their families. In addition to the pain and distress associated with hospitalization, psychological interventions address the anxiety and depression that affect the lives of heart patients and their families.

Coping with Cancer

In Chapter 10, we met Victoria, who had been treated for non-Hodgkin's lymphoma when she was 16 years old. Her diagnosis and treatment had been very stressful, not only for Victoria but for her parents and three siblings. After her initial inpatient treatment, she took part in 3 months of intensive and then 6 months of less intensive chemotherapy. The hospital in which she received treatment was over 500 miles from her home, and transportation to the hospital was one of those sources of stress for her family. The nausea that she experienced as one of the side effects of the chemotherapy prohibited flying, so her parents drove her to the appointments and then brought her home. This arrangement was time-consuming, requiring the entire family to concentrate on Victoria and her treatment, often to the neglect of other family members' needs.

Victoria could not attend school, where she had been a popular and outgoing student, but she took part in a home schooling program so that she continued to earn high school credits. Being isolated from her friends and alone at home all day was one of the more distressing aspects of the 6 months of less intensive therapy. Victoria believes that the experience changed her into a more introspective and less outgoing person.

Her friends were uncertain about how to treat her. Having a peer with a potentially fatal illness was something beyond their experience, and the awkwardness they felt caused them to avoid her. Victoria thought that her boyfriend would also be alienated by her illness, but he was not, and their relationship continued throughout her treatment and afterward.

Victoria's family experienced all the aspects of a family in crisis, but they coped with the crisis and supported Victoria and her treatment. This support was important to Victoria, who had always been close to her family and felt distant from her friends during her treatment. As the experts (Moos, 1984) recommend, Victoria and her family managed to find some positive aspects to her illness, and the family maintained their closeness throughout her treatment.

The American Cancer Society (1998) estimated that more than 1.25 million people in the United States were diagnosed with cancer in 1998. Most of those people experienced feelings similar to those of Victoria, who was not only fearful and anxious but also angry. Indeed, the diagnosis of cancer nearly always has a significant psychological impact on the patient. Helping people cope with their emotional reactions to this diagnosis and preparing them for the negative side effects of some cancer treatments are important jobs for psychology-oriented health care providers.

Psychological Impact of Cancer

Although some cancer patients suffer from psychosocial problems as a result of their illness, serious distress and depression are not universal. The percentage of patients suffering from psychological problems depends on how these problems are defined. Most cancer patients experience some depression after receiving a diagnosis of cancer, but when clinical depression is used as a criterion, the prevalence among cancer patients may not be any greater than it is among other hospitalized patients. For example, only about 6% of cancer patients in one study (Derogatis et al., 1983) were clinically depressed. When other psychosocial problems are considered along with depression, the role of emotional disturbances in cancer increases, with 47% experiencing some sort of psychiatric disorder. Chronic mild distress and anxiety were the most common of the problems. Although the majority of cancer patients do not experience serious psychological problems (Telch & Telch, 1985), many experience some problems.

Problems Associated with Cancer Treatments

Currently, nearly all medical treatments for cancer have negative side effects that may add stress to the lives of cancer patients. These therapies include surgery, radiation, chemotherapy, hormonal treatment, and immunotherapy. The first three are the most common and also the most stressful.

Barbara Andersen (1998) reported that psychological interventions can effectively reduce distress and pain in patients undergoing treatment for cancer. Cancer patients who undergo surgery are likely to experience distress, rejection, and fears, and often receive less emotional support than other surgery patients. Postsurgery stress leads to lower levels of immunity, which may prolong rate of recovery and increase vulnerability to other disorders. Radiation and chemotherapy also have severe side effects. Many patients who receive radiation therapy anticipate their treatment with fear and anxiety, fearing the loss of hair, burns, nausea, vomiting, fatigue, and sterility. Most of these conditions do occur, so patients' fears are not unreasonable. However, patients are seldom adequately prepared for their radiation treatments, and thus their fears and anxieties may exaggerate the severity of these side effects.

Chemotherapy is also frequently accompanied by unpleasant side effects that precipitate stressful reactions in cancer patients. At least half of cancer patients treated with chemotherapy experience nausea, fatigue, depression, weight change, hair loss, sleep problems, and loss of appetite (Burish, Meyerowitz, Carey, & Morrow, 1987). Sexual problems are also common, regardless of the cancer site, and 70% of women interviewed 3 years after chemotherapy had decreased or no sexual interest, and 85% of men in treatment for Hodgkin's disease had lost their sexual drive.

Victoria described her chemotherapy treatments as "terrible." Some of the procedures were painful, and the side effects made Victoria feel helpless and out of control. During the course of her chemotherapy treatments, Victoria experienced nausea and vomiting. She lost her appetite and all interest in eating, so she lost 30 pounds. Her hair fell out, and she experienced a significant loss of coordination and a decreased ability to concentrate. Years later, she believes that she has still not regained her former ability to concentrate. Many cancer patients have similar unpleasant experiences during chemotherapy.

Not only do many patients become nauseated by chemotherapy, but some experience anticipatory nausea; that is, they become conditioned to nausea by certain sights and smells that precede the treatment. Several psychological interventions have demonstrated some success in controlling anticipatory reactions (Andersen, 1989), including hypnosis, progressive muscle relaxation with guided imagery, systematic desensitization, diversion of attention, and biofeedback.

Stress in Former Cancer Patients

More than half of all cancer patients survive at least 5 years (U.S. Department of Health and Human Services

[USDHHS], 1998a) and many show no physical signs of the disease during that time (Burish et al., 1987). However, many of these people continue to manifest psychological reactions to cancer. Cancer patients in remission often suffer from stress and other psychological problems for years before they are able to resume a normal lifestyle (Burish et al., 1987). The longer the remission, the more likely it is that the patients will be able to experience a quality of life comparable to their lives before cancer. However, many former cancer patients remain anxious about recurrence and carefully monitor every physical symptom for signs of cancer. Victoria was especially frightened about a relapse during the two years after she was pronounced to be in remission. As the years passed, her fears decreased, but she is still anxious about the possibility of recurrence.

Paradoxically, some patients become accommodated to their treatment and find returning to normal functioning to be quite difficult. Some patients become distressed after they leave the protective environment of the hospital. Similarly, parents of leukemia patients in one study became more anxious at the time that their children's chemotherapy was over. "Leaving treatment meant a loss of security and decreased social support. Possibly, treatment also provided a sense of increased control by giving patients an active means of trying to control the cancer." (Burish et al., 1987, p. 162)

Few follow-up studies have investigated the effects of cancer beyond 5 years after treatment, but one study that did (Byrne et al., 1989) investigated the patterns of marriage and divorce in adults who had survived cancer between 5 and 15 years earlier, when they were children or adolescents. The former cancer patients were less likely to be married than the controls, and those who married had slightly shorter marriages. However, individuals who had survived cancers of the central nervous system accounted for most of the difference, and the marriage patterns among former cancer patients who had tumors in other sites were similar to those of people who had not developed cancer during childhood or adolescence. This study measured only one aspect of adjustment after childhood cancer, but this aspect is an important index of normal adjustment. The results indicate that cancer did not prevent most of these people from marrying and that their marriages were comparable in length to those of people who had no history of cancer.

Psychological Treatment for Cancer Patients

We have seen that the diagnosis of cancer is frequently experienced as a major crisis and that it often leads to anger, depression, anxiety, and other emotional reactions. Each of these feelings is likely to have harmful effects, not only on the patient's psychological health but also on relationships with family members and the medical staff. For this reason, individual or group psychotherapy or a combination can be important in cancer treatment programs.

Psychologists have helped cancer patients learn techniques such as relaxation training to reduce pain, insomnia, and nausea; self-instruction, to talk to themselves in a constructive rather than a negativistic manner; and problem-solving skills, to enhance their sense of personal control (Telch & Telch, 1985). Many of these coping strategies are directed at reducing the deleterious effects of such medical interventions as chemotherapy, surgery, and radiation; several strategies are effective, including deep muscle relaxation to alleviate postchemotherapy nausea. Techniques aimed at increasing personal control through problem-solving seem less effective.

Some researchers (Dunkel-Schetter & Wortman, 1982; Wellisch, 1981) have emphasized the advantages of social support groups as part of the treatment for cancer patients. Discussions about fears, anxieties, and uncertainties faced by all cancer patients may be easier in a group of people with similar problems. Cancer patients may feel they do not wish to burden friends and families with the additional emotional difficulties that would arise from an open discussion of their illness. As a result, friends and family members may

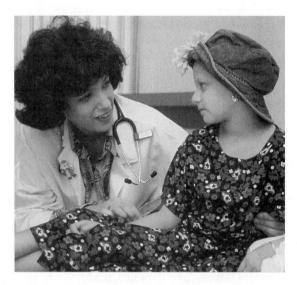

Children with cancer have problems and concerns that differ from adult cancer patients.

withdraw emotionally and physically, leaving cancer patients with less social support at a time when their need for support has increased. Support groups for cancer patients are generally aimed at increasing social support and reducing emotional distress. Studies on several such groups have indicated their effectiveness in helping cancer patients manage their emotional reactions. In addition, several studies have found that patients who participate in such groups lived longer than those who received only medical care.

David Spiegel and his colleagues (Spiegel, 1993; Spiegel, Bloom, & Yalom, 1981; Spiegel, Kraemer, Bloom, & Gottheil, 1989) have studied the beneficial effects of support groups on emotional adjustment and survival in breast cancer patients. The support groups met twice weekly for 1 year. One group included a supportive environment in which the women were free to express negative emotions, and the other included a similar support group plus hypnosis. After 12 months patients in both support groups were less tense, depressed, fatigued, and phobic than the untreated participants. In addition, patients in the hypnosis support group experienced significantly lower levels of pain than those who received either support group therapy alone or no treatment. The support group experience was also associated with extended survival, with the women in support groups living an average of 18 months longer than those who received only medical treatment.

A similar study with malignant melanoma patients (Fawzy et al., 1993) showed that patients who participated in the group showed improved coping ability and fewer recurrences of their cancer compared to a group that had received only medical care. Six years after their initial treatment, only 3 of the 34 patients in the therapy group had died, compared to 10 of the 34 patients in the comparison group. Therefore, psychosocial interventions may show double benefits of helping cancer patients cope with their illness and increasing survival time.

Young cancer patients have special coping problems. First, young children with cancer are typically removed from the secure environment of home and family, their source of both physical and social support. Parents often have added emotional and financial burdens, which may have a negative impact on their relationship with the child. Indeed, parents experience residual emotional effects from their children's cancer that resembled posttraumatic stress disorder (Kazak et al., 1997). In addition, chronically ill children may believe they are to blame for their condition, reasoning that they have done something bad to cause their own cancer. Returning to a normal routine as soon as possible, including resuming schoolwork, benefits these children.

Adolescent cancer patients have some of the same needs as younger children, but they have additional problems concerning newly formed sex roles and autonomy. The uncertainties about the future that affect all cancer patients make vocational choice and possible marriage and family life special issues for adolescents with cancer. In addition to an uncertain future, adolescent cancer patients are even more strongly affected than adults by the physical changes that often accompany cancer treatment (Wellisch, 1981). The loss of a limb, scars from surgery, or hair loss from chemotherapy can be a frightening experience, a threat to self-esteem, an assault to self-confidence, and an impediment to peer acceptance.

Victoria had no surgery and thus no scars, but her hair fell out, and her peers treated her differently, all of which were distressing. Her parents arranged for home schooling in the attempt to keep her occupied and to allow her to continue her education. This strategy was wise, because it allowed Victoria to graduate with her high school class and to be prepared to go to college. She never believed that she was going to die, so she was anxious to engage in activities that would allow her to continue her life and be as normal as she could during her treatment.

Patients frequently feel socially obligated to appear cheerful and optimistic. Because cancer patients face many uncertainties about their treatment and prognosis, they may feel especially burdened to express an optimism they may not feel (Dunkel-Schetter & Wortman, 1982). The dishonesty of appearing optimistic and striving for a cheerful acceptance of cancer may be more harmful than beneficial. For example, cancer patients who fight angrily against their disease tend to live longer than those who passively accept their fate (Pettingale, Morris, Greer, & Haybittle, 1985). Therefore, an honest expression of negative feelings may be both emotionally and physiologically healthy for cancer patients. However, pessimism, hopelessness, and depression are negative feelings that are not healthy. A sense of hope—a fighting spirit—can be beneficial in recovering from all diseases.

In Summary

The diagnosis of cancer may sound like a death sentence to some, but an increasing number survive this illness. Pain is a frequent problem with cancer patients, with about two-thirds suffering from severe pain. Cancer patients frequently suffer depression, marital stress, and other emotional and psychological disorders as well, but these experiences are not inevitable, and some evidence suggests that they are only slightly elevated in cancer patients.

The standard medical treatments for cancer—surgery, chemotherapy, and radiation—all have negative side effects that often produce added stress. These side effects include changes in body image, loss of hair, nausea, fatigue, and sterility. Psychological interventions, including relaxation, individual psychotherapy, and support groups can help patients cope with the unpleasant side effects of cancer.

Adjusting to Diabetes

Dawn was diagnosed with **diabetes mellitus** when she was 4 years old. She has no clear memories of life without diabetes, and no facet of her life has been unaffected by the disease. She remembers being ostracized by other children during elementary school because they were afraid that playing with her would make them sick, too. She hid her condition during junior high and high school, but her attempts to fit in led her to neglect her diabetes regimen.

The Physiology of Diabetes

Before examining the psychological issues in the management of diabetes, let's look more closely at the physiology of the disorder. The **pancreas**, located below the stomach, produces different types of secretions. The **islet cells** of the pancreas produce several hormones, two of which, glucagon and insulin, are critically important in metabolism. **Glucagon** stimulates the release of glucose and therefore acts to elevate blood sugar levels. The action of **insulin** is the opposite. Insulin decreases the level of glucose in the blood by causing tissue cell membranes to open so glucose can enter the cells more freely. Disorders of the islet cells result in difficulties in sugar metabolism. Diabetes mellitus is a disorder caused by insulin deficiency.

If the islet cells do not produce adequate insulin, sugar cannot be moved from the blood to the cells for use. Excessive sugar accumulates in the blood and also appears in abnormally high levels in the urine. If unregulated or poorly regulated, diabetes may cause coma and death.

The two types of diabetes mellitus are (1) insulin-dependent diabetes mellitus (IDDM), also known as juvenile-onset diabetes or Type I diabetes, and (2) noninsulin dependent diabetes mellitus (NIDDM), also known as adult-onset diabetes or Type II diabetes. Type I diabetes is an autoimmune disease that occurs when the person's immune system attacks the insulin-making cells in the pancreas, destroying them (Roberts, 1998). This process usually occurs before age 30 and leaves the person without the capability to produce insulin and thus dependent on insulin injections. Type II diabetes appears during adulthood, typically when a person is past the age of 30. Type II diabetes affects ethnic minorities disproportionately, and those who develop this disease are often overweight and poor (Fisher et al., 1997; USDHHS, 1998b). The characteristics of both types of diabetes are shown in Table 11.1. Both require lifestyle changes in order for the patient to adjust to the disease and to minimize health complications. Diabetes is one of the chronic disorders that require daily monitoring and relatively strict compliance to both medical and lifestyle regimens.

The administration of insulin can control the most severe symptoms of insulin deficiency but it does not cure the disorder. Nor do insulin injections mimic the normal production of insulin. Lack of insulin prevents the blood sugar level from being regulated by the body's control mechanisms. This inability to regulate blood sugar often causes diabetics to have other health problems. Elevated levels of blood sugar seem to be involved in the development of (1) damage to the blood vessels, leaving diabetics prone to cardiovascular disease (diabetics are twice as likely as other people to have hypertension and to develop heart disease); (2) damage to the retina, leaving diabetics at risk for blindness (diabetics are 17 times as likely to go blind as nondiabetics); and (3) kidney diseases, leaving diabetics prone to renal failure. In addition, diabetics, compared with nondiabetics, have more than double the risk of cancer of the pancreas (Everhart & Wright, 1995). Dawn experienced damage to her retinas at age 17, and the laser surgery left her vision permanently impaired. She is not blind, as her doctors feared she would be, but she has no night vision, and she can focus

Table 11.1

Characteristics of insulin-dependent and noninsulin-dependent diabetes mellitus

Insulin-dependent	Noninsulin-dependent
Onset occurs before age 30	Onset occurs after age 30
Patients are underweight	Patients are overweight
Patients experience frequent thirst and urination	Patients experience frequent thirst and urination
Affects equal numbers of men and women	Affects more women
Has no socioeconomic correlates	Affects more poor than middle-class people
Requires insulin injections	Requires no insulin injections
Carries risk of kidney damage	Carries risk of cardiovascular damage
Accounts for 5% of diabetics	Accounts for 95% of diabetics

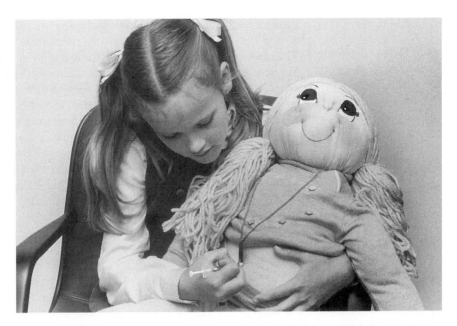

Learning to inject insulin in one of the skills that children with Type I diabetes must master.

only if given time. These visual impairments prevent her from qualifying for a driver's license.

The Impact of Diabetes

The diagnosis of any chronic disease produces an impact on patients for two reasons: first, the emotional reaction to having a lifelong incurable disease; and second, the adjustments to lifestyle required by the disease. For diabetes that begins during childhood, both children and their parents must come to terms with the child's loss of health (Kovacs et al., 1990) and the management of the disorder, which includes careful restrictions in diet, insulin injections, and recommendations for regular exercise. Dietary restrictions include careful scheduling of meals and snacks as well as adherence to a set of allowed and disallowed foods. Diabetics must test their blood sugar levels at least once (and possibly several times) per day, drawing a blood sample and using the testing equipment correctly. The results guide diabetics to appropriate levels of insulin injections. These in-

jections are also a daily requirement and can be a source of fear and stress. Regular medical visits, which may frighten the children and create scheduling difficulties for the parents, are also part of the regimen.

Dawn did a poor job of taking care of herself when she was a teenager. She learned to give herself insulin injections when she was 6 years old, and her compliance with this aspect of her care has always been good. Eating was a problem. She never developed a taste for sweets, so avoiding them was not difficult, but she was always a finicky eater and did not like to eat three meals a day. She found skipping meals easy and saw it as a good strategy for losing weight. However, one diet put her in the hospital because of a very low blood sugar level.

Noninsulin-dependent (Type II) diabetes often does not require insulin injections, but this type of diabetes does require lifestyle changes and oral medication. African Americans, Hispanic Americans, and Native Americans are at higher risk for Type II diabetes than are European Americans (US-

DHHS, 1998b), and being overweight is a risk for all groups. Indeed, gaining weight increases, and losing weight decreases, the risk for Type II diabetes (Colditz, 1995). Therefore, a frequent component of treatment is weight loss. Type II diabetics must deal with dietary restrictions and attend to their schedule of oral medication. Diabetes often affects sexual functioning in both men and women, and diabetic women who become pregnant often have problem pregnancies. Type II diabetes is more likely to cause circulatory problems, leaving adult-onset diabetics prone to cardio-vascular problems, which is their leading cause of death.

Some diabetics deny the seriousness of their condition and ignore the need to restrict diet and take medication. Others become aggressive, and they either direct their aggression outward and refuse to comply with their treatment regimen or they turn their aggression inward and become depressed. Finally, many diabetics become dependent and rely on others to take care of them, thus taking no active part in their own care. All these reactions can interfere with the management of blood sugar levels and lead to serious health complications, including death.

Dawn was able to deny the seriousness of her condition until she experienced kidney failure at age 22. She was put on kidney dialysis, and eventually received a kidney transplant. In the hospital, she became aware of the dangers of her condition in a way that she had never been before. Not only did she understand that she might die, but the possibility of nerve damage and amputation of a limb made her more vigilant about self-care. Now she monitors her blood sugar at least three times a day, eats regularly, and gives herself appropriate insulin injections.

Health Psychology's Involvement with Diabetes

Health psychologists are involved in both researching and treating diabetes. Research efforts have concentrated on the ways that diabetics understand and conceptualize their illness, the effect of stress on glucose metabolism, the dynamics of families with diabetic children, and the factors that influence patient compliance with medical regimens. Health psychologists orient their efforts toward improving compliance with medical regimens so diabetics can control their blood glucose levels and minimize health complications.

Stress has been hypothesized to play two roles in diabetes: as a possible cause of diabetes and as a factor in the regulation of blood sugar in diabetics (Wertlieb, Jacobson, & Hauser, 1990). The role of stress as a factor in blood glucose levels is clearer than any causal role stress may play in precipitating diabetes. For example, an active stressor such as solving math problems produced more effect on the blood glucose level of diabetics than did a passive stressor such as viewing a gory movie. Not all the diabetics showed blood glucose changes in response to stress, but more than half of them did. A longitudinal study (Goldston, Kovacs, Obrosky, & Iyengar, 1995) examined the role of stress in metabolic control for school-age children with Type I diabetes. The extent to which stressful negative events disrupted the children's life was a strong predictor of metabolic control, but *number* of negative stressful life events made little or no contribution to blood glucose regulation. Dawn sees stressful negative events as major problems in her management of her condition. She has trouble staying on her regimen when she is having trouble with her boyfriend. These researchers speculated that even positive life events, such as an outstanding personal achievement, can affect metabolic control.

Another line of research concerns diabetic patients' understanding of their illness and how their understanding affects their behavior. Both patients and health care workers assume that patients recognize the symptoms of high and low blood glucose levels, and these perceptions are important in the management of diabetes. Symptom perception, however, is not as accurate as everyone assumes (Gonder-Frederick, Cox, Bobbitt, & Pennebaker, 1986). For example, 58% of the diabetics had inaccurate beliefs about high blood glucose levels and 42% had inaccurate beliefs about low levels. These patients were more likely to have *beliefs* that suggested problems than they were to have problems; that is, their reports of symptoms were false alarms. Patients also overlooked symptoms that indicated problems, but the tendency toward false alarms was the more frequent error. The women in the study were more vigilant in both correctly and incorrectly perceiving symptoms, whereas the men were more likely to miss symptoms. These results suggest that education for diabetics does not succeed in teaching symptom perception.

Compliance of diabetics with their treatment regimen is quite poor (Harris & Lustman, 1998; Johnson, Freund, Silverstein, Hansen, & Malone, 1990; Johnson, Tomer, Cunningham, & Henretta, 1990; Orme & Binik, 1989), and this problem is of primary concern to psychologists involved in providing care for diabetics. Innovative approaches such as self-monitoring of blood glucose levels (Wysocki, 1989; Wysocki, Green, & Huxtable, 1989) have been less successful than expected because patients fail to use the information they gather to alter their treatment. Patients tended to ignore the measured values and to estimate that their treatment needs were less than they actually were, exhibiting unrealistic optimism and cognitive distortions.

More promising results have come from a study (Ratner, Gross, Casas, & Castells, 1990) that demonstrated the effect of hypnosis on compliance with a diabetic treatment regimen. The only change in management strategy was the use of hypnosis. The participants were adolescents, a group that is especially poor at complying with diabetic treatment regimens. The adolescents who had been hypnotized showed blood glucose and hemoglobin values consistent with compliance. Although hypnosis diverges from the traditional management strategy for diabetes, this study suggests that the technique may be helpful in enhancing compliance even with adolescent diabetics.

The role of health psychology in diabetes management is likely to expand, because behavioral components can add to the effectiveness of educational programs for diabetic patients. Education alone is not adequate in helping diabetics follow their regimen (Goodall & Halford, 1991). Because situational factors such as stress and social pressure to eat the wrong foods affect adherence, programs with a behavioral skills training component might be a valuable addition to diabetes management training. Problem-solving skills have been shown (Toobert & Glasgow, 1991) to improve diabetics' adherence to diet, exercise, and blood glucose testing. Such behavior-oriented management programs can teach diabetics skills that help them to maintain a healthier lifestyle.

In Summary

Diabetes mellitus is a chronic disease that results from failure of the islet cells of the pancreas to manufacture sufficient insulin, affecting blood glucose levels and producing effects in many organ systems. The disease can become apparent in either childhood or adulthood, but the juvenile-onset variety is typically more serious, and such patients require insulin injections to survive. Diabetics must maintain a strict regimen of diet, exercise, and insulin supplements to avoid the serious cardiovascular, neurological, and renal complications of the disorder.

As with other chronic diseases, a diagnosis of diabetes mellitus produces distress for both patients and their families. Health psychologists have studied the factors involved in adjusting to the disorder and those that affect compliance with the necessary lifestyle changes. Adolescent diabetics are especially likely to be poor at adherence, but the technique of self-monitoring blood glucose level has not been effective in enhancing adherence. Skills and problem-solving training programs have shown more success in helping diabetics manage their disorder.

Dealing with HIV and AIDS

Glenn Burke had always wanted to play baseball, and he had enough skill to become a major league player. From 1976 to 1979, he was a gifted outfielder for the Los Angles Dodgers and Oakland

Athletics and played for the Dodgers in the 1977 World Series. Burke's promising career was never fulfilled—not because he lacked ability but because players, managers, and general managers suspected that he was gay, and they made his life as a ballplayer miserable. Burke *was* gay, but he did not acknowledge his sexual orientation openly until 2 years after he left baseball. He was also an African American, and the combination of being gay and being African American probably cut short his baseball career. Prejudice in organized baseball in the late 1970s was so strong that the Dodgers offered to pay Burke for an expensive honeymoon—if only he would get married. After he was traded to the Oakland Athletics, Billy Martin, the controversial manager of the Athletics (as well as several other teams) told Burke, "I don't want no faggot on my team," and the team promptly refused to sign Burke to an extended contract.

After his baseball career came to a premature end, Burke continued to have difficulties. He spent some time in San Quentin prison and more time as a homeless person on the streets of San Francisco. Eventually he contracted AIDS, but he fought hard against the disease and survived many months longer than doctors had predicted. After developing AIDS-related illnesses and losing nearly 100 pounds from his once-powerful athletic frame, he died in May 1995 at the age of 42. Unlike many gay men who develop AIDS, Burke reconciled with his family and was cared for by his sister during his final months.

AIDS is a disorder in which the immune system loses its effectiveness, leaving the body defenseless against bacterial, viral, fungal, parasitic, cancerous, and other opportunistic diseases. Immune deficiency itself is not fatal, but without the immune system, the body cannot protect itself against the many organisms that can invade it and cause damage. (For a more complete discussion of the immune system and its function, see Chapter 6). The danger from AIDS comes from the opportunistic infections that start when the immune system no longer functions effectively. In this way

AIDS is similar to the immune deficiency in children who have been born without immune system organs and are susceptible to a variety of infections. AIDS is the result of exposure to a contagious virus, the **human immunodeficiency virus (HIV)**. Presently, two variants of the human immunodeficiency virus have been discovered; HIV-1, which causes most AIDS cases in the United States, and HIV-2, which is responsible for most AIDS cases in Africa, although some HIV-2 cases have appeared in the United States. The progression from HIV infection to AIDS varies, and a few HIV-infected people have remained free of AIDS symptoms for many years.

Incidence and Mortality Rates for HIV/AIDS

AIDS appears to be a relatively new disease, first recognized in 1981. Some scientists (Corbitt, Bailey, & Williams, 1990; Froland et al., 1988) believe that the disease dates at least to the 1950s, and isolated cases of AIDS in humans may be thousands of years old. The current HIV epidemic originated in African chimpanzees (Gao et al., 1999) and probably occurred because the chimpanzees were hunted for food. Although the virus is not deadly in these chimpanzees, it is in humans. During the 1980s, both the number of new cases and the number of deaths from AIDS increased rapidly until HIV infection became one of the 10 leading causes of death in the United States. Currently, however, death rates from AIDS are declining sharply, and AIDS is no longer one of the 10 leading causes of death (USDHHS, 1998b).

In 1992, the Centers for Disease Control and Prevention (CDC, 1992) revised its definition of HIV infection so that incidence figures from 1993 and subsequent years are not directly comparable to earlier figures. This new and expanded definition includes adolescents and adults who are infected with HIV and who have a very low CD4+ T-lymphocyte cell count (formerly called helper T-lymphocytes). This new definition also added three clinical conditions to the AIDS classification:

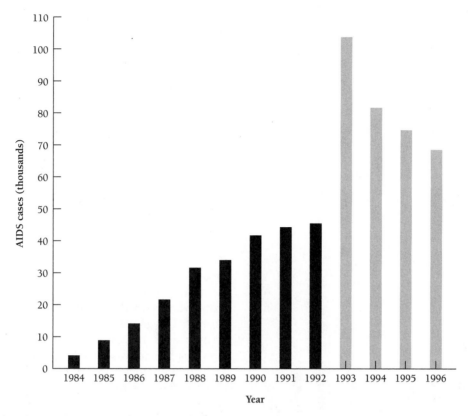

Figure 11.1   Incidence of AIDS cases by year, United States, 1984 to 1997.   *Source:* Data from *Statistical Abstracts of the United States, 1997* (117th ed., p. 141), by U.S. Bureau of the Census, 1997, Washington, DC: U.S. Government Printing Office. NOTE: Data for 1993 to 1997 are based on the expanded definition of AIDS and are not comparable to earlier data.

pulmonary tuberculosis, recurrent pneumonia, and invasive cervical cancer.

The changed definition has the advantages of uniformity and simplicity, but it distorted the incidence of the disease for the early 1990s. The number of cases in 1993 appears to double the 1992 number (see Figure 11.1), but this count includes the large backlog of people who, in previous years, would not have been classified as having AIDS. As Figure 11.1 shows, AIDS cases began a steady decline after 1993.

As the incidence of AIDS steadily declined, mortality from this disease dropped even more. From 1996 to 1998, the mortality rates for AIDS

in the United States dropped by 47%, a decrease far greater than that of any other leading cause of death. Figure 11.2 shows that the number of deaths from AIDS declined sharply after 1993. HIV-infected individuals are living longer because of drug therapies, early detection, and lifestyle changes. Combinations of antiretroviral drugs have changed the course of HIV infection, slowing the progression of infection and prolonging lives (Kelly, Otto-Salaj, Sikkema, Pinkerton, & Bloom, 1998). In addition, several strategies adopted by HIV patients may prolong their lives (Folkman, 1993). Giving up unhealthy habits such as smoking, drinking alcohol, and taking illicit drugs;

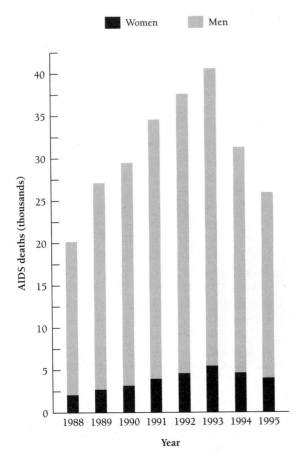

Figure 11.2   Death rates from AIDS by gender, United States, 1988 to 1997. *Source:* Data from *Statistical Abstracts of the United States, 1994* (114th ed., p. 97), by U.S. Bureau of the Census, 1995, Washington, DC: U.S. Government Printing Office; and *Statistical Abstracts of the United States, 1997* (117th ed., p. 100), by U.S. Bureau of the Census, 1995, Washington, DC: U.S. Government Printing Office.

becoming more vigilant about their health; and exercising more control over their treatment can help infected persons live longer and healthier lives.

The HIV and AIDS Epidemics

Once considered by some to be a gay man's disease, AIDS is no longer a threat only to men who have sex with other men. An analysis of people in-fected with HIV reveals at least four distinct epidemics of the infection in the United States (USD-HHS, 1998b), and each of these epidemics has changed over the past several years. Historically, the prominent epidemic affected men who had sex with men. This epidemic accounted for many of the first U.S. cases of AIDS, and gay men were the target of interventions to change their risky behavior. Male-male sexual contact is still the leading source of HIV infection, but this mode of transmission is now declining, and only about half of HIV transmissions are presently due to male-male sexual contact (USDHHS, 1998a).

A second epidemic affects injection drug users, with the number of these cases declining slightly. A third epidemic includes transmission through heterosexual contact, and this number is increasing. A fourth epidemic occurs through transmission from women to their children during the birth process. This mode of transmission has decreased sharply with the advent of antiretroviral medication for pregnant women who are HIV positive.

Although incidence of HIV is declining for most modes of transmission, it is rising rapidly for male-female sexual contact, with women much more likely than men to be infected through this method. Of those cases for which transmission can be determined, heterosexual contact accounted for only about 2% to 3% of all HIV infections in 1985, but by 1996, male-female sexual contact accounted for 15% to 20% of all HIV infections. Moreover, as of 1996, women accounted for 20% of all AIDS cases, compared with only 6% in 1985 (USDHHS, 1998a). As of 1995, women accounted for about 16% of AIDS deaths, but because they now make up about 20% of AIDS cases, the proportion of women to men dying of AIDS will continue to increase. Women are vulnerable to HIV infection primarily through two routes of transmission: heterosexual contact, which accounts for about half of all cases of AIDS in women, and injection drug use, which accounts for more than 40% of the cases. The third most frequent category is heterosexual contact with an injection drug user—a practice that makes classification difficult. However, women infected through this third mode have contracted the AIDS virus either through heterosexual contact or injection drug use, so these two methods of transmission currently are responsible for almost all AIDS cases among women (USDHHS, 1998a).

Minority ethnic groups have been affected disproportionately, especially by the epidemics affecting heterosexuals and injection drug users. In 1996, African Americans became the largest segment of the population with HIV, with 43% of HIV infections. European Americans accounted for 36% of the cases and Hispanic Americans 20%. The number of those infected through injection drug use has fallen, but heterosexual transmission has increased, especially among minority women. As of 1996, African American women made up more than 60% of women with AIDS, and AIDS continued to be the leading cause of death for African American women between the ages of 25 and 44 years (USDHHS, 1998b). The trend toward declining rates of HIV infection has not occurred for minorities as rapidly as for Whites.

Age is also a factor in HIV infection. The birth process is one mode of transmission, so some infants and children are HIV infected, but only about 1% of AIDS cases are younger than 13. Young adults are more likely to be infected than other age groups, largely due to their risky behaviors (Rosenberg & Biggar, 1998). For these young adults, gender and ethnicity factors apply: Most of the infected young adults are men, and ethnic minorities are disproportionately affected. People over age 50 are less likely to be infected than younger adults, but when infected, they tend to develop AIDS more rapidly and to get more opportunistic infections (CDC, 1998a).

Symptoms of HIV and AIDS

HIV progresses over a decade or more through four stages, but people vary greatly in the length of time at each stage. During the first stage of HIV infection, symptoms are not easily distinguishable from those of other diseases. Within a week or so

of infection, people frequently experience fever, sore throat, skin rash, headache, and other mild symptoms (McCutchan, 1990). This relatively short first period of 1 to 8 weeks is typically followed by a latent period that may last as long as 10 years during which infected people are asymptomatic or experience only minimal symptoms. During the third stage, patients typically have a cluster of symptoms including swollen lymph nodes, fever, fatigue, night sweats, loss of appetite, loss of weight, persistent diarrhea, white spots in the mouth, and painful skin rash. During the final stage, the patients' CD4+ T-lymphocyte cell count drops to 200 or less per cubic millimeter of blood (healthy people have a CD4+ count of 1,000). As their immune system begins to lose its defensive capacities, patients become susceptible to various opportunistic infections involving the lungs, gastrointestinal tract, nervous system, liver, bones, and brain. Symptoms include greater weight loss, general fatigue, fever, shortness of breath, dry cough, purplish bumps on the skin, and AIDS-related dementia. At this point, HIV becomes full-blown AIDS, from which no person has ever recovered.

The diseases associated with HIV and AIDS are caused by a variety of agents, including viruses, bacteria, fungi, and parasites. The supply of CD4+ T-lymphocytes is depleted, so the immune system no longer has a mechanism for fighting infections within cells. The AIDS virus damages or kills the part of the immune system that fights *viral* infections, leaving no way for the body to fight HIV. But HIV does not destroy the antibodies that the immune system has already manufactured, so the immune system response that occurs through antibodies circulating in the blood remains intact. Therefore, being HIV positive does not often cause a person, for example, to develop infections with the bacterium that causes strep throat or the virus that causes influenza. Most HIV-infected people have antibodies to fight against these common agents. Instead, HIV results in infection from otherwise rare organisms, which leads to such diseases as *Pneumocystis carinii* pneumonia, Kaposi's sarcoma, tuberculosis, and toxoplasmic encephalitis.

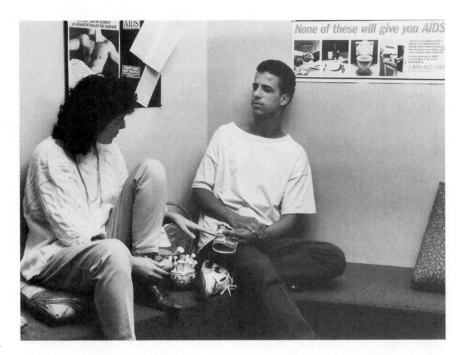

Interventions to change risky behaviors are currently the most effective way to decrease the transmission of HIV.

The Transmission of HIV

Although HIV is an infectious organism with a high fatality rate, the virus is not easily transmitted from person to person. The main routes of infection are from person to person during sex, from mother to child during pregnancy or birth, and from direct contact with blood or blood products (Glasner & Kaslow, 1990). Concentrations of HIV are especially high in the semen and blood of infected people. Therefore, contact with infected semen or blood is a risk. Other body fluids do not contain such a high concentration of HIV, making contact with saliva, urine, or tears much less of a risk. No evidence exists that any sort of casual contact spreads the infection. Eating with the same utensils or plates or drinking from the same cup as someone who is infected does not transmit HIV, nor does touching or even kissing someone who is infected. Insect bites do not spread the virus, and even being bitten by someone

who is infected will not infect the person who is bitten.

People most at risk for HIV infection are those affected by causes of the four epidemics—male-male sexual contact, injection drug use, heterosexual contact, and transmission from mother to baby during birth. Each of the groups affected by these four epidemics experiences somewhat different risks.

Male-Male Sexual Contact In the early years of AIDS, men who had sex with men made up the majority of AIDS cases. In recent years, HIV infection rates have decreased among gay and bisexual men, but this group still remains the largest risk group. Among gay and bisexual men, unprotected anal intercourse is an especially risky behavior, particularly for the receptive partner. Because the delicate lining of the rectum is often damaged during anal intercourse, the receptive person is at

WOULD YOU BELIEVE...?

It's Not Safe to Stay in the Closet

Would you believe that gay men who are infected with HIV and who conceal their sexual orientation experience a more rapid decline in health? Individuals vary in how rapidly the HIV virus progresses after infection. Some variation occurs according to (1) mode of transmission; (2) characteristics of the strain of the virus; (3) characteristics of the host, such as age and immune system function before infection; and (4) psychosocial factors, including concealment of sexual orientation.

In a group of HIV positive gay men, those who concealed their sexual orientation developed AIDS symptoms more rapidly and died earlier than those who were more open about their sexual orientation (Cole, Kemeny, Taylor, Visscher, & Fahey, 1996). Furthermore, the rapidity of progression was related to how strongly the men concealed their sexual orientation—the more "closeted," the faster HIV progressed. This progression was unrelated to demographic characteristics, health practices, or sexual behavior. Men who concealed their homosexuality most, compared with those who concealed least, experienced a 1.5- to 2-year faster progression of HIV. The magnitude of this difference is comparable to the effect of using versus not using some types of antiretroviral therapy!

Being "in the closet" or "out of the closet" is an important factor in the lives of gay men. Concealment of sexual orientation allows gay men to avoid the social censure that often accompanies being openly gay, but it also requires misrepresentation and effort to maintain this facade. In this study (Cole et al, 1996), few of the gay men were completely in the closet, but some were much more so than others. For example, some men were in the closet at work but not with their friends. These men needed to conceal a very relevant aspect of their lives for a large portion of the day. This type of inhibition might have some impact on health, thus affecting HIV progression (Cole et al., 1996).

Inhibiting significant factors about themselves might affect physiological mechanisms, including the immune system. This route is one possible explanation for the relationship between concealment and HIV progression. Others include reluctance to be identified as gay, which also might cause delays in seeking treatment for HIV infection; such delays could, of course, affect the progression of the infection.

A complicating factor is sensitivity to social censure. Gay men who conceal their sexual orientation might do so to avoid the censure that often accompanies coming out of the closet. This rejection-sensitivity is related to HIV progression (Cole, Kemeny, & Taylor, 1997): Rejection-sensitive men who concealed their sexual orientation did not accelerate their HIV progression. Therefore, gay men who are HIV positive may accelerate the progression of their infection if they stay in the closet or if they come out, depending on how sensitive they are to social censure.

---

high risk if his partner is infected with HIV. The damaged rectum makes an excellent route for the virus to enter the body, and infected semen has a high concentration of HIV. Unprotected oral sex with an infected partner is also a risky practice because HIV can enter the body through any tiny cut or other lesion in the mouth.

Condom use has become common among older gay men, but many younger ones engage in unsafe sexual practices, especially after using alcohol or other drugs (Penkower et al., 1991). Heavy drinking, heavy drug use, and being 35 or younger are each significantly related to this unsafe practice. These same three variables also predict number of sexual partners, willingness to have anonymous sex, and failure to use condoms. Unprotected sex has an attraction for some gay men, an attraction that can overcome knowledge of the risks posed by this behavior (Kelly & Kalichman, 1998). Risk-taking individuals may engage in a variety of dangerous behaviors, including use of intoxicants and unprotected sex. In addition, the use of intoxicants can cloud people's ability to make wise decisions about potentially dangerous sexual practices.

Injection Drug Use   Another high-risk behavior is the sharing of unsterilized needles by injection drug users, a practice that allows the direct transmission of blood from one person to another. Injection drug use is the second most frequent source of HIV infection in the United States (USD-HHS, 1998a). Use of injection drugs persists in spite of people's knowledge that sharing needles is a risky behavior (Loxley & Hawks, 1994). Some injection drug users continue in this behavior under certain situations, for example, when intoxicated or when there is no immediate access to sterile drug equipment.

This mode of transmission accounts for a greater percentage of infected African Americans and Hispanic Americans than European Americans (USDHHS, 1998a). Also, a higher percentage of infected women than men were exposed to the virus through this route. Several behavioral factors are related to HIV infection for women who inject drugs, including the number of sex partners and whether or not they traded sex for money or drugs (Astemborski, Vlahov, Warren, Solomon, & Nelson, 1994). Women who trade sex for injection drugs are at high risk for HIV infection from two sources—unsafe sex with a partner who injects drugs and use of contaminated needles. However, the greater of the two risks is from sex with drug-using partners (Freeman, Rodriguez, & French, 1994). As noted earlier, heterosexual contact is the source of the only HIV epidemic currently increasing in the United States.

Heterosexual Contact   Heterosexual contact is the leading source of HIV infection in Africa (Eckholm & Tierney, 1990) and the fastest growing source in the United States (USDHHS, 1998b).

African Americans and Hispanic Americans are disproportionately represented among those infected through heterosexual contact, and women from these two ethnic backgrounds are in greater danger than men from heterosexual contact.

This gender asymmetry comes from ease of transmission during sexual intercourse: Male to female transmission is eight times more likely than female to male transmission (Padian, Shiboski, Glass, & Vittinghoff, 1997). Although men are susceptible to HIV through sexual contact with women, their risk is quite small. Indeed, HIV is not easily transmitted through heterosexual sex; however, the presence of sexually transmitted diseases is an important factor, because several sexually transmitted diseases cause genital lesions, allowing the HIV virus to enter the blood.

Regular use of condoms provides a high level of safety for heterosexual men and women. A prospective study (de Vincenzi, 1994) of HIV-negative men and women who had a relationship with an infected partner showed that none of the HIV-negative partners who used condoms consistently for vaginal and anal intercourse tested positive for HIV. For those couples who used condoms inconsistently, 10% became HIV positive. In addition, having heterosexual contact with multiple partners places people at a relatively high risk for HIV infection (Avins et al., 1994). Unsafe sexual behaviors are related to drug use among heterosexual men and women as they are with gay and bisexual men. Those who use alcohol, cocaine, or marijuana are less likely to use condoms (Lowry et al., 1994). Factors that reduce condom use increase risks for transmission of HIV.

Transmission during the Birth Process   Another group at risk for HIV infection includes children born to HIV-positive women. This transmission tends to occur during the birth process. Children infected with HIV during the birth process suffer a variety of developmental disabilities including intellectual and academic impairment, psychomotor dysfunction, and emotional and behavioral difficulties (Levenson & Mellins, 1992). In addition, many of these children are born to mothers who ingested drugs during pregnancy and are thus put at further risk for developmental difficulties.

Knowledge of HIV positive status does not deter young women from becoming pregnant (Murphy, Mann, O'Keefe, & Rotherram-Borus, 1998). Between 15% and 30% of children born to HIV positive women are infected, but this percentage can be cut to 8% or less if the pregnant woman receives prenatal treatment with antiretroviral drugs. Therefore, seeking prenatal care is critically important for HIV positive women who become pregnant, and early prenatal care is responsible for much of the decline in this version of the epidemic.

Psychologists' Role in the HIV Epidemic

Psychologists have an increasingly important role in combating the HIV epidemic. During the early years of the epidemic, psychologists were involved in both primary and secondary prevention efforts. Primary prevention includes changing behavior to decrease HIV transmission. Secondary prevention includes helping people who are HIV positive to live with the infection, counseling people about being tested for HIV, helping patients deal with social and interpersonal aspects of the disease and helping patients adhere to their complex treatment program. Much of the recent improvement in length of survival of HIV infected patients rests with the effectiveness of drug treatments, and psychologists' knowledge concerning adherence to medical regimens is now relevant to managing HIV infection.

Encouraging Protective Measures   Except for infants born to HIV-infected mothers, most people have some control in protecting themselves from the human immunodeficiency virus. Fortunately, HIV is not easily transmitted from person to person, making casual contact with infected persons a low risk. People can protect themselves against infection with HIV by changing those behaviors that are high risks for acquiring the infection—

namely, having unprotected sexual contact or sharing needles with an infected person. The majority of people in the United States, Canada, and Europe who are infected have become so in one of these two ways. Limiting the number of sex partners, using condoms, and avoiding shared needles are three behaviors that will protect the largest number of people in the United States and Canada from HIV infection.

However, other protective measures may be applicable for some people. Health care workers who participate in surgery, emergency care, or other procedures that bring them into contact with blood should be careful to prevent infected blood from entering their body through an open wound. For example, dentists and dental hygienists now wear protective gloves, and health care workers are taught to adhere to a set of standard protective measures.

The tendency to base judgment on appearances can be dangerous when it comes to HIV infection. Because HIV infection typically has a long asymptomatic incubation period, people can be contagious and still appear healthy. Choosing sex partners based on the appearance of health can be very risky. Even with the widespread concern about AIDS and infection with HIV, many people continue to engage in high-risk behaviors. Alcohol and other noninjection drugs are often linked to unsafe sexual practices. In addition to research cited earlier, two studies have shown that some people at risk often appear oblivious of any personal threat from the disease. A study that asked adolescents about their high-risk sexual behaviors (Biglan et al., 1990) showed that engaging in one type of high-risk sexual behavior was associated with engaging in other high-risk behaviors. For example, adolescents who had sex with multiple partners whom they do not know very well were also not likely to use condoms. Moreover, these high-risk sexual behaviors were related to other health-risk behaviors such as smoking and drinking. Another study (Kelly et al., 1990) revealed that 37% of the patrons of gay bars reported engaging in unprotected anal intercourse and having unrealistic beliefs about the potential danger of HIV. Those who avoided this high-risk behavior were more likely to attribute safety to their own behavior (as opposed to luck, chance, or fate), be more knowledgeable about high-risk practices, have fewer sex partners, be older, consider safety an accepted norm in their social contacts, and be more realistic about their own risk.

Many people who engage in high-risk behaviors do so as part of a pattern of taking risks. Thus, psychological programs constructed to change high-risk sexual behaviors must consider the optimistic bias, naive beliefs, or disregard for safety among people who are at greatest risk.

Helping People with HIV Infection   People who believe they may be infected with HIV, as well as those who know that they are, can benefit from various psychological interventions. People with high-risk behaviors may have difficulty deciding whether to be tested for HIV; psychologists can provide both information and support for these people. A significant minority of gay and bisexual men, injection drug users, and a larger proportion of heterosexual men and women with multiple partners and inconsistent use of condoms have never been tested for HIV. People in this last group may be unaware of their risk and deny a need to be tested. Because HIV infection has a long incubation period, at-risk heterosexual men and women may contaminate others for years before they learn they have HIV.

The decision to be tested for HIV has both benefits and costs (Folkman, 1993). The benefit, of course, is that people can find out their serostatus as soon as possible. A positive HIV test can lead to early treatment, which can prolong a person's life. Another potentially positive benefit of early testing is the reduction or elimination of behaviors that place others at risk. Many, but not all, gay and bisexual men reduce risky sexual behaviors, and most inform their primary partner of the results of testing. However, some research (Ickovics et al., 1998) indicated that women's sexual behavior tends not to change as a result of HIV testing.

What are the costs of receiving an HIV-positive test result? Does such information increase anxiety, depression, anger, and psychological distress? This news is distressing, and women who are tested are more anxious and depressed than women who are not, even before learning of their serostatus (Ickovics et al., 1998). In a large national sample of men and women (Fleishman & Fogel, 1994), more than 40% of persons with AIDS were diagnosed with clinical depression, a percentage considerably higher than that reported in other studies. Some people who react with severe psychopathology may have existing problems (Folkman, 1993), but the existence of a serious psychiatric disorder decreases the quality of life for those who are HIV positive (Holmes, Bix, Meritz, Turner, & Hutelmyer, 1997).

Coping processes can affect the amount of distress experienced by those who learn they are HIV positive, and psychological interventions can reduce their distress. Avoidant coping, such as denying reality or clinging to illusory hope, is associated with high levels of psychological distress. Active coping, including problem solving and seeking social support, is related to better adjustment. Cognitive behavioral stress management interventions have been successful in boosting positive coping and increasing social support (Lutgendorf et al., 1998), indicating that psychological interventions have a place in HIV management.

Psychologists can also help HIV patients adhere to the complex medical regimens designed to control HIV infection (Kelly et al., 1998). A combination of drug treatments became common in 1996 after its effectiveness became apparent. Patients typically take at least three different antiretroviral medications; they often take other drugs to combat side effects of the antiretroviral drugs as well as drugs to fight opportunistic infections. These regimens can include as many as a dozen drugs, all of which must be timed precisely. When patients do not follow the schedule, the effectiveness diminishes. Psychologists can help patients adhere to this schedule as well as facilitate their self-management skills.

In Summary

Acquired immune deficiency syndrome (AIDS) is the result of depletion of the immune system after infection with the human immunodeficiency virus (HIV). When the immune system fails to defend the body, a number of diseases may develop, including bacterial, viral, fungal, and parasitic infections that are uncommon in people who have functioning immune systems.

HIV progresses into AIDS through four stages, but throughout most of the time, an HIV-positive person has few or no symptoms and may unknowingly infect others with the virus. For this reason, frequent blood tests for people in high-risk categories are essential to control the spread of AIDS. The modes of transmission of HIV are behavioral, with receptive anal intercourse and the sharing of needles for intravenous drug injection the two behaviors that have spread the infection to the most people in the United States. Unprotected heterosexual contact with an infected partner accounts for an increasing proportion of people with HIV, the majority of whom are women and belong to ethnic minorities. The number of babies infected with HIV is decreasing because new antiretroviral drug therapies sharply decrease transmission from an infected mother during the birth process.

Psychologists use a variety of interventions to help patients reduce high-risk behaviors, to cope with their illness, to manage their symptoms, and to adhere to the complex drug regimens have improve survival. In addition, psychologists provide counseling services for those seeking to be tested and for those whose tests reveal infection. These programs not only encourage protective behaviors but also emphasize the role of positive health in combating AIDS.

Living with Alzheimer's Disease

Alzheimer's disease, a degenerative disease of the brain, is a major source of impairment among older people, affecting nearly half the people over 85 in the United States (Plaud, Mosley, & Moberg, 1998). Medical researchers identified the brain abnormalities that underlie Alzheimer's disease in the late 19th century. In 1907, a German physician, Alois Alzheimer, reported on the relationship between autopsy findings of neurological abnormalities and psychiatric symptoms before death. Shortly after his report, other researchers began to call the disorder Alzheimer's disease.

Although Alzheimer's patients show behavioral symptoms of cognitive impairment and memory loss, the disease can be diagnosed definitively only through autopsy. A microscopic examination of the brain of those with Alzheimer's disease reveals "plaques" and tangles of nerve fibers in the cerebral cortex and hippocampus. These tangles of nerve fibers are the physical basis for Alzheimer's disease.

The underlying mechanisms in the development of the disease are not yet completely understood, but research has identified two different forms of the disease: one that occurs before age 60 and the other that occurs after age 65. The early-onset type is quite rare, representing less than 1% of all Alzheimer's patients (Mayeux & Schupf, 1995). Early-onset Alzheimer's seems to be due to a genetic defect, and at least three different genes have been implicated on chromosomes 1, 14, and 21 (Daly, 1998).

The late-onset type seems to be related to apolipoprotein E, a protein involved in cholesterol metabolism (Goedert, Strittmatter, & Roses, 1994). One form of apolipoprotein, the E4 form, increases the risk for developing the tangles of neurons that are characteristic of Alzheimer's disease by about three times (Farrer et al,, 1998), and the E2 form may offer some protection. Other factors that are unidentified also contribute to the development of the disease. This research on the physiology underlying Alzheimer's disease offers the promise of identifying the causes of this disease and suggests the possibility of treatment for those at risk and perhaps even for those with the disease.

The incidence of Alzheimer's disease rises sharply with advancing age (Hebert et al., 1995).

Denis Evans and colleagues (Evans et al., 1989) found that more than 10% of all people over age 65 showed symptoms that indicated a probable diagnosis of Alzheimer's disease. These people showed signs of serious cognitive, language, and memory deficits. This study also showed a strong association between age and Alzheimer's disease, with only 3% of the people between ages 65 and 74 demonstrating symptoms of the disease; 18.7% of the people between ages 75 and 84 manifesting symptoms; and 47.2% of their sample over age 85 showing symptoms of Alzheimer's disease. The increase does not continue, however, and people who have not developed symptoms of Alzheimer's disease by their mid-80s are less likely to do so than people in their 70s (Ritchie & Kildea, 1995). The high number of people over 85 years old who have symptoms of probable Alzheimer's disease presents a pessimistic picture for the aging population in developed countries, where Alzheimer's is likely to become a large public health problem (Brookmeyer, Gray, & Kawas, 1998).

Because the symptoms of Alzheimer's include a number of behavior problems that are also symptoms of psychiatric disorders, the disease can be difficult to diagnose. These symptoms include memory loss, language problems, agitation and irritability, sleep disorders, suspiciousness and paranoia, incontinence, and sexual disorders (Plaud et al., 1998). These behavioral symptoms can be the source of much distress to the patients as well as to their caregivers. The most common psychiatric problem among Alzheimer's patients is depression. As many as 20% of Alzheimer's patients exhibit symptoms of clinical depression and an additional 30% to 50% suffer from depressed mood (Mulsant, Pollock, Nebes, Hoch, & Reynolds, 1997). Depression is especially common among people in the early phases of the disease and in early-onset Alzheimer's. Those people who retain much awareness of their problems find their deterioration distressing and respond with a feeling of helplessness and depression.

The memory loss that characterizes Alzheimer's disease may first appear in the form of small, ordinary failures of memory, but the memory loss progresses to the point that Alzheimer's patients fail to recognize family members and forget how to perform even routine self-care (Rabins, 1989). In the early phases of the disease, patients are usually aware of their memory failures, making this symptom even more distressing. This chapter opened with the case of Sylvia, who was typical of many Alzheimer's patients in that she became angry with herself for not being able to recall people's names and for forgetting words in the middle of a sentence. She knew that she should be able to say the right name or word, a situation that sparked frustration and fury.

Sylvia's language problems highlight a related cognitive deficit. The inability to utter the intended word is quite common among Alzheimer's patients. Sometimes patients substitute other words for the one they intended, but the substitutes are not always good matches, posing communication problems. This language disability can lead to frustration and, if patients withdraw from attempts to communicate, it can promote isolation.

Patients with Alzheimer's disease often exhibit symptoms of agitation, irritability, and even violence. Sylvia was no exception. A gentle, even passive woman during the first 80 years of her life, she frequently became aggressive and threatening as her disease progressed. She accused Brenda of mistreating her and on one occasion cut up all her old photos of Brenda. In some cases, Sylvia's explosive agitation was related to her memory failure. Sometimes she would have an explosive outburst while getting dressed because she had forgotten how to complete the task and had become confused and frustrated. At other times she would become angry because her daily routine had been disrupted and she was uncertain about how she should behave.

The common symptoms of paranoia and suspiciousness may also relate to cognitive impairments. Alzheimer's patients may forget where they have put belongings and, because they cannot find their possessions, accuse others of taking them. However, suspicious and accusatory behaviors are not limited to misplaced belongings. Like many Alzheimer's patients, Sylvia concentrated her suspicions and accusations on her primary caregiver, leading Brenda to become resentful and emotionally distressed.

Although difficulties in staying asleep are common among older adults, Alzheimer's patients have even more severe problems than their peers. As a result, these patients tend to wander at all times of the day and night (Rabins, 1989). This behavior can disturb those who sleep in the same house and provide opportunities for the patients to injure themselves. After Brenda and Bob moved Sylvia into their house, this problem became so serious that they were required to retain a "sitter" to watch Sylvia at night. The sitter was instructed to gently lead Sylvia back to her bedroom whenever she roamed around at night.

Incontinence and sexual disorders are acutely distressing problems to both the patients and their caregivers. Incontinence is very common in patients with advanced cases of Alzheimer's disease. In the year before she died, Sylvia lost all control over her bowel movements. Even more distressing to Brenda, she seemed also to have lost her awareness of normal excretory functions and showed no appreciation for her daughter's extra work in cleaning her. Also distressing to Brenda was her mother's inappropriate sexual behavior, a common disorder among Alzheimer's patients. Sylvia would sometimes masturbate in public and use obscene language, behaviors that were totally uncharacteristic of her earlier life. A pattern of behavioral symptoms, such as Sylvia's, is strong indication of Alzheimer's disease and the only means of diagnosis before autopsy.

Helping the Patient

Presently, no cure for Alzheimer's disease exists; the most effective treatment for the disease would be one that prevented or reversed the degeneration of neurons in the brain. Incurability and untreatability are two different things, and the physical symptoms and other accompanying dis-

orders of Alzheimer's disease can be treated, but not cured. Treatment approaches include drugs for delaying the progression of cognitive deficits, neuroleptic drugs for reducing agitation and aggression, and the use of music and pets to relax Alzheimer's patients. However, none of these techniques is very effective (Rabins, 1996).

In addition to these interventions, several researchers have advocated behavioral approaches in treating Alzheimer's patients. An analysis of the antecedents of patients' problem behaviors allows modification of the environment of Alzheimer's patients so they can adjust better to their lives (Plaud et al., 1998). By identifying the events that precede problem behaviors, family members can eliminate or reduce those events and thus perhaps decrease patients' undesirable behaviors. Changes include alterations in the environment and in the patient's behaviors. For example, patients with awareness of their memory loss can learn to write notes as a way of keeping track of the important things in their lives. For those who get lost in their own homes, labeling the doors can be helpful.

The Progressively Lowered Stress Threshold model is an alternative approach for dealing with dementias (Hall, 1994). This approach divides symptoms into cognitive or intellectual problems, affective or personality changes, losses in the ability to plan, and lowering of stress thresholds that cause episodes of dysfunctional behavior. This model holds that dysfunctional episodes are caused by stresses such as fatigue, changes in environment or routine, inappropriate levels of stimulation, performance demands that exceed capability, and physical stressors. This model provides an assessment of behavior problems and allows for interventions to minimize dysfunctional episodes by helping caregivers to structure the environment, establish a routine for the patients, minimize fatigue, and identify pain. For example, for patients who yelled throughout the day, 60% had previously unnoticed fractures that caused them considerable pain. This behavioral management program offers a way to approach the care of patients with Alzheimer's disease so as to allow them prolonged periods of functioning while providing their caretakers with a way to approach the demands of caring for a person with diminishing capabilities.

Although none of these therapies can cure Alzheimer's disease, most help control undesirable behaviors and alleviate some of the distressing symptoms of the disease. Any treatment that can delay symptoms of Alzheimer's disease can make significant differences in the number of cases and in the costs of management (Brookmeyer et al., 1998). In the early phases of Alzheimer's disease, both patients and their families are distressed by its symptoms, but as the patients worsen and lose awareness, the stress of Alzheimer's becomes more severe for the family.

Helping the Family

As with other chronic illnesses, Alzheimer's disease affects not only patients but also their families. For Alzheimer's disease, however, the symptoms of the illness are particularly distressing to the families (Cohler, Groves, Borden, & Lazarus, 1989). The memory impairments are disturbing, because patients may fail to recognize their spouses and children. Cognitive impairments lead to changes in personality, and the one affected no longer seems like the same person. The suspiciousness that Alzheimer's patients frequently manifest can lead to accusations that hurt family members, and Alzheimer's patients who are violent upset normal family functioning. Families tend to find dangerous or embarrassing behaviors especially distressing (Barrett, Ford, Stewart, & Haley, 1994). In addition to this emotional burden, the problems of taking care of an Alzheimer's patient greatly disrupt family routine.

For instance, arguments between Brenda and Bob increased during the time Sylvia lived with them. Brenda neglected her own appearance, became absorbed in her caregiving duties, and lost interest in sexual relations with Bob. Before Sylvia's illness, Brenda and Bob shared interests in the law, movies, books, and traveling. Although she could

have arranged to do so, during the 3 years her mother lived with them, Brenda never took a vacation or even went to a movie.

In the United States, the caregiver role is occupied mostly by women (Cohler et al., 1989; Pearlin, Turner, & Semple, 1989), and an unmarried woman has the greatest likelihood of becoming the primary caretaker for Alzheimer's patients (Modesti & Tryon, 1994). The National Long-term Care Survey (Stone, Cafferata, & Sangl, 1987) showed that family caregivers are usually the patients' wives or daughters. For Alzheimer's patients with spouses who are able to provide care, the caregiving falls to the spouse, and men as well as women fill this role. These spouses may not be able to provide the necessary care with ease because as older adults, the spouses may be in poor health themselves. Therefore, adult children often become involved in caregiving, sometimes by assisting one parent to provide care for the other. Daughters and daughters-in-law are called on to help more often than sons or sons-in-law, whose assistance is typically in the form of helping their wives or sisters (Cohler et al., 1989). The gender inequity also exists in the assistance that adult children provide to parents who are caregivers, with men receiving more assistance in caring for their wives than women receive in caring for their husbands.

Not only must people who care for Alzheimer's patients have the time and energy for this task, but they must also take care of their other obligations as well. Often the demands of caring for an Alzheimer's patient conflict with job or career; family members are usually not free to leave jobs because caregiving is an economic as well as an emotional strain. Many families exhaust their financial and emotional resources to provide care for an Alzheimer's patient (Pearlin et al., 1989).

In some ways, Brenda was more fortunate than the typical caregiver. Bob's income was sufficient, and Brenda was able to suspend her career to care for her mother. Brenda could have continued with her career and hired a full-time nurse, but she felt that she should be the one to provide care.

Brenda's feelings were typical of caregivers for Alzheimer's patients (Cohler et al., 1989).

Alzheimer's caregivers frequently experience feelings of loss for the relationship that they once shared with the patient. This sense of loss may be similar to bereavement, only the person is still alive (Pearlin et al., 1989). During her times alone, Brenda found herself reminiscing more and more about her childhood and the pleasant times she enjoyed with her mother. She knew that Sylvia would never regain the loving personality that marked her earlier life. The woman Brenda once knew no longer lived in her mother's body, and she grieved over her loss.

Caregivers experiencing the stress and strain of their role exhibit a number of symptoms of their own distress, including fatigue, frustration, helplessness, grief, shame, embarrassment, anger, and depression (Soukup, 1996). Anger is a common problem with Alzheimer's caregivers. Spouses become angry and frightened when they realize that they are faced with years of a deteriorating relationship. Caregivers who are adult children are often sandwiched between helping an Alzheimer's parent and taking care of children, and this strain can lead to anger, fatigue, depression, and loss of sleep (Soukup, 1996).

The chronic stress of caregiving makes these individuals of interest to psychoneuroimmunologists, who have studied how this chronic stress affects the immune system (Cacioppo et al., 1998; Kiecolt-Glaser et al., 1991; Kiecolt-Glaser & Glaser, 1989; Kiecolt-Glaser, Glaser, et al., 1987). A comparison of caregivers of Alzheimer's patients with a matched control group (Kiecolt-Glaser, Glaser, et al., 1987) showed that the caregivers were more distressed, exhibited a poorer immune response, and developed more infectious illnesses. In addition, the level of impairment of the Alzheimer's patient was related to the level of distress in the caregiver; the more impaired patients had more distressed caregivers. These results indicate that the chronic stress of providing care for Alzheimer's patients lowers immune system functioning and increases vulnerability to infectious illness.

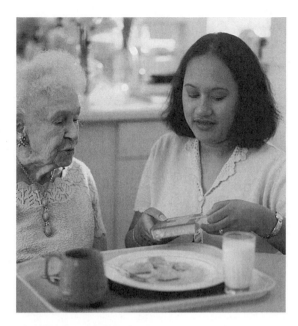

Caring for an Alzheimer's patient can produce high levels of stress, making caregivers vulnerable to illness.

The type of support caregivers receive from *their* friends and family can affect their immune systems (Kiecolt-Glaser, Dyer, & Shuttleworth, 1988). Caregivers who received positive support had better immune functioning than those who received little support or negative support, such as criticism of how they provided care. The people who received negative support from friends and family showed the poorest immune functioning of anyone in the study. This finding emphasizes how important it is that caregivers for Alzheimer's patients receive support and assistance in coping.

Cognitive-behavioral therapies can help caregivers manage their negative emotions (Plaud et al., 1998). In addition, support groups can help people who care for Alzheimer's patients. Participation in a group that encourages an open, honest sharing of feelings, including negative feelings, can provide support that families may not be able to give. This additional support may be needed because of the strain imposed on the family and

BECOMING HEALTHIER

1. If you are the primary caregiver to someone who is chronically ill, don't ignore your own health—both physical and psychological. Regularly schedule some time for yourself.

2. If you have Type I diabetes, don't try to hide your illness from your friends. Although you have a chronic disease, you can live a long and productive life, but you must adhere faithfully to a life-long regimen that includes diet, insulin injection, and regular exercise. If you live with someone with diabetes, offer social and emotional support, and encourage that person to stick with required health practices.

3. If you are the primary caregiver to someone with HIV or AIDS, seek social and emotional support through groups specifically convened to offer such support. The white pages of your telephone book lists numbers to call for information.

4. If you are a caregiver to someone with Alzheimer's disease, take regular breaks. (You have friends who can assume caregiver duties for short periods.) Look for an Alzheimer's support group in your community and attend meetings as frequently as possible.

friends of the patient, people who would otherwise be the main sources of support. Support groups can also be sources of information about caring for the patients and about community resources that provide respite care.

In Summary

Alzheimer's disease is a progressive, degenerative disease of the brain that affects cognitive functioning, especially memory. Other symptoms include language problems, agitation and irritability, paranoia and suspiciousness, sleep disorders, depression, incontinence, and sexual problems. These symptoms are also indicative of some psychiatric disorders and make Alzheimer's disease distressing to both patients and caretakers.

Increasing age is a risk factor for Alzheimer's disease, with nearly half the people over 85 exhibiting symptoms. Several different gene sites have been identified in connection with this disease.

Drug treatments intended to slow the progress of the disease have limited effectiveness, and treatment is largely oriented toward managing the negative symptoms and helping family caregivers

cope with the stress. Management of symptoms can include changing the environment to make care less difficult. Treatment may also be desirable for those who provide care to Alzheimer's patients, because a high percentage of these caregivers experience stress and stress-related problems, depression being the most common. Individual therapy or increased social support from an Alzheimer's support group can help the caregivers and families of Alzheimer's patients cope with the stress of providing care.

Answers

This chapter addressed six basic questions:

1. **What is the impact of chronic illness?**

   Unlike acute diseases, chronic illnesses can persist for years and affect not only the afflicted person but friends and family members as well. Long-term chronic illnesses frequently bring about a crisis in people's lives, change the way people see themselves, produce financial hardship, and disrupt family dynamics. Support groups and programs designed by health psychologists help people cope with the emotional problems associated with chronic illness, problems that traditional medical care often overlooks.

2. **What is involved in cardiac rehabilitation programs?**

People who survive a heart attack and those who undergo cardiac surgery typically engage in a cardiac rehabilitation regimen that consists of medication, smoking cessation, regular exercise, and a recommendation for a low-fat, low-salt diet. Cardiac rehabilitation programs may also include components to help patients (and their spouses) deal with the anxiety, depression, and sleep disturbances that are common after heart problems.

3. **How can patients be helped in coping with cancer?**

The standard medical treatments for cancer—surgery, chemotherapy, and radiation—all have negative side effects that often produce added stress due to changes in body image, loss of hair, nausea, fatigue, and sterility. Psychological interventions, including relaxation, individual psychotherapy, and support groups can help patients cope with the unpleasant side effects of cancer.

4. **What is involved in adjusting to diabetes?**

Diabetes, both insulin-dependent (Type I) and noninsulin-dependent (Type II), requires changes in lifestyle, including constant monitoring and compliance with the treatment regimen. Treatments include insulin injections for Type I diabetics and adherence to careful dietary restrictions, scheduling of meals, avoidance of certain foods, regular medical visits, and routine exercise for all diabetics. Health psychologists, using cognitive-behavioral techniques, can help diabetics adhere to treatment regimens.

5. **How can HIV infection be managed?**

Infection with the human immunodeficiency virus (HIV) depletes the immune system, leaving the body vulnerable to acquired immune deficiency syndrome (AIDS) and a variety of opportunistic infections. Four different populations in the U.S. have been affected by HIV epidemics; (1) men who have sex with men, (2) injection drug users, (3) heterosexuals, and (4) children born to HIV positive mothers. Psychologists are involved in the HIV epidemic by encouraging protective behaviors, counseling infected people to help them cope with living with a chronic disease, and helping patients adhere to complex medical regimens that have changed HIV infection to a manageable chronic disease.

6. **What is the impact of Alzheimer's disease on patients and their families?**

Alzheimer's disease is a brain disease that produces memory loss, language problems, agitation and irritability, sleep disorders, suspiciousness, wandering, incontinence, and loss of ability to perform routine care. Alzheimer's disease has genetic components, but age is the main risk, with the prevalence doubling for every decade after age 65. Medical treatments have limited effectiveness, and the main management strategies consist of interventions to allow patients longer periods of functioning and counseling and support groups for family members, who frequently experience more stress than the patient.

Glossary

diabetes mellitus A disorder caused by insulin deficiency.

glucagon A hormone, secreted by the pancreas, that stimulates the release of glucose, thus elevating blood sugar level.

human immunodeficiency virus (HIV) A virus that attacks the human immune system, depleting the body's ability to fight infection; the infection that causes AIDS.

insulin A hormone that enhances glucose intake to the cells.

islet cells The part of the pancreas that produces glucagon and insulin.

pancreas An endocrine gland, located below the stomach, that produces digestive juices and hormones.

Suggested Readings

Cousins, N. (1983). *The healing heart: Antidote to panic and helplessness.* New York: Norton.

Norman Cousins describes his heart attack and his recovery in this readable, personal book about living with heart disease. Cousins's approach was unorthodox, but his advice led to an optimistic view of the process of recovery and coping.

Heston, L. L., & White, J. A. (1991). *The vanishing mind: A practical guide to Alzheimer's disease and other dementias.* New York: Freeman.

This practical book provides valuable information for family members and other caregivers who deal with Alzheimer's disease and other dementias.

Holland, J. C., & Lewis, S. (1993). Emotions and cancer: What do we really know? In D. Goleman & J. Gurin (Eds.), *Mind/body medicine: How to use your mind for better health* (pp. 85–109). Yonkers, NY: Consumer Reports Books.

In addition to examining the evidence on emotions and cancer in a nontechnical format, Holland and Lewis review various adjunct therapies for cancer, including psychotherapy, imagery, and support groups. They also give advice for coping with cancer and for helping someone with cancer deal with the emotional and physical problems of the disease.

Kelly, J. A., Otto-Salaj, L. L., Sikkema, K. J., Pinkerton, S. D., & Bloom, F. R. (1998). Implications of HIV treatment advances for behavioral research on AIDS: Protease inhibitors and new challenges in HIV secondary prevention. *Health Psychology, 17,* 310–319.

Jeffrey Kelly and his colleagues review the changed and changing field of HIV research and treatment. This article not only discusses the changes in medical treatment for HIV infection but also describes how involvement for psychologists has increased as HIV becomes a more manageable chronic illness.

Taylor, S. E., & Aspinwall, L. G. (1993). Coping with chronic illness. In L. Goldberger & S. Breznitz (Eds.), *Handbook of stress: Theoretical and clinical aspects* (2nd ed., pp. 511–531). New York: Free Press.

Shelly Taylor and Lisa Aspinwall summarize the research on coping with chronic illness, including the stresses that accompany chronic illness, the variety of coping strategies that people use to deal with such illnesses, and interventions to help people cope more effectively.

 Ward, E. M. (1997, December). Dealing with diabetes: Diet and exercise hold key to control. *Environmental Nutrition, 20,* 1–2.

This readable article reviews the disease of diabetes and provides information about how to control blood glucose and the importance of doing so. Available through InfoTrac College Edition by Wadsworth Publishing Company.

CHAPTER 12

Preventing Injuries

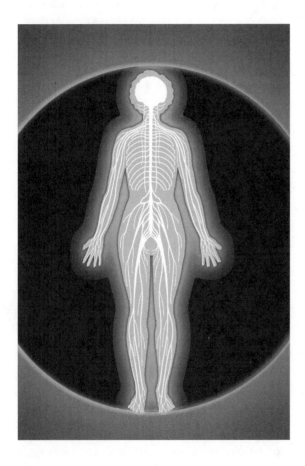

QUESTIONS

This chapter focuses on six basic questions:

1. How can adults make children's world safer?

2. What can young people do to reduce their chances of unintentional injuries?

3. What unintentional injuries are most likely to affect adults?

4. What are some of the strategies for reducing unintentional injuries?

5. What are the major types and the impact of intentional injuries?

6. How can intentional injuries be reduced?

JAMES: DRINKING, DRIVING, AND FIREARMS

James, a European American college student, acknowledges that he took many safety risks in his 23 years and feels lucky that he was not injured seriously. James grew up in a small Southern town where drinking alcohol was a primary recreation for him and his friends, and many of his risks involved alcohol, motor vehicles, firearms, or some combination of the three. When he was in high school, James and his friends drank heavily on weekends. A group of them played a game that involved one member of the group riding on the top of the cab of James's truck in order to shoot whatever came into the headlights. The person who was shooting was strapped to the top of the cab to prevent him from falling, but some falls did occur. One resulted in a broken leg, so the group decided to stop playing that game.

James continued to take risks, including driving after he had been drinking. He says that he had a drinking problem during high school, but that he never hesitated to drive. His drinking habits have changed since he started college; he drinks much less but continues to drive after drinking. Although he knows the risks, he doesn't believe that these risks apply to him because he changes his driving behavior after he has been drinking; that is, he avoids busy streets and drives more slowly. He has had one crash while he was driving drunk, but that crash resulted in only a minor injury. James has not experienced any major injury despite his many risks.

James likes guns and owns both handguns and hunting rifles. Indeed, he carries a firearm in his truck and has done so ever since high school. He knows the risks involved with guns, and he is more cautious with firearms than he is with driving after drinking. He knows the proper safety procedures for handling guns and insists that his friends observe these procedures. He acknowledges that drinking makes people less safety conscious and slows their reflexes, but he still feels that he is careful with firearms. However, James knows that having a gun in his truck can be a risk—once a friend became angry at another person and wanted the gun from James's truck to shoot that person. James talked his friend out of it, but the inci-

dent made James aware that having a gun might be a danger even if he was not going to use the firearm himself.

Although James has taken a great many risks, he sees those risks more clearly now than during the incidents. He now considers himself very lucky to have experienced only minor injuries, but he believes that his precautions concerning driving slowly after drinking and his training in firearm safety have contributed to his escape from injury. He has taken more chances than many people, but his beliefs concerning precautions are similar to those of many people. His belief that he will escape the negative consequences of risky behavior fits into the framework of optimistic bias (Weinstein, 1980), in which one believes that negative events will happen to others more often than to oneself. Taking protective measures is also a common strategy to decrease perceived hazards (Norris, 1997). Most people take some type of precaution to avoid injury or crime victimization. Unfortunately, most people also put themselves at risk in some ways, and, like James, they may not acknowledge that their behavior is a major health risk.

Research indicates that unhealthy habits tend to be related, just as healthy behaviors also tend to go together. A relationship exists between health-risking behaviors and health-enhancing behaviors of 10th to 12th graders (Hawkins, 1992). High school students who engaged in such unhealthy behaviors as smoking, carrying a weapon, and driving while drinking were less likely to use seatbelts, eat a healthy diet, get adequate sleep, or have healthy dental habits.

Before 1970, psychologists, like nearly everyone else, referred to unintentional injuries as *accidents,* a term with connotations of chance, fate, or inevitability (Williams & Lund, 1992). During the 1970s and 1980s, physician William Haddon, Jr. (Haddon, 1970, 1972, 1980) began to change the way psychologists and many others looked at unintentional injuries. Rather than viewing them simply as a consequence of unavoidable human error, health psychologists now see unintentional injuries as resulting from a complex of conditions, including individual behaviors, dangerous environmental conditions, and lack of tough legislation and enforcement. Health psychologists are concerned in each of these three areas with unintentional injuries at the various developmental stages.

✓ **CHECK YOUR SAFETY RISKS**

Check the items that apply to you.

If you do not have a young child in your home, go to Item 7.

❏ 1. Children in my home seldom or never wear helmets when they ride a bicycle or use a skateboard.

❏ 2. In my home, cleaning materials, chemicals, or poisons are stored in an unlocked cabinet under the sink.

❏ 3. In my home, a child under the age of 2 sleeps in the top bunk of a bunk bed.

❏ 4. In my home, a child under the age of 2 sometimes is left unattended in a high chair.

❏ 5. Children in my home sometimes go swimming without an adult supervisor.

❏ 6. I allow young children to ride in the front seat of a car.

❏ 7. I keep a loaded gun in my home.

❏ 8. I seldom or never use a seatbelt when driving or riding in a motor vehicle.

❏ 9. I sometimes drive after having more than two drinks.

❏ 10. I sometimes ride with someone who has been drinking.

❏ 11. I sometimes ride a bicycle or motorcycle without a helmet.

❏ 12. I usually ride my bicycle on the left side of the road, facing oncoming traffic.

❏ 13. I sometimes smoke in bed.

❏ 14. While swimming I have sometimes dived into a body of water without knowing exactly what was in the water.

❏ 15. I sometimes ride a bicycle after drinking.

❏ 16. I sometimes play sports after drinking.

Each of these items represents a common safety risk, but many other behaviors and situations can be dangerous. Although potential harm cannot be avoided completely, most safety rules do not greatly restrict one's freedom nor limit one's enjoyment of leisure-time activities.

Unintentional Injuries

Unintentional injuries are the fourth leading cause of death in the United States, accounting for about 4% of all deaths. However, fatalities from unintentional injuries have been declining in recent years (Ventura, Anderson, Martin, & Smith, 1998). From 1965 to 1995, the death rate from unintentional injuries dropped by almost 50% (see Figure 12.1). Nevertheless, unintentional injuries remain the leading cause of death in the United States for all groups up to age 35 and account for more than 40% of all deaths among young people 15 to 24 years of age (USBC, 1998).

The primary causes of death from unintentional injuries are motor vehicle crashes, which account for almost half of all unintentional deaths. Figure 12.1 shows a continuous decline in the *rate* of death from motor vehicle injuries from 1965 to 1995. Despite large increases in the number of

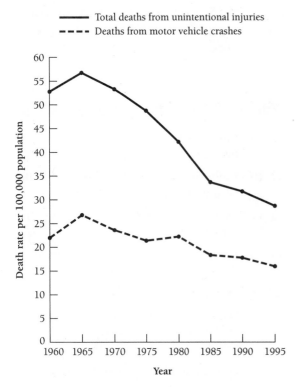

Figure 12.1   Deaths from unintentional injuries (total and motor vehicle-related) per 100,000 of U.S. population, 1960–1995.   *Source:* Data from *Statistical Abstracts of the United States, 1973,* (p. 61); *1988* (p. 77); and *1997* (p. 94), by U.S. Bureau of the Census, Washington DC: U.S. Government Printing Office.

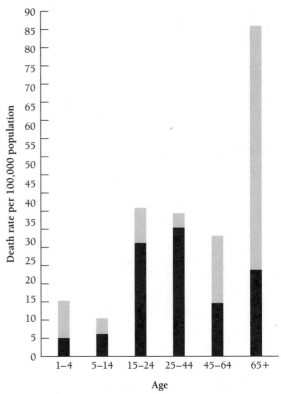

Figure 12.2   Deaths from unintentional injuries by age, per 100,000 of U.S. population, 1995. (Motor vehicle deaths are shown in black.)   *Source:* Data from "Report of Final Mortality Statistics, 1995," by R. N. Anderson, K. D. Kochanek, & S. L. Murphy, 1997, *Monthly vital statistics report,* Vol. 45, No. 11, Table 7.

drivers and the number of miles driven, the *total number* deaths from motor vehicle crashes steadily dropped from almost 55,000 in 1970 to 42,000 in 1993 (USBC, 1979, 1998). The use of seatbelts and airbags, better built cars, and safer roads have each contributed to this decline. However, since 1993, there has been a slight upturn in total fatalities, an increase that parallels a relaxation of speed limits on highways and roads.

Gender and age are factors in motor vehicle deaths. Men have more than twice the rate of motor vehicle deaths as women (USBC, 1998). Figure 12.2 shows that children have the lowest rate of death from motor vehicle injuries and that

the rates rise sharply for adolescents and adults under the age of 45 (Anderson, Kochanek, & Murphy, 1997).

In addition to the large number of fatalities from unintentional injuries, even larger numbers of people suffer nonfatal injuries every year. Nonfatal injuries are responsible for increased health care costs, lost work and school days, disability, and pain. Clearly, violent death and injury are major health problems in the United States, and health psychologists have been involved in strategies to reduce their number (Saldana & Peterson, 1997; Williams & Lund, 1992).

Although all age groups are vulnerable to unintentional injuries, the pattern of death and injury varies with the different developmental stages.

Childhood

Unintentional injuries are the leading cause of death for children in the United States, accounting for nearly 40% of all deaths among children under age 15 (Anderson et al., 1997). However, because children of this age have a relatively low death rate, the number of young children killed unintentionally is much lower than it is for adolescents or older people (see Figure 12.2).

Unintentional injuries to children are often caused by the unsafe acts of adults or an environment made unsafe by adults. The most frequent fatal injuries are from motor vehicle crashes, the major cause of unintentional injuries at every age. Figure 12.2 shows that for children 1 to 4 years of age, about one-third of unintentional fatalities stem from motor vehicle crashes, and for children 5 to 14, more than half the deaths from unintentional injuries are due to motor vehicle crashes. The majority of automobile-related injuries to children under age 5 result from an adult's failure to properly restrain an infant or toddler in the back seat of a car (Saldana & Peterson, 1997). Unfortunately, several infants and young children in the front seat of a car have been killed or seriously injured by the deployment of passenger-side airbags, but nearly all these injuries could have been avoided by properly restraining children in the *back* seat (National Highway Traffic Safety Administration, 1993–1996).

Drownings are the second leading cause of children's deaths from unintentional injuries, and not all drownings occur in a swimming pool. For children under the age of five, bathtubs and large buckets filled with water are potentially deadly containers. For older children, swimming pools are the most common place for drownings, and warm weather states such as California, Arizona, and Florida have more than their share of swimming pool drownings (Saldana & Peterson, 1997).

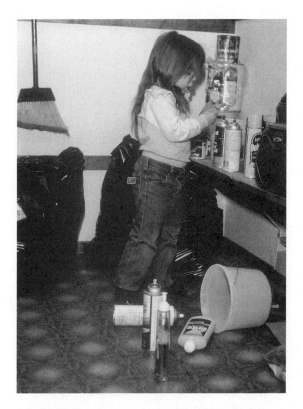

Homes include a number of safety hazards for young children.

Children are also killed and injured by burns, most of which result from house fires. Many house fires are due to adults' smoking, but children are often the victims. Smoking is the leading cause of fire-related deaths and the second leading cause of fire-related injuries (Miller, 1993). More than 3,600 people die each year and 18,000 receive nonfatal injuries from residential fires (CDC, 1998b), and children under the age of five have an increased risk of death from residential fires; the younger the child, the greater the risk. As with most childhood injuries, burns are much more common among boys than girls (Saldana & Peterson, 1997).

Other causes of childhood unintentional injuries include falls, suffocations, poisonings, and bicycle mishaps. Falls contribute significantly to childhood unintentional injuries. Children under age 4 can be severely injured or killed by falling relatively short distances, such as from a bunk bed, a swing, or an open window. Suffocation is the second leading cause of death from unintentional injuries for children under the age of 1 year and is the fourth leading cause of death among children 1 to 4 years old (Saldana & Peterson, 1997). Poisoning deaths have decreased for young children in recent years, largely because of the increased use of child-resistant containers. Nevertheless, thousands of children become ill each year from exposure to dangerous chemicals. For each poisoning death for a child under age six, there are 20,000 calls to poison control centers (Saldana & Peterson, 1997). Finally, unintentional bicycle injuries result in more visits to emergency rooms than any other injuries. Bicycle injuries are related to both age and gender; the number of deaths and injuries increases up to early adolescence, with boys between the ages of 10 and 14 having the highest rates (Saldana & Peterson, 1997). The majority of bicycle fatalities are due to head injuries, and many of these could have been prevented by the proper use of bicycle helmets. (We discuss use of helmets later in the section on prevention of injuries.)

Youth

The passage from childhood to adolescence in the United States carries with it a greatly increased risk of death from unintentional injuries, especially those resulting from automobile crashes. Figure 12.2 shows that death rates from unintentional injuries in 1995 quadrupled as individuals moved from childhood to adolescence and young adulthood. Mortality from motor vehicle crashes increased more than fivefold from ages 5–14 to ages 15–24. The primary reason for this jump, of course, is that young people are beginning to drive and also to ride with other neophyte drivers. Like James, adolescents are also likely to drive after drinking alcohol or to ride with someone who has been drinking. Moreover, nearly half the teenager

deaths from motor vehicle crashes occur during the nighttime hours and more than half take place on weekends (Lescohier & Gallagher, 1996). In addition, teenagers are the age group least likely to use seatbelts (Saldana & Peterson, 1997).

Because they are a leading killer of young people, injuries are responsible for more lost years of life than any other source. For example, each death through heart disease equals 13 lost years, and each cancer-related death accounts for 16 lost years of life, but each death due to unintentional injury subtracts an average of 35 years from life expectancy (USBC, 1998). Just as older people could reduce their risk of heart disease and cancer by changing their behavior, young people could decrease their risk of unintentional injuries and add to their life expectancy by altering their behavior. Most deaths among high school students are the result of behaviors that contribute to either unintentional or intentional injuries.

Among behaviors that lead to unintentional injuries are not using seatbelts, not using bicycle and motorcycle helmets, driving after drinking, and riding with a driver who has been drinking. Laura Kann and her associates (Kann et al., 1998) reported that nearly 20% of students in grades 9 to 12 rarely or never used seatbelts while riding in a car or truck driven by someone else and that male students were less likely than female students to use seatbelts. Of students who had ridden a motorcycle during the past year, 36% rarely or never wore a motorcycle helmet. Kann et al. also found that 88% of those who had ridden a bicycle rarely or never used a helmet. During the month preceding the survey, more than one-third of students had ridden with a driver who had been drinking alcohol.

Some gender and ethnic differences appear in frequency of behaviors contributing to unintentional injuries (Kann et al., 1998), but there were more similarities than differences among the various groups. Table 12.1 shows that high school boys are less likely to use seatbelts than high school girls and more likely to drive after drinking, and James and his friends exemplified these

Table 12.1 Percentage of high school students who participated in behaviors that contribute to unintentional Injuries, by gender and ethnicity—United States, youth risk behavior survey, 1997

Ethnic group	Rarely or never used seatbelts	Rarely or never used motorcycle helmets	Rarely or never used bicycle helmets	Rode with a driver who had been drinking	Drove after drinking alcohol
White	17%	34%	87%	37%	19%
Female	11	30	87	35	14
Male	22	37	87	40	23
Black	31	45	96	34	9
Female	29	51	95	30	5
Male	34	42	96	37	14
Hispanic	20	55	92	43	18
Female	17	53	91	41	11
Male	23	56	92	45	24
Total	19	36	88	37	17
Female	15	32	98	35	12
Male	23	38	88	38	21

Source: "Youth Risk Behavior Surveillance—United States, 1997," by L. Kann, S. A. Kinchen, B. I. Williams, J. G. Ross, R. Lowry, C. V. Hill, J. A. Grunbaum, P. S. Blumson, J. L. Collins, & L. J. Colbe, 1998, *Morbidity and Mortality Weekly Report, 44,* No. SS-3, p. 35.

behaviors. However, boys and girls are quite similar with regard to other dangerous behaviors. Also, African American students engaged in each of these risky behaviors somewhat more frequently than European American youth, especially in their reluctance to wear seatbelts or use motorcycle helmets. Hispanic American students were somewhat less likely than other students to wear motorcycle helmets and more likely to have ridden with a driver who had been drinking. Nevertheless, different ethnic groups are quite similar in risk-taking behaviors (see Table 12.1). For example, a very high percentage of high school students in all three ethnic groups rarely or never wore a bicycle helmet. This survey reveals that young people, regardless of gender or ethnicity, are willing to engage in a variety of risky behaviors.

Automobile crashes are by far the leading cause of fatal and nonfatal injuries among adolescents and young adults. For young people 15 to 24, nearly 77% of fatalities from unintentional injuries are due to motor vehicle crashes (see Figure 12.2). Alcohol has been identified in nearly half the motor vehicle deaths involving teenagers, despite more severe penalties for drunken driving. At the same blood alcohol level, teenager drivers are much more likely than adult drivers to have fatal automobile crashes (Lescohier & Gallagher, 1996). Figure 12.2 shows that the people with the highest rates of death from motor vehicle crashes are 15 to 44 years of age—the age groups that report the highest number of alcohol-impaired driving episodes (Liu et al., 1997). Alcohol's major contribution to motor vehicle injuries and fatalities among young people comes from two sources: greater risk-taking behavior and impaired psychomotor functioning (Honkanen, 1993).

Besides alcohol, another major contributor to motor vehicle injuries is failure to wear seatbelts, and young men have the lowest rate of seatbelt use. Studies in the late 1980s consistently demonstrated that seatbelts save lives. Seatbelt use cuts

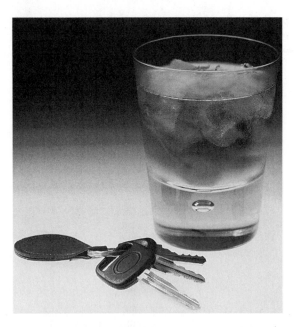

Alcohol is a significant contributor to motor vehicle crashes.

the probability that a person will die in a motor vehicle accident by 30% to 50% (Wagenaar, Maybee, & Sullivan, 1988); seatbelts are effective in preventing fatal injuries irrespective of the occupant's age, size of vehicle, travel speed, type of road, type of crash, time of year, or geographical area (Evans, 1987).

Alcohol is also a strong contributor to unintentional bicycle fatalities and injuries for young people. Indeed, for adolescents and young adults, alcohol is involved in nearly as high a percentage of bicycle-associated fatal injuries as it is in automobile fatalities. One study (Li & Baker, 1994) found that almost one-third of fatally injured bicyclists 15 years old or older tested positive for alcohol, and nearly one-fourth were legally intoxicated. Again, young men were more likely than young women to test positive for blood alcohol. More than half the legally intoxicated bicyclists killed were between 25 and 34 years of age, and even among fatally injured bicyclists 15 to 19 (not yet old enough to purchase alcohol legally), nearly one in seven had a positive BAC.

A case-control study in Finland (Olkkonen & Honkanen, 1990), where bicycling is an important mode of transportation, showed that intoxicated bicyclists had a more than tenfold risk of accidental injury compared with bicyclists who had not been drinking. This study also revealed that bicycle injuries were more likely to result from falling than from collisions. In other words, drunk bicycle riders seem to need neither another vehicle nor a fixed object (other than the road) to injure themselves.

Besides alcohol, failure to use bicycle helmets is an important contributor to unintentional injuries. In the United States, more than 600,000 bicyclists a year are injured badly enough to require medical attention, more than 1,300 die of various injuries while riding a bicycle, and nearly 90% of those who received fatal head injuries could have survived if they had been wearing protective helmets (Sacks, Holingreen, Smith, & Sosin, 1991). Nearly 90% of the fatalities resulted from collisions with motor vehicles; most of the victims were male, and about half were children or adolescents. If only half the bicyclists had complied with helmet use, more than 1,000 lives would have been saved between 1984 and 1988.

Death rates from drowning also increase through late childhood and early adolescence, reaching a peak at age 18. Gender and ethnicity play a role in drowning deaths; young men are 10 times more likely than young women to die from drowning, and African American youth are three times more likely to drown than European American youth (Lescohier & Gallagher, 1996). Alcohol, which is involved in about 40% of drowning deaths, is a dangerous companion to water in at least two ways; it impairs judgment and it reduces dexterity (Schwartz, 1993). James and his friends often went swimming after they had been drinking, and he remembers jumping into water of unknown depth while he was drunk. The next day, he realized how dangerous his behavior was, but drinking and the social situation contributed to his risky behavior.

Gunshot wounds are another source of death and injury for young people. In the United States, most deaths from gunshot wounds are intentional—people aim to shoot others or themselves. Nevertheless, a sizable number of deaths from firearms are unintentional. In the United States, more than 40% of households with children between 3 and 17 have some sort of firearm, and 23% have one or more loaded guns ("Poll," 1998). The availability of firearms in the United States results in nearly 500 deaths per year from unintentional gunshot wounds, and most of these deaths are of young people between ages 10 and 19 (Lescohier & Gallagher, 1996). Regardless of intention, firearms are the second leading cause of deaths in every age category from 10 to young adulthood (Fingerhut, 1993). For youths 15 to 19 years old, more than half the unintentional fatalities from firearms were either hunting related or the result of playing with a gun (Lescohier & Gallagher, 1996). Neither James nor any of his friends experienced a firearms injury, and James believes that his awareness of the dangers and his caution when handling guns contributed to this outcome.

Although falls, bicycle mishaps, drowning, and gunshot wounds are responsible for most nonmotor vehicle fatalities among young people, sports-related injuries account for far more emergency room visits and more hospitalizations than any other category of unintentional injury. Sports injuries are seldom fatal, but each year an estimated 2.6 million people seek emergency room treatment because of a sports injury, and nearly all these people are teenagers or young adults. In any given year, about 6% of 16- and 17-year-olds are treated for a sports-related injury. As with other unintentional injuries, boys and men have more sports-related injuries than girls and women— adolescent boys are about twice as likely as girls to suffer a sports injury, and that ratio moves to about 3 to 1 for older adolescents (Lescohier & Gallagher, 1996).

Adulthood

Whereas the passage from childhood to youth is marked by a vast increase in unintentional fatal injuries, the transition from youth to adulthood brings about little change in a person's risk. As people advance from adolescence and young adulthood to mature adulthood, they have a trifle lower overall risk of unintentional fatalities but a slightly higher risk of motor vehicle fatalities (see Figure 12.2). Between the ages of 25 and 44, motor vehicle crashes account for 90% of all fatal unintentional injuries. However, as adults pass middle age, their risk of motor vehicle fatalities drops sharply, and their risk of death from other unintentional injuries begins a steep ascent. Figure 12.2 shows that adults 45 to 64 years old are much less likely than younger adults to die in a motor vehicle crash but are much more likely to die from another type of unintentional injury (Anderson et al., 1997).

As noted earlier, deaths from motor vehicle crashes have declined during the past 25 years, despite the addition of many more drivers and considerably more miles driven. Besides improved roads and safer cars, the use of seatbelts and airbags has brought down the number of motor vehicle fatalities. In addition, seatbelts can reduce nonfatal injuries to both drivers and front seat passengers. Data on nearly 900 front seat passenger car occupants (Conn, Chorba, Peterson, Rhodes, & Annest, 1993) showed that about half of them were not wearing seatbelts at the time of a crash. Those not wearing seatbelts tended to be younger and to have been drinking at the time of the crash. Looking at all passenger cars, front seat occupants not wearing seatbelts were more than four times as likely as those who were wearing seatbelts to suffer serious injury. For small cars, the difference was much less, but for large cars the chances of a serious injury were 10 times greater for front seat occupants who were not wearing seatbelts. The evidence is clear that using seatbelts lowers one's chance of serious injury in almost all types of motor vehicle crashes. Airbags have also helped reduce motor vehicle deaths (Ferguson & Lund, 1995), and some evidence exists that airbags are somewhat more effective than seatbelts in reducing driver deaths (Zador & Ciccone, 1993). In addition, passenger-side airbags save the lives of many adults in frontal and other crashes (Braver, Ferguson, Greene, & Lund, 1997).

For adults, alcohol is involved in a significant number of motor vehicle as well as nonmotor vehicle injuries. One study (Cherpitel, 1994) examined a large number of casualty patients admitted to emergency rooms in several hospitals. Nearly 10% of the patients were legally intoxicated at the time of admission, and many of these had a blood alcohol content at or above .10. Moreover, many of the patients who were legally drunk at the time of admission had a history of heavy drinking as well as at least one other alcohol-related event that required a prior emergency room visit. For both men and women, however, the risk of injury increases with as little as one drink a day (Cherpitel, 1995).

Older adults have higher mortality rates from unintentional injuries than younger and middle-aged ones (see Figure 12.2). Unintentional injuries are only the seventh leading cause of death among people age 65 and older (Anderson et al., 1997), but, as Figure 12.2 shows, the rate of unintentional fatalities among older people is more than twice as great as it is for any other age range. People age 65 and older have higher rates of motor vehicle deaths than any age group except the ages 15 to 24 and 25 to 44, but these deaths make up only one-fourth of all unintentional deaths among people over 65. Older people die from many of the same unintentional injuries that kill children, especially falls and fires. Children under the age of five have an increased risk of death from residential fires, but older people have an even greater risk. After the age of 65, the death rate from residential fires rises sharply as people age. Older people are at an increased risk from residential fires for two possible reasons—infirmity, which can make escape more difficult, and diminished cognitive functioning, which can lead to cooking devices left unattended or improperly used (CDC, 1998b). In addition to falls and fires, older people often die from complications of medical procedures and misuse of legal drugs and medicines.

In contrast to children and older people who suffer most of their unintentional injuries at home, adults of other age groups are most often injured in the workplace, and both gender and ethnic background influence the frequency of workplace injuries. African Americans and men of all ethnic backgrounds are at a higher risk than European Americans and women, largely because they have more hazardous jobs. An examination of all occupation-related deaths in North Carolina over a 15-year period (Loomis & Richardson, 1998) revealed that African Americans had a 36% greater risk of fatal unintentional job-related injuries than European Americans. In this analysis, African American men had the greatest risk (10.9 per 100,000 person-years) followed by White men (7.87), African American women (0.45), and White women (0.30). If African Americans and European Americans worked at the same jobs, the gap in occupation-related deaths would almost disappear. The gap, however, would not completely vanish, and African American men would still have a slightly higher mortality rate than European American men, a difference that is difficult to explain (Loomis & Richardson, 1998).

An investigation of job-related deaths revealed that 83% were from unintentional traumatic injuries, 14% from homicide, and the remainder were from undetermined causes (Loomis, Richardson, Wolf, Runyan, & Butts, 1997). For female workers, however, work-related homicide equaled all unintentional injuries combined. This study also found that for men, car crashes were the leading cause of death on the job, followed in order by falling objects, machinery, and falls. The most dangerous industries were those that traditionally exposed more men than women to hazardous work, namely, construction, trucking, agriculture, and logging. In addition, older workers and African Americans had higher rates of on-the-job deaths than younger workers or European Americans.

Hazardous industries such as construction, transportation, manufacturing, and agriculture place workers in dangerous conditions, but work conditions are not the only contributor to unintentional injuries on the job; attitudes toward safety also affect injury risk (Cohen & Colligan, 1997). The attitudes of both workers and man-

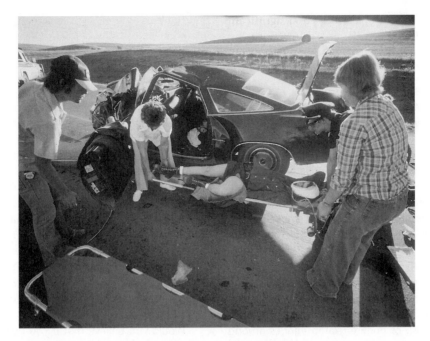

Automobile crashes continue to be the leading cause of both fatal and nonfatal injuries in the United States.

agers are important in creating a workplace atmosphere that can increase or decrease the risk for injuries. When managers place workers under time pressure to perform hazardous tasks, safety precautions become a lower priority, thereby increasing the chances of injury. Workers contribute to unsafe behaviors when they maintain the attitude that safety practices are for "wimps" and impinge on their freedom to do their job. These attitudes create a climate of disdain for safety measures that increases risk.

Workers and managers can create opportunities for injury by failing to understand the extent of danger that exists in the workplace and by adhering to beliefs in worker autonomy (Eakin, 1997). Although a business may involve dangerous chemicals, heavy lifting, or hazardous machinery, both managers and workers tend to underestimate the danger. This underestimation is another version of optimistic bias, the belief that bad things will not happen.

Even when danger is acknowledged, managers often believe that safety is the workers' (and not the manager's) responsibility (Eakin, 1997). This belief leads managers to provide safety equipment or procedures but not to provide training or to ensure enforcement of procedures for its use. When injuries occur, such managers blame their employees. Workers who are aware of hazards may not take appropriate precautions because they believe that the hazards are part of the work or that safety procedures are too much trouble. This attitude is consistent with the view that "accidents happen" and are beyond personal control.

However, this fatalistic attitude is being replaced by a more effective approach to worksite injuries, one that emphasizes the responsibility of managers, unions, and employees (Baker, Israel, & Schurman, 1996; Stout, Jenkins, & Pizatella, 1996). During the decade of the 1980s, worksite deaths declined by 37%, and much of this decline was due to injury prevention programs that focused

WOULD YOU BELIEVE...?

Smoking Creates Risks for Unintentional Injuries

Would you believe that smokers have far more unintentional injuries than nonsmokers—even though many of the injuries have nothing to do with fires? Interestingly, research shows that smokers have significantly more nonfire-related unintentional injuries than nonsmokers. Among the injuries are those related to motor vehicle crashes, occupational injuries, and suicide. Jeffery Sacks and David Nelson (1994) reviewed the literature and found that smokers, compared with nonsmokers, have a 50% increased risk of motor vehicle crashes and are more than twice as likely to be injured on the job. In addition, smokers have a much greater chance of committing suicide than nonsmokers.

Sacks and Nelson discussed several reasons for the increased risk of nonfire-related injuries among smokers. First, some evidence suggests that carbon monoxide or nicotine from cigarettes may be associated with reduced night vision as well as increased errors in driving judgment, either of which could increase the risk for unintentional injury.

Second, the relationship between smoking and nonthermal injuries is complicated by smoking's association with a number of other factors, any one of which may relate to increased unintentional injuries. These confounding factors include increased alcohol and drug consumption, lower educational and socioeconomic status, decreased levels of social support, and reduced use of seatbelts and other safety devices.

A third explanation for smokers' elevated risk of injuries is their increased risk of smoking-related illnesses, such as cardiovascular disease and cancer. Sudden heart ailments can precipitate a motor vehicle crash, and both cardiovascular disease and cancer may contribute to depression and thus to suicide. In addition, Sacks and Nelson cited evidence that medication for these two diseases can increase the risk of unintentional injury.

Fourth, and perhaps most important, is that smokers are more likely to become distracted by the act of lighting a cigarette or by dropped embers. Also, smoke may obscure one's vision by causing eye irritations, eye blinking, and coughing—all of which may increase one's risk of injury. This explanation probably accounts for much of smokers' increased risk of injuries from motor vehicle crashes and some of their elevated risk for occupational injuries. *However, smokers who work on jobs where smoking is prohibited still have more occupational injuries than nonsmokers!* Thus, if you smoke but work at a job that does not permit smoking, you nevertheless have a greater chance of being injured than if you did not smoke.

Would you believe that if you quit smoking you may have an increased risk of unintentional injuries on the day you quit? Beginning with the assumption that nicotine withdrawal leads to a deterioration of mood and cognitive functioning, Andrew Waters, Martin Jarvis, and Stephen Sutton (1998) hypothesized that workers would have a higher risk of unintentional injury on No Smoking Day (NSD) in the United Kingdom. (No Smoking Day is held the second Wednesday of March and is equivalent to the Great American Smokeout held every November in the United States.) Waters et al. then compared the number of nonfatal unintentional injuries reported on NSD with the numbers for the two preceding Wednesdays and the two subsequent Wednesdays. As predicted, they found a significantly greater number of injuries on NSD than on either the two previous or the two following Wednesdays. This finding suggests that nicotine withdrawal is closely related to an increase in nonfatal injuries. Would you believe that smokers and smokers trying to quit both have more than their share of unintentional injuries?

on education, enforcement, and safer workplace environments (Stout et al., 1996). The percent of decline varied by gender, ethnic background, and type of industry. Men had a slightly greater decline in occupational death rates than women, and African Americans, compared with European Americans, experienced a much larger drop in job-related deaths. These differences would be expected because, by the end of the decade, men and African Americans were less likely to be assigned to hazardous working conditions. With regard to industry, the most dangerous ones (mining, construction, transportation, and agriculture/forestry/fishing) at the beginning of the decade generally enjoyed the greatest gains in safety by the end of the decade. This report concluded that:

> We must continue to challenge the common public perception that occupational injuries are random "accidents." Quite the contrary, most fatal occupational injuries are preventable. Employers and employees must take the responsibility of evaluating their workplaces and implementing appropriate measures to prevent injuries and deaths. (Stout et al., 1996, p. 76)

In Summary

Unintentional injuries are the fourth leading cause of death in the United States and the leading cause of death among young people. About half of all fatal unintentional injuries are due to motor vehicle crashes—the leading cause of unintentional injuries for all age ranges. Children under the age of 15 have the lowest death rates from unintentional injuries. Besides motor vehicle crashes, children die from drownings, fires, falls, suffocation, poisoning, and bicycle injuries. For young adults, motor vehicle crashes account for more than four out of five unintentional deaths. The other deaths are largely from falls, bicycle mishaps, drowning, and gunshot wounds. Alcohol is a major contributor to many unintentional injuries among adolescents and young adults. The most common sources of unintentional injuries

to adolescents and young adults are sports, but sports-related injuries have a very low mortality rate. For adults, motor vehicle crashes account for a very high proportion of deaths from unintentional injuries. Older adults have the highest death rate from unintentional injuries, and tend to die from motor vehicle crashes, falls, fires, and complications following medical procedures. In all age groups, African American adults have a higher mortality rate from unintentional injuries than European American adults. Much, but not all, of the difference for adults is a result of African Americans working in more hazardous jobs. Many unintentional injuries on the job are a consequence of both managers and workers underestimating the potential hazards of the workplace.

Strategies for Reducing Unintentional Injuries

During the past 25 years, psychologists have played an increasingly important role in developing and implementing strategies for reducing unintentional injuries. Death rates from unintentional injuries have been going down and much of this decline is due to interventions aimed at (1) changing individual behaviors, (2) changing the environment, or (3) changing the law.

Changing the Individual's Behavior

Changing an individual's behavior is one component of a comprehensive program to reduce unintentional injuries. Most of the emphasis on reducing unintentional injuries through changes in the individual's behavior has centered on home safety, workplace safety, motor vehicle safety, and bicycle safety. In all four areas, however, individually oriented interventions have been, at best, only moderately successful.

Strategies to Prevent Home Injuries Psychologist Lizette Peterson and her colleagues (Peterson,

Gillies, Cook, Schick, & Little, 1994; Peterson, & Schick, 1993; Saldana & Peterson, 1997) have been concerned with reducing injuries to children, especially those that occur in the home. The most effective interventions to reduce children's injuries are directed at parents. Peterson and Brenda Schick (1993) trained both children and their mothers in setting rules of safe behavior. Using a behavior analysis approach suggested by B. F. Skinner (1953), Peterson and Schick examined minor unintentional injuries experienced by second-grade children with respect to the injuries' antecedents, the event itself, and the consequences of the event. Using this analysis as a guide, Peterson and Schick developed categories of rules for injury prevention. Their analysis revealed that most of the injuries could have been avoided if children had followed such basic rules as "Don't walk backwards," "Don't run with anything in your mouth," or "Don't touch, taste, or smell medicines or cleaners." This strategy holds some promise of reducing unintentional injuries to children, provided parents are willing and able to implement such a program.

Injuries from falls in the home are a serious threat to the health of many older persons, but strategies to change individual behavior have not been a very effective means of reducing these unintentional injuries. Strategies have included relaxation therapy, reflective safety tape, assertiveness training, exercise, and safety information (Steinmetz & Hobson, 1994). One study (El-Faizy & Reinsch, 1994) compared an experimental group of older adults who received an educational intervention with a control group that did not receive such information. Both groups received a home safety assessment that included ways of making the home safer. Although the participants in the educational intervention group gained *information* regarding the benefits of the proposed changes, they did no better than people in the control group in implementing safety precautions. Similarly, a study of older members of the Kaiser Permanente health maintenance organization found that a comprehensive program emphasizing home

safety, exercise, and risky behaviors reduced the number of falls by only 7% (Hornbrook et al., 1994). Moreover, this study reported that the participants' chances of avoiding falls serious enough to require medical treatment were not significantly improved by the intervention. Results from these studies suggest that interventions aimed at changing behavior of individuals are not, by themselves, sufficient to reduce unintentional injuries in the home.

Strategies to Prevent Workplace Injuries The preferred strategy for reducing workplace injuries is changing the environment rather than changing individual behavior (Hofmann & Stetzer, 1996). Providing a safer workplace and creating a workplace climate that encourages safety are more certain approaches than attempting to change individual behavior, but workers' behavior is an important and modifiable factor in workplace safety. Protective clothing does not work when it remains on the rack; ventilation systems do not work unless activated; alarms that have been disconnected to eliminate their annoying noise fail to alert workers of dangers.

Training workers and enforcing safety procedures can reduce workplace injuries by changing individual behavior. Workers cannot behave safely without knowledge and skills that allow them to recognize and avoid dangers on the job (Cohen & Colligan, 1997). Therefore, worker education is one strategy to prevent workplace injuries, and this approach shows some success. Unfortunately, even workers who know what is safe do not always behave accordingly. Pressure to complete tasks and a workplace climate that disdains safety can prevent even knowledgeable and well-trained workers from adhering to safety procedures. Training alone is not sufficient. Developing a workplace climate that values safety is a more important step in creating safer workplaces (Eakin, 1997).

Techniques to personalize workplace safety add to the effectiveness of training (Cohen & Colligan, 1997). For example, workers are often reluctant to comply with safety practices related to long-term injury, such as wearing earplugs to prevent hearing loss. A program that showed workers the results of hearing tests on days when they wore earplugs versus days when they did not dramatically increased compliance with the requirement to wear earplugs.

When workers receive feedback about safety performance, their behavior improves (Cohen & Colligan, 1997). Many safety training procedures involve only a single training session. One session can provide information and training that prompts behavior changes, but these changes may disappear as workers revert to older behavior patterns. Feedback can help sustain the changes by providing reminders and monitoring new behaviors. The addition of incentives for desirable performance can be even more effective. That is, when principles of behavior modification are applied to safety behaviors, those behaviors increase in frequency. Therefore, procedures that are capable of changing individual behavior also apply to workplace safety-related behaviors.

Strategies to Prevent Motor Vehicle Injuries

Much of the decline in motor vehicle deaths is due to safer cars and roads, but socially oriented programs and a variety of interventions aimed at changing the behavior of individuals have also contributed to this decline.

One individually oriented strategy for reducing alcohol-related traffic injuries is the designated driver approach, whereby one person is supposed to abstain from alcohol and be responsible for driving and the overall safety of others in the party. Although this concept has been part of the social norm for a number of years, controversy still exists as to its effectiveness in reducing traffic-related injuries. Some research suggests that participation in a designated driver program does not affect enjoyment of the social occasion for either the passengers or the driver (Shore, Gregory, & Tatlock, 1991). However, other research (Glascoff, Knight, & Jenkins, 1994) indicated that many designated drivers do not remain abstinent and that alcohol consumption by passengers increased when they had a designated driver. Some observers (DeJong & Wallack, 1992) have argued that powerful economic interests (bars, restaurants, and the alcohol industry) are behind the designated driver concept and that these programs may encourage some underage adolescents to binge drink. In addition, the designated driver program has deflected attention away from the consequences of drunk driving and from the social, environmental, and economic factors that influence alcohol consumption.

Strategies to Prevent Bicycle-Related Injuries

Fatal and nonfatal bicycle injuries continue as an important health problem in the United States. Would greater use of bicycle helmets reduce the number of deaths and severe head injuries? Evidence suggests that bicycle helmets help save lives and protect against severe head and facial injuries. One study (Thompson, Rivara, & Thompson, 1996) compared bicyclists treated in emergency rooms for head injuries with bicyclists treated for all other injuries and found that, regardless of the bicyclist's age or type of helmet worn, use of a helmet significantly reduced the number of head injuries, brain injuries, and severe brain injuries, especially in collisions with motor vehicles. This same research group (Thompson, Nunn, Thompson & Rivara, 1996) also found that bicycle helmets helped prevent severe facial injuries to the upper and middle face, but not the lower face. Another team of investigators (Sacks et al., 1991) estimated that if all bicyclists would wear helmets, fatal head injuries could be cut by nearly 90% Unfortunately, however, only about 12% of high school students regularly wear helmets while riding bicycles (Kann et al., 1998). This situation suggests that more effective interventions are needed to help prevent bicycle-related injuries.

One intervention to reduce bicycle injuries has been counseling or advising by a physician. This

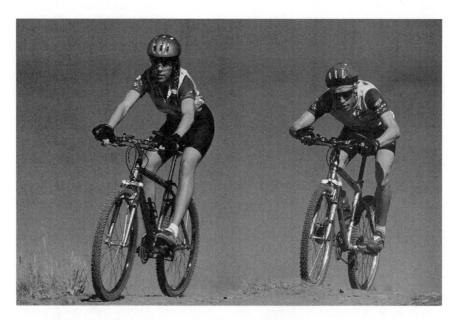

Strategies to increase helmet use are effective in reducing bicycle injuries.

strategy, however, has been only marginally successful, perhaps because physicians are less likely to stress injury prevention than illness prevention (Moser, McCance, & Smith, 1991). Physician counseling with children on the importance of wearing bicycle helmets does not seem to increase use of helmets, even though a very high percentage of pediatricians report that they discuss bicycle helmet use with their patients. A follow-up study (Cushman, James, & Waclawik, 1991) found that children whose families received physician counseling plus take-home pamphlets were no more likely to have purchased helmets than was a control group whose families received neither the counseling nor the pamphlets.

How can physicians get children to wear bicycle helmets? Carol Runyon and Desmond Runyon (1991) offered several suggestions. First, they acknowledged that educational programs do not work. Second, they suggested that an effective campaign must focus on changing children's beliefs regarding the magnitude of the risk for serious head injury and the effectiveness of helmets

in preventing those injuries. Next, they proposed that interventions must also address the "nerd" factor—that is, reduce children's beliefs that bicycle helmets are "nerdy" looking. In addition, they called for increased availability of low-cost helmets that look attractive to children. To be effective, Runyon and Runyon contended, campaigns should be repeated in different contexts, using a variety of media.

Some research findings support these suggestions. For example, one study (Frank, Bouman, Cain, & Watts, 1992) indicated that changes in beliefs regarding the seriousness of injuries can lead to changes in safety-oriented behaviors, and another (Sacks et al., 1991) reported that bicycle helmets, if worn by all cyclists, could save 500 lives and prevent 1,500 head injuries a year. In addition, poor helmet design and being derided by one's peer group (the "nerd factor") can be barriers to bicycle helmet use (Stevenson & Lennie, 1992). This finding supports the theory of reasoned action and the theory of planned behavior (see Chapter 3), both of which suggest that behavior follows intentions, and intentions are, in part, shaped by subjective norms. Thus, if children believe that their peers regard bicycle helmets as fashionable (the social norm), they are more likely to wear them. As for cost, an affordable price contributes more to the purchase of helmets than does physician counseling (Cushman et al., 1991). Another study (Farley, Haddad, & Brown, 1996) used a variety of strategies to increase bicycle helmet use among children 5 to 12 years old. The strategies included educational activities designed to change attitudes and beliefs regarding helmet use, discount coupons to purchase helmets, and reinforcement for wearing helmets. Some of these young cyclists were exposed to the intervention while others were not. Children in cities that received the intervention increased bicycle helmet use from a very low rate of 1.3% to 33% after 4 years. During this same time, children in the control cities also increased their use of helmets but not as much as children in the exposed cities.

Thus, theory and research have combined to provide effective strategies for increasing helmet use. However, the problem of implementing these tactics on an individual basis remains a huge hurdle to the regular use of bicycle helmets. As with other unintentional injury topics, changing the environment or enacting and enforcing legislation may be more efficient means of reducing fatal and nonfatal injuries.

Changing the Environment

A second strategy for reducing unintentional injuries is to make changes in the environment. Such an approach includes building safer cars and roads, manufacturing better bicycle and motorcycle helmets, and making the home and workplace safer. Although some of the changes may require new legislation, others have been and can be made without changing laws. For example, no law mandates that smoke alarms be placed in every residence. Yet state and local health departments, aided by mass advertising and information campaigns, have helped placed smoke alarms in 94%

of U.S. households, and the presence of these alarms has cut residential fire-related deaths in half (CDC, 1998b). Also, people's demand for safer cars was an incentive for automobile manufacturers to build cars with seatbelts and airbags long before legislation mandated passive restraints. Similar environmental changes can be effective means of reducing unintentional injuries.

An example of modifying the environment was reported by one research team (Paul, Sanson-Fisher, Redman, & Carter, 1994) that trained volunteers to go into the homes of people with young children and check for unsafe conditions. More than three of every four homes had multiple safety hazards, but after residents became aware of these hazards, they made significant reductions in the number of dangerous environmental conditions. A more comprehensive approach (Davidson et al., 1994) targeted major hazards in 5- to 16-year-old children's environment. This program, conducted in Harlem and called the Safe Kids/Healthy Neighborhoods Injury Prevention Program, included such environmental interventions as (1) renovating playgrounds; (2) involving children and adolescents in safe, supervised activities, such as dance, art, sports, and carpentry; (3) conducting injury and violence prevention classes; and (4) providing bicycle helmets and other safety equipment. In a comparison of injuries during and after the intervention and injuries from the preceding years, the targeted age group showed a decline of 44%, indicating that a comprehensive program to alter specific environmental conditions can successfully reduce the rate of injury.

However, when people must make a major effort or a substantial financial commitment toward a safer environment, multifaceted community interventions are less successful. A comprehensive injury prevention program in an African American community in Philadelphia (Schwarz, Grisso, Miles, Holmes, & Sutton, 1993) consisted of (1) making simple modifications in the home such as providing smoke detectors, water thermometers, night lights, poison prevention supplies, and emergency telephone numbers; (2) inspecting the home to inform residents of hazards and ways to eliminate or reduce them; and (3) educating residents about specific injury prevention practices. After 12 months, residents in the intervention homes had more knowledge of injury prevention and had more safety supplies available than did residents in the control homes. However, the investigators found no difference between the intervention group and the control group in home hazards that required a major effort to correct. These results agree with those of other studies (Hsu & Williams, 1991), which suggest that lack of money and lack of control over one's environment lead to an inability to comply with many injury-prevention strategies that call for changes in one's environment.

Changing the Law

In general, legal interventions that require safety have been more effective than either educational programs or environmental manipulations (Zador & Ciccone, 1993). Children now live in a safer environment because of laws that require protective action or prohibit the manufacture of hazardous products that can kill or injure children. Children are injured and die from motor vehicle crashes more often than from any other cause, and legislation has been aimed at this problem. In the United States, all 50 states and all territories have laws that mandate protection of children in motor vehicles (National Safe Kids Campaign, 1997). These laws vary in their requirements and enforcement, but the existence of laws increases the use of restraints, which in turn decreases the rate of injury and death to children riding in vehicles. Since 1988, deaths from motor vehicle crashes have decreased among children.

Laws that prohibit the manufacture of hazardous products can also decrease risks to children. During the 1960s and 1970s, many children suffocated inside abandoned refrigerators because there was no way to open the door from the inside. Since passage of the Refrigerator Safety Act, which banned products that could not be opened from the inside, childrens' deaths from asphyxia-

tion have been nearly eliminated (Durlak, 1997). Similarly, the Poison Prevention Packaging Act of 1970, which mandated that dangerous household substances such as aspirin, paint solvent, and prescription drugs be sold in special packaging, has cut the number of children's deaths from poisoning to one fourth the previous rate. Laws banning cribs that could strangle infants and clothes that could easily catch fire have saved the lives of many children (Peterson & Gable, 1997). The decreasing rate of children's deaths from unintentional injuries closely parallels the passage of safety legislation designed to protect children.

Laws mandating the use of bicycle helmets have also been effective in preventing head injuries. The frequency of helmet use among children in grades four, seven, and nine changed in connection with the passage of laws (Dannenberg, Gielen, Beilenson, Wilson, & Joffe, 1993). In this survey, one Maryland county passed a mandatory helmet law and coupled it with an educational safety campaign. A second county received only the educational intervention, and a third county received very little educational information. After the law was passed, helmet use rose from 11% to 37% in the first county, from 8% to 13% in the county that received an extensive educational intervention, and from 7% to 11% in the third county. Differences in helmet use between the second and third counties were not significant, indicating again that educational campaigns are not effective. Although the law was more effective than education alone, the majority of children in the first county still did not routinely wear helmets. Those who did were more likely to have friends who wore helmets, to believe that the law was good, and to use car seatbelts. Interestingly, having a previous injury or having a friend who was injured while riding a bicycle did not contribute to a child's use of a helmet. This study suggests that laws can increase injury-prevention behaviors, but that many people will continue to engage in unsafe behaviors.

Laws have also decreased unintentional injuries in adults. In 1970, the Occupational Safety and Health Administration (OSHA) was founded to prevent injury and illness among U.S. workers (OSHA Facts, 1998). This regulatory administration is part of the U.S. Department of Labor and employs inspectors to ensure compliance with workplace safety regulations, and its staff helps employers develop safety and health programs. OSHA recognizes businesses that have excellent safety programs, and these businesses serve as models for others. The substantial decreases in accidental death and injury for workers after rigorous enforcement goes into effect (Stout et al, 1996) point to the effectiveness of such an approach to increasing safety.

Laws that require seatbelt use have also had a positive impact on the rate of injuries and deaths from automobile crashes (National Highway Traffic Safety Administration [NHTSA], 1998). Many countries adopted laws requiring seatbelt use before the United States did (Robertson, 1983), but 49 of 50 states and all territories now have such laws (NHTSA, 1998). Seatbelt use reduces fatalities between 40% and 50% and diminishes the extent of injury. Laws requiring seatbelt use have increased use to over 60%. Another legal intervention that has increased vehicle safety is the requirement that new vehicles be equipped with driver and passenger airbags, which went into effect for cars with model year 1998 and for trucks for model year 1999. Airbags decrease fatalities by 30% but pose hazards for adults who are not properly seated or are not belted into their seats correctly (Braver, Ferguson, Greene, & Lund, 1997). In addition, airbags are a risk for children riding in the front seat, leading to the recommendation that children younger than 12 should not ride in the front seat of a vehicle. Despite these risks, airbags significantly decrease the risk to drivers and adult passengers during crashes, and the laws and regulations mandating their inclusion have been effective in decreasing risk.

Increasing the legal drinking age led to a decline in alcohol-related motor vehicle injuries (Saldana & Peterson, 1997). However, laws aimed at punishing such unsafe behaviors as driving too fast or driving while intoxicated are not very effective unless the punishment is quite severe. In contrast, legislation that increases the certainty of punishment, that mandates seatbelt use, or that increases liquor and beer taxes has been an effective mode of reducing drunk driving fatalities.

Presently, interventions aimed at the individual, the environment, and the law, combined with severe penalties for noncompliance, offer the most promise in preventing unintentional injuries.

In Summary

Interventions for reducing unintentional injuries can be aimed at changing the individual's behavior, changing the environment, or changing legislation. Change in individual behavior is a goal of strategies to prevent home injuries, workplace injuries, motor vehicle injuries, and bicycle-related injuries. Programs to prevent home injuries frequently target children and older people, but most of these programs have not been very successful. Changing worker behavior is not the preferred strategy for creating safer workplaces, but some interventions have prompted workers to use safety equipment and procedures. Strategies, such as having a designated driver, that attempt to reduce motor vehicle fatalities by emphasizing individual behavior have been only marginally successful. Also, individualized approaches to increasing bicycle helmet use are not very effective, but when the cost of helmets goes down and their social acceptance goes up, adults and children are more likely to buy and use them.

Strategies to alter the environment are generally more successful than those that attempt change through individual interventions. Environmental changes include building safer cars and roads, making the home and neighborhood safer, and providing safer equipment for workers.

Laws, too, can have an impact on reducing unintentional injuries. Laws requiring child protection in motor vehicles, child-proof medicine containers, flame-retardant clothing, refrigerators that open from the inside, and the use of automobile seatbelts and bicycle helmets have saved many lives and prevented thousands of serious injuries.

Intentional Injuries

Unintentional injuries are the leading cause of death for people in the United States below age 35, but intentional injuries are also among the leading causes of death for this age group. Both suicide and homicide are among the top 10 leading causes of death for children and youth, and many young people suffer nonfatal injuries as a result of the violent acts of others. Violence is a more common cause of injury and death in the United States than in other industrialized nations (Acierno, Resnick, & Kilpatrick, 1997), with violent crimes occurring at a rate of about 8 per 1,000 people. The settings for violence and its effects differ over the lifespan.

Childhood

Childhood is a period during which mortality rates are low. Children between ages 5 and 9 years have the lowest death rate for any age group (National Center for Injury Prevention and Control, 1998). Their risks are the highest for unintentional injuries, but children are also in danger from intentional violence, most often at the hands of their parents. Child maltreatment is by no means a recent phenomenon (ten Bensel, Rheinberger, & Radbill, 1997), but the identification of child battering as a social problem did not occur on a national level until the 1960s. Treating infants with skull and long bone fractures led pediatricians and radiologists to recognize that these injuries were caused by beatings. Evidence began to accumulate that such beatings were common and a major source of injury for infants and children.

Injuries at different ages during childhood have varying consequences, but some consequences exist for all children (Kempe, 1997). One common result of intentional injuries is that abused children may be vigilant and feel threatened in a variety of situations. Abused children also tend to be fear-

ful about rejection, abandonment, and additional abuse. Mistrust and poor self-esteem are problems common to abused persons of all ages. Problems in the nurturing relationship lead abused children to be thwarted in their attempts to seek nurturance. These children often display aggressive behavior, have poor ability to express emotions, and have poor cognitive and problem-solving skills—problems that may last a lifetime.

Infancy is a time during which children are particularly vulnerable. Abuse is the leading cause of death for infants after the perinatal period, making the first year of life the most dangerous single year during childhood (Zeanah & Scheeringa, 1997). Figure 12.3 shows the death rate for homicide at all ages; infants die of intentional injury more often than children at other ages. Children injured during infancy are at risk for permanent damage to their nervous systems, which can lead to cognitive and developmental problems (Kempe, 1997). In addition, abuse can prevent the formation of subsequent nurturing relationships. Adults who abuse children were almost always abused themselves, but not all people who were abused during childhood become abusers; many grow up to become good parents by forming other relationships during childhood, relationships that allow them to feel valued and safe in some ways. However, children who do not form such relationships are at high risk to become abusers themselves.

Abuse can prevent children from accomplishing some of the developmental tasks of young childhood (Kempe, 1997), including forming attachments to others (usually parents), seeing themselves as separate individuals, and developing physical, cognitive and language skills. Abuse during early childhood can impede the development of these tasks and impair children's ability to get along with their age-mates and to do well in school.

School-aged children and adolescents who are abused may exhibit symptoms of psychopathology or behavior disorders (Kempe, 1997). Physical abuse may continue during middle childhood, but it is not as likely to be initiated at this age as is sexual abuse. Girls between ages 10 and 13 are partic-

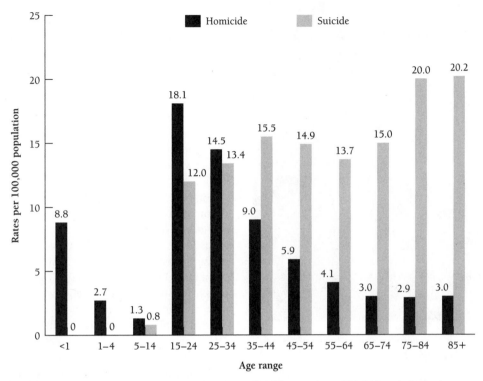

Figure 12.3 **Homicide and suicide rates over the lifespan (per 100,000 population).**
Source: Data from *Health United States, 1998.* Tables 47 (pp. 250–252) and 48 (pp. 253–255), by Department of Health and Human Services, 1998, (DHHS publication No. PHS 98-1232), Washington, DC: U.S. Government Printing Office.

ularly vulnerable to sexual abuse (Bagley & King, 1990), but boys are also victims. Biological parents are not nearly as likely to be perpetrators of sexual abuse as they are of physical abuse, but stepfathers and boyfriends are more frequent perpetrators, along with other male family members and adults in positions of trust.

Children are also exposed to violence in their communities, and children in poor urban neighborhoods are particularly vulnerable (Jenkins & Bell, 1997). The dramatic increase in youth violence that began during the late 1980s affected children, who were often witnesses to violence in their communities and schools. Surveys of inner-city children reveal that between one-fourth and one-half have witnessed shootings, muggings, or stabbings, and as many as 30% reported that they

have been mugged or threatened with a weapon. Older children and adolescents are even more likely to be witnesses and victims of such violence. In many cases, those who witness violence are acquainted with both the victims and the assailants, making the experience more traumatic. Children exposed to violence can develop posttraumatic stress disorder (PTSD) and other stress-related and anxiety problems.

Youth

Violence is a more pervasive problem for adolescents and young adults than for children, and adolescents between ages 16 and 19 have the highest rates of criminal victimization of any age group (Jenkins & Bell, 1997). Unlike children, adolescents

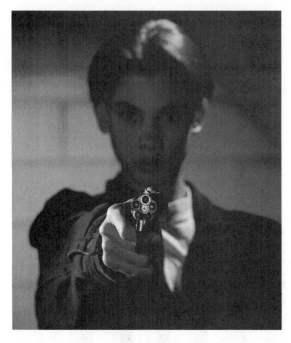

Access to guns is a significant factor in the deadliness of violence among youth.

are frequent perpetrators of violence. In addition to homicide, suicide is ranked among the leading causes of death, beginning with 10-year-olds. Figure 12.3 shows the dramatic increase in both homicide and suicide beginning at age 15.

Neither homicide nor suicide rates reveal the full picture of violence: Between 100 and 400 assaults occur for each homicide (Garbarino & Kostelny, 1997), and 8 to 10 suicide attempts exist for each suicide death (Ruzicka, 1995). In a survey of high school students (Kann et al., 1998), almost 46% of boys and 26% of girls had been in a physical fight during the previous 12 months; 4% of all students had to seek medical help for injuries sustained in a fight. This same survey found that 27% of girls and 15% of boys had seriously considered attempting suicide, and nearly 8% of all students had made at least one attempt at suicide. The types and settings for youth violence are varied, and some young people are at much higher risk than others.

Being young and living in the United States are two conditions that place many people at risk for violence. Compared with other age groups and other countries, young people who live in the United States have an increased risk of intentional injury or death (Garbarino & Kostelny, 1997). In addition, economic factors, ethnic background, and gender all influence risks for being involved in violence either as a perpetrator or as a victim. Poor mental health, drug use, and problems at school are associated with violent behavior (Ellickson, Saner, & McGuigan, 1997). Poverty is a risk factor, and living in a poor neighborhood is often synonymous with living in a high-crime neighborhood (Greenberg & Schneider, 1994). Poverty tends to be associated with ethnic minority status in the United States, putting ethnic minority youth at increased risk (but also elevating the risk for all people living in these neighborhoods). Young men are more likely to be both perpetrators and victims of physical violence than young women. Those factors combine to put young African American men at particularly high risk for homicide.

Young African American men are much more likely to die from homicide than any other segment of U.S. society, including young European American men and African Americans in other age groups. For example, the death rate from homicide by firearms is nearly 10 times higher among male African Americans ages 15 to 44 than it is for male European Americans of the same age (USBC, 1998). For all age groups, African Americans are nearly eight times more likely to be victims of murder than European Americans. Figure 12.4 contrasts the homicide rates by ethnicity and gender of victims from 1980 to 1996. Note the sharp decrease in homicide for both genders and both ethnic groups in recent years after a peak in the early 1990s. Despite widespread publicity about growing violence, homicide rates are actually decreasing, but the rates for young African American men continue to be much higher than for other groups.

Gender is also a factor in assaults, with young women at higher risk for sexual assault and young men at increased risk for other assaults (Acierno et

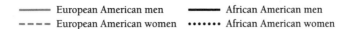

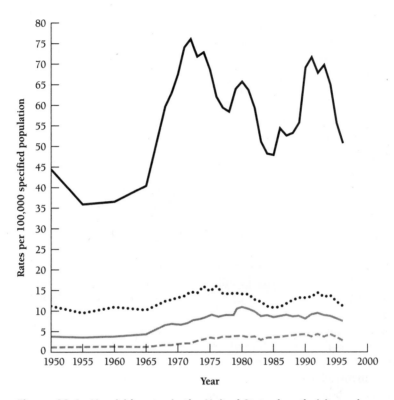

Figure 12.4   Homicide rates in the United States by ethnicity and gender of victim, 1980 to 1996.   *Source:* Data from *Statistical Abstracts of the United States 1995* (115th ed., p. 204), by U.S. Bureau of the Census, 1995, Washington, DC: U.S. Government Printing Office; and from *Health, United States, 1998*, (pp. 250–252), by U.S. Department of Health and Human Services, 1998, Washington, DC: U.S. Government Printing Office.

al., 1997). Between half and two-thirds of all sexual assaults occur before the victims reach age 18, making late childhood and adolescence a vulnerable time. Unfortunately, those who have been victimized are at increased risk for future incidents. Ethnicity is also a factor, with non-Hispanic European American women at higher risk than Hispanic American or African American women. The official reports of rape do not capture the magnitude of the problem, because a large majority of victims of sexual assault do not report the incident to police and are thus not counted in the official crime statistics. When they are forced to have sex, men are even less likely than women to report to authorities. Perhaps as few as 16% of sexual assaults are reported to police, but about half of all rape victims experience either minor or serious physical injury as a result of the sexual assault. In addition to physical injury, assault and rape increase the risk for mental health problems that are related to suicide (Cohen, Spirito, & Brown, 1996).

Access to weapons contributes to the increased deadliness of violence among adolescents. In 1997, about 18% of high school students reported that they had carried a gun, knife, or club during the 30 days preceding the survey (Kann et al., 1998), but this represents a drop from 1993 when one-fourth of high school students reported carrying a weapon to school (Kann et al., 1995). In high-violence neighborhoods, the percentages are higher. Nearly half of inner-city 7th- and 8th-grade boys in one survey (Webster, Gainer, & Champion, 1993) carried knives and one-fourth carried guns. Among 7th- and 8th-grade girls, 37% carried a knife. Although adolescents report that they believe their schools are dangerous and they are in need of self-protection, these junior high school students carried guns more for aggressive purposes than for defensive reasons.

Easy access to firearms is a factor in homicide and suicide among young people: Firearms are used in a majority of homicides and suicides among youth (O'Donnell, 1995). Federal laws prohibit gun sales to adolescents, but they have access to firearms through family and friends as well as through theft. Young people with behavior problems are more likely than other adolescents to carry a gun, and over three-fourths of young people with guns are involved in gangs, drugs, or other illegal activities. About 30% of adolescents with guns have used them to shoot at someone.

Weapon-related violence received a great deal of publicity due to six shootings in U.S. public schools during 1997 and 1998 (Witkin, Tharp, Schrof, Toch, & Scattarella, 1998). The children who committed these shootings gained access to a variety of guns, which are more plentiful than in years past. With easy access to guns, adolescents who are troubled and angry can fantasize about revenge, and the publicity over each shooting makes this action attractive to others, promoting additional shootings. The school shootings brought publicity, but school violence has been a topic of concern to educators for years. Bringing weapons to school has been one focus of this concern, but fights without weapons have been the most common type of school violence during recent school years (National Education Association, 1998). The

publicity generated by the shootings has given a boost to strategies to reduce school violence.

The increased access to weapons has not only led to an increase in homicide and assault-related injuries among teenagers, but it has also contributed to suicide attempts among young people (Resnick et al., 1997). The risk factors for suicide attempts among youth are similar to risk factors for other age groups—easy access to weapons, alcohol and drugs, feelings of isolation, lack of social support, and low self-esteem. Also, junior high and high school students who lack a sense of being connected to family or school are at significantly increased risk for suicide attempts. In young people, estrangement from family and trouble in romantic relationships can lead to the feelings of isolation that are related to suicide attempts (Lester, 1994). Being gay or bisexual also increases the suicide risk for young men (Remafedi, French, Story, Resnick, & Blum, 1998). Because youth suicide produces so many years of lost life, many prevention strategies are aimed at this age group.

Adulthood

Intentional violence is also a cause of injury and death for adults, but the context of this violence shows some differences from that of violence in youth. As Figure 12.3 shows, suicide becomes a more common cause of death than homicide beginning at age 25; the number of suicides increases and homicides decreases. Violence in the streets and workplace has an impact on adults, but homes are more dangerous (Carden, 1994). Domestic violence is a major cause of injury and death, and partner violence and elder abuse are the two varieties of domestic abuse that affect adults. In addition, intentional injuries occur in the workplace as well as on the streets and in homes. Therefore, adulthood is a period during which intentional violence continues to be a source of death and injury.

The same social and economic factors that influenced violence in youth continue to have an impact on adults. Income level, ethnicity, and gender relate to risk of victimization. These factors converge in inner-city neighborhoods, putting poor African American men at increased risk for street violence. Men are more likely than women to be murder victims for all income levels and all ethnicities (Bureau of Justice Statistics, 1998b), but adults over age 25 are less than half as likely to be murdered as youth between ages 18 and 25 (Bureau of Justice Statistics, 1998a). Street violence becomes less of a risk for adults, but violence at home remains a major problem.

The scope of domestic violence in the United States remains unclear because no national survey of the problem exists (Chalk & King, 1998). Estimates are based on reported cases, and many incidents go unreported. A survey of women (in Acierno et al., 1997) revealed that only 46% of women who had been severely physically assaulted reported the incident to police. Therefore, official reports of cases of intentional injury underestimate the problem.

Early publicity on domestic violence focused on husbands who physically abused their wives, but research soon appeared indicating that women also initiated partner violence. In a representative sample of young adults in New Zealand (Magdol et al., 1997), women were more likely to be perpetrators of violent acts than men, although serious violence was unusual for either. For severe domestic violence, men were more common perpetrators than women. This finding is consistent with other research (Hale-Carlsson et al., 1996; Kurz, 1997) showing that women are more likely to be injured as a result of partner abuse.

Michael Johnson (1995) argued that domestic violence can be divided into two types. He called one type common couple violence, which fits into the pattern of conflicts in which an argument escalates into a fight. The physical violence can be minor, but when it becomes serious, women are more likely than men to be injured. Johnson termed the other type of domestic violence *patriarchal terrorism,* which describes a situation in which a man dominates his family by using phys-

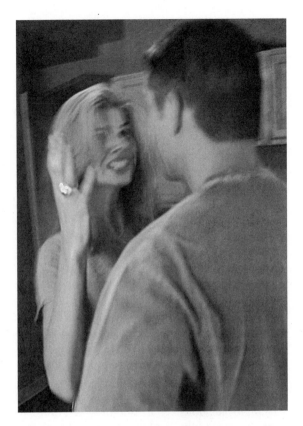

Domestic disagreements can escalate into domestic abuse.

ical force as well as other control strategies. This description is consistent with that of the severely violent men in the study of young adults in New Zealand (Magdol et al., 1997) and is also consistent with findings that many men who beat their wives are also likely to abuse their children (Kurz, 1997). This pattern of domestic violence is an extension of male dominance in families and results in injury and death to both women and children. In summary, women are more likely than men to be homicide victims as a result of domestic violence and more likely to be injured or killed by an intimate partner than by a stranger.

Availability of weapons is also a factor in domestic violence and suicide (Bailey et al., 1997). Having a loaded gun in the house is a way to turn an argument into a homicide. Because shooting is one of the most effective methods of killing oneself, having a gun also increases the odds that a suicide attempt will be completed. Thus, having a gun in the house increases the risk of both homicide and suicide. Other factors that relate to suicide are a history of mental illness and living alone (Bailey et al., 1997).

Domestic violence can spill out into the workplace. A number of homicides have occurred when angry spouses entered a workplace and attacked or killed their partners as well as others who happened to be present (Solomon, 1998). Other workplace violence incidents involve angry employees or former employees who threaten, harm, or kill supervisors or coworkers. These two types of violence may be related, and perpetrators of domestic violence are at increased risk for workplace violence as well (Brownell, 1996). Workplace violence does not come "out of nowhere," and both corporate policy and workers' behavior can be predictors of violent outbursts. For example, insensitive discipline and terminations and a failure to set limits on harassment and intimidation can lead to employee violence. In addition, a failure to take the possibility of violence seriously can endanger managers and human resources personnel (Caudron, 1998).

The gender difference in risk for violence applies to suicide: Men are more likely to commit suicide than women, especially at younger ages. Suicide rates vary a great deal among countries (Ruzicka, 1995). For example, Hungary has the highest rate and Greece the lowest. In most developed countries, suicide rates increased during the past 15 years. The United States has a suicide rate in the lower half of the distribution of countries, similar to the rates in Canada and Japan. In the United States, variation occurs among ethnic groups, and Native Americans have the highest suicide rates, followed by European Americans (USD-HHS, 1998a). African Americans, Hispanic Americans, and Asian Americans commit suicide only about half as often.

Alcohol is connected to suicide and suicide attempts in people of nearly every age. One study (Eckardt et al., 1981) found that alcohol was involved in as many as 30% of all suicide attempts. This finding does not mean that alcohol caused many attempts; some people may decide to kill themselves while sober and then use alcohol as an anesthetic. However, an inability to control alcohol consumption is related to one's chances of attempting suicide. For example, 40% of alcoholic women have attempted suicide (Gomberg, 1989), whereas fewer than 9% of nonalcoholic women have attempted to take their own lives. Moreover, problem drinkers are from 2 to 15 times more likely to succeed at committing suicide than light drinkers or nondrinkers. (Eckardt et al., 1981). This association does not mean that use of alcohol is responsible for suicides; the relationship could be due to general feelings of despair and hopelessness that lead some people to both abuse alcohol and to attempt suicide.

Suicide also varies with age. Youth suicide has gained a great deal of publicity, but adults are even more likely to commit suicide. Suicides among older adults account for a lower percentage of their deaths but only because older people have higher rates of death from other causes. Figure 12.3 shows that suicide rates are higher for middle-aged adults than for youth and even higher among older people. Indeed, individuals over age 85 have the highest suicide rate of any age category.

Older people are also at risk for violence from others, which can come from family caregivers in the home or from professional caregivers in institutions. Elder abuse includes physical, psychological, sexual, or financial abuse or neglect of older people (Chalk & King, 1998). This type of domestic violence is less common than child abuse or partner violence but still constitutes a substantial problem.

Being in need of care puts older people at risk for emotional, physical, and possibly financial dependence on others, who may be abusive or neglectful. Risk factors for elder abuse include functional impairment and cognitive disability as well as age and poverty (Lachs, Williams, O'Brien, Hurst, & Horwitz, 1997). Caring for elders who are poor or who are functionally or cognitively impaired places burdens on caregivers that may be overwhelming. Thus, factors that make caregiving more stressful increase the risk for abuse. In addition, lack of awareness of the specific needs of older people can contribute to neglect.

Elder abuse is a significant risk for older people. Indeed, one study (Lachs et al., 1997) showed that abuse posed as high a mortality risk as hypertension or other diseases. Abused older persons were at twice the risk as those who were not abused. Like other types of domestic violence, elder abuse can be difficult to diagnose because the abused person depends on the abuser and may be reluctant to complain to authorities. In addition, physicians may not be alert to the possibility of abuse or reluctant to intervene.

In Summary

Intentional violence is a problem that affects people throughout the lifespan. For children, homicide is one of the leading causes of death, and violence is a major source of injury. This violence can come from abuse by parents and from exposure to community violence. Abuse not only causes injury, but can also prevent children from accomplishing developmental tasks such as forming close relationships and learning problem-solving skills. In addition to physical abuse, children are at risk for sexual abuse, with girls at higher risk than boys.

Youth violence extends to perpetration as well as victimization. Several types of violence affect youth, including community violence, school violence, sexual assault, homicide, and suicide. Young men are at higher risk than young women for all types of violence except sexual assault. In addition to gender, several risk factors combine to put young African American men living in inner-city neighborhoods at a sharply increased risk for assault and homicide in both their communities and their schools. Availability of firearms is one factor that relates to the deadliness of violence. Several well-publicized school shootings highlighted the easy availability of guns for youth, but school violence was a problem years before these incidents brought the problem to public attention. Access to firearms also relates to suicide risk for youth.

Adults are also in jeopardy from violence. Two types of domestic violence—partner abuse and elder abuse—affect adults. In addition, adults experience violence in their communities and workplaces. People in intimate relationships behave violently toward each other, but women are the targets of the most severe attacks and suffer more injuries than men from partner abuse, and the availability of firearms can turn partner abuse into homicide. Community violence rates are lower for adults than for adolescents, but suicide rates increase with increasing age. Elder abuse can occur in the form of physical, emotional, or financial abuse or neglect of the elderly. Thus, all age groups are at risk for various types of intentional violence.

Strategies to Reduce Intentional Injuries

Strategies for reducing intentional injuries include interventions aimed at changing individual behavior, the environment, and the law. The interventions tend to be aimed at specific problems, and some strategies for reducing intentional injuries combine changes in individual behavior, the environment, and the law. Indeed, changes in all three will be necessary to make substantial progress in reducing intentional injuries. Joyce Osofsky (1997) contended that individual efforts to reduce various types of violence must be supplemented by a national campaign in the media to "change the image of violence from one that is acceptable, even admired, to something disdained and considered unacceptable" (p. 326). Such a strategy would go beyond any of the three approaches to changing public opinion. In the United States—the most violent of the developed countries—this suggestion seems warranted.

Domestic Violence

Three types of domestic violence—child abuse, partner violence, and elder abuse—have been targets of three types of interventions. Child abuse prevention differs from partner violence interventions and both differ from programs aimed at elder abuse. One overarching problem with all domestic abuse programs is the lack of evaluation for their effectiveness. According to the report (Chalk & King, 1998) of a special committee assembled to evaluate domestic violence interventions, services are fragmented by jurisdiction and specialty, and evaluations for effectiveness are not routine. Therefore, many programs with intuitive appeal may not have supporting evidence for their effectiveness.

Child Abuse Programs   Interventions for child abuse are aimed at both parents and children. The programs for parents include legal interventions to restrain violence or to remove the child from an abusive environment, as well as programs to help parents do a better job. Other programs are intended to minimize the harm that violence has done to children who have been abused. In addition, legal strategies focus on compulsory reporting of suspected child abuse.

Some programs have targeted high-risk parents, attempting to prevent initial incidents of abuse (Chalk & King, 1998; Murray, Guerra, & Williams, 1997). Factors that contribute to risk include poverty, young age, and a history of abuse, either as a victim or as a perpetrator. Programs may consist of parent support in the form of education or support groups, home visits, and mental health counseling. All of these approaches take the form of changing the individual behavior of abusive or potentially abusive parents. Follow-up

evaluation has demonstrated that these interventions are beneficial for the mother-child relationship and for these children's early development.

Preserving the family by changing dysfunctional family interactions has been the goal of many social service interventions. This goal may not be realistic unless interventions are long term (Chalk & King, 1998). Children may be safer in another setting than in a preserved yet still abusive family. However, placing an abused child in foster care or a group home may not be sufficient, because the experience of violence has already produced damage. Children placed in alternative living environments need services to help them recover from the violence that prompted their placement.

One type of abuse prevention aimed at changing children's behavior is sexual abuse prevention. The goal of these programs, which are often school based, is to change the individual behavior of children so that they escape sexual abuse (Chalk & King, 1998). They provide information to children on how to behave in potentially abusive situations. Children are taught to flee from people or situations in which a person tries to touch them sexually and to tell about such attempts. Evaluations for these programs are largely lacking, but some evidence indicates that children retain the knowledge they gain, including the notion that they should flee from an abuse situation.

Changes in the law have made reporting of child abuse mandatory for health care and education professionals. The rationale is that, by requiring physicians, psychologists, nurses, counselors, and teachers to report suspicious cases, children can be protected from escalating violence. No evidence yet exists for the effectiveness of mandatory reporting (Chalk & King, 1998), and these laws may have unexpected and negative consequences for children.

In summary, the interventions aimed at changing parents' behavior and teaching children to avoid and report sexual abuse have some effect, but the demonstrated effects are small on what is a large problem. Changing the environment is not

BECOMING SAFER

1. If you have young children in your home, you can make their lives safer by adopting a few basic rules and following these rules consistently.

2. Always properly buckle your seatbelt when riding in a motor vehicle.

3. Never ride a bicycle, motorcycle, or skateboard without a helmet.

4. Don't drive after drinking even a small amount.

5. Never ride with a driver who has been drinking.

6. Don't keep a loaded firearm in your residence or clean a firearm unless you are certain that it is not loaded.

7. Don't ride a bicycle, play sports, or work with machinery after you have been drinking.

8. Follow safety rules at work even if your co-workers ignore them.

9. Do not endorse violence as a way to deal with problems with children, in relationships, or in school.

10. If you are a victim of violence, get out of the situation and seek help so that you can recover psychologically as well as physically.

11. If you feel tempted to injure someone in your care, join a support group to learn strategies for coping with this stressful situation.

12. Learn to recognize suicidal cognitions in yourself and others and seek help.

---

a strategy used to prevent child abuse, and changing the law has not proven to be effective in decreasing risks of violence to children.

Partner Abuse Interventions Strategies for reducing partner abuse focus on caring for victims and preventing additional incidents. These strategies fall into two groups: social services and legal interventions. The majority of social services programs are shelters to which abused women can escape (Chalk & King, 1998). These shelters offer a range of services such as counseling, job training, legal advice, and housing assistance. Evaluation of the effectiveness of shelters is almost impossible because each shelter serves different clients and offers somewhat different programs. Some research (Chalk & King, 1998) indicates that women who go to shelters are less likely to be victims of violence than those who do not, and the presence of shelters can help to realize that escape is possible.

Legal interventions are also used to decrease partner violence. Legal strategies include protective orders to keep batterers away from their partners, mandatory arrest and prosecution, and legal reporting requirements. Protective orders can be good short-term solutions to partner abuse, but studies that evaluate their effectiveness are lacking (Chalk & King, 1998), and protective orders are typically part of a legal response that involves arrest and prosecution.

Incidents of partner violence prompt mandatory arrest in some states and many jurisdictions; this strategy is the most common legal intervention (Mills, 1998). Mandatory arrest and prosecution laws or policies appeared as a result of pressure on police departments that had responded to domestic violence with too little concern and had held the view that these incidents were not important instances of violent crime. Some evidence suggests that mandatory arrest deters further violence, but the policy can also create unwanted effects and possibly even increase violence in some cases (Mills, 1998). Mandatory prosecution has not been studied as extensively, but one study (Davis, Smith, & Nickles, 1998) found that mandatory prosecution was no more effective than mandatory arrest in deterring additional domestic violence.

Legal reporting requirements are not very effective in reducing partner violence, because those responsible for reporting are reluctant do so. Less than 15% of physicians questioned female assault victims about partner abuse, and few women who sought emergency room services for physical assault were referred for additional services (Acierno et al., 1997). In addition, physicians did not want to question women about domestic abuse because such inquiries would be personal and distressing and would make physicians responsible for taking additional action. This attitude is a barrier to identifying and decreasing partner abuse.

Another barrier is the acceptance of violence that Osofsky (1997) mentioned. Nearly 3 million married couples do some type of violence to each other each year (Sorenson, Upchurch, & Shen, 1996). Furthermore, many people find such behavior acceptable, at least under some circumstances. A survey of American couples (Straus, Gelles, & Steinmetz, 1980) found that 25% of wives and over 30% of husbands considered violence an acceptable way to resolve some disputes. This attitude is a major barrier to reducing partner violence.

Reducing Elder Abuse   Programs for reducing elder abuse are less common and less frequently evaluated than other types of domestic abuse programs (Chalk & King, 1998). In many ways, efforts to reduce abuse of older people parallel approaches to curbing child abuse; both concentrate on protecting individuals who cannot protect themselves, and both use social and legal interventions.

All states in the United States have some protective services oriented toward older people (Chalk & King, 1998). Such services investigate cases of suspected abuse or neglect combined with case management that include medical, educational, and legal services. These services may have either the older people or their caregivers as the targets. Caregivers for Alzheimer's disease are one such targeted group, and support groups and respite care can help caregivers cope with the stress of providing care for older patients with dementia.

Services to older people include assistance with the things that would allow them to live independently and care for themselves. None of these programs have evaluations that would allow an assessment of effectiveness.

Legal interventions include mandatory or voluntary reporting laws in most states in the United States, protective orders, arrest and prosecution, legal counseling, and appointment of guardians (Chalk & King, 1998). These procedures may be comparable in effectiveness to the child abuse statues upon which they are based, but no evaluations exist for these relatively new changes in the law.

Creating Safer Workplaces

Although unintentional injuries are common in the workplace, two types of intentional workplace violence pose hazards. One type is an extension of partner abuse and occurs when domestic disputes are carried into the workplace. Cases in which a person enters a workplace and injures or kills his or her partner make headlines, but these dramatic cases represent only a small part of the workplace violence that spills over from the home. This abuse diminishes productivity, creates workplace tension, and adds to health care costs.

The realization that domestic violence has workplace implications led Polaroid Corporation to start a women's group for battered employees (Solomon, 1998). The group helped women get out of their abusive situations and put the company in a position to respond to the other type of workplace violence: threats to workers by employees or former employees. The Polaroid Corporation's attention to domestic violence is unusual for a large business, but responding to potential violence in employees has become a task of modern corporations. An increasing number of companies have developed policies and procedures to deal with violent situations.

Current recommendations (Barrett, Riggar, & Flowers, 1997) include a variety of strategies to prevent workplace violence. Identifying employees who may be violent is difficult, but preemployment screenings can identify those with a history of harassing or violent behavior. Businesses should complete a risk assessment that includes an examination of the physical work environment as well as of the workplace climate for situations that promote risk (Barrett et al., 1997). The physical environment can provide opportunities for intruders to hide or can allow easy access to employees, both of which can increase risk of violent attacks. Managers and supervisors who allow hostile interactions of others or initiate such interactions create a hostile working environment, which increases risks of violence from frustrated, angry employees in their organization. Supervisors who are authoritarian and insensitive in handling discipline or layoffs increase the possibility for violence among former employees.

Companies should formulate a plan for dealing with dangerous employees, develop a reasonable grievance procedure to defuse employee anger; safeguard against dismissed employees; and protect potential targets such as supervisors, managers, and human resources personnel. Sending clear messages to employees that threats of violence are unacceptable is another precaution. This last recommendation is consistent with discouraging violence in all aspects of society.

Violence prevention represents one type of workplace wellness program, and many companies have started multimodal programs to create a healthier workforce. Improved health has become a goal for companies that wish to reduce employee turnover, increase productivity, and contain company health care costs (Kizer, 1987). Preventing unintentional injuries is a common component of workplace wellness programs, but workplace wellness, safety, and violence prevention programs are rarely coordinated (Baker et al., 1996). These programs have some target behavior interventions that are common to disease as well as injury prevention, including interventions aimed at smoking, alcohol and substance abuse, and stress management. Comprehensive, coordinated programs could be cost efficient as well as effective in promoting worker health and safety.

Legal regulations have also taken aim at workplace violence. The Occupational Safety and Health Administration (1996) issued guidelines for prevention of violence in the workplace for workers in health care and social service settings. These regulations encourage employers to develop violence-prevention plans for their employees. Included in the regulations are components requiring worksite analysis, safety and health training, management commitment to safer workplaces, and control of hazards. In summary, attempts to prevent workplace violence focus on changing individual behavior, altering the environment, and enacting laws to control workplace violence.

Reducing Community and School Violence

Violence in the community and the school affect young people in two ways—as victims and as perpetrators. Changing the behavior of a large segment of the population seems an overwhelming task, but violence of all types decreased in the late 1990s (USBC, 1997). These decreases are probably not due to any program efforts, because no large-scale coordinated efforts have targeted community violence. Some programs have undertaken the strategies of changing individual behavior, the environment, and the law.

Programs that attempt to change individual behavior can have some indirect violence-reducing effects; these include strategies that target risk factors for violence rather than aggressive behavior itself (Stiffman, Earls, Dore, Cunningham, & Farber, 1996). For example, programs for parents at high risk for child abuse can decrease youth violence by keeping children from modeling the violence they experience (Murray et al., 1997). Programs aimed at alcohol and drug use can also decrease violence because use of these substances often increases aggression. Programs aimed specifically at youth include conflict resolution programs, mentoring, and psychological and peer counseling (Stiffman et al., 1996).

Conflict resolution programs often appear as part of the school curriculum and teach problem-solving skills as well as violence prevention. One such program is Responding in Peaceful and Positive Ways (RIPP) based on social learning theory and administered in the school system (Meyer & Northup, 1997). This intervention consists of 25 sessions that teach problem solving and alternative ways to resolve or avoid conflicts. An evaluation of this program indicated positive effects in self-esteem, fewer injuries due to violence, and a lower school suspension rate. The changes in individual behavior seem to produce positive effects for decreasing violence.

Providing mentors who furnish positive role models may also be effective in combating violence (Murray et al., 1997). Programs such as Big Brothers/Big Sisters provide children with adult mentors who form nurturing relationships with the children. This type of mentoring program can help decrease the use of violence to solve interpersonal problems, but programs that help young people prepare for, obtain, and keep jobs are more successful.

Job training and access to jobs can be part of a successful strategy for reducing violence by changing the environment (Stiffman et al., 1996). In some communities, the most attractive employment options involve illegal activities, and offering meaningful alternatives can be a powerful deterrent to crime. Other community changes include recreational programs, such as midnight basketball, and street monitoring, such as Neighborhood Watch.

Altering the environment can also help to decrease school violence (National Education Association, 1998). In addition to attempting to change children's behavior, alterations in building arrangement can eliminate opportunities for fights. Wooded areas on or near campuses can give intruders the opportunity to approach unobserved, and secluded wings or classrooms give students chances to begin fights without being interrupted. Some schools have hired consultants to perform safety "audits" in which dangerous features of the school environment are located and changed.

Changing the law is another strategy designed to reduce youth violence in schools and communities. Legal approaches include removing violent youth from communities, restricting access to weapons, and arrest and incarceration. Residential treatment programs for violent youth are not a new approach, but the latest version is the "boot camp" in which young offenders are placed in military-type programs. The history of the residential treatment approach has not shown a great deal of effectiveness, despite its widespread use (Stiffman et al., 1996). Youth who participate in such programs commit additional crimes at a high rate. Thus, incarceration has not demonstrated its effectiveness in deterring youth crime.

Restricting weapons is an important component of reducing community and school violence; this approach has shown more promise of decreasing violence than residential programs or incarceration (Stiffman et al., 1996). A growing belief that access to firearms posed a serious threat to school safety led the U.S. government to pass a public law in 1994 mandating a "zero tolerance" policy toward weapons in schools (Pipho, 1998). The goal of this legislation was to decrease the number of guns in schools, and the law included several mandated penalties for bringing guns or explosives into school. Although case-by-case exceptions are allowed under the law, expulsion for one year is the required penalty for most weapons violations. The recency of the legislation means that no assessment of its effectiveness has been done, but other strategies to restrict firearms access have been effective in decreasing injuries and deaths (Stiffman et al., 1996).

Cutting Suicide Rates

Suicides occur in all age groups from preadolescence to old age, but the people most often targeted for intervention are adolescents, young adults, and elderly people. Different factors relate to suicide at different ages, and effective suicide prevention strategies take into account these differences.

Many high schools have suicide-prevention programs, including mental health teams for counseling at-risk students, written formal suicide policies, and programs for training teachers and counselors to identify and work with threats of suicide (Malley, Kush, & Bogo, 1994). Other components of school-based interventions include training parents to identify problems in their children and teaching students to identify and report problems to responsible adults (Kalafat, 1997). Indeed, the most emphasized component of school-based programs is teaching students to identify their own and others' suicidal contemplations and to report them to teachers or counselors. This may be difficult for adolescents, who have a tendency to rely on peers rather than adults.

An evaluation of a school program (Kalafat & Elias, 1994) compared a group of 10th-grade students who had participated in such classes with a group of controls. Students who had taken part in the intervention classes gained more knowledge about suicidal peers and had more favorable attitudes toward helping troubled schoolmates than did the controls. Assessing long-term benefits of suicide prevention programs is difficult, but some evidence indicates that school-based programs can be effective. One study (Kalafat, 1997) found that a county with a suicide prevention program had a lower suicide rate than the state average. No causal conclusions can be drawn from these results, but the differences suggest that a widely implemented school-based program can be effective.

An intervention available to all age groups is the telephone hot line service that allows suicidal people to call suicide prevention centers and talk to trained volunteers. However, a meta-analysis of studies over a 70-year period indicated that traditional hot line services had little or no effect on the rate of suicide for people who call (Dew, Bromet, Brent, & Greenhouse, 1987).

A more effective telephone-based approach was developed in Italy and oriented toward older people. It differed from the traditional hot line in that trained workers contacted older people at risk for suicide (De Leo, Carollo, & Dello Bueno, 1995). This two-faceted service, called Tele-Help/Tele-Check, provided older people with a portable alarm system so they could call any time of the day or night if they needed help (Tele-Help). The second aspect of this service (Tele-Check) consisted of trained staff members making contact with older clients twice a week to monitor their medical and psychological condition and to offer emotional support. Although Tele-Help/Tele-Check is not solely a suicide prevention program, the service was effective in reducing suicides. During a 4-year period, only one person in the intervention community committed suicide compared with an expected rate of more than seven. This study suggests that when older people receive emotional and social support, they feel less despair and alienation and have more reason to live.

Another suicide reduction strategy is to limit access to firearms (Cohen, Spirito, & Brown, 1996). Use of firearms to commit suicide has increased, and a majority of completed suicides involves firearms. For young people, suicide is often an impulsive action, and access to a gun makes the chances of death more likely. Restricting access to firearms, especially loaded guns, can be beneficial. Training or mandating parents to take precautions with their firearms as well as using other strategies to limit access may be helpful. Access to firearms is not the only limiting factor in suicide: restricting access to drugs can also make suicide more difficult. Limiting the number of pills per prescription for sedatives reduced the number of suicides in Australia (in Cohen et al., 1996). It must be remembered, however, that although limiting access to firearms or drugs can have a preventive effect for impulsive suicide attempts, determined people will still use other methods.

The more successful suicide prevention programs, then, provide social support and combat isolation, both in young people and in older people. Another way to cut suicide rates is to restrict access to means of doing violence to oneself so that an impulsive urge to die will not turn into a completed suicide.

In Summary

Violence prevention strategies work by changing individual behavior, the environment, or the law. In addition, changing the social acceptability of violence would decrease violence on many levels. Domestic violence interventions are aimed at decreasing child, partner, and elder abuse through all three strategies. Because abused children can grow into people who do violence to others, reducing parental violence can reduce societal violence in the long run. Some commonalities exist among interventions for all types of domestic violence, including help for stressed caregivers, alternative living arrangements for the abused, and laws that mandate arrest and prosecution. Evaluations of the effectiveness of interventions for domestic violence are largely lacking.

Reducing workplace violence may include strategies to reduce domestic violence, because partner abuse may occur in a workplace, endangering the partner as well as other employees and even customers. Other violence-reduction strategies are aimed at preventing angry employees or former employees from committing violence in the workplace.

Community and school violence are more difficult to reduce than domestic or workplace violence, but violent crimes have decreased during the late 1990s. Conflict resolution programs in schools can help students deal with others in nonviolent ways, and mentoring and jobs programs are among the more successful approaches. Reducing access to firearms can also decrease community and school violence.

Strategies to prevent suicide must focus on factors that relate to suicidal behaviors in various age groups, but social isolation and depression are factors in suicide at all ages. Programs directed toward identifying and alleviating such factors as depression, alienation, and despair probably offer some promise for reducing suicide rates, and re-

ducing access to the means of suicide can also prevent impulsive suicide attempts.

Answers

This chapter addressed six basic questions:

1. **How can adults make children's world safer?**

    Adults can make children's world safer by following several basic, nonrestrictive rules: (1) Don't allow children under the age of five to ride in the front seat of a motor vehicle. Restrain young children in the back seat. (2) Supervise young children while they are taking a bath, sitting in a highchair, or using a knife or scissors. (3) Don't store chemicals, cleaning supplies, or poisons in areas accessible to children. (4) Don't permit children to swim without adult supervision.

2. **What can young people do to reduce their chances of unintentional injuries?**

    Young people can reduce their chances of unintentional injuries by following several basic rules: (1) Use seatbelts while driving or riding in a motor vehicle. (2) Don't drive after drinking or ride with someone who has been drinking. (3) Never ride a bicycle or use a skateboard without a helmet. (4) Don't ride a bicycle or participate in sports after drinking. (5) Don't play with or clean a firearm that has some possibility of being loaded.

3. **What unintentional injuries are most likely to affect adults?**

    The leading unintentional injury to adults is motor vehicle crashes, but seatbelts and airbags can help many people survive these crashes. Alcohol is involved in nearly half of motor vehicle fatalities among adults, but it is also a factor in many other unintentional injuries. Many adults are injured or killed in the workplace, with men being far more vulnerable than women and African Americans somewhat more vulnerable than European Americans.

4. **What are some of the strategies for reducing unintentional injuries?**

   Strategies for reducing unintentional injuries can be divided into three areas of focus—those aimed at (1) changing the individual's behavior, (2) changing the environment, and (3) changing the law. Attempts to change individual behavior through education, lectures, or advice is not very effective. Changing the environment is somewhat more effective than attempts to change an individual's behavior. Examples of changing the environment include building safer cars and roads and making changes in the home and neighborhood. Laws that mandate use of seatbelts and the manufacture of flame-retardant children's clothes, child-proof medicine containers, and refrigerators that open from the inside have reduced unintentional injuries to adults and children.

5. **What are the major types and the impact of intentional injuries?**

   Intentional violence is a problem that affects people throughout the lifespan, but children and youth are more frequent targets of assault and homicide than middle-aged or older people. Child abuse can have lifelong effects for victims, creating a cycle of violence that produces violent adolescents and adults. Youth violence extends to perpetration as well as victimization, and youth are involved in community violence, school violence, sexual assault, homicide, and suicide. Young African American men are at a particularly high risk. Adults are also in jeopardy from violence. Two types of domestic violence—partner abuse and elder abuse—affect adults. In addition, adults experience violence in their communities and workplaces as well as suicide.

6. **How can intentional injuries be reduced?**

   Violence prevention strategies work to change individual behavior, the environment, or the law. In addition, a societal change in the acceptability of violence would decrease violence on many levels. Domestic violence interventions are aimed at decreasing child, partner, and elder abuse through all three strategies, by providing support for stressed caregivers, alternative living arrangement for the abused, and legal requirements for arrest and prosecution of offenders. Reducing workplace violence requires strategies to reduce domestic violence that spills over into the workplace and plans for dealing with angry employees or former employees. Conflict resolution programs in schools can help students deal with others in nonviolent ways; creating mentoring experiences and jobs in the community can help at-risk individuals; and reducing access to firearms can also decrease community and school violence. Strategies to prevent suicide must focus on suicidal behaviors in various age groups, but programs directed at reducing social isolation and depression offer some promise for reducing suicide rates. Reducing access to the means of suicide can also prevent impulsive suicide attempts.

Suggested Readings

Carden, A. D. (1994). Wife abuse and the wife abuser: Review and recommendations. *Counseling Psychologist, 22,* 539–582.

This report reviews nearly 200 publications on wife abuse and presents theories that might explain why some people become spouse abusers. Carden also presents a profile of the abuser and suggests possible strategies to prevent domestic violence.

Saldana, L., & Peterson, L. (1997). Preventing injury in children: The need for parental involvement. In T. S. Watson & F. M. Gresham (Eds.), pp. 221–238. *Handbook of child behavior therapy.* New York: Plenum Press.

Psychologists Lisa Saldana and Lizette Peterson discuss the variety of unintentional injuries to children and offer strategies for reducing these injuries.

Stiffman, A. R., Earls, F., Dore, P., Cunningham, R., & Farber, S. (1996). Adolescent violence. In R. J. DiClemente, W. B. Hansen, & L. E. Ponton (Eds.), *Handbook of adolescent health risk behavior* (pp. 289–312). New York: Plenum Press.

Arlene Stiffman and her colleagues review research on all forms of adolescent violence and its impact on adolescents and on society. In addition, they discuss the challenge of prevention and approaches to reducing interpersonal, community, and school violence.

Rembolt, C. (1998). Making violence unacceptable. *Educational Leadership, 56,* 32–38.

This article discusses the problem of school violence and some of the approaches to prevention, including changing students' behavior and modifying the environment. Available through InfoTrac College Edition by Wadsworth Publishing Company.

Williams, A. F., & Lund, A. K. (1992). Injury control: What psychologists can contribute. *American Psychologist, 47,* 1036–1039.

This brief article provides some background to the injury control field and discusses the role of psychologists in injury reduction.

CHAPTER 13

Smoking Tobacco

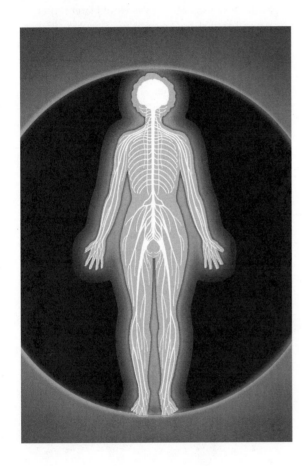

QUESTIONS

This chapter focuses on five basic questions:

1. How does smoking affect the respiratory system?

2. Who chooses to smoke and why?

3. What are the health consequences of tobacco use?

4. How can smoking rates be reduced?

5. What are the effects of quitting?

LISA: WISHING TO QUIT SMOKING

Lisa, a 31-year-old African American office manager, has been smoking for 9 years. Neither of her parents smoked, and as a teenager, Lisa was never tempted to try smoking. After working in an office for about 3 years, one day Lisa had a particularly unpleasant argument with a co-worker in another office. When she returned to her office, she was still angry. She asked her friend, Karen, for a cigarette. Lisa smoked just one that day and did not inhale. About 10 days later, after another altercation with the same co-worker, she stormed back to her office and almost demanded a cigarette from Karen. Again, she smoked just one, but the next morning she stopped at a convenience store and bought a pack of cigarettes. At first, she smoked just two a day—one at work and one in the evening after work.

Gradually, Lisa increased the number of cigarettes she smoked per day. After about a year, she was up to a pack a day, a number that she maintains at present. Interestingly, she has never purchased cigarettes by the carton, reasoning that quitting would be easier if she did not have several unused packs around her apartment. Twice Lisa has made serious attempts to stop smoking. The first time was about 2 years ago when she asked her doctor for a prescription for the nicotine patch. That procedure was partially successful—she quit for 4 months. When she began smoking again, she returned almost immediately to one pack a day. About a year later, she tried for a second time to quit—this time on her own. Once again she was partly successful, but she refrained from cigarettes for only 3 weeks. Why did she go back to smoking after wanting to quit and succeeding at doing so? Lisa says that one day she got angry at her boss, and she knew if she didn't do something to occupy her hands and mouth she might do or say something she would later regret.

When Lisa first began smoking, people were permitted to smoke in her building. When the building became smoke free, Lisa would step outside to smoke, or she would smoke while running errands between one building and another. The prohibition against smoking in her building neither reduced nor increased the number of cigarettes Lisa smokes at work.

Lisa believes that she is at greater risk for cancer than other people because she had cancer when she was 12 years old. Lisa's attitude of vulnerability is therefore different from that of most smokers who think that smoking is generally unhealthy but who nevertheless believe that other smokers are at greater risk for cancer and heart disease than they are. This chapter summarizes the level of those risks, the risks for other tobacco products, the nonlethal hazards of smoking, the dangers of passive smoking (environmental tobacco smoke), the prevalence of smoking in the United States, the reasons why people smoke, and some methods of preventing and reducing smoking. First, though, we briefly review the effects of smoking on the respiratory system, the body system most immediately affected by smoking.

Smoking and the Respiratory System

Through respiration, oxygen is taken into the body and carbon dioxide is expelled. This process draws air deep into the lungs, and with the air can come other particles that may damage the lungs. Smoking routinely introduces a variety of particles into the lungs, and several diseases are associated with smoking.

Functioning of the Respiratory System

The exchange of oxygen and carbon dioxide occurs deep in the lungs. To get air into the lungs, the **diaphragm** and the muscles between the ribs (intercostal muscles) contract, increasing the volume within the chest. As the space inside the chest increases, the pressure within the chest falls below atmospheric pressure, and air is forced into the lungs by that pressure.

Check the items that apply to you.

❑ 1. I have smoked more than 100 cigarettes in my life.

❑ 2. I currently smoke more than five cigarettes a day.

❑ 3. I currently smoke more than a pack of cigarettes a day.

❑ 4. I currently smoke more than two packs of cigarettes a day.

❑ 5. I am a smoker who believes that the health risks of smoking have been exaggerated.

❑ 6. I am a smoker who believes that smoking is probably harmful, but I plan to stop smoking before those effects can harm me.

❑ 7. I don't smoke cigarettes, but I do smoke at least one cigar a day.

❑ 8. I don't smoke cigarettes, but I do smoke my pipe at least once a day.

❑ 9. I smoke cigars because I believe that they carry a very low risk for heart disease and cancer.

❑ 10. I smoke a pipe because I believe that pipe smoking is not very harmful.

❑ 11. I live with someone who is a heavy smoker.

❑ 12. I use smokeless tobacco (chewing tobacco) on a daily basis.

Each of these items represents a health risk from tobacco products, which account for about 400,000 deaths a year in the United States, mostly from heart disease, cancer, and chronic obstructive pulmonary disease. Count your check marks to evaluate your risks. As you read this chapter, you will see that some of these items are more risky than others.

Figure 13.1 traces the flow of air into the lungs. The nasal passages, pharynx, larynx, trachea, bronchi, and bronchioles conduct air into the lungs. These passages have little ability to absorb oxygen, but in the process of inhalation, the air is warmed, humidified, and cleansed. Millions of **alveoli**, located at the ends of the bronchioles, are the site of oxygen and carbon dioxide exchange. Each tiny alveolus in the lungs is like a bubble, giving the lungs a spongy appearance. The alveoli have thin walls (only one cell in thickness) that allow the easy exchange of gases.

Air rich in oxygen is drawn into the lungs and reaches the alveoli. Blood that has circulated through the body travels back to the heart and then back to the lungs. This blood has a high carbon dioxide content and a low oxygen content. In the lungs, the blood circulates to the capillaries that surround each alveolus, where an exchange of carbon dioxide and oxygen occurs based on differences in diffusion pressures. The blood, now oxygen rich, travels back to the heart and is pumped out to all areas of the body.

During exhalation, the diaphragm and the muscles between the ribs relax. The air in the alveoli is compressed, and the increased pressure forces the air out of the lungs by the same route through which it entered. The expelled air contains a great deal of carbon dioxide and little oxygen. Not all air leaves the lungs during exhalation, and each breath mixes new air with air that remains in the lungs.

Air is an excellent medium for the introduction of foreign matter into the body. Airborne particles potentially move into the lungs with every breath. Protective mechanisms in the respiratory system, such as sneezing and coughing, expel some of the dangerous particles. Noxious stimulation in the nasal passages may activate the sneeze reflex, whereas stimulation in the lower respiratory system promotes the cough reflex.

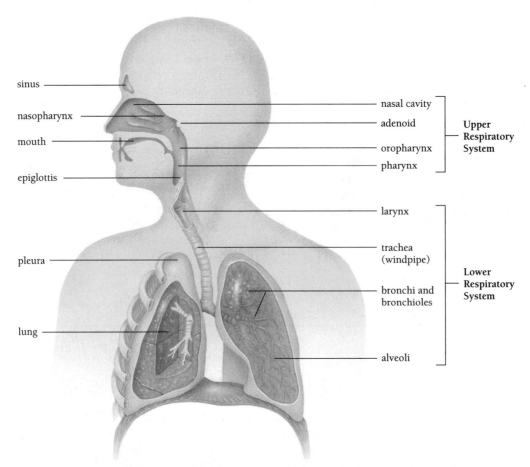

sinus

nasopharynx

mouth

epiglottis

pleura

lung

nasal cavity

adenoid

oropharynx

pharynx

Upper
Respiratory
System

larynx

trachea
(windpipe)

bronchi and
bronchioles

Lower
Respiratory
System

alveoli

Figure 13.1   Respiratory system.   *Source: Introduction to Microbiology* (p. 525), by J. L. Ingraham & C. A. Ingraham, 1995, Belmont, CA: Wadsworth. Copyright © 1995 by Wadsworth Publishing Company. Reprinted by permission.

Another protective mechanism in the respiratory system is called the **mucociliary escalator.** Diffusion of gases requires a moist environment, and the respiratory system is kept moist by its mucous membrane lining. In the nasal cavity, pharynx, and bronchi, the lining of the respiratory system contains **cilia,** tiny hairlike structures. The cilia and mucous membranes form the mucociliary escalator. Mucus is secreted in the respiratory system, and the beating of the cilia moves the mucus toward the pharynx, where it is usually swallowed or coughed out. This transport mechanism cleanses the system of inhaled particles, providing an important defense against dangerous particles.

Several respiratory disorders are of interest to health psychologists. All kinds of smoke, as well as other types of air pollution, increase mucus secretion in the respiratory system but decrease the activity of the cilia, thus decreasing the efficiency of the mucociliary escalator. As mucus builds up, people cough to get rid of the mucus, but coughing may also irritate the bronchial walls. Irritation and infection of the bronchial walls may damage the cilia and destroy tissue in the bronchi. The formation of scar tissue in the bronchi, irritation or infection of bronchial tissue, and coughing are characteristics of **bronchitis,** one of several chronic obstructive pulmonary diseases that are

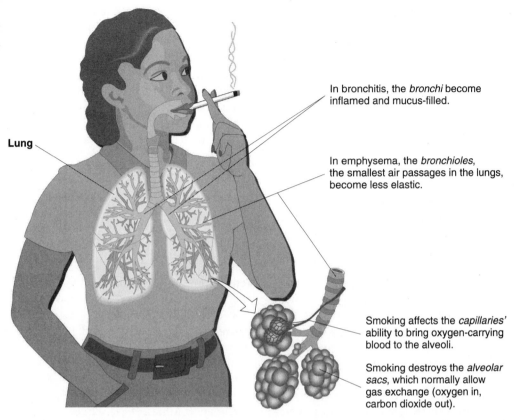

In bronchitis, the *bronchi* become inflamed and mucus-filled.

In emphysema, the *bronchioles*, the smallest air passages in the lungs, become less elastic.

Lung

Smoking affects the *capillaries'* ability to bring oxygen-carrying blood to the alveoli.

Smoking destroys the *alveolar sacs*, which normally allow gas exchange (oxygen in, carbon dioxide out).

Figure 13.2 How smoking affects the lungs. *Source: An Invitation to Health* (7th ed., p. 493), by D. Hales, 1997, Pacific Grove, CA: Brooks/Cole. Copyright © 1997 by Brooks/Cole Publishing Company. Reprinted by permission of Wadsworth Publishing Co.

the third leading cause of death in the United States.

The most common of the chronic obstructive pulmonary diseases is acute bronchitis, which is caused by infection and usually responds quickly to antibiotics. When the irritation persists and the mechanism underlying the illness continues, it can become a chronic problem. Cigarette smoke is the major cause of chronic bronchitis, but environmental air pollution and occupational hazards may also underlie chronic bronchitis.

Another chronic obstructive pulmonary disease is **emphysema,** a disorder that develops when scar tissue and mucus obstruct the respiratory passages, bronchi lose their elasticity and collapse, and air is trapped in the alveoli. The trapped air breaks

down the alveolar walls, and the remaining alveoli become enlarged. Both damaged and enlarged alveoli have reduced surface area for the exchange of oxygen and carbon dioxide. Damage also obstructs blood flow to the undamaged alveoli, and so the respiratory system becomes restricted. The loss of efficiency in the respiratory system means that respiration delivers a limited amount of oxygen. People with emphysema usually cannot exercise strenuously, and even normal breathing can become impossible for them.

Chronic bronchitis, emphysema, and lung cancer are all diseases of the respiratory system associated with the inhalation of irritating, damaging particles. Figure 13.2 shows how smoke can damage the lungs, producing bronchitis and emphysema.

Cigarette smoking is of particular interest to health psychologists because it is a voluntary behavior that can be avoided, whereas air pollution and occupational hazards are social problems not under direct personal control. Thus, smoking is the target for much negative publicity and for interventions for change, but what specifically makes inhaled smoke dangerous?

What Components in Smoke Are Dangerous?

The processed tobacco in cigarettes contains at least 2,550 compounds, and burning increases the number to over 4,000 (USDHHS, 1989). But which of these components in cigarette smoke might be dangerous? Nicotine is the pharmacological agent that underlies addiction to cigarette smoking (Kluger, 1996), but is nicotine the main culprit responsible for the adverse health effects of smoking? Can nicotine cause coronary heart disease, cancer, ulcers, bronchitis, and emphysema? What does this drug do in the body?

Nicotine is a stimulant drug, an "upper." It affects both the central and the peripheral nervous systems. Certain central nervous system receptor sites are specific for nicotine; that is, the brain responds to nicotine, as it does to many drugs. But smoking is a particularly effective means of delivering drugs to the brain. Nicotine, for example, can be found in the brain 7 seconds after having been ingested by smoking—twice as fast as via intravenous injection. The half-life of nicotine, the time it takes to lose half its strength, is 30 to 40 minutes. Addicted smokers rarely go more than this length of time between "fixes."

When nicotine is delivered to the brain, catecholamines, neurotransmitters that include epinephrine and norephinephrine, are released. These substances act as stimulants, increasing cortical arousal, which can be measured by an electroencephalograph (EEG). In addition, smoking releases beta-endorphins, and the pleasurable effects of smoking may be due to the release of these opiates produced by the body (Pomerleau, Fertig, Seyler, & Jaffe, 1983). Nicotine also increases the metabolic

level, which explains the tendency for smokers to be thinner than nonsmokers (Perkins, Epstein, Marks, Stiller, & Jacob, 1989). Cigarette smoking may also account for the finding that thinness is associated with mortality—thin smokers are at an increased risk for death, but thin people who do not smoke are not at an elevated risk (Sidney, Friedman, & Siegelaub, 1987).

The term *tars* describes the water-soluble residue of tobacco smoke condensate, which is known to contain a number of compounds identified or suspected as **carcinogens**—that is, agents that may cause cancer. Mortality from smoking-related diseases decreases with decreasing tar yields (Tang et al., 1995), but the problem in evaluating the role of tars in cigarette smoke is that tars and nicotine vary together in commercially available cigarettes. Some cigarettes are high in both, although the trend is toward cigarettes that are relatively low in both. Currently, no commercially available cigarettes are low in tars and high in nicotine, even though such a product might have advantages. For low-nicotine cigarettes, smokers increase their smoking rate (Maron & Fortmann, 1987) and inhale more deeply (Herning, Jones, Bachman, & Mines, 1981), exposing themselves to more of the dangerous tars. Thus, there may be few health advantages to low-yield cigarettes.

Several other by-products of tobacco smoke are suspected of being health risks. **Acrolein** and **formaldehyde** belong to a class of irritating compounds called **aldehydes**. Formaldehyde, a demonstrated carcinogen, disrupts tissue proteins and causes cell damage. **Nitric oxide** and **hydrocyanic acid** are gases generated in smoking tobacco that affect oxygen metabolism and thus could be dangerous.

In Summary

The respiratory system allows oxygen to be taken into the lungs, where an exchange with carbon dioxide occurs at the level of the alveoli. Along with air, other particles can enter the lungs; some of these particles can be harmful. Cigarette smoke can cause damage to the lungs, and smokers are prone to bronchitis, an inflammation of the bronchi. Cigarette smoke contributes heavily to the development of chronic obstructive pulmonary diseases such as chronic bronchitis and emphysema.

Several chemicals, either within the tobacco itself or produced as a by-product of smoking, can cause organic damage. Although nicotine in large doses is extremely toxic, its precise harmful effects on the average smoker are difficult to assess. This difficulty exists because the level of nicotine in commercial cigarettes varies with the level of tars, another class of potentially hazardous substances. Thus, determining what specific components of smoke connect to which sources of illness and death is difficult.

A Brief History of Tobacco Use

When Christopher Columbus and other early European explorers arrived in the Western hemisphere, they found that the Native Americans had a custom considered odd by European standards: The natives carried rolls of dried leaves, which they set afire, and then they "drank" the smoke. The leaves were, of course, tobacco. Those early European sailors tried smoking, liked it, and soon became quite dependent on it. Although Columbus disapproved of his sailors using tobacco, he quickly recognized that "it was not within their power to refrain from indulging in the habit" (Kluger, 1996, p. 9). Within a century, smoking and the cultivation of tobacco spread around the world, and no country where people have learned to use tobacco has ever successfully barred the habit (Brecher, 1972).

Smoking was a habit that grew rapidly in popularity among Europeans, but it was not without its detractors. Elizabethan England adopted the use of tobacco, although Elizabeth I disapproved, as did her successor, James I. Another prominent Elizabethan, Sir Francis Bacon, spoke against tobacco and the hold it exerted over its users. Many objections to tobacco were of a similar nature—namely, that people who became addicted to it often spent money on it even though they could not afford to purchase it. Because of its scarcity, tobacco was expensive: In London in 1610, it sold for an equal weight of silver.

In 1633, the Turkish Sultan Murad IV decreed the death penalty for subjects who were caught smoking. He then conducted "sting" operations on the streets of his empire and beheaded those vulnerable people who were seduced to use tobacco (Kluger, 1996). From the early Romanoff empire in Russia to 17th-century Japan, the penalties for tobacco use were also severe. Still the habit spread. In the Spanish colonies, smoking by priests during Mass became so prevalent that the Catholic Church forbade it. In 1642 and again in 1650, tobacco was the subject of two formal papal bulls, but in 1725 Pope Benedict XIII annulled all edicts against tobacco—he liked to use snuff, that is, ground tobacco.

Over the centuries, tobacco has been used in a variety of forms, including snuff, pipes, cigars, and cigarettes. Cigarettes (shredded tobacco rolled in paper) were not popular until the 20th century, although some soldiers smoked them during the U.S. Civil War. However, cigarette smoking was not widespread during the last half of the 19th century because many men considered it rather effeminate. Ironically, cigarette smoking was not socially acceptable for women either, and few women smoked during this period. Cigarette smoking became more popular during the 1880s when ready-made cigarettes came on the market. Gradually, people came to prefer factory-made cigarettes to those they had to roll themselves.

The widespread adoption of cigarette smoking was aided in 1913 by the development of the "blended" cigarette, a mixture of the air-cured Burley and Turkish varieties of tobacco mixed with flue-cured Virginia tobacco. This blend provided a cigarette with a pleasing flavor and aroma that was also easy to inhale. Cigarette smoking became increasingly popular during World War I, and during the 1920s, the age of the "flapper," cigarette smoking started to gain popularity among women.

From the time of Columbus until mid-19th century, tobacco did not lack enemies, but no one had tried to ban it for scientific or medical reasons.

Historically, the assault on tobacco had come from people who damned it on moral, social, xenophobic, or economic grounds (Kluger, 1996). The tobacco industry continued to grow despite (or perhaps because of) the fact that many in authority had condemned the use of tobacco for one or more of these reasons. It was not until the mid-1960s that the scientific evidence on the dangerous consequences of smoking became widely recognized.

During the 1940s and 1950s, it was not uncommon for physicians to smoke and to recommend the practice to their patients as a method of relaxation and stress reduction. Tobacco companies, of course, used a variety of techniques to increase smoking rates. Besides multiple advertising approaches, they provided free cigarettes to soldiers during World War II and continued to give away free samples after the war. At that time, only a few people suspected that smoking might have negative health consequences, so the choice to smoke was a common one.

Choosing to Smoke

Unlike many health hazards, smoking is a voluntary behavior, making any negative consequences avoidable. In the recent history of the United States, the choice to smoke has become less and less common. Several different factors relate to the individual choice to smoke or not.

Who Smokes and Who Does Not?

The profile of smokers differs from that of nonsmokers in gender, ethnicity, personal beliefs and behaviors, and educational level. In addition, changes have occurred over time, with the per-

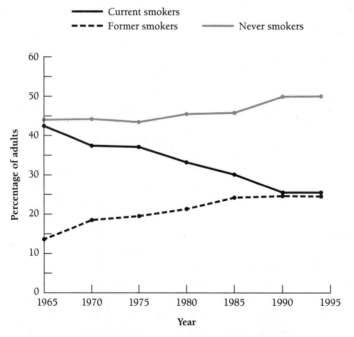

Figure 13.3 Percentage of current, former, and never smokers among adults, United States, 1965–1994. *Source:* CDC. (1998d). "Percentage of adults who were current, former, or never smokers, + overall and by race, Hispanic origin, age, and education, National Health Interview Surveys, selected years—United States, 1965-1994." Tobacco Information and Prevention Source, www.cdc,gov/tobacco

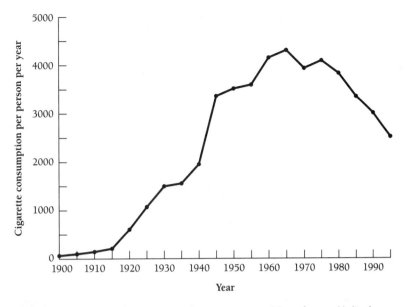

Figure 13.4 **Cigarette consumption per person 18 and over, United States, 1900–1995.** *Source:* "Surveillance for Selected Tobacco use Behaviors— United States, 1900–1994," by G. A. Giovino et al., 1994, *Morbidity and Mortality Weekly Report, 43,* No. SS-3, pp. 6–7; and the National Center for Health Statistics, 1995, p. 273, *Health, United States.* Hyattsville, MD: U.S. Government Printing Office.

centage of smokers decreasing since the 1960s. Currently, about 25% of the adults in the United States are classified as smokers (CDC, 1998d). This percentage represents millions of smokers, but it also means that three of every four adults in the United States are nonsmokers. About one-fourth of the adult population are cigarette smokers, one-fourth are former smokers, and one-half have never smoked. Figure 13.3 shows trends in smoking rates since 1965 when almost 45% of adults in the United States smoked and only about 14% were former smokers (CDC, 1998d).

In 1964, the U.S. Surgeon General issued a report spelling out the adverse effects of smoking on health (U.S. Public Health Service [USPHS], 1964). Beginning in 1967 each package of cigarettes had to carry a warning of the potential danger of smoking, and in 1970, cigarette advertising was banned from television. Coincidental with these warnings, smoking rates have declined in the United States. The highest rate of per capita cigarette consumption in the U.S. was in 1966, or 2 years

after the first Surgeon General's report on the dangers of smoking. Since that time the per capita consumption has steadily decreased. Figure 13.4 shows the per capita consumption of cigarettes in the United States from 1900 to 1995. However, this per capita decrease has not meant financial ruin for tobacco companies (see the Would You Believe . . . ? box).

In 1965, more than half of all adult men in the United States were smokers, but only about 34% of adult women smoked. Since that time, both men and women have begun to smoke less, but the rate of smoking for men has declined more sharply than the rate for women, nearly equalizing the percentages of male and female smokers. Figure 13.5 shows these trends. Note that the 25-year steady decline in smoking rates for both men and women leveled off during the 1990s. Two factors are behind this leveling off: First, the National Center for Health Statistics (1994) changed its definition of current smoker to include people who smoke only "some days" or have smoked at least 100 lifetime

WOULD YOU BELIEVE...?

Tobacco Sales Are Doing Fine

Would you believe that tobacco companies are prospering and will likely continue to prosper, despite a decrease in smoking among middle aged and older adults in the United States? Although U.S. tobacco companies seem to have lost some recent major legal battles, their future financial health appears much stronger than the future physical health of their regular customers.

Two recent trends give the tobacco industry reason for optimism. First, their promotion of cigarettes to adolescents is apparently paying dividends. John Pierce and his associates (Pierce, Choi, Gilpin, Farkas, & Berry, 1998) surveyed adolescents who had no susceptibility to smoking when first interviewed. After 3 years, more than half these young people could name a favorite cigarette advertisement, and having a favorite commercial was a good predictor of who would begin smoking. Pierce et al. estimated that 34% of experimentation with cigarettes was due to advertising, a figure that would translate to more than 700,000 new smokers each year.

A second reason for optimism in the tobacco industry lies in the expanding markets in Africa, Eastern Europe, and Asia. Richard Kluger (1996) has remarked that in these areas, smoking is regarded as a sign of being up-to-date, "an emblem of advancement, fashion, savoir-faire, and adventure as projected in images beamed and plastered everywhere by its makers" (p. xii). To Kluger the situation is ironic in that "the more evidence accumulated by science on the ravaging effects of tobacco, the more lucrative the business has become and the wider the margin of profit" (p. xii). In Kluger's interesting and informative book, *Ashes to Ashes,* he notes that many governments in emerging nations have, themselves, become addicted to cigarettes because of the taxes they receive from cigarette sales.

The nations of the former Soviet Union present an alluring potential market to American and British tobacco companies. Although the people in the former Soviet bloc have been longtime smokers, their consumption had traditionally been limited to inferior-tasting cigarettes manufactured in outmoded domestic factories that could not keep up with a growing demand. Despite a shortage of creature comforts, the people of the former Soviet Union continued their strong appetite for tobacco products.

Into this potentially lucrative market rode the Marlboro man, dispatched by his parent, Philip Morris. This longtime American tobacco company proceeded to renovate old factories, build new ones, and spend a total of $1.5 billion during the first 4 years after the Soviet breakup (Kluger, 1996). Their investment, of course, has reaped dividends. Thanks to the former Soviet countries and other Eastern European nations, Philip Morris's international sales have increased by 10% a year, easily compensating for any erosion of the U.S. market (Kluger, 1996).

As appealing as the countries of Eastern Europe appear, China presents an even larger prize to Western tobacco companies. The number of current smokers in China is not precisely known, but Kluger (1996) estimated the number at 300 million—about one-quarter of the population and about 30% of the world's smoking population. However, unlike governments of the former Communist countries of Eastern Europe, the Chinese government has been more reluctant to open its doors to foreign tobacco and has actively sought to reduce smoking among its people by restricting cigarette advertising and putting health warnings on cigarette packs. Undaunted, Philip Morris has taken a patient course of action. It has sponsored a national soccer league, presented U.S. style television shows, and displayed other forms of advertising, even "though the average Chinese couldn't get near the product" (Kluger, 1996, p. 721). Only time will tell if these tactics will be successful, but given the history of tobacco companies, it seems safe to predict that these efforts will eventually pay off.

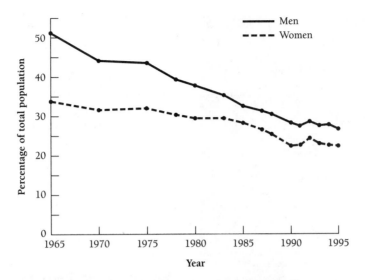

Figure 13.5 **Percentages of adult male and female cigarette smokers, United States, 1965–1995.** *Source:* Centers for Disease Control and Prevention. (1998d). National Health Interview Surveys, selected years—United States, 1965–1994. Tobacco Information and Prevention Source, www.cdc,gov/tobacco

cigarettes, thus including more people as smokers. Second, smoking among high school students has increased since 1990 (Johnston, O'Malley, & Bachman, 1998).

The recent increase in adolescent smoking is due in part to the change in definition of current smoker, but more young people have begun daily smoking each year since the new definition (CDC, 1998c), suggesting that the rising smoking rates among teenagers is not merely a reflection of the new definition. Daily smoking rates for both male and female adolescents declined from 1975 to 1987, but more recently, both boys and girls have begun to smoke more. In the senior class of 1975, boys and girls smoked at about the same rates— 27% and 26%. By 1987 daily use had dropped to 16% for male and 20% for female adolescents (CDC, 1998e), but in the 1990s, smoking increased among high school students. In 1997, 22% of both male and female high school seniors were daily smokers, and 36% had smoked within the month before the survey (CDC, 1998f).

The percentages of adolescent smokers vary with ethnicity, but the recent trend toward higher smoking rates is constant for all ethnic groups. European American adolescents have the highest rate of smoking at 40%, but 22% of African American and 34% of Hispanic American adolescents smoked in 1997 (CDC, 1998f). Ethnicity is also a factor in adult smoking rates (USDHHS, 1998d). African Americans (27%) smoke at a higher rate than European Americans (26%), Hispanic Americans (19%), and Asian Americans (15%), but Native Americans (39%) have the highest smoking rate for any ethnic group.

What personal characteristics and behaviors predict smoking? For college students, several psychological and demographic factors relate to smoking (Emmons, Wechsler, Dowdall, & Abraham, 1998). These include being dissatisfied with education, being unhappy, living in a coed dorm, valuing parties, having multiple sex partners, using marijuana, binge drinking, and having a negative view of religion. These personal characteristics

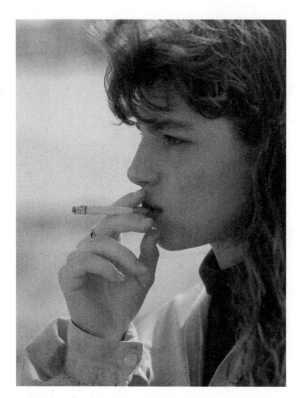

More adolescents are beginning to smoke on a regular basis.

and behaviors suggest that smokers are somewhat discontented and tend to take social risks.

In 1965, gender was the factor most strongly associated with smoking, but as seen in Figure 13.5, the rates of smoking for women and men are now quite similar. Currently, the best predictor of smoking is educational level: The more years of school people have attended, the less likely they are to smoke. Moreover, the *rate* of decline has been steeper for college graduates than for high school dropouts. Figure 13.6 shows not only the inverse relationship between smoking and education but also the steeper decline for college graduates. For young adults age 18 to 24, however, socioeconomic level seems to be the best predictor. More than 75% of young men and 60% of young women in low socioeconomic homes smoke (Winkleby, Robinson, Sundquist, & Kraemer, 1999).

Why Do People Smoke?

Despite widespread publicity linking cigarette smoking to a variety of health problems, millions of people continue to smoke. That fact is puzzling because many smokers themselves acknowledge the potential dangers of their habit. The question of why people smoke can be divided into two separate ones. Why do people begin to smoke and why do they continue? Answers to the first question are difficult because most young people are aware of the hazards of smoking. The best answer to the second question seems to be that different people smoke for different reasons, and the same person may smoke for different reasons in different situations.

Why Do People Start Smoking? Most young people are aware of the hazards of smoking (Zuckerman, Ball, & Black, 1990), yet many of them begin smoking each year. Why do young people start smoking after they have learned of the dangers of this practice? One possible explanation is that many young smokers have an optimistic bias and believe that those dangers do not apply to them and that they can easily quit (Williams & Clarke, 1997). Because teenagers tend to be oriented to the present, threats about the long-term health hazards of smoking are neither an effective way to persuade them not to begin smoking nor a good strategy to convince them to stop.

Howard Leventhal and Paul Cleary (1980) hypothesized that teenagers may begin smoking for any one of three different reasons: tension control, rebelliousness, or social pressure. Many teenagers start smoking because cigarettes are associated with the image of rebelliousness and independence (Mittelmark et al., 1987). Another hypothesized reason for starting to smoke is social pressure. Some teenagers are especially sensitive to social pressure and may start smoking if they have friends who smoke (Leventhal & Cleary, 1980). A great deal of research evidence supports this contention. Indeed, having friends who smoke is a strong predictor of experimentation with cigarettes (Mittelmark et al., 1987). In addition, the perceived smoking behavior of friends was a strong predictor of smoking onset in teenagers. Peers influence teenage smokers to continue by offering cigarettes; teenagers who smoked received 26 times more offers of cigarettes than teenagers who were nonsmokers (Ary & Biglan, 1988). One study (Stanton, Mahalski, McGee, & Silva, 1993) showed that "image" was an important reason for smoking among 11-year-olds, and that peers, relaxation, and pleasure were other reasons young adolescents gave for smoking. In addition, peer and parental smoking influences young adolescents not only in the use of tobacco but also in the use of alcohol and marijuana (Hansen et al., 1987).

Not all peer groups are equally in favor of smoking (Mosbach & Leventhal, 1988). Junior high school students identified four different peer groups with varying acceptance of smoking. The "dirtballs" were boys who smoked, used other drugs, were poor students, and had other personal or school-related problems. The "hotshots" were mainly girls who were popular and successful students, and the "jocks" were mainly boys who were interested in organized sports. The last group, the "regulars," were students who did not belong to any of these groups and were typical students. Mosbach and Leventhal found that the "dirtballs" and the "hotshots" made up only 15% of their sample but accounted for 56% of the smokers. The attitudes and attractions of smoking differed in the two groups. The "dirtballs" were typically smokers before they entered junior high school and were attracted to one another and the behavior of the group because of the satisfaction of excitement and danger. The "hotshots," on the other hand, experimented with smoking during junior high school because of peer pressure and a need for acceptance and excitement. Unlike the "dirtballs," who were unconcerned with the dangers of smoking, these girls were worried about smoking's hazards. This study explored the complexities of peer pressure and peer acceptance in the initiation and maintenance of smoking in young adolescents. Its findings demonstrate that the motivations of teenagers differ with respect to smoking and suggest

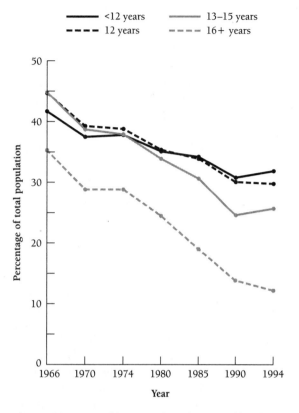

Figure 13.6 Smoking rates by educational level, United States, 1966–1994. *Source:* "Percentage of adults who were current, former, or never smokers, + overall and by race, Hispanic origin, age, and education, National Health Interview Surveys, selected years—United States, 1965–1994." Tobacco Information and Prevention Source, www.cdc,gov/tobacco

that smoking prevention efforts must be varied to succeed with young adolescents.

The evidence on the influence of social surroundings and smoking has led to a consensus on the importance of situational factors. The 1989 U.S. Surgeon General's report (USDHHS, 1989) suggested that situational factors are more important than personality factors in the initiation of smoking. Teenagers with smoking parents are more likely to start, although some controversy exists over which parent is more critical as an influence. Those with older siblings who smoke are also more likely to start. Teenage boys who start smoking are very likely to have friends who smoke, and teenage girls who start are likely to have boyfriends who smoke.

Many young women and girls (especially Whites and Hispanics) begin smoking as a means of weight control. A survey of mostly European American, upper-middle class students in grades 7 to 10 (French, Perry, Leon, & Fulkerson, 1994) found that weight concerns were related to smoking initiation for girls but not for boys. Girls were most likely to begin smoking if they had two or more eating disorder symptoms, a history of attempts at weight loss during the past year, a fear of weight gain, or a strong wish to be thin. Girls who reported any one of these behaviors or concerns were about twice as likely as other girls to be current smokers.

Once young people begin to smoke, they quickly become dependent on the habit. The Centers for Disease Control and Prevention (CDC, 1994b) surveyed young smokers 10 to 22 years old and found that nearly two-thirds of these young people who had smoked at least 100 cigarettes during their lifetime reported that "It's really hard to quit," but only a small number of young people who had smoked fewer than 100 lifetime cigarettes gave this response. In addition, nearly 90% of young people who smoked more than 15 cigarettes a day found quitting to be very hard. These results suggest that once people have smoked about 100 cigarettes or have increased their daily cigarette consumption to more than 15 per day, they have become dependent on smoking and will have great difficulty quitting.

Why Do People Continue to Smoke? Research into why people smoke suggests that no single explanation is satisfactory and that different people probably smoke for different reasons. Much of this research can be traced to theoretical work by Silvan S. Tomkins (1966, 1968), who hypothesized four different types of smoking behavior: habitual, positive affect, negative affect, and addictive.

Habitual smokers are those who smoke with little awareness and little reward. These smokers probably began smoking either to increase positive affect or to reduce negative affect, but they continue as a matter of habit. Often they are unaware that they have lit a cigarette. *Positive affect* smokers seek to increase stimulation, to bring about a feeling of relaxation, or to gratify sensorimotor needs. *Negative affect* smokers, on the other hand, smoke to reduce feelings of anxiety, distress, fear, guilt, and so forth. Theoretically, negative affect smokers should smoke more during periods of stress and less while relaxed. Lisa, our case study, seems to be a negative affect smoker. She started smoking as a reaction to an emotional confrontation with a co-worker, then, after quitting for 3 weeks, she relapsed when she became angry with her boss. Unlike habitual smokers, *addictive* smokers are not only aware of smoking but are also keenly conscious of the fact that they are *not* smoking. They usually know how long it has been since their last cigarette and how long it will be before their next one. Addictive smokers are those who never leave home or office without first checking their supply of cigarettes. They often keep several extra packs available in case of emergency.

Research has tended to support Tomkins's notion that types of smoking behavior are somewhat separate and distinct. Studies using factor analysis (Ikard, Green, & Horn, 1969; Zuckerman, Ball, & Black, 1990) have confirmed different reasons for smoking, but the number of factors has varied in these studies. These additional factors do not invalidate the notion that smoking has various motivations; rather, they suggest that smoking is a complex behavior.

Because smokers tend to have different reasons for smoking, smoking cessation programs should be tailored to fit the individual smoker (Leventhal & Avis, 1976). Using Tomkins's original model, three different mechanisms can be identified that sustain smoking behavior: pleasure-taste, addiction, and habit. In one experiment, Howard Leventhal and Nancy Avis drastically altered the taste of cigarettes by dipping them in vinegar and allowing them to dry. These adulterated cigarettes were much less attractive to smokers who had scored high on the pleasure-taste scale than to smokers who scored high on the addiction scale, confirming the importance of taste for these smokers. Smokers who scored high on the addiction scale smoked as many of the bad-tasting cigarettes as of the regular ones. Smokers who scored high on the habit scale were affected by orders to keep a record of their smoking, but the pleasure-taste smokers were not. High-addiction smokers also behave in accordance with their motivation for smoking: They experienced more distress than those scoring low on the addiction scale.

Thus, it seems that people smoke for at least four or five basic reasons. Some smoke for relaxation and pleasure; some smoke as a reaction to negative emotion; some smoke as a reaction to environmental cues, such as alcohol or other people smoking; and some seem to be nicotine-dependent and must smoke to avoid the unpleasant symptoms of nicotine withdrawal.

In addition, many people continue to smoke because they have an *optimistic bias* that leads them to believe that they personally have a lower risk of disease and death than do other smokers. When asked about chances of living to be 75 years old, people who had never smoked and those who were former and light smokers estimated fairly accurately (Schoenbaum, 1997). Heavy smokers, on the other hand, greatly overestimated their chances of living to age 75. This optimistic bias extends to specific diseases (Ayanian & Cleary, 1999). More than 60% of heavy smokers failed to acknowledge their increased risk for heart disease, and more than 50% failed to accept their heightened risk for cancer.

In conclusion, people probably smoke for a variety of reasons and these reasons either singly or in combination are strong enough to outweigh the effects of their knowledge of the hazards of cigarette smoking—knowledge that is attenuated by an optimistic bias.

Models to Explain Smoking Behavior

Several theoretical models have been proposed to explain smoking behavior. This section looks at two of these models: the nicotine addiction model and the social learning model. To be useful, these models should be able to predict who will begin to smoke and who will continue.

The Nicotine Addiction Model The nicotine addiction model holds that people continue to smoke to maintain an adequate level of nicotine and to prevent withdrawal symptoms from occurring. The model thus offers a better explanation for maintenance of the smoking habit than for its initiation.

If the nicotine addiction model is valid, smokers should smoke a greater number of low-nicotine than of high-nicotine cigarettes. Stanley Schachter (1980) tested this hypothesis by supplying heavy, long-duration smokers with cigarettes that alternately, over several weeks, were high or low in nicotine. The cigarettes all looked the same, and the participants did not know how much nicotine they would be ingesting. The different nicotine levels made a difference in smoking rates for every participant. On the average, they smoked 25% more low-nicotine than high-nicotine cigarettes. In another experiment in the series, Schachter measured the number of puffs taken from low- and high-nicotine cigarettes. Smokers took more puffs from low-nicotine cigarettes than from ones high in nicotine. Both experiments indicated that smokers are able to regulate the amount of nicotine they ingest, even when that amount is not directly related to the number of cigarettes smoked.

The nicotine addiction model does not explain why people start to smoke or why some people smoke and others do not. It also fails to explain why some people are light smokers and others smoke heavily. If nicotine were the only reason for smoking, then other modes of nicotine delivery should substitute fully for smoking. Evidence, however, indicates that other delivery methods are not entirely satisfactory to smokers. Experiments with administering nicotine through the nicotine patch (Kenford et al., 1994), intravenously (Lucchesi, Schuster, & Emley, 1967), and with nicotine chewing gum (Hughes, Gust, Keenan, Fenwick, & Healey, 1989) indicate that, although smokers may decrease smoking when nicotine is available through other modes, they still find it difficult to

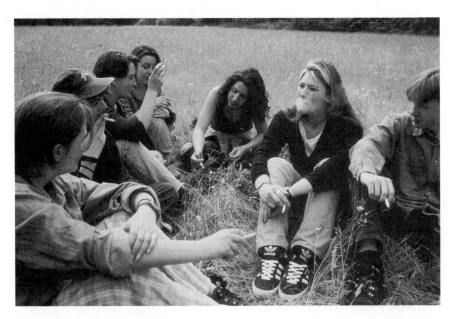

Acceptance into a social group can be a powerful source of reinforcement for adolescents, increasing the pressure to begin smoking.

stop smoking. Also, smokers prefer cigarettes with nicotine to those without, but if only nonnicotine cigarettes are available, smokers will still smoke them (Jarvik, 1977). Although nicotine may play a role in the maintenance of smoking, these findings indicate that something other than nicotine is involved.

The Social Learning Model A second model of smoking is based on social learning theory. According to this model, people learn patterns of behavior (including smoking) because those behaviors are reinforced in some manner (Bandura, 1977; Rotter, 1982; Skinner, 1953). How can smoking become acquired behavior, given that many smokers report negative consequences of their initial attempts at smoking? One's first cigarette is often followed by coughing, dizziness, watering eyes, and even nausea. Why would anyone continue a behavior that is associated with so many negative consequences? The answer is that for those who do continue (and many do not), the reinforcement value of smoking outweighs all these negative aspects.

Most smokers begin smoking during adolescence, a time when peer pressure is often quite strong. Also, most who begin at a young age smoke their first cigarettes in the presence of peers. The positive reinforcement of being accepted or of being "cool" may easily outweigh the unpleasant aspects of one's first attempt at smoking. In addition, initial smoking may be negatively reinforcing if it removes unpleasant stimuli, such as the fear of being regarded as unpopular or an outsider. Also, many people do not inhale when they first begin to smoke, thus avoiding many of the aversive stimuli. In any event, some form of positive consequences outweighs the aversive effects of first inhalation of smoke.

With practice, the aversive consequences of smoking decrease so that there are few, if any, immediate negative effects of smoking. This situation is potentially dangerous, because beginning smokers do not feel the long-range negative effects on their health. They maintain the smoking habit because it continues to relieve tension or to be reinforcing in other ways.

Social learning theory is able to explain the initiation of smoking and also offers a suitable explanation of why people continue to smoke. Once smokers become addicted, they must continue to smoke to receive the rewarding effects of a stimulant drug and especially to avoid the aversive effects of withdrawal.

In Summary

The rate of smoking in the United States has slowly declined since the mid-1960s. The historical trend for men to smoke at a higher rate than women has begun to change, and presently only a slightly higher percentage of men than women smoke. Ethnic background is a factor in smoking for both adolescents and adults, with Native Americans having the highest smoking rate. African American adults smoke more than European American adults, but as adolescents, Whites have heavier smoking rates. Hispanic Americans and Asian Americans smoke at lower rates. Currently, educational level has become a better predictor of smoking status than gender, with more highly educated people smoking at a much lower rate than those with less education.

Describing who smokes is easier than explaining why people smoke, but reasons for smoking can be divided into questions concerning why people begin to smoke and why they continue to smoke. Most smokers begin as teenagers, at a time when peer pressure is especially strong. Young people recognize the dangers of smoking but do so anyway as part of a risk-taking, rebellious style of life. This question about why people continue is a difficult one and has not been fully answered. However, several theoretical models have been proposed, including the nicotine addiction model and the social learning model. The first explains smoking behavior as a chemical addiction, whereas the social learning model suggests that smokers may begin smoking to gain peer approval or to avoid social ostracism, but once they start, they continue to avoid the aversive stimuli connected with withdrawal symptoms. A combination of the nicotine addiction and social learning models

yields a useful explanation for both the initiation and the maintenance of the smoking habit.

Health Consequences of Tobacco Use

Cigarette smoking is the single deadliest behavior in the history of the United States, and it is the largest preventable cause of death and disability. As the 20th century drew to a close, tobacco use was responsible for about 400,000 deaths yearly, or more than 1,000 deaths a day. Presently, about one of every five deaths in the United States is related to the individual's choice to use tobacco products (CDC 1993). Although most of those deaths are from heart disease, cancer, and chronic obstructive pulmonary disease, about 1,400 people a year die from fires begun by cigarettes (CDC, 1993). Smoking cigarettes while drinking alcohol produces a number of fatal and nonfatal burns every year, but smoking by itself contributed more to those fires than drinking by itself (Ballard, Koepsell, & Rivara, 1992). Heavy smokers were nearly four times as likely as nonsmokers to be injured or killed in a residential fire. In addition to adults killing themselves by smoking, they also contribute to the deaths of more than 1,700 infants a year by forcing them to breathe environmental tobacco smoke (CDC, 1993).

What Is the Evidence?

Is the evidence for the negative health consequences of tobacco merely correlational or has a causal link been established? Although experimental studies are lacking, sufficient evidence from descriptive investigations has firmly established a cause and effect relationship between cigarette smoking and several deadly diseases, namely heart disease, lung cancer, and chronic obstructive pulmonary disease. As we saw in Chapter 2, scientists can attribute causation from descriptive studies, provided seven criteria are met; that is, they can assume a cause and effect when: (1) a *dose-response* relationship exists between smoking and the likelihood of developing a disease; (2) the incidence of the disease drops for people who quit smoking; (3) smoking *precedes* the disease; (4) plausible biological explanations exist for the link between smoking and disease; (5) a vast number of studies have consistently found an association between smoking and disease; (6) the strength of this association has been substantial, with some of the highest relative risks in all of health and medicine; and (7) the evidence for a causal relationship between smoking and disease is based on well-designed studies. As noted in Chapter 2, scientists have found evidence to support each of these seven criteria, thus offering strong evidence that smoking causes both heart disease and lung cancer. This chapter briefly summarizes some of that evidence and provides support for a link between cigarette smoking and chronic obstructive pulmonary disease.

Evidence for the harmful effects of tobacco use began to emerge as early as the 1930s, and by the 1950s, the relationship between cigarette smoking and lung cancer, coronary heart disease, and emphysema was well established (Kluger, 1996; Wynder, 1997). Despite this established link, many scientists and health professionals were still smoking during the 1950s and early 1960s, and they tended to exhibit an *optimistic bias* with regard to their own risk; that is, they believed that negative consequences of smoking would affect others but not them (Weinstein, 1984). But as a consequence of that bias, a full 10 years were lost in the fight against this deadly behavior. According to epidemiologist Ernst Wynder (1997):

> If the health professions with the support of government forces had taken on this issue forcefully when the first indicating reports were published the decline in cigarette smoking that we have now finally observed among men in most industrialized countries would have occurred much earlier: the incidence of many of the tobacco-related diseases from which our society suffers today would have been reduced. (p. 692)

The causal relationship between cigarette smoking and disease in Western nations is now so solidly established that almost no scientists are currently investigating the association. However, some recent research on the health effects of smoking in China has emerged, and results of these studies indicate that Chinese smokers have a risk of dying from lung cancer, heart disease, and chronic obstructive pulmonary disease that is quite similar to the risk for U.S. smokers (Chen, Xu, Collins, Li, & Peto, 1997; Lam et al., 1997). At their present rate of smoking, an estimated 2 million Chinese will die of smoking-related causes each year (Chen et al., 1997).

In the United States and other Western nations, most current research on smoking explores other smoking-related issues, for example, the effects of environmental tobacco smoke and the association between cigarette smoking and such nonlethal disorders as cognitive dysfunction, visual problems, rapid aging, and male impotence. We look at this research later, but first we present data on the relationship between smoking and the three leading causes of death in the United States—cardiovascular disease, cancer, and chronic obstructive pulmonary disease.

Smoking and Cardiovascular Disease   Cardiovascular disease (including both heart disease and stroke) is not only the leading cause of death in the United States but it is also the primary cause of cigarette-related deaths. More than 850,000 people die of cardiovascular disease in the United States every year, and more than one-fifth of these deaths, or 180,000 a year, are due to smoking (USDHHS, 1995).

What is the level of risk for cardiovascular disease among people who smoke? In general, research suggests that the relative risk is about 2.0 (CDC, 1993), which means that people who smoke cigarettes are twice as likely to die of cardiovascular disease than people who do not smoke. The risk is slightly higher for men than for women, but both male and female smokers have a significantly increased chance of both fatal and nonfatal heart attack and stroke (Colditz et al., 1988).

What is it about smoking that might contribute to cardiovascular disease? Some evidence suggests that cigarette smoking increases the progression of atherosclerosis by as much as 50% during a 3-year period (Howard et al., 1998), speeding the formation of plaque within the arteries. In addition, nicotine itself may contribute to heart disease. This drug, which is the principal pharmacological agent in tobacco, has a stimulant effect on the nervous system, activating the sympathetic division of the peripheral nervous system. Under nicotine stimulation, heart rate, blood pressure, and cardiac output increase, but skin temperature decreases and blood vessels constrict. This combination of increased heart rate and constricted blood vessels places increased strain on the cardiovascular system and thus may elevate smokers' risk of coronary heart disease.

Smoking and Cancer Cancer is the second leading cause of death in the United States, and smoking plays a role in the development of several cancers, especially lung cancer. Although about 80% of smoking-related cancer deaths are from lung cancer, smoking may also be responsible for deaths from cancers of the lip, oral cavity, pharynx, esophagus, pancreas, larynx, trachea, urinary bladder, and kidney (CDC, 1993).

Both female and male smokers have an extremely high relative risk of about 9.0 for lung cancer (Lubin, Richter, & Blot, 1984; Schoenberg, Wilcox, Mason, Bill, & Stemhagen, 1989). This risk is the strongest link established to date between any behavior and a major cause of death. More than 150,000 people die each year from smoking-related cancers, and about 120,000 of these are from lung cancer (USDHHS, 1998a).

During the 1990s and about 20 to 25 years after cigarette consumption began to decline (see Figure 13.4), lung cancer deaths also began to level off. However, from 1950 to 1989 lung cancer deaths rose sharply, a trend that lagged about 20 to 25 years behind the rapid rise in cigarette consumption. Could the rise in lung cancer deaths before 1990 have been due to environmental pollution or some other factor? Evidence from one prospective study (Thun, Day-Lally, Calle, Flanders, & Heath, 1995) strongly suggested that neither pollution nor any other non-smoking factor was responsible for the increase in lung cancer deaths from 1959 to 1988. Although lung cancer deaths for smokers rose significantly during this period, lung cancer deaths among nonsmokers remained about the same, indicating that indoor/outdoor pollution, radon, and other suspected carcinogens had little or no effect on lung cancer mortality. These results, along with those from earlier epidemiological studies, strongly suggest that cigarette smoking is the primary contributor to lung cancer deaths.

Smoking and Chronic Obstructive Pulmonary Disease Chronic obstructive pulmonary disease (COPD) is currently the third leading cause of death in the United States, and cigarette smoking accounts for more than four of every five deaths from this disease (USDHHS, 1998b). Chronic obstructive pulmonary disease includes a number of respiratory and lung diseases; the two most common are chronic bronchitis and emphysema. Since 1980, mortality rates from COPD have increased faster than for any other major cause of death except HIV infection. By the 1990s, deaths from COPD had risen to about 85,000 a year, and the death rate was 40% higher than it was two decades earlier (USDHHS, 1998b). Reasons for this increase are not completely clear, but the risk for COPD increases with cigarette smoking (Gross, 1994).

Chronic obstructive pulmonary disease is relatively rare among nonsmokers. Only 4% of male nonsmokers and 5% of female nonsmokers receive a diagnosis of COPD (Whitemore, Perlin, & DiCiccio, 1995), with 85% of COPD mortality in men and 60% of COPD deaths among women attributable to smoking. Nonsmokers who live with spouses who smoke are at slightly increased risk for chronic obstructive pulmonary disease.

In summary, the three leading causes of death in the United States are also the three principal smoking-related causes of death. The U.S. Public

Health Service has estimated that about half of all cigarette smokers will eventually die from their habit (USDHHS, 1995).

Other Effects of Smoking

In addition to heart disease, cancer, and chronic obstructive pulmonary disease, a number of other diseases and disorders have been linked to smoking. For example, smoking is related to the recurrence of ulcers (Gugler, Rohner, Kratochvil, Branditätter, & Schmitz, 1982; Sontag et al., 1984); to diseases of the mouth, including periodontal disease (Ismail, Burt, & Eklund, 1983); and to diminished physical strength, poorer balance, and more impaired neuromuscular performance (Nelson, Nevitt, Scott, Stone, & Cummings, 1994). Smokers are also more likely than nonsmokers to develop the common cold (Cohen, Tyrrell, Russell, Jarvis, & Smith, 1993); to experience problems with cognitive functioning (Launer, Feskens, Kalmjin, & Kromhout, 1996), and to experience accelerated facial wrinkling, making them appear older than nonsmokers of their age (Ernster et al., 1995; Grady & Ernster, 1992). Smokers are more likely to suffer from two age-related problems: hearing loss (Cruickshanks et al., 1998) and macular degeneration, a serious visual impairment (Christen, Glynn, Manson, Ajani, & Buring, 1997; Klein, Klein, & Moss, 1998; Seddon, Willett, Speizer, & Hankinson, 1997)

Female smokers have about twice the chance of developing ovarian cysts than nonsmoking women (Holt et al., 1994), and women who smoke at least one pack of cigarettes a day have a deficit in bone density that is sufficient to increase the risk of bone fractures (Hopper & Seeman, 1994). Adolescent girls and boys who smoke five or more cigarettes daily have slower growth of lung function than adolescents who do not smoke (Gold, Wang, Wypij, Speizer, Ware, & Dockery, 1996). Finally, male smokers may receive a double dose of undesirable effects from cigarettes. Smoking not only may make them older and less attractive in appearance (Ernster et al., 1995), but it also increases their chances of becoming sexually impotent (Mannino, Klevens, & Flanders, 1994).

Smokers are also ill more often than nonsmokers, and the effects of these illnesses are not limited to individual smokers. Society, too, pays a price. The Public Health Service estimated that smoking-related illnesses in 1996 cost the nation $50 billion in direct costs and another $50 billion in indirect costs (CDC, 1998g). The frequency of acute illness among smokers is significantly higher than among nonsmokers, and both women and men who smoke lose far more workdays than those who do not (USDHHS, 1989). In addition, young people who smoke are less physically fit, more prone to coughing spells, and more likely to develop early atherosclerotic lesions than their counterparts who do not smoke (CDC, 1994a). In summary, smokers have a much higher mortality rate than nonsmokers, suffer from more nonfatal illnesses, and are more likely to develop chronic illnesses that eventually kill them.

Cigar and Pipe Smoking

Are cigar and pipe smoking as hazardous as cigarette smoking? The tobacco used in pipes and cigars differs somewhat from the tobacco used to make cigarettes, but pipe and cigar tobacco is similarly carcinogenic. The risk to pipe and cigar smokers, however, is not as elevated as it is for cigarette smokers because pipe and cigar smokers do not inhale as much smoke as cigarette smokers do.

As noted earlier, one study (Lubin et al., 1984) found that the relative risk for people who smoked only cigarettes was about 9.0, indicating that cigarette smokers were nine times more likely than nonsmokers to die from lung cancer. In comparison, people who smoked only cigars had a risk of 2.9 and those who smoked only pipes had a 2.5 elevation in their risk for lung cancer. However, the combination of cigars or pipes with cigarettes dramatically increased the relative risk for lung cancer. The combination of cigars and cigarettes yielded a rate of 6.9, whereas the combination of pipes and cigarettes raised the relative risk to 8.1, a rate nearly as high as for cigarettes alone (Lubin et al., 1984). These researchers found no elevation in risk for lung cancer for either cigar or pipe smokers who never inhaled. Cigar and pipe smoking may be less hazardous than cigarettes, but they are not safe. Furthermore, the risks associated with cigar smoking have spread with its resurgence in popularity. Cigar smoking has more than doubled since the 1980s, increasing among both genders and within all ages, ethnic backgrounds, income groups, and educational levels (Hyland, Cummings, Shopland, & Lynn, 1998).

Passive Smoking

Many nonsmokers find the smoke of others to be a nuisance and even irritating to their eyes and nose. But is this **passive smoking**, also known as **environmental tobacco smoke (ETS)** or secondhand smoke, harmful to the health of nonsmokers? In the 1980s, some evidence began to accrue that passive smoking might be a health hazard. Specifically, passive smoking has been linked to lung cancer, heart disease, and a variety of respiratory problems in children.

Passive Smoking and Lung Cancer   Research on the excess risk for lung cancer for passive smokers reveals a slight but consistent relationship between nonsmokers' exposure to the smoke of others and their likelihood of developing lung cancer. One review found a statistically significant but only slightly elevated relative risk of about 1.3 for lung cancer in people exposed to ETS (Wu, 1990). Studies have examined people with spouses who smoke (Fontham et al., 1994) and those who work in smoke-filled environments (Kabat, Stellman, & Wynder, 1995) to determine the risks of this type of smoke exposure. These studies have found either a slightly elevated risk or no additional risk for lung cancer. Level of exposure may be a factor (Siegel, 1993), and those with higher levels of exposure are at increased risk. However, nonsmokers exposed to ETS may have other characteristics that place them at risk for lung cancer (Matanoski, Kanchanaraksa, Lantry, & Chang, 1995). For example, nonsmoking wives exposed to ETS, compared with those not exposed, tend to be older, have less education, live in a larger city,

consume more alcohol, eat less nutritious foods, and consume fewer dietary vitamin supplements. Each of these factors carries some risk of poorer health and some may contribute to a higher risk of lung cancer.

These studies suggest that passive smoking may contribute to a slight additional risk for lung cancer, possibly as high as 20% to 30%. Relative risks of this magnitude should be interpreted with reference to the prevalence of the disease within the comparison group—in this case, nonsmokers who are not exposed to cigarette smoke. Because lung cancer in this comparison group is quite rare, an elevated risk of 20% or 30% for nonsmokers exposed to environmental tobacco smoke does not add a great number of nonsmokers to the lung cancer mortality rates. In summary, environmental tobacco smoke may contribute slightly to lung cancer rates, but evidence for any direct, independent contribution remains extremely weak.

Passive Smoking and Breast Cancer   Until recently, researchers noted a paradox involving smoking and breast cancer. That is, studies of active smoking and breast cancer generally showed a *weaker* relationship than those of passive smoking and breast cancer. How could exposure to the environmental smoke of other people place a woman at a greater risk than if she were an active smoker?

The answer seems to be that most of the earlier studies on smoking and breast cancer included passive smokers in the nonsmoker comparison group. If passive smoking is a strong risk, then including passive smokers in the comparison group would diminish the difference in breast cancer rates between active and passive smokers. Recent studies addressed this issue by comparing active smokers with a group exposed to neither active nor passive smoking. One study (Morabia, Bernstein, Héritier, & Khatchatrian, 1996) found a strong dose response relationship between active smoking and breast cancer when comparing smokers with an unexposed reference group. More pertinent to our present discussion, this study found that being exposed to environmental tobacco smoke for an equivalent of 2 hours a day for 25 years tripled a woman's chances of developing breast cancer. A more recent study (Lash & Aschengrau, 1999) found that passive smokers, compared with women who have never actively nor passively smoked, doubled their risk of breast cancer. The risk was even stronger for women exposed to passive smoking before age 12. However, women who were first exposed to environmental tobacco smoke after the age of 12 had a much lower but still significant risk. These studies suggest that passive smoking may be nearly as strong a risk for breast cancer as active smoking, but clearly more research is needed on this issue.

Passive Smoking and Heart Disease   Whereas relatively few nonsmokers die each year of lung cancer from passive smoking, a large number die from heart disease as a result of exposure to environmental tobacco. The excess risk of heart disease for passive smokers may be only about the same as the relative risk for lung cancer; that is, about 1.2 to 1.3 (Werner & Pearson, 1998). Nevertheless, even a small elevated risk for heart disease translates into thousands of deaths each year in the United States because a large number of people in the comparison group (which consists of nonsmokers who are not exposed to ETS) die of coronary heart disease. Altogether, passive smoking probably kills less than one-tenth as many people through lung cancer as it does through heart disease (Steenland, 1992).

How does passive smoking contribute to heart disease? Some evidence suggests that exposure to environmental tobacco speeds up atherosclerosis (Calermajer et al., 1996; Howard et al., 1998). This contribution to heart disease death is significant: Of the 30,000 to 60,000 people who die from ETS per year in the United States, about 75% of the deaths are from heart disease (Werner & Pearson, 1998).

Exposure to environmental tobacco smoke presents a much greater relative risk of death from heart disease than from lung cancer. With both illnesses, however, the risk from passive smoking is far less than the risk from active smoking. One

study (Sandler, Comstock, Helsing, & Shore, 1989) found the increases in the all-cause mortality rates were 1.17 for men and 1.15 for women, rates that are only slightly above those of nonsmokers who are not exposed to environmental tobacco smoke.

Passive Smoking and the Health of Children   Infants are possibly the people at greatest risk from environmental tobacco, and some of that risk is for death. One early study (Haglund & Cnattingius, 1990) found that infants whose mother smoked were more likely than other infants to die of sudden infant death syndrome (SIDS). A more recent study (MacDorman, Cnattingius, Hoffman, Kramer, & Haglund, 1997) looked at the effects of maternal smoking on SIDS and found a dose-response relationship; that is, the more cigarettes mothers smoked, the greater their infants' risk for sudden death. When mothers smoked one to nine cigarettes per day during pregnancy, their infants' chances of SIDS were doubled, but when mothers smoked 10 or more cigarettes daily, their infants' risk for sudden infant death was about three times greater than the risk of infants of nonsmoking mothers. Although maternal smoking reduces fetal birth weight and low birth weight increases the likelihood of infant death, this study found that lowered birth weight contributed very little to the relationship between maternal smoking and SIDS.

Among nonlethal problems faced by infants of parents who smoke are a greater incidence of bronchitis and pneumonia (USDHHS, 1984) an increased risk of asthma and lower respiratory tract illnesses (Stoddard & Miller, 1995), exacerbated existing cases of asthma (Chimonczyk et al., 1993), low birth weight (Ahluwalia, Grummer-Strawn, & Scanlon, 1997; Martin & Bracken, 1986), and childhood cancers (John, Savitz, & Sandler, 1991). However, the negative effects of environmental tobacco smoke diminish as children pass the age of 2 years (Wu, 1990).

In summary, passive smoking has been associated with sudden infant death and a number of respiratory problems in children under 2 years of age. Moreover, some evidence exists that ETS may be a risk factor for other health conditions in young children.

Smokeless Tobacco

Smokeless tobacco includes snuff and chewing tobacco, forms of tobacco that were more popular during the 19th century than at present. Currently, the segment of the U.S. population most likely to use smokeless tobacco is young White men. A survey of high school students (Kann et al., 1998) found that 21% of European American boys but less than 2% of the girls had used smokeless tobacco during the previous 30 days. This same survey found much lower rates for Hispanics and African Americans. Who are these young male users of smokeless tobacco? Gender and ethnic background aside, the people most likely to use smokeless tobacco are those who also smoke cigarettes, are involved in organized athletics, do not come from two-parent homes, and see friends and older family members using this form of tobacco (Tomar & Giovino, 1998). The finding that users of smokeless tobacco are more likely than nonusers to participate in organized sports is an interesting one; professional athletes may be models for this behavior or the ploy of marketing smokeless tobacco at sporting events may be successful. The segment of the population most likely to use smokeless tobacco—young White males— nearly all believe that smokeless tobacco can cause cancer, but this belief has almost no effect on their use of the product (Tomar & Giovino, 1998).

Health risks of smokeless tobacco include cancer of the oral cavity, periodontal disease, high cholesterol, and heart disease. One study (Tucker, 1989) found that people who used smokeless tobacco were 2.5 times more likely to have high cholesterol levels than those who did not use tobacco, and a 12-year follow-up of male Swedish construction workers (Bolinder, Alfredsson, England, & de Faire, 1994) showed that use of smokeless tobacco more than doubled the risk of cardiovascular mortality for men 35 to 54 years of age. The risks of smokeless tobacco are probably not as great as those of cigarette smoking; nevertheless, chewing tobacco has significant health hazards.

In Summary

The health consequences to tobacco use are multiple and serious. Smoking is the number one cause of preventable death in the United States, causing about 400,000 deaths a year, mostly from cardiovascular disease, lung cancer, and chronic obstructive pulmonary disease. But smoking also carries a risk for nonfatal diseases and disorders, such as ulcers, periodontal disease, loss of physical strength and bone density, respiratory disorders, cognitive dysfunction, facial wrinkling, sexual impotence, hearing loss, and macular degeneration.

Many nonsmokers are bothered by the smoking of others, and young children have an excess risk of respiratory disease from passive smoking. Research suggests that environmental tobacco smoke does not contribute substantially to death from lung cancer, but it may be responsible for several thousand deaths a year from cardiovascular disease.

Like cigars and pipes, smokeless tobacco is probably somewhat safer than cigarette smoking, but no use of tobacco is safe. Teenagers who use smokeless tobacco tend to believe that this form of tobacco is much safer than cigarette smoking, but the use of smokeless tobacco is associated with increased rates of oral cancer and periodontal disease and may be related to coronary heart disease.

Interventions for Reducing Smoking

In view of the evidence that cigarette smoking is potentially life threatening, people should have ample motivation to refrain from smoking—either to quit or never to begin. However, considering the positive and negative reinforcement offered by smoking, overcoming the temptation to start and especially breaking an established smoking habit can be expected to be quite difficult. Interventions designed to reduce smoking rates can be

BECOMING HEALTHIER

1. If you do not smoke, don't start. College students are still susceptible to the pressure to smoke if their friends are smokers. The easiest way to be a nonsmoker is to stay a nonsmoker.

2. If you smoke, don't fool yourself into believing that the risks of smoking do not apply to you. Examine your own optimistic biases regarding smoking. Do not imagine that smoking low-tar and low-nicotine cigarettes makes smoking safe. Research indicates that these cigarettes are about as risky as any others.

3. If you smoke, quit. Even if you feel that quitting will be difficult, make an attempt to quit. If your first attempt is not successful, try again. Research indicates that people who keep trying are very likely to succeed.

4. If you have tried to quit on your own and have failed, look for a program to help you. Remember that not all programs are equally successful. Research indicates that the most effective programs combine some psychological techniques with nicotine replacement therapy.

5. The best cessation programs allow for some individual tailoring to meet personal needs. Try different techniques until you find one that works for you.

6. If you are trying to quit smoking, find a supportive network of friends and acquaintances to help you stop and to boost your motivation to quit. Avoid people who try to sabotage your attempt to quit, and be cautious in going to places or engaging in activities that have a high association with smoking.

7. Cigar smoking has undergone a resurgence in popularity. Cigar and pipe smoking are not as dangerous as cigarette smoking, but remember that no level of smoking is safe.

8. No level of tobacco exposure is safe. Exposure to environmental tobacco smoke is not nearly as dangerous as smoking, but it is not safe, either. Smokeless tobacco use also carries a number of health risks.

9. If you smoke, do not expose others to your smoke. Young children are especially vulnerable, and smoking parents can minimize the risks of respiratory disease in their children by keeping smoke away from their children.

---

divided into those that deter people (usually adolescents) from beginning and those that encourage current smokers to stop.

Deterring Smoking

Information alone is not an effective way to change behavior. Adolescents pay little attention to the health warnings that appear on cigarette packages, so these legally mandated warnings are not an effective means of informing adolescents about the dangers of smoking (Cecil, Evans, & Stanley, 1996). In addition, smoking prevention programs that use lectures, posters, pamphlets, articles in school newspapers, and so forth are almost universally ineffective in preventing young people from starting to smoke (Thompson, 1978).

Why are these attempts at deterring smoking ineffective? Perhaps it is because many young smokers possess an optimistic bias. This unrealistic attitude is common among college-age smokers, who rated themselves as no different from the average college student for their risk of developing lung cancer (Brannon & Papadimitriou, 1985). They rated their risk of heart disease and bronchitis/emphysema as somewhat lower than that of the average college student. Because smoking elevates the chances of developing all three disorders, these self-ratings were unrealistically optimistic. A later study with younger participants found that sixth graders also had an optimistic bias concerning several health and environmental risks, including smoking (Whalen et al., 1994).

Psychological procedures aimed at buffering young adolescents against the social pressures to smoke have been more effective than educational programs. These techniques, usually called "inoculation" programs, are based on the same psychological concepts as the stress inoculation programs discussed in Chapter 8. These programs typically expose adolescents to social pressures to smoke, but they also arm them with techniques to refuse such pressure. Such programs are based on the notion that young adolescents can be "inoculated" against pressures emanating from parents, older siblings, and peers who model smoking behavior, as well as from the media (including tobacco advertisements) that encourage cigarette smoking. This social pressure is analogous to a disease, and the therapy program is comparable to inoculation because it intervenes with small amounts of the disease rather than trying to cure an established disorder.

Several teams of researchers have had some success in deterring teenagers from smoking by using other young people as models. One program developed by Richard Evans and his colleagues (Evans, 1976; Evans et al., 1981; Evans, Smith, & Raines, 1984; Wills, Pierce, & Evans, 1996) used films in which other teenagers were depicted using persuasive communication to counter arguments in favor of smoking. In these films, the teenage models are shown encountering and resisting social pressure to smoke and also transmitting information regarding the immediate and the long-term negative consequences of smoking. Evans et al. (1981) reported promising results for this approach in a 3-year follow-up of a program conducted in the Houston public schools. Participation in the program appeared to give young adolescents the skills to be more successful at resisting urges to begin smoking.

A similar program (Murray, Richards, Luepker, & Johnson, 1987) found that a peer-led program designed to build skills to counteract social pressure to smoke was successful in restraining smoking,

both immediately and at a 2-year follow-up. After 4 years, some effects for the program persisted (Murray, Davis-Hearn, Goldman, Pirie, & Luepker, 1988), but long-term follow-up data have not been so positive. A 6-year follow-up of a smoking prevention program that used the social influence model (Flay et al., 1989) found no differences in smoking rates during the senior year in high school for children who had received the experimental intervention during the sixth grade and those who had received the regular health education program.

However, when buffering techniques are combined with an intensive community-wide anti-smoking campaign directed at adults, long-term positive results are possible. Seventh-grade students living in communities that had adopted intensive anti-smoking programs also experienced a psychological intervention that included training in resisting social pressure to smoke (Vartiainen, Paavola, McAlister, & Puska, 1998). Comparison students received no intervention and lived in communities with no unusual media campaigns. After 15 years—well into young adulthood—both male and female participants who had received interventions were smoking at significantly lower rates than those in the control communities, suggesting that this combination can produce long-term gains.

Quitting Smoking

A second method of reducing smoking rates is for current smokers to quit. Although quitting smoking is not easy, millions of Americans have done so during the past 35 years. Currently, there are about as many former smokers in the United States as there are smokers—about one-fourth of the adult population are in each category, and about one-half have never smoked (CDC, 1998d).

Like adolescents when they contemplate starting to smoke, many long-term smokers who are considering quitting possess an optimistic bias. Moreover, those who quit but then relapse tend to decrease their perception of smoking's dangers (Gibbons, Eggleston, & Benthin, 1997). Also, current smokers are less likely than those who never smoked or former smokers to believe that smoking causes lung cancer and emphysema, or that smoking is generally harmful to health (Brownson et al., 1992).

An Australian study (Chapman, Wong, & Smith, 1993) showed significant differences between smokers and ex-smokers in 11 of 14 beliefs about smoking. Smokers were more likely than ex-smokers to have positive beliefs about smoking, such as that no strong evidence exists linking smoking and cancer, that most lung cancer is caused by things other than smoking, and that smoking fewer than 20 cigarettes per day is safe. Furthermore, the smokers failed to believe that smokers have more than their share of heart disease, stroke, bronchitis, poor circulation, coughing, and breathlessness. Once again, optimistic bias seems to be one factor contributing to the difficulty of quitting.

Consistent with these findings is evidence (Gibbons, Eggleston, & Benthin, 1997) that former smokers who relapse decrease their perception of smoking's risk. Interestingly, relapsers with high self-esteem are even less likely to see cigarette smoking as personally harmful. High self-esteem relapsers may experience some dissonance when they resume smoking and may try to handle that dissonance by changing their attitude toward smoking. Indeed, relapsers with high versus low self-esteem tended to rationalize that smoking is not all that bad. This finding suggests that people with high self-esteem may be more likely than those with low self-esteem to experience optimistic bias concerning personal risks and may find quitting quite difficult.

Besides an optimistic bias, another factor contributing to the difficulty of quitting smoking is its addictive qualities. Most people who both smoke and drink alcohol consider smoking to be a more difficult habit to break. People seeking treatment for alcohol or drug dependence who also smoked were asked which would be most difficult to quit—their problem substance or tobacco (Kozlowski et al., 1989). A majority of these people reported that cigarettes would be more difficult to quit. Nevertheless, a growing number of people have quit smoking, which indicates that the de-

cline in smoking rates (as shown in Figure 13.3) is due not merely to fewer people starting to smoke but in large part to increased cessation rates. Many of these people have quit on their own, but others have found assistance through formal therapy programs.

Quitting without Therapy   Most people who have quit smoking have done so on their own, without the aid of formal cessation programs. In order to understand this process, Stanley Schachter (1982) surveyed two populations: the psychology department at Columbia University and the resident population of Amaganset, New York. In questioning these people about their success in quitting smoking, Schachter found a success rate of over 60% for both groups, with an average abstinence length of more than 7 years. Surprisingly, nearly a third of the heavy smokers who quit said they had no problems in quitting. Schachter interpreted the high success rate, even for heavy smokers, as evidence that quitting may be easier than the clinic evaluations indicate. He suggested that people who attend clinic programs are those who have, for the most part, failed in attempts to quit on their own. In addition, he hypothesized that the clinic success rates of 20% to 30% represent success for each program, with those who fail in one program going on to another in which they may also have about a 20% to 30% chance for success. Schachter's data suggest that those who try to quit on their own largely succeed and never attend a clinic. Thus, people who attend clinics are an atypical group, self-selected on the basis of previous failure. These people, therefore, do not represent the general population of smokers, and failure rates based on clinic populations may be too high.

Schachter also found that people who had been heavy smokers reported that they found it more difficult to quit and had more unpleasant effects from quitting than did light smokers. However, no difference appeared in success rates between heavy and light smokers. Later studies (Cohen et al., 1989; Coambs, Li, & Kozlowski, 1992) reported that, among younger smokers, light smokers were more likely than heavy smokers to quit, whereas among older smokers, heavy smokers were more successful at quitting, perhaps because older smokers may have experienced some serious health problems.

Nicotine Replacement Therapy People who have not been able to quit on their own often seek help from outside sources. Formal cessation programs include nicotine replacement therapy, psychological interventions, and a combination of the two. The two most common nicotine replacement therapies are the nicotine patch and nicotine gum. Both work by providing nicotine-addicted smokers with a substitute for the nicotine they formerly obtained by smoking cigarettes. Nicotine patches, which resemble large bandages, work by releasing a small, continuous dose of nicotine into the body's system. People move from larger dose to smaller dose patches until they are no longer dependent on nicotine. With nicotine gum, ex-smokers receive small amounts of nicotine through chewing—a behavior that may guard against the unwanted weight gain that often follows smoking cessation. Presently, both the patch and nicotine gum are available over the counter—that is, without a physician's prescription. How effective are these nicotine replacement therapies?

In 1996, the Agency for Health Care Policy and Research (AHCPR) addressed questions concerning the treatment of tobacco dependence, nicotine addiction, and clinical practice. The AHCPR, consisting of a panel of scientists, clinicians, consumers, and researchers reviewed all English-language research published between 1975 and 1994 and suggested guidelines to clinicians, smoking cessation specialists, and health care administrators, insurers, and purchasers. Both the full report (Fiore et al., 1996) and a summary (Smoking Cessation Clinical Practice Guideline Panel and Staff, 1996) provide comprehensive information on the effectiveness of nicotine replacement therapy as well as on psychological interventions. Other researchers and clinicians (Tsoh et al., 1997; Wetter et al., 1998) have used the guidelines from this panel to help psychologists and other clinicians work with smokers who wish to quit.

After reviewing the evidence, the AHCPR identified only the nicotine patch and nicotine gum as effective pharmacological aids in smoking cessation. Moreover, the panel suggested that one or the other of these forms of nicotine replacement should be offered in any cessation program. A recent review (Tsoh et al., 1997) reported that nicotine gum produced about 17% to 18% success versus 9% for placebo gum, whereas the nicotine patch was slightly more effective—about 22% versus about 9% for a placebo patch. When combined with the drug bupropion, the patch does even better, producing a 35% quit rate after 1 year (Jorenby et al., 1999).

Although the effectiveness of the patch and the gum are similar, the AHCPR (Fiore et al., 1996) recommended the patch over the gum because compliance problems are fewer. On the other hand, the gum seems to have an advantage in helping control the weight gained by many ex-smokers. However, research reviewed by the panel found that nicotine gum provides only temporary help in controlling weight. Ex-smokers using the gum maintain weight better than those using the patch, but once they stop using the gum they gain about as much as if they had never used it (Fiore et al., 1996).

Neither the nicotine patch nor nicotine gum is without potential side-effects. The AHCPR panel cautioned against the use of either by pregnant women, unless the beneficial effects of quitting clearly outweigh the potential risk of nicotine replacement. Also, people with recently diagnosed heart attack should not use the patch or the gum. In addition, the patch causes mild skin reactions in nearly half of the users, and the gum can cause mouth soreness, hiccups, and jaw ache. Other possible side effects of nicotine replacement methods include nausea, light headedness, and sleep disturbances (Tsoh et al., 1997).

In summary, nicotine replacement therapy is more effective than a placebo, but nicotine replacement alone will help less than 20% of smokers quit (Wetter et al., 1998). The effectiveness of both the nicotine patch and nicotine gum is enhanced when combined with various psychological approaches to smoking cessation.

Psychological Approaches Psychological approaches aimed at smoking cessation typically include a combination of strategies, such as behavior modification, cognitive-behavioral approaches, contracts made by smoker and therapist in which the smoker agrees to stop smoking, group therapy, social support, relaxation training, stress management, "booster" sessions to prevent relapse, and other treatment approaches.

Most psychologists working with smoking cessation problems begin with some implicit or explicit theory, such as one or more of the models we discussed in Chapter 3. For example, they may use the transtheoretical model of James Prochaska (Prochaska et al., 1994) to assess a smoker's readiness to give up smoking. Smokers at the precontemplation stage have no intention to quit and therefore are not yet good candidates for psychological interventions. If smokers at this level are simply ignorant of the hazards of cigarettes, the practitioner can provide valid information to help them move to the next (contemplation) stage, at which they are aware of the problem and may consider quitting sometime in the future. Expensive psychological interventions aimed at smokers at the precontemplation stage yield very low rates of effectiveness and high rates of wasted effort (Lichtenstein et al., 1996; Tsoh et al., 1997).

One psychological technique recommended by the AHCPR panel members is practitioner support. Their review found a 15% cessation rate for programs with strong provider support compared with only a 9% success rate for those with no ongoing contact. Supportive practitioners are in a position to increase smokers' *self-efficacy;* that is, their belief that they can execute the behaviors necessary to stop smoking. One method of enhancing a smoker's self-efficacy is verbal persuasion. A therapist can explain that millions of people have successfully stopped smoking. Indeed, half of all living people who have ever smoked have quit. Another avenue of verbal persuasion would be to inform smokers who have been unsuccessful with their first or second quit attempts that most people succeed after three at-

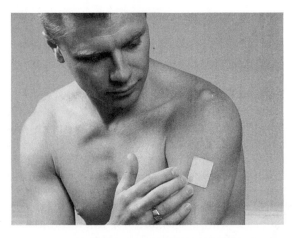

Nicotine patches in a multimodal program can be effective in helping people quit smoking.

tempts (Tsoh et al., 1997). However, information communicated through verbal persuasion has a limited influence on self-efficacy. The strongest source of self-efficacy is previous successful performance. Thus, the therapist may be able to point to earlier successes in quitting, even if the smoker had quit for only a short time. If smokers can quit once, they can quit again.

A related approach is to encourage smokers to inform family and friends of their intentions to quit, a technique designed to give them a larger base of social support. Smokers also can be taught that changes in their environment can reduce cues to smoke; smokers can throw away their cigarettes, avoid places and events where others are smoking, and reduce consumption of alcohol, tea, colas, or other drinks associated with smoking. They can be taught that stress, arguments, and negative mood are associated with desire to light up a cigarette. These stressful situations cannot be entirely avoided, but other cognitive and behavioral strategies to distract attention from smoking cues can be taught. Therapists can train smokers to use such relaxation techniques as deep breathing, visual imagery, progressive muscle relaxation, and self-hypnosis. (We discussed these and other forms of stress management in Chapter 8.) Smokers effectively trained in stress-coping skills are more likely to quit than those who have not learned these techniques (Fiore et al., 1996).

Both individual and group counseling can be successful in helping people to quit smoking (Wetter et al., 1998). Psychologists, physicians and nurses can be effective providers, but effectiveness is positively related to the amount of contact between client and therapist. The increased costs of intensive interventions are offset by their improved effectiveness. Programs that include more sessions tend to be more effective than programs with fewer sessions, but increases beyond about seven sessions merely increases cost, not effectiveness. The most effective programs include both a counseling component and a nicotine-replacement component. These elements are both effective, and the combination of the two improves outcomes.

Who Quits and Who Does Not?

Another issue is the question of who quits smoking and who does not. What factors relate to smoking cessation? Investigators have examined several factors that may answer this question, including gender, weight concern, social support, perceived health benefits, and confidence that one can quit.

Are men more likely than women to quit smoking? Because men have had higher quit rates than women over the past 35 years, many observers assumed that women have more difficulty quitting than men. Although some evidence exists to support this idea, the reason may be that female smokers who try to quit have more obstacles to overcome. Some research (Bjornson et al., 1995) suggests that these gender differences could be explained by baseline differences; that is, at the beginning of the study, women were *less* likely (1) to be married, (2) to have made a previous attempt to quit, (3) to have made longer quit attempts, and (4) to be heavy smokers. Also, women were *more* likely to live with other smokers. Regardless of gender, each of these factors is associated with poorer quit rates. In other words, women generally have more obstacles to overcome in trying to quit smoking.

Some research suggested that women were more likely to fail in cessation programs, but evidence for this is somewhat complex (Fortmann & Killen, 1994). First, women were more likely to volunteer to participate in such programs—possibly they were simply going along with a friend. Second, once women expressed a genuine interest in quitting, they were as likely as men to quit. Third, although women had more difficulty during the first 24 hours, after that time they had the same quit rates as men. In summary, women may be more willing to make quit attempts and may be less successful during the first 24 hours, but they are equal to men in avoiding relapse once they have quit.

Does a supportive social network of nonsmokers help people quit smoking? Cessation programs are more effective in maintaining abstinence when spouses of participants are trained to offer support to the partner who is trying to quit. In contrast, having a greater than average number of smokers in one's social network is a hindrance to maintaining abstinence (Mermelstein, Cohen, Lichtenstein, Baer, & Kamarck, 1986). Similarly, pregnant women who smoke are more like to quit if their partners are nonsmokers or if they receive support from their partners (McBride et al., 1998).

Do smokers who abuse alcohol find it harder to quit smoking than smokers who do not? Clinical psychologists have long recognized the strong relationship between smoking and drinking, but until recently there has been little research on how quitting one affects quitting the other. Some evidence now suggests that smokers with drinking problems are much less likely than those with no history of alcohol abuse to quit smoking. On the other hand, problem drinkers who are able to stop drinking, compared with problem drinkers who continue to drink, are three times as likely to quit smoking (Breslau, Peterson, Schultz, Andreski, & Chilcoat, 1996).

Does a diagnosis of heart disease or cancer influence a person's likelihood of quitting smoking? Recent hospitalization and recently diagnosed heart disease are both positively related to cessation rates, but a diagnosis of cancer does not seem to prompt people to quit, possibly because those people believe that it is too late to benefit from quitting (Freund, D'Agostino, Belanger, Kannel, & Stokes, 1992).

Finally, is smoking cessation related to smokers' self-efficacy for quitting smoking—that is, their level of confidence that they have the ability to do what is necessary to quit and to maintain abstinence? One study (Condiotte & Lichtenstein, 1982) measured self-efficacy before, during, and after involvement in smoking control programs and found that smokers' feelings of self-efficacy predicted who would relapse, how soon they would relapse, and in what situations they were likely to relapse. In addition, people high in self-efficacy were more likely than inefficacious participants to reestablish abstinence following a slip.

In another study (DiClemente, 1981), self-efficacy scores were better predictors of smoking cessation than either demographic data or smoking history. For example, factors that did *not* differentiate between abstainers and recidivists were age, educational level, socioeconomic status, age at beginning smoking, cigarettes smoked per day, number of prior attempts to quit, longest previous abstinence, or number of years smoking. In this study, only self-efficacy predicted success at quitting.

Relapse Prevention

The problem of relapse is not unique to smoking. Relapse rates similar to those for smoking have also been found in the treatment of alcohol and heroin addiction (Hunt, Barnett, & Branch, 1971). The high rate of relapse after smoking cessation treatment prompted G. Alan Marlatt and Judith Gordon (1980) to examine the relapse process itself. For many people who have been successful in quitting, one cigarette precipitates a full relapse, complete with feelings of total failure. Marlatt and Gordon termed this phenomenon the *abstinence violation effect*. They incorporated strategies into their treatment to cope with patients' despair when they violate their intention to remain abstinent. By training patients that one "slip" does not

constitute relapse, Marlatt and Gordon buffer them against a full relapse. Slips are common even among people who will eventually quit. One-fourth of successful self-quitters slip at one time or another (Hughes et al., 1992). Thus, a single slip should not discourage people from continuing their effort to stop smoking.

Self-quitters have very high relapse rates. One study (Hughes et al., 1992) found that two-thirds of smokers who quit on their own had relapsed after only 2 days and 92% had resumed smoking after 6 months. In formal smoking cessation programs that include relapse prevention, failure rates are not quite so high—about 70 to 80%.

The AHCPR guidelines (Fiore et al., 1996) suggest several procedures for preventing relapse and strongly recommend they be incorporated into all cessation programs. First, therapists should review reasons for relapse, such as fear of weight gain, unpleasant withdrawal symptoms, negative mood or depression, and lack of social support for cessation. Once these factors have been identified, therapists can work to reduce or eliminate them. For example, for smokers who fear gaining weight, the practitioner can inform them that the health benefits of quitting smoking are far greater than any health problems that might accompany weight gain. (We discuss smoking cessation and weight gain later.) For smokers who are depressed, the therapist can provide individual or group counseling. For those suffering prolonged withdrawal symptoms, the therapist can recommend nicotine replacement therapy. For smokers needing more social support, the intervention can include making follow-up telephone calls and enlisting encouragement from the ex-smoker's family and friends. These and other techniques can reduce relapse rates (Tsoh et al., 1997), but they do not keep most people who have quit smoking from starting again. Thus, relapse remains a problem even in programs designed to cope with it.

In Summary

Smoking rates can be reduced either by preventing people from starting or by getting current smokers to quit. One successful approach to preventing young people from starting is the "inoculation" method, in which teenagers are given information to buffer them against the persuasive arguments of peers and media. These behavioral interventions—which include peer influence, training in refusal skills, and practice at making decisions—have had some success in deterring young people from smoking. How can people quit smoking? Because giving up nicotine may result in withdrawal symptoms, many successful cessation programs include nicotine replacement in the form of a nicotine patch or nicotine gum. Both are more effective than a placebo, but without counseling, neither can claim high success rates. By combining nicotine replacement with psychological interventions, quit rates become higher—perhaps as high as 30%. In addition, millions of people have stopped smoking on their own. Men are more likely to be successful at quitting than women, perhaps because women face more barriers when they try to quit. In addition, self-efficacy is related to successful quitting. Many people are able to quit for 6 months to 1 year, but the problem of relapse remains serious. Programs aimed at this relapse problem can be successful, but cessation programs need to address the issue of relapse.

Effects of Quitting

When smokers quit, they experience a number of effects. Some of the effects are the health benefits that smokers consider when they quit. However, another effect is the weight gain that many smokers fear and that may deter some smokers from quitting.

Quitting and Weight Gain

Both smokers and former smokers generally agree that quitting smoking may mean unwanted weight gain (Chapman, et al., 1993). Are such concerns justified? Indeed, the possibility exists that the overall increase in weight for U.S. residents is attributable to the number of smokers who have quit

and gained weight. One analysis (Flegal, Troiano, Pamuk, Kuczmarski, & Campbell, 1995) indicated that quitting smoking does not account for the majority of the increases in overweight among U.S. residents, but it is a factor. Former smokers tend to gain weight, and those who quit are significantly more likely to become overweight compared with those who continue to smoke.

The weight gain associated with quitting is typically modest, about 9 pounds for men and 11 for women (Flegal et al., 1995). Women tend to be more concerned than men about weight gain (Pirie, Murray, & Luepker, 1991), but they should also consider that they will probably gain weight even if they don't quit smoking. A study of cardiovascular risk factor changes during menopause (Burnette, Meilahn, Wing, & Kuller, 1998) showed that women who quit smoking gained about 11 pounds during the first year after menopause, but both nonsmokers and those who continued to smoke gained more than 5 pounds during this same period. Although women are generally more concerned about weight gain than are men, the total weight gain after smoking cessation is about the same for women and men (Nides et al., 1994); however, this similar figure reflects a higher percentage for women, who are typically slighter than men.

More optimistic findings came from a study reporting that weight gain following smoking cessation can be temporary (Chen, Horne, & Dosman, 1993). The mean body mass index was highest in ex-smokers, lowest in smokers, and intermediate in those who had never smoked. However, for female ex-smokers, both body mass index and body weight decreased significantly with years of smoking cessation. Men experienced a nonsignificant trend in the same direction. Former smokers are heaviest about 2 years after quitting, after which time their weight matches that of those who have never smoked.

Besides gender, what other factors relate to weight gain after smoking cessation? A long-term follow-up of a national sample of former smokers (Williamson et al., 1991) found that people who had the most trouble with weight gain were African

Americans (both men and women), heavy smokers, smokers under age 55, and women with children.

Does physical activity curtail weight gain in people who quit smoking? Research from the Nurses' Health Study (Kawachi, Troist, Robnitzky, Coakley, & Colditz, 1996) revealed that women who increased their level of exercise after quitting smoking gained less weight than women who quit but did not become more physically active. These findings suggest that the health of female smokers is enhanced if they quit smoking, and that if they are worried about weight, a moderate exercise program can probably hold down any excess gain to a few pounds.

The extra weight gained by former smokers—men and women—does not negate the health benefits of smoking cessation. Quitting smoking is much more beneficial to health than maintaining lower weight. Although menopausal women who quit smoking gained more than twice as much weight as nonsmokers and continuing smokers (Burnette et al., 1998), they improved their cardiovascular risk factors, in part by raising HDL. Adopting other healthy behaviors such as an improved diet can boost health and extend life (Grover, Gray-Donald, Joseph, Abrahamowicz, & Coupal, 1994), but this extension is days to months. Quitting smoking can extend life by several years. The health benefits of quitting outweigh the health risks of weight gain.

Health Benefits of Quitting

Can longtime cigarette smokers improve their health and add years to their life by quitting? One estimate suggests that the average reduction in life expectancy for smokers is 5 to 8 years, depending on the amount of smoking (Fielding, 1985). Can smokers regain some of their life expectancy by quitting? How long must ex-smokers remain abstinent before they reverse the detrimental effects of smoking?

The 1990 report of the Surgeon General summarized studies indicating that former light smokers (fewer than 20 cigarettes a day) who were able to abstain for 16 years had about the same rate of mortality as people who had never smoked (USDHHS, 1990). This encouraging finding was true for both women and men (see Figure 13.7). For women who were heavy smokers (more than 20 cigarettes a day), the benefits of quitting were substantial, especially after the third year of abstinence. Women who were light smokers seemed to have benefited almost immediately from quitting, and by the 16th year of abstinence they had the same mortality rate as women who had never smoked. So Lisa, the smoker described in the introduction to this chapter who smokes 20 cigarettes or fewer a day, could eventually reduce her risk of death to a level about equal to what it would have been if she had never smoked.

Figure 13.7 shows that men who are heavy smokers have a risk of death about 2 times greater than those who have never smoked. But those who quit show a steady reduction in mortality rate after the first year of abstinence if they have not already developed some smoking-related condition. After 16 years without smoking, men reduce their mortality risk to about half that of current smokers and only slightly more than that of nonsmokers. Men who were formerly light smokers do even better after 16 years of abstinence; they have about the same relative risk as men who have never smoked. For those with cancer, heart disease, or stroke, the benefits of quitting do not show up until after 3 years of abstinence, perhaps because many sick people quit in the years immediately before they die.

Longtime smokers who quit reduce their chances of dying from heart disease much more than they lower their risk of death from lung cancer. Several studies show that cigarette smokers who quit can eventually reduce their risk of cardiovascular disease to that of a nonsmoker, but their risk of cancer, especially lung cancer, remains elevated. For example, men who quit smoking for 30 years had only a very slightly elevated risk of coronary heart disease, but these same men had nearly a threefold risk for lung cancer (Ben-Shlomo, Smith, Shipley, & Marmot, 1994). How-

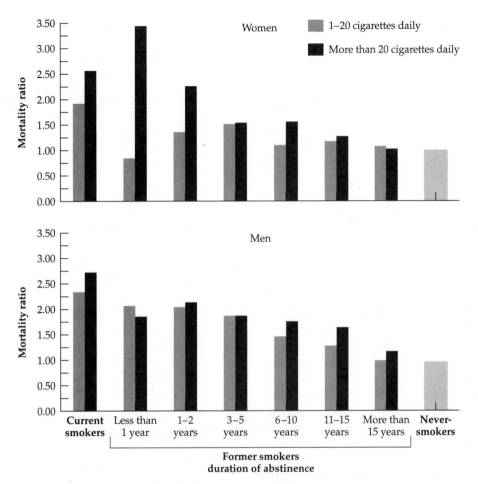

Figure 13.7 Overall mortality ratios for current and former smokers compared with never smokers, by sex and duration of abstinence. *Source: The Health Benefits of Smoking Cessation: A Report of the Surgeon General* (p. 78), by U.S. Department of Health and Human Services, 1990 (DHHS Publication No. CDC 90-8416), Washington, DC: U.S. Government Printing Office.

ever, this increased risk of lung cancer for former smokers was less than one-fourth the risk of men who continued smoking. Thus, men who quit smoking for 30 years reduce their risk of both cardiovascular disease and lung cancer, but their risk for lung cancer remains substantially higher than that of men who have never smoked. Women also reduce their risks by quitting. The excess risk of stroke disappears in middle-aged women who stop smoking, regardless of the number of cigarettes

they had smoked, the age at which they had started, or the presence of other stroke risk factors (Kawachi et al., 1993). These studies suggest that by quitting smoking, both male and female smokers can reduce their risk of cardiovascular disease to that of nonsmokers, although they may never completely erase their elevated risk of lung cancer. Thus, never starting to smoke is healthier than quitting, but quitting, though seldom easy, can pay off.

In Summary

Many smokers fear that if they stop smoking they will gain weight, but the evidence shows that the average weight gain for most men and women is relatively modest—about 9 to 11 pounds. Even excessive weight gain is far less risky than continuing to smoke. On a more positive note, stopping smoking improves health and extends life expectancy. Some evidence suggests that after smokers have quit for 16 years, their all-cause mortality rate may return to that of nonsmokers, although they may continue to have an excess risk for lung cancer mortality.

Answers

This chapter addressed five basic questions.

1. **How does smoking affect the respiratory system?**

   The respiratory system allows for the intake of oxygen and the elimination of carbon dioxide. Cigarette smoke drawn into the lungs eventually damages the lungs, and chronic bronchitis and emphysema are two chronic pulmonary diseases related to smoking. Tobacco contains several thousand compounds, including nicotine, and smoking exposes smokers to tars and other compounds that contribute to heart disease and cancer.

2. **Who chooses to smoke and why?**

   About one-fourth of all U.S. adults smoke, about one-fourth are former smokers, and about one-half have never smoked. Men and women now smoke in about equal numbers. Educational level has replaced gender as the best predictor of smoking—higher education is associated with lower smoking rates. Most smokers start as adolescents, and one motivation is that smoking is part of a risk-taking, rebellious style that is attractive to some adolescents. No conclusive answer exists for why people continue to smoke, but the nicotine addiction model hypothesizes that smokers need to maintain levels of this addictive drug, and the social learning model suggests that starting to smoke is part of a peer pressure or peer approval process.

3. **What are the health consequences of tobacco use?**

   Smoking is the number one cause of preventable death in the United States, causing about 400,000 deaths a year, mostly from cardiovascular disease, lung cancer, and chronic obstructive pulmonary disease. Smoking also carries a risk of nonfatal diseases and disorders such as ulcers, periodontal disease, loss of physical strength and bone density, respiratory disorders, cognitive dysfunction, facial wrinkling, sexual impotence, and macular degeneration. Passive smoking does not contribute substantially to death from lung cancer, but environmental tobacco smoke raises young children's risk of respiratory disease and adults' risk of cardiovascular disease. Smokeless tobacco is probably somewhat safer than cigarette smoking, but the use of smokeless tobacco is associated with increased rates of oral cancer and periodontal disease and may be related to coronary heart disease.

4. **How can smoking rates be reduced?**

   One way to reduce smoking rates is to prevent people from starting. One such program is the "inoculation" method in which teenagers are given information to buffer them against the persuasive arguments of peers and media. Most people who quit do so on their own without any formal cessation program, but relapse is a problem for these smokers. Nicotine replacement in the form of a nicotine patch or nicotine gum can be a useful component in smoking cessation, but use of nicotine replacement alone is not a very successful approach. Behavioral techniques can be effective in helping people quit; the addition of such techniques to nicotine replacement treatment can boost the effectiveness of cessation programs.

5. What are the effects of quitting?

Many smokers fear weight gain upon quitting, and a modest gain (9 to 11 pounds) is common. Nevertheless, gaining weight is not as hazardous to a person's health as continuing to smoke. Quitting improves health and extends life, but returning to the risk level of nonsmokers for cardiovascular mortality can take 16 years or longer, and most ex-smokers retain some elevated risk for lung cancer.

Glossary

acrolein A yellowish or colorless, pungent liquid produced as a by-product of tobacco smoke; one of the aldehydes.

aldehydes A class of organic compounds obtained from alcohol by oxidation and also found in cigarette smoke; they cause mutations and are related to the development of cancer.

alveoli Small, saclike structures at the end of the bronchioles; the sites of oxygen and carbon dioxide exchange.

bronchitis Any inflammation of the bronchi.

carcinogen A substance that induces cancer.

cilia Tiny, hairlike structures lining parts of the respiratory system.

diaphragm The partition separating the cavity of the chest from that of the abdomen.

emphysema A chronic lung disease in which scar tissue and mucus obstruct the respiratory passages.

environmental tobacco smoke (ETS) The smoke of spouses, parents, or co-workers to which nonsmokers are exposed; passive smoking.

formaldehyde A colorless, pungent gas found in cigarette smoke; it causes irritation of the respiratory system and has been found to be carcinogenic; one of the aldehydes.

hydrocyanic acid A poisonous acid produced by treating a cyanide with an acid; one of the products of cigarette smoke.

mucociliary escalator The mechanism by which debris is moved toward the pharynx.

nitric oxide A colorless gas prepared by the action of nitric acid on copper and also produced in cigarette smoke; it affects oxygen metabolism and may be dangerous.

passive smoking The exposure of nonsmokers to the smoke of spouses, parents, or co-workers; environmental tobacco smoke.

Suggested Readings

Gilbert, D. G. (1995). *Smoking: Individual differences, psychopathology, and emotion.* Washington, DC: Taylor & Francis.

In this book, Gilbert discusses the relationship between smoking and emotion, gender differences in the effects of tobacco use, and the association between personality and smoking behavior.

Husten, C.G., Warren, C. W., Crossett, L., & Sharp, D. (1998). Trends in tobacco use among high school students in the United States, 1991–1995. *Journal of School Health, 68,* 137–140.

This article summarizes recent trends in tobacco use among high school students, including the recent increase in cigarette smoking. Available through InfoTrac College Edition from Wadsworth Publishing Company.

Kluger, R. (1996). *Ashes to ashes; America's hundred-year cigarette war, the public health and the unabashed triumph of Philip Morris.* New York: Knopf.

Kluger presents a lengthy but fascinating account of the story of tobacco, the attempts to discourage its use, and the ultimate victory of the tobacco industry.

Pomerleau, O. F. (1980). Why people smoke: Current psychobiological models. In P. O. Davidson & S. M. Davidson (Eds.), *Behavioral medicine: Changing health lifestyles* (pp. 94–112). New York: Brunner/Mazel.

This review of the leading theories of tobacco use includes a summary of relevant research.

CHAPTER 14

Using Alcohol and Other Drugs

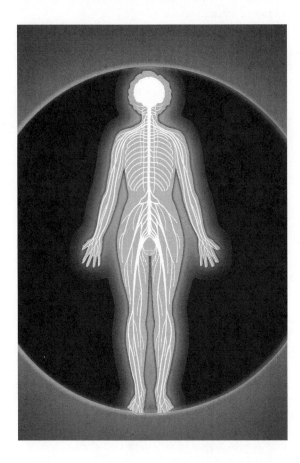

QUESTIONS

This chapter focuses on six basic questions:

1. What are the major trends in alcohol consumption?
2. What are the health effects of drinking alcohol?
3. Why do people drink?
4. How can people change problem drinking?
5. What problems are associated with relapse?
6. What are the health effects of other drugs?

CHAD: A SOCIAL DRINKER AGAIN

Chad, a European American college senior, classifies himself as a social drinker because he drinks only in social situations or when he is out with friends. He usually has just one drink per day and never more than four drinks. A year ago, however, his consumption was much higher. At that time, he was a member of a fraternity and frequently went out with his friends and drank heavily. About two or three times a year, he would get "stupid, falling down drunk," usually as a celebration for some occasion such as the completion of mid-term exams.

Being part of a college fraternity shaped Chad's drinking habits. Unlike the majority of his peers in high school, he had no interest in experimenting with alcohol. In fact, he had a very negative attitude toward drinking, an attitude that started to change when he began to drink. His first experience with alcohol was just before his 18th birthday, when some friends took him out and got him drunk on beer. Although this episode resulted in a terrible hangover, Chad did not develop negative feelings about drinking.

As a freshman in college, Chad joined a fraternity, where drinking was a major part of the social life. Although he did not drink as much as many of his fra-

ternity brothers, he began to drink at the fraternity house and at local clubs and bars. When one of the fraternity brothers had drunk too much, the other members would try to keep him from doing anything too embarrassing and to get him back to the fraternity house safely. Occasionally, Chad was the one in need of help, but more often, he provided assistance.

During college, Chad's level of alcohol consumption escalated to frequent moderate drinking combined with occasional binges. Presently, however, his drinking has decreased—partly because his fraternity has been dissolved but mostly because his last binge resulted in a "blackout" in which he did not remember the socially embarrassing behavior that got him thrown out of his favorite club. As a consequence of his embarrassment, he resolved never to get drunk again. However, he continues to be a light social drinker.

Chad believes that his reduction in drinking was the result of a natural process of "settling down." He has also noticed that his younger classmates and friends seem to be drinking less, mostly as a result of a change that increased the legal drinking age from 18 to 21.

Alcohol Consumption—Yesterday and Today

Is Chad's assessment of his drinking patterns accurate—is he a social drinker, or does he have problems associated with alcohol? Is his drinking typical for college students? What drinking patterns present problems? This chapter includes answers to these questions, but first, we examine the history of drinking.

A Brief History of Alcohol Consumption

The use of alcohol is not something that can easily be traced; it was discovered worldwide and repeatedly, dating back beyond recorded history. The yeast that is responsible for producing alcohol is

airborne, and fermentation occurs naturally in fruits, fruit juices, and grain mixtures. Producing beverage alcohol requires no sophisticated technology, and there is evidence that most ancient cultures used beverage alcohol. Ancient Babylonians discovered both wine (fermented grape juice) and beer (fermented grain), as did the ancient Egyptians, Greeks, Romans, Chinese, and Indians. Pre-Columbian tribes in the Americas also used fermented products.

Ancient civilizations also discovered drunkenness, of course. In several of those countries, such as Greece, drunkenness was not only allowed but practically required on certain occasions, but these occasions were limited to festivals. This pattern resembles present-day practices in the United States, where drunkenness is condoned at some

Check the items that apply to you.

❑ 1. I have had five or more drinks of beer, wine, or liquor in one day at least once during the past month.

❑ 2. I have had five or more alcoholic drinks on the same occasion on at least five different days during the past month.

❑ 3. When I drink too much I sometimes don't remember a lot of the things that happened.

❑ 4. I sometimes ride with a driver who has been drinking.

❑ 5. On at least one occasion during the past year I drove a motor vehicle after having more than two drinks.

❑ 6. I frequently drive after having one or two drinks.

❑ 7. I sometimes ride a bicycle after having a couple of drinks.

❑ 8. I sometimes play sports after having a couple of drinks.

❑ 9. Some of my friends or family have told me that I drink too much.

❑ 10. I have tried to cut down on my drinking, but I never seem to succeed.

❑ 11. At least once in my life I have tried to completely quit drinking, but I was not successful.

❑ 12. I believe that the best way to enjoy many activities (such as a dance or a football game) is to drink alcohol.

❑ 13. After waking up with a hangover, I sometimes have a drink to feel better.

❑ 14. There are some activities that I perform better after drinking.

Each of these items represents a health risk from misusing alcohol, increasing your risk for diseases and unintentional injuries. Count your check marks to evaluate your risks. As you read this chapter, you will learn that some of these items are more risky than others.

parties and celebrations. Most societies condone drinking alcohol but not drunkenness, except on certain occasions.

Distillation was discovered in ancient China, and refined in 8th-century Arabia. Because the process is somewhat complex, the use of distilled spirits did not become widespread until they were commercially manufactured. In England, fermented beverages were by far the most common form of alcohol consumption until the 18th century, when England encouraged the proliferation of distilleries to stimulate commerce. Along with cheap gin came widespread consumption and widespread drunkenness. However, intoxication from distilled spirits was confined mostly to the lower and working classes; the rich drank wine, which was imported and thus expensive.

In colonial America, drinking was much more prevalent than it is today. Men, women, and children all drank, and it was considered acceptable for all to do so. This practice may not seem consistent with our present-day image of the Puritans, but nevertheless the Puritans did not object to drinking. Rather, they considered alcohol one of God's gifts. Indeed, in those years alcohol was often safer than unpurified water or milk, so the Puritans had a legitimate reason to condone the consumption of alcoholic beverages. What was not acceptable to them was drunkenness. They believed that alcohol should, like all things, be used in moderation. Therefore, the Puritans established severe prohibitions against drunkenness but not against drinking.

The 50 years following U.S. independence marked a transition in the way early Americans

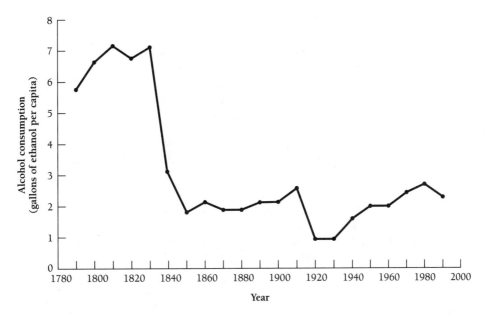

Figure 14.1 U.S. consumption of all alcoholic beverages, 1790–1993, ages 15 and older.
Source: From *The Alcoholic Republic: An American Tradition* (p. 9), by W. J. Rorabaugh, 1979, New York: Oxford University Press. Copyright © 1979 by Oxford University Press. Reprinted by permission. Also from *Ninth Special Report to the U.S. Congress on Alcohol and Health,* by NIAAA, 1997, Washington, DC: U.S. Government Printing Office.

thought about alcohol (Critchlow, 1986). An adamant and vocal minority came to consider liquor a "demon" and to totally abstain from its use. Similar attitudes arose in Britain (McMurran, 1994). This attitude was mostly limited to the upper and upper-middle classes. Later, abstention came to be an accepted doctrine of the middle class and people who aspired to join the middle class. Intemperance in drinking alcohol thus became associated with the lower classes, and "respectable" people, especially women, were expected not to be heavy drinkers.

Temperance societies proliferated throughout the United States during the mid-1800s. However, the term is a misnomer: The societies did not promote *temperance*—that is, the moderate use of alcohol. Rather, they advocated *prohibition,* the total abstinence from alcohol. Temperance societies held that liquor weakened inhibitions; loosened desires and passions; caused a large percentage

of crime, poverty, and broken homes; and was powerfully addicting, so much so that even an occasional drink would put one in danger. Figure 14.1 shows a dramatic decrease in per capita alcohol consumption in the United States after 1830, a decrease due directly to the spread of the temperance (prohibition) movement. Note also the more recent decline in consumption since about 1980.

In response to the growing temperance movement, both the demographics and the location of drinking changed. Drinking became associated with the lower and working classes. Rather than being consumed in a family setting or a respectable tavern, alcohol became increasingly confined to saloons, which were patronized largely by urban industrial workers (Popham, 1978). Portrayed by the temperance movement as the personification of evil and moral degeneracy, saloons served as a focus for growing Prohibitionist sentiment.

Prohibitionists were finally victorious in 1919 with the ratification of the 18th Amendment to the Constitution of the United States. This amendment outlawed the manufacture, sale, or transportation of alcoholic beverages and lowered per capita consumption drastically (as shown in Figure 14.1). This amendment was not popular and created a large illegal market for alcohol. The growing unpopularity of Prohibition resulted in the 21st Amendment, which repealed the 18th Amendment and ended Prohibition in 1934. Figure 14.1 shows that after the repeal of Prohibition, alcohol consumption rose sharply. Although the current per capita consumption of alcohol is considerably higher than during Prohibition, it is less than half the rate reached during the first 3 decades of the 19th century.

The Prevalence of Alcohol Consumption Today

About 50% of the adults in the United States are classified as current drinkers (defined as having at least one drink during the past 30 days), about 15% engage in binge drinking (five or more drinks on the same occasion at least once during the past 30 days), and a little more than 5% are heavy drinkers (five or more drinks on the same occasion on at least five different days during the past month) (U.S. Department of Health and Human Services [USDHHS], 1998c). These drinking rates—shown in Figure 14.2—continue a 20-year decline in alcohol consumption in the United States and are consistent with data indicating that per capita consumption of alcohol has dropped since 1980.

The frequency of drinking and the prevalence of heavy drinking are not equal for all demographic groups in the United States. Rather, drinking varies by ethnic background, age, gender, and educational level. European Americans tend to have higher rates of drinking than either African Americans or Hispanic Americans. About 55% of European Americans are current drinkers, whereas only 42% of Hispanic Americans and 40% of African Americans are classified as current drinkers. Among

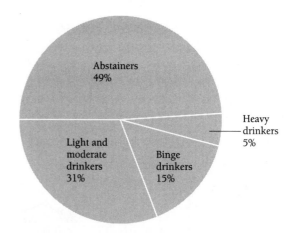

Figure 14.2 Alcohol consumption by type of drinker, adults, United States, 1997. Source: *Preliminary results from the 1997 National Household Survey on Drug Abuse* (DHHS publication No. SMA 98-3251), by U.S. Department of Health and Human Services (USDHHS), 1998, Washington, DC: U.S. Government Printing Office.

both European Americans and Hispanic Americans, about 16% of adults engage in binge drinking. However, only 10% of African American adults are binge drinkers. Hispanic Americans, despite having a significantly lower rate of drinking than European Americans, have a slightly higher rate of heavy drinking—6.3% to 5.7%. African Americans have the lowest rate of heavy drinking (3.8%), just as they have the lowest rate of current and binge drinking (USDHHS, 1998c).

Age is another factor in drinking. Adults age 21 to 39 have the highest rates of drinking, but young adults age 18 to 25 have the highest rates of binge drinking and heavy drinking. Nearly half of the drinkers age 18 to 25 are binge drinkers and about one in five are heavy drinkers (USDHHS, 1998c). Many of Chad's friends were binge drinkers and Chad, too, had several episodes of binge drinking during his earlier years at college. Binge drinking can lead to a variety of hazards (especially for inexperienced drinkers), such as intoxication, poor judgment, and impaired coordination. Certain situations promote binge drinking, and college students are at particular risk. Chad chose to binge drink on "special occasions," such as homecoming or after mid-term and final exams. One study of drinking at a college festival found that binge drinking was common and that legal drinking age had little impact on binge drinking (Corcoran, 1994). Indeed, heavy drinkers tend to hold an optimistic bias (Hansen, Raynor, & Wolkenstein, 1991), believing that their drinking is not likely to cause them problems.

Among adolescents 12 to 17, current use of alcohol dropped dramatically after the legal age for buying alcohol was raised to 21 in most states: In 1979, one half the adolescents in this age group were current users, but by 1992, only one of five were current drinkers, a rate that has remained relatively stable since 1992 (USDHHS, 1998c). Although binge drinking is still common among college and high school students, the percentage of students who engage in this drinking pattern is going down. Among male high school seniors, for example, binge drinking has declined from more than 50% during the early 1980s to less than 40% during the early 1990s. For female high school students, binge drinking also decreased by about 10 percentage points for this period—from a little over 30% to just above 20% (Cronk & Sarvela, 1997).

Why are young people drinking less? One possibility is that they are replacing alcohol with illicit drugs. However, the evidence for this hypothesis is somewhat mixed. A report by Lloyd Johnston and his colleagues (Johnston, O'Malley, & Bachman, 1998) showed only a slight or no increase in high school students' use of most illicit drugs from 1991 to 1997. However, during this same period, use of marijuana among high school students rose sharply, giving some support to the view that high school students may be replacing alcohol with marijuana.

Alcohol consumption rates are lowest among older adults (USDHHS, 1998c). This situation may be due more to heavy drinkers dying younger than to older drinkers moderating their drinking habits as they age. Indeed, studies that have followed the same people over time (NIAAA, 1988; Stall, 1986) have found only a small decrease in alcohol consumption as people become older.

Gender and educational level are also related to alcohol consumption. Compared with women, men are more likely to be current drinkers (58% to 45%), binge drinkers (23% to 8%), and heavy drinkers (9% to 2%) (USDHHS, 1998c). These percentages suggest that men have more problems with binge and heavy drinking than do women. Educational level is another predictor of drinking behavior. In Chapter 13, we saw that the more education people have, the less likely they are to smoke cigarettes. With alcohol, however, the reverse is true: The more years of schooling, the greater the likelihood that people drink alcohol. In 1997, more than two-thirds of college graduates were defined as current drinkers, whereas only 38% of people with less than a high school education were current drinkers. However, high school dropouts are just as likely as college graduates to be binge drinkers and more likely to be heavy drinkers (USDHHS, 1998c), suggesting either that college graduates drink more wisely than high school dropouts or that they are less honest in reporting their drinking habits.

In Summary

People have been consuming alcohol since before recorded history, and people have probably abused alcohol for almost as long. In most ancient societies—as well as modern societies—alcohol in moderation was condoned, but alcohol abuse and drunkenness were condemned.

Alcohol consumption per capita reached a peak in the United States during the first 3 decades of the 19th century. From about 1830 to 1850, consumption dropped dramatically due to the efforts of early prohibitionists. Presently, alcohol consumption in the United States is going down among nearly all ethnic and age groups. Only about 50% of adults are current drinkers, about 30% are light or moderate drinkers, 15% are binge drinkers, and 5% are heavy drinkers. European Americans have higher rates of alcohol consumption than Hispanic Americans and African Americans, adults 21 to 39 consume more than other age groups, and college graduates are much more likely to be drinkers than high school dropouts, who nevertheless are more likely to be heavy drinkers.

The Effects of Alcohol

Essentially the same thing happens to alcohol when you drink it as when you do not—it turns to vinegar (Goodwin, 1976). In the body, two enzymes turn alcohol into vinegar, or acetic acid. The first enzyme, **alcohol dehydrogenase**, is located in the liver and has no other known function except to metabolize alcohol. Alcohol dehydrogenase breaks down alcohol into aldehyde, a very toxic chemical. **Aldehyde dehydrogenase** converts aldehyde to acetic acid.

The process of metabolizing alcohol produces at least three health-related outcomes (1) an increase in lactic acid, which correlates with anxiety attacks; (2) an increase in uric acid, which causes gout; and (3) an increase of fat in the liver and in the blood.

The specific alcohol used in beverages is called **ethanol.** Like other alcohols, ethanol is a poison. But cases of alcohol poisoning are rare and almost always involve inexperienced drinkers who have drunk very large amounts of distilled liquor in a very short time, often on a "dare." Chad reported that "funneling," putting a funnel in someone's mouth and pouring liquor into the funnel, was sometimes practiced at his fraternity. This method of drinking can provide so much liquor so rapidly that it can be lethal. Otherwise, ingesting beverage alcohol is self-limiting: Intoxication usually yields to unconsciousness, preventing lethal poisoning.

Men and women are not equally affected by drinking alcohol. One factor is the difference in body weight; a 120-pound person is more strongly affected by three ounces of alcohol than a 220-pound person. But body weight is not the only factor. Women are more strongly affected by alcohol because of differences in the absorption of alcohol into the blood (Frezza et al., 1990), and these dif-

ferences may make women more vulnerable to the effects of alcohol regardless of body weight.

Among the problems associated with drinking are alcohol's ability to produce tolerance, dependence, withdrawal, and addiction. Although these concepts can be applied to many drugs, a consideration of the relevance to alcohol is necessary in evaluating alcohol's potential hazards.

Tolerance is a term applied to the effects of a drug when, with continued use, more and more of the drug is required to produce the same effect. Drugs with high tolerance potential are dangerous because people who build up tolerance need to take more of the drug to produce the effect they want and expect. If this amount is progressively larger, any dangerous effects or side effects of the drug become more of a hazard. Alcohol is a drug with generally moderate tolerance potential, but it seems to affect people differentially. For some, heavy use of alcohol for an extended period is required before noticeable tolerance begins to develop. For others, tolerance can develop within a week of moderate daily consumption. With increased tolerance comes an increased risk of the physical damage that alcohol can cause.

Dependence is separate from tolerance, and it too is a term that can be applied to many drugs. Dependence occurs when a drug becomes so incorporated into the functioning of the body's cells that it becomes necessary for "normal" functioning. If the drug is discontinued, the body's dependence on that drug becomes apparent and **withdrawal** symptoms develop. These symptoms are the body's signs that it is adjusting to functioning without the drug. Dependence and withdrawal are physically determined and are manifested in physical symptoms. Generally, withdrawal symptoms are the opposite of the drug's effects. Because alcohol is a depressant, withdrawal from it produces symptoms of restlessness, irritability, and agitation.

The combination of dependence and withdrawal is often described as **addiction.** Addictive drugs are those that produce dependence and, when discontinued, result in withdrawal. Many drugs produce notoriously unpleasant withdrawal, and alcohol is one of the worst. How difficult the process is depends on many factors, including the length of use and the degree of dependence. In some cases, withdrawal from alcohol can be life threatening, with mortality rates estimated as high as 5% to 10% (Lerner & Fallon, 1985). Usually, the first symptom to appear is tremor—the "shakes." Sleep difficulties are also common. In those severely addicted, **delirium tremens** occurs, with hallucinations and disorientation. Convulsions may also occur during withdrawal, a process that usually lasts between 2 days and a week. The physical dangers are so severe that the process is often completed in a special facility devoted to alcohol treatment.

Tolerance and dependence are independent properties. A drug may produce tolerance but not dependence; also, a person can develop dependence on a drug that has little or no tolerance potential. In addition, some drugs have both a tolerance and a dependence potential. Some research (Zinberg, 1984) even indicates that tolerance and dependence are not inevitable consequences of taking drugs. Not everyone who drinks alcohol does so with sufficient frequency and in sufficient quantity to develop a tolerance, and most drinkers do not become dependent.

Some people speak of "psychological" dependence, but this term has little scientific meaning beyond the notion that some activities, including drinking alcohol, become part of one's habitual manner of responding. Giving up the activity is accomplished only through much difficulty because the person has become habituated to it. Psychological dependence could be extended to many behaviors that are difficult to change, such as gambling, overeating, jogging, or even watching television.

Hazards of Alcohol

Alcohol produces a variety of hazards, both direct and indirect. *Direct hazards* are harmful physical effects due to alcohol itself, exclusive of any psy-

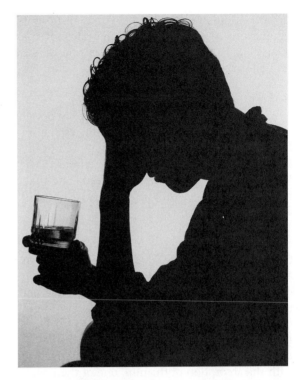

The indirect effects of alcohol pose more dangers than the direct physiological effects.

chological, social, or economic consequences. *Indirect hazards* include harmful consequences that result from psychological and physiological impairments produced by alcohol.

Direct Hazards   Although alcohol affects almost every organ system in the body, liver damage is the main health consideration for long-term, heavy drinkers. With heavy drinking (more than five or six drinks a day), fat accumulates in the liver, resulting in its enlargement. If this level of drinking continues, blood flow through the liver becomes blocked, liver cells die, and a form of hepatitis develops. The next stage is **cirrhosis**, the accumulation of nonfunctional scar tissue in the liver. Cirrhosis, an irreversible condition, is a major cause of death among alcoholics, yet not all alcoholics develop it. Moreover, people with no history of alcohol abuse may also develop liver cirrhosis (Gordon & Kannel, 1984), but cirrhosis is significantly associated with heavy alcohol use (Klatsky & Armstrong, 1992) and is one of the leading causes of death in the United States. For reasons not yet clearly understood, mortality from cirrhosis has steadily declined since 1973.

Chronic alcohol abuse is also a factor in developing several other disorders, including respiratory illness and severe neurological damage. Critically ill respiratory patients who are also chronic alcohol abusers have a much higher death rate than respiratory patients with no history of alcohol abuse (Moss, Bucher, Moore, Moore, & Parsons, 1996). Prolonged, heavy drinking is also implicated in the development of a neurological dysfunction called **Korsakoff syndrome** (also known as Wernicke-Korsakoff syndrome). Korsakoff syndrome is characterized by chronic cognitive impairment, severe memory problems for recent events, disorientation, and an inability to learn new information. Alcohol is related to the development of this syndrome through its interference with the absorption of thiamin, one of the B vitamins (Martin, Adinoff, Weingarter, Mukherjee, & Eckardt, 1986). Heavy drinkers can experience thiamin deficiency, which is worsened by their typically poor nutrition. Alcohol accelerates the progression of thiamin-related brain damage, and when this process has started, vitamin supplements do not reverse the progression. Moreover, most alcoholics do not receive treatment until the process is at an irreversible stage.

Although heavy, prolonged drinking is a risk factor for Korsakoff syndrome, light to moderate consumption does not seem to lead to cognitive impairment. Indeed, some research even suggests that older women may benefit cognitively from some daily intake of alcohol. Several studies (Hebert et al., 1993; Launer, Feskens, Kalmjin, & Kromhout, 1996) have found that low to moderate alcohol consumption among older people has no detrimental effect on such cognitive functions as immediate recall, word fluency, and memory for faces. A recent study from France (Dufouil, Ducimetiere, Apérovitch, 1997) found that men 49 to 71 years old who drank one to five or more

drinks a day suffered no increased cognitive impairment than a comparison group of abstainers. Surprisingly, when these researchers looked at women, they found that those who averaged up to four drinks per day had better overall cognitive scores than a comparable group of abstainers. Clearly, these puzzling results call for much more research on the effects of moderate alcohol consumption on cognitive abilities of older women and men.

Does alcohol contribute to the development of cancer? Research evidence on this issue is not entirely clear due to the confounding effects of cigarette smoking in many heavy alcohol users (Popham, Schmidt, & Israelstam, 1984), but prolonged drinking seems to be implicated in cancer of the liver, esophagus, nasopharynx, and larynx (Driver & Swann, 1987). In the Framingham study, deaths from all cancers were only slightly related to heavy consumption of alcohol in men and not at all related in women (Gordon & Kannel, 1984). No evidence from that study showed that light or moderate drinking significantly increased the chances of dying from cancer.

Alcohol presents some risk for breast cancer in women. Some inconsistency of results existed in early studies, in part because of relatively small sample size. Also, research from different countries has not produced consistent results. To evaluate the risk of alcohol on breast cancer, Stephanie Smith-Warner and her associates (Smith-Warner et al., 1998) conducted a pooled analysis of six large cohort studies. This analysis included more than 320,000 women in Canada, the Netherlands, Sweden, and the United States. Smith-Warner et al. found a very slight increase in breast cancer for women who consumed about one drink a day, but for those who drank about 2.5 drinks daily, the risk increased to about 40% above the risk for women who did not drink. This analysis was sufficiently large to determine that the type of drink— beer, wine, or liquor—made no difference. All were equally related to breast cancer; that is, women consuming two to five drinks a day of any alcoholic beverage had a relative risk for breast cancer of about 1.4. Interestingly, this analysis revealed no additional risk for women who drank more heavily, probably because the number of women who consume more than five drinks a day and who also develop breast cancer is not sufficient to detect any added risk.

Alcohol also affects the cardiovascular system, but the effects may not all be negative. (The next section looks at the possible positive effects of moderate alcohol consumption on cardiovascular functioning.) Heavy, chronic drinking, however, does have a direct and harmful effect on the cardiovascular system. In large doses, alcohol reduces oxidation of fatty acids (the heart's primary fuel source) in the myocardium. The heart directly metabolizes ethanol, producing fatty acid ethyl esters that impair functioning of the energy-producing structures of the heart. Alcohol also can depress the myocardium's ability to contract, which can lead to abnormal cardiac functioning. In addition, alcohol consumption is related to increased systolic blood pressure, especially among African American women and men, although this association may be due to high levels of stress that contribute both to alcohol consumption and to increased blood pressure (Curtis, James, Strogatz, Raghunathan, & Harlow, 1997).

Alcohol has a direct and hazardous effect on pregnancy and the developing fetus in two basic ways. First, very heavy alcohol consumption reduces fertility (Greenwood, Love, & Pratt, 1983). Several possible reasons exist for infertility in women who are chronic, heavy users of alcohol. Excessive alcohol consumption produces amenorrhea, cessation of the menstrual cycle, which may be caused either by cirrhosis or by a direct effect of alcohol on the pituitary or the hypothalamus. Another possible reason for infertility is vitamin deficiency, especially a lack of thiamin (Greenwood et al., 1983).

The second direct, hazardous effect of excessive drinking during pregnancy is that it increases the risk of **fetal alcohol syndrome** (FAS). FAS affects many infants of mothers who drank excessively during pregnancy. This syndrome includes specific facial abnormalities, growth deficiencies, central nervous system disorders, and mental retardation. The disorder has increased during recent years,

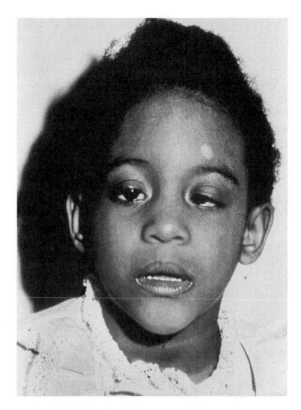

Facial abnormalities, growth deficiencies, central nervous system disorders, and mental retardation are symptoms of fetal alcohol syndrome.

climbing from an incidence of 1.0 per 10,000 births in 1979 to 6.7 per 10,000 births in 1993 (CDC, 1995). Although heavy drinking is the main contributor to fetal alcohol syndrome, heavy smoking, stress, and poor nutrition are also involved, and combinations of these factors are not unusual in heavy drinkers.

What about moderate and even light drinking during pregnancy? Light to moderate drinking is not likely to cause fetal alcohol syndrome, but significant decreases in cognitive functioning have been observed in children of mothers who drank three or more drinks per day during pregnancy (Larroque et al., 1995). Slightly less alcohol consumption by pregnant mothers can lead to other health problems for the child. For example, children born to women who average two drinks a day have a lower average birth weight, and this condition, although not itself a danger, is related to many risks for newborns. Also, women who drink as little as four drinks a week show an increased risk of spontaneous abortion. Children of women who drank moderately during pregnancy showed somewhat slower reaction times and greater distractibility (Streissguth, Barr, Kogan, & Bookstein, 1996). Even small amounts of alcohol, especially during the early months of pregnancy, have a direct and hazardous effect on the developing fetus, at least for many women (Coles, Smith, Lancaster, & Falek, 1987).

Indirect Hazards In addition to these direct physiological damages, alcohol consumption is associated with several indirect hazards. Most of the indirect dangers arise from alcohol's effects on aggression, judgment, and attention. Alcohol also affects coordination and alters cognitive functioning in ways that contribute to increased chances of unintentional injury not only to the drinker but also to nondrinkers who live with a drinker (Rivara et al., 1997).

The most frequent and serious indirect hazard of alcohol consumption is the increased likelihood of unintentional injuries, the fifth leading cause of death in the United States and the leading cause of death for people under age 45. A dose-response relationship exists between alcohol consumption and unintentional fatal injuries; that is, the greater the number of drinks consumed per occasion, the greater the incidence of fatalities from unintentional injuries. People who consume five or more drinks per occasion are about twice as likely to die from unintentional injuries as people who drink fewer than five drinks per occasion, and people who consume nine or more drinks are more than three times as likely to die from injuries (Anda, Williamson, & Remington, 1988).

Motor vehicle crashes account for the largest number of alcohol-related fatalities. In the United States, more than 40,000 people die each year from injuries resulting from motor vehicle crashes, and about 40% of those deaths (about 16,000 per year) are related to alcohol-impaired

driving (Liu et al., 1997). A recent self-report survey of adults in 49 states and the District of Columbia (Liu et al., 1997) found that alcohol-impaired driving was most frequent among young men 21 to 34 years old, but it was almost as common among men 18 to 20 who were not yet old enough to purchase alcohol legally. The survey also found that European Americans were most likely to report incidences of driving after drinking, followed by Hispanic Americans and African Americans in that order.

Alcohol consumption can also lead to more aggressive behavior for some drinkers. Both laboratory experiments and crime statistics have shown a relationship between alcohol and aggression. A review of laboratory studies (Taylor & Leonard, 1983) concluded that moderate and high doses of alcohol produce aggression in about 30% of drinkers. In a naturalistic situation, both a threat of harm and actual physical injury can prompt aggression among heavy drinkers (Taylor, Gammon, & Capasso, 1976). In addition, people exposed to others who urge aggression (as opposed to restraint) are more likely to act aggressively (Taylor & Leonard, 1983). Aggression, therefore, is not an inevitable or simple consequence of the pharmacological effects of alcohol but rather a response that may occur in certain situations and with certain individuals.

Similarly, alcohol may increase crime, at least in some cases. Two early studies (Mayfield, 1976; Wolfgang, 1957) on the relationship between alcohol and crime indicated that either the victim or the offender or both had been drinking in two-thirds of the homicides studied. Not only are people who commit homicides likely to be drinking, but consuming alcohol also relates to increased chances of being a crime victim. These relationships, however, do not demonstrate a *causal* relationship between alcohol and crime. In addition, the majority of crimes are committed by people who are *not* alcohol dependent, and the majority of alcohol abusers do *not* commit crimes.

Chad and his fraternity brothers were aware of the possible injuries that might result from binge drinking. They tried not to drive while drunk and to take care of each other, but they did not designate a nondrinking driver. Instead, the designated driver role fell to the least intoxicated person. The fraternity members were not exempt from hazards; one member was killed in an automobile crash and one committed suicide while drinking and playing Russian roulette. Chad says that these tragedies did not slow the rate of drinking in the fraternity.

Finally, drinking alcohol can influence people's decision-making ability in sexual situations. Problem drinkers (Avins et al., 1994) and non-problem drinkers (Stall, McKusick, Wiley, Coates, & Ostrow, 1986) both tend to be less likely to use safe sex procedures when they drink alcohol. Also, high school students who use alcohol, compared with those with no substance use, tend to have more sexual partners and to be less likely to use condoms (Lowry et al., 1994). (We discussed alcohol-related unsafe sex practices more fully in Chapter 11.)

Benefits of Alcohol

Is it possible that drinking might be *good* for you? This question was raised as a result of several early studies (Room & Day, 1974; Stason, Neff, Miettinen, & Jick, 1976) that reported a U-shaped or J-shaped relationship between alcohol consumption and mortality. In other words, light to moderate drinkers (one to five drinks per day) had the best prospects for good health, whereas nondrinkers and heavy drinkers had the greatest risk. Later evidence from several longitudinal studies supported the findings that light or moderate drinking was positively related to both reduced mortality and lower risk of disease. These early studies prompted further research, which has consistently found some health benefits for light to moderate levels of alcohol consumption.

Reduced Mortality A group of researchers (Klatsky, Friedman, & Siegelaub, 1981) at the Kaiser-Permanente health facility conducted a longitudinal study of alcohol and mortality. This study followed more than 2,000 European American and African American men and women for 10 years and charted their mortality rates in relation to their drinking habits. The participants were divided into four groups: (1) nondrinkers, (2) those reporting two or fewer drinks per day, (3) those reporting three to five drinks per day, and (4) those reporting more than six drinks per day. Light drinkers (those reporting two or fewer drinks per day) had the lowest mortality rate. Nondrinkers had a mortality rate comparable to that of moderate drinkers, and both had mortality rates 50% higher than those of the light drinkers. Heavy drinkers (people who reported drinking over six drinks per day) fared worst, with a mortality rate double that for light drinkers. Cancer, cirrhosis, accidents, and respiratory conditions all contributed to this increase in mortality.

Additional research in studies of both the general population and selected populations has confirmed that drinking can be beneficial. The Alameda County study (Berkman, Breslow, & Wingard, 1983), the Framingham study (Friedman & Kimball, 1986), a study conducted in Australia (Cullen, Knuimon, & Ward, 1993), and another report from Japan (Kitamura et al., 1998) found that moderate-drinking men had a survival advantage, although the relationship for women was not so clear. However, a study of female nurses (whose drinking habits were similar to those of U.S. women in general) showed that compared with nondrinkers, women who consumed 3½ to 18 drinks per week had a reduced risk of death, especially from cardiovascular disease (Fuchs et al., 1995). Women who drank more than 18 drinks per week, however, had an increased risk of death from other causes, such as breast cancer and cirrhosis.

The decrease in mortality associated with drinking seems to be due to decreases in coronary heart disease rather than stroke (Maclure, 1993), although some recent research (Sacco et al., 1999) has found that up to two drinks a day can cut one's risk for stroke in half. Until recently, a U-shaped relationship has generally emerged between amount of alcohol consumed and likelihood of death from all cardiovascular diseases; that is, abstainers and very heavy drinkers were at greatest risk, whereas light and moderate drinkers had the lowest rate of death from cardiovascular disease. Another study (Rehm, Bondy, Sempos, & Vuong, 1997) showed that men were protected from heart disease and death from heart disease by light, moderate *and* heavy drinking. Only after consumption rose above 42 drinks a week were these men at a greater risk than were abstainers. This and other reports strongly suggest that moderate consumption of alcoholic beverages can reduce one's risk of death, especially from coronary heart disease.

Does the type of alcoholic drink make a difference for mortality risk? Because some early research indicated that wine—and specifically red wine—protected people from cardiovascular disease, some physicians have recommended wine but not beer or spirits to their patients. However, there is limited evidence to suggest that wine has any special properties beyond those offered by ethanol itself. A number of recent studies (Marques-Vidal, Ducimetiere, Evans, Campou, & Arveiler, 1996; Parker et al., 1996; Rehm et al., 1997) have found no differences in type of alcohol, suggesting no particular advantage for wine over beer and liquor.

What factors could account for this negative relationship between light to moderate levels of drinking and coronary heart disease? Several suggestions have been made, but the most likely explanation involves high-density lipoprotein (HDL). Specific subfractions of high-density lipoprotein known as HDL_2 and HDL_3 are negatively associated with coronary heart disease. If consumption of alcohol contributes specifically to the elevation of HDL_2 and HDL_3, then moderate or heavy drinking should offer protection against heart disease. Several reports (Gaziano et al., 1993; Linn et al., 1993) have indicated that drinking is related to elevations of HDL and to decreased risk for heart attack.

Increases in HDL may not be the only means by which alcohol consumption protects against heart disease. One study (Jackson, Scragg, & Beaglehole, 1992) found that even recent consumption of alcohol tends to protect against heart attack; that is, people who had consumed alcohol during the past 24 hours had a lower risk of both fatal and nonfatal heart attack than those who had not drunk alcohol. Because HDL levels cannot increase so rapidly, this finding indicated that some other mechanism also contributes to alcohol's protective qualities. Alcohol may also protect against blood clots (Ridker, Vaughan, Stampfer, Glynn, & Hennekens, 1994), thus guarding against heart attacks. Furthermore, this protective factor changes quickly, providing some protection against heart attack within hours of consumption (Ridker et al., 1994).

In summary, the reduced mortality associated with light to moderate levels of drinking is largely attributable to decreased coronary heart disease fatalities, which offsets other sources of mortality, such as cirrhosis and accidents. The decrease in CHD mortality seems to be due to increases in high-density lipoprotein and possibly to decreased tendency to form internal blood clots.

Other Benefits of Alcohol   If moderate drinking has a beneficial effect on mortality rates, could it also be related to better health? Investigators in the Alameda County study (Camacho & Wiley, 1983) found that moderate alcohol consumption (17 to 45 drinks per month) was most closely associated with good health scores. Abstention was negatively related to subsequent health, and heavy drinkers, especially women, reported somewhat lower health scores than the average. However, heavy drinkers were not as unhealthy as the nondrinkers, suggesting that drinking is related to overall physical health.

People who drink may also have better mental health than those who abstain due to the buffering effects of drinking on stress. Some evidence shows that drinkers who are under stress are less likely to be depressed than abstainers under similar stress (Lipton, 1994). However, a U-shaped relationship seems to exist between drinking and depression, so people who drink heavily have higher levels of depression than light and moderate drinkers (Lipton, 1994).

In addition, alcohol may increase bone mineral density in both women and men and thus provide some protection against bone fractures. The Framingham study, (Felson, Zhang, Hannan, Kannel, & Kiel, 1995) looked at alcohol consumption in a group of older people and found that women who drank seven or more ounces of alcohol per week had higher bone mineral density than women who were light drinkers or nondrinkers. For men, consumption of 14 ounces or more per week was associated with higher bone mineral density, although the difference for men was not as great as it was for women. Lesser amounts of alcohol intake did not improve levels of bone mineral density (Felson et al., 1995).

The conclusion is that drinkers not only have a lower mortality rate than abstainers but are sick less often, are less depressed, and have stronger bones is controversial (see box, Would You Believe . . . ?)

In Summary

Alcohol consumption has both harmful and beneficial effects on one's personal health. In addition, it has some negative indirect effects on society that reach beyond an individual's physical health. The direct hazards of prolonged and heavy drinking include cirrhosis of the liver and a brain dysfunction called Korsakoff syndrome. In addition, some evidence suggests that alcohol may contribute to the development of some cancers. Also, heavy drinking during pregnancy increases the risk of fetal alcohol syndrome, a serious disorder that often includes growth deficiencies and severe mental retardation. In addition, alcohol is a risk factor for many types of violence, both criminal and accidental. The level of alcohol consumption necessary to increase the risk is not as high as the level necessary to produce legal intoxication, but the more heavily people drink the more likely they will be involved in accidents and violent crimes. Finally, alcohol consumption may also lead to poor decisions regarding sexual behavior.

The principal positive aspect of alcohol consumption is its buffering effect against mortality and morbidity from heart disease, probably by increasing HDL and possibly by reducing blood clotting. Other benefits of light to moderate drinking may include lower levels of depression and increased bone mineral density.

Why Do People Drink?

Those trying to understand drinking and alcohol abuse have proposed several models to explain behavior related to alcohol consumption. These models go beyond the pharmacological effects of alcohol and even beyond the research findings to integrate and explain drinking. To be useful, a model for drinking behavior must address at least three questions. First, why do people start drinking? Second, why do most people maintain moderate rather than excessive drinking levels? Third, why do some drink so much as to develop serious problems?

Until the 19th century, drinking was well accepted in the United States and Europe but drunkenness was unacceptable under most circumstances. This attitude makes drinking the norm, thus requiring no explanation for it, but leaves drunkenness unexplained. Two models have been proposed to explain drunkenness: the moral model and the disease model (McMurran, 1994).

The moral model appeared first, holding that people have free will and choose their behaviors, including excessive drinking. Those who do so are, thus, either sinful or morally lacking in the self-discipline necessary to moderate their drinking. The moral model of alcoholism began to fade in the late 19th century, when the medical model started to gain prominence. Unacceptable behaviors that were formerly seen as moral problems became medical problems and thus subject to scientific explanation and medical treatment. The medical model of alcoholism conceptualized problem drinking as symptomatic of underlying physical problems, and the notion that alcoholism is hereditary grew from this view. The first form of this hypothesis took the view that a "constitutional

WOULD YOU BELIEVE...?

What Your Doctor Never Told You about Alcohol

Would you believe that drinking may be good for you, but health care professionals are reluctant to admit it? Addiction authority Stanton Peele (1993) contended that medical investigators, public health officials, and health educators are uneasy about research findings concerning alcohol's beneficial health effects. He suggested that the United States has been so influenced by what he called the "temperance mentality" that medical authorities have trouble accepting their own findings about alcohol. "A cultural preoccupation with alcoholism and the negative effects of drinking works against frank scientific discussions in the United States of the advantages for the cardiovascular system of alcohol consumption" (Peele, 1993, p. 805).

Medical authorities have spent so much time forming arguments for the negative effects of alcohol that they have trouble acknowledging that it might also have positive effects. For example, Shari Linn and her colleagues (1993) studied a representative sample of the U.S. population to determine the relationship between high-density lipoprotein (HDL) and alcohol consumption. They found such a relationship for both European Americans and African Americans even after controlling for other factors that influence HDL. These researchers were left with the finding that drinking increases HDL, which has been shown to relate to lowered cardiovascular risk. However, they did not conclude that people at risk for heart disease should increase their alcohol consumption. Instead they said, "Even if there is a causal association between alcohol consumption and higher HDL cholesterol levels, it is suggested that efforts to reduce coronary heart disease risks concentrate on the cessation of smoking and weight control" (Linn et al., 1993, p. 811). In making these conclusions, they ignored their own findings.

Peele contended that the negative effects of alcohol dominate discussions at professional conferences and meetings. Researchers—often despite their own research findings—are eager to condemn and reluctant to recommend drinking, an obvious bias among these scientists. No official medical organization in the United States has made a recommendation concerning the positive effects of drinking alcohol. Peele pointed out that the benefits of light to moderate drinking are similar to those obtained by following a low-fat diet in decreasing the risk for coronary heart disease, yet many medical groups have made official statements concerning the wisdom of adopting a low-fat diet, and none have recommended moderate drinking.

The first official statement about the benefits of light drinking came in 1996 from a joint committee of the Agriculture Department and the Department of Health and Human Services (Nestle, 1997). The acknowledgment that light drinking may lower the risk of heart disease appears in the 1996 version of the *Dietary Guidelines for Americans,* but these guidelines continue to caution against drinking other than with meals and more than one drink per day for women and two for men.

Scientific evidence accumulated during the 1980s suggesting that moderate drinking might improve cardiovascular disease risk, but recommendation against drinking continued in the 1990 revision of the *Guidelines* due to the personal beliefs of the Surgeon General and the pressure brought on him by organizations opposed to drinking (Nestle, 1997). The changes in the *Guidelines* came about as a result of mounting scientific evidence and political pressure, this time from the liquor industry. This pressure was fueled by the "French paradox," the lower level of cardiovascular disease in France despite a high-fat diet, and the benefits were allegedly due to drinking red wine. As we have seen, however, red wine has no particular advantage over any other type of alcohol as a protection against cardiovascular disease (Marques-Vidal et al, 1996; Nestle, 1997; Parker et al., 1996; Rehm et al. 1997).

The current version of the dietary *Guidelines* allows for the possibility that drinking can be a positive health habit, but the move from Prohibition to moderation has not occurred throughout the medical establishment.

weakness" ran in families and that this weakness produced alcoholics.

Problem drinking does run in families, but the relative contributions of heredity and environment remain unknown. Most authorities agree that both genetic and environmental influences play a role in shaping alcohol abuse. Children of problem drinkers are more likely than children of nonproblem drinkers to abuse alcohol as well as other drugs (USDHHS, 1997). These children grow up in an environment marked by marital discord, tolerance for early initiation of alcohol use, and lack of parental warmth and communication. Such an environment combined with an inherited vulnerability for alcohol abuse greatly increases a child's likelihood of becoming a problem drinker (USDHHS, 1997). However, most children reared in this type of environment are resilient enough to resist those environmental effects and do not become problem drinkers (Ohannessian, Stabenau, & Hesselbrock, 1995). How can investigators learn about the relative effects of environment and heredity on the development of problem drinking?

To determine the contribution of genetic factors, researchers typically study either twins or adopted children or both. Twin studies ordinarily involve measuring the degree of agreement between pairs of identical twins, with comparisons in the amount of agreement between pairs of fraternal twins. If identical twins are more similar to each other than fraternal twins are, the difference is assumed to be due to genetics. Indeed, research (USDHHS, 1997) generally shows a closer concordance of problem drinking for identical twins than for fraternal twins. This greater concordance between identical twins supports the idea of at least some genetic component in alcohol abuse.

A second test of a hereditary factor in alcohol abuse is the study of adopted children. Adoption studies investigate the frequency of alcohol abuse in adoptees one of whose biological parents was alcoholic. Donald Goodwin and his colleagues (Goodwin, Schulsinger, Hermansen, Guze, & Winokur, 1973) conducted such a study in Denmark and found some support for a hereditary component for alcoholism, but questions concerning the definition and diagnosis criteria have resulted in less than clear support.

Studies in Sweden with adopted men (Cloninger, Bohman, & Sigvardsson, 1981) and adopted women (Bohman, Sigvardsson, & Cloninger, 1981) showed that men with both an environmental and a genetic risk had the greatest likelihood of developing either mild or severe drinking problems. However for men with moderate drinking problems, genetics was clearly more influential than social factors. These studies suggest that understanding the relative influence of biological, psychological, and social factors for alcohol abuse is a complex problem, with few clear-cut answers. All these influences play a role, and the people most likely to become alcohol dependent are those who are at risk for each of these factors (Begleiter & Kissin, 1996).

Like many personal characteristics, alcohol dependence is a complex issue, with no easy answers regarding its genetic components. Stanton Peele (1993) warned against accepting a simple version of hereditary influences on drinking:

> Whatever people may inherit that heightens susceptibility to alcoholism operates over years as a part of the long-term development of alcohol dependence. Moreover, a large majority of children of alcoholics do not become alcoholic, and the majority of alcoholics do not have alcoholic parents. (p. 809)

The Disease Model

The disease concept of alcoholism is a variation of the medical model, holding that people with problem drinking have the disease of alcoholism. Throughout history, isolated attempts have been made to describe alcohol intoxication as a disease brought about by the physical properties of alcohol, but not until the late 1930s and early 1940s did this view begin to become popular. In psychiatric and other medically oriented treatment programs in the United States, the disease model still predominates, but it is less influential in psychologically based treatment programs and in treatment programs in Europe and in Australia.

The disease model of alcoholism was elevated to scientific respectability by the pioneering work of E. M. Jellinek (1960), who identified several different types of alcoholism and described various characteristics of these types. The two most common types are **gamma alcoholism**, or loss of control once drinking begins, and **delta alcoholism**, or the inability to abstain. Jellinek's disease model, however, has been criticized as being too restrictive and simplistic (Edwards, 1977).

The Alcohol Dependency Syndrome Dissatisfaction with Jellinek's disease model led Griffith Edwards and his colleagues (Edwards, 1977; Edwards & Gross, 1976; Edwards, Gross, Keller, Moser, & Room, 1977) to advocate the alcohol dependency syndrome, which rejects the term *alcoholism* and the notion that problem drinking is a disease. The word *syndrome* adds flexibility to the disease model by suggesting a group of concurrent behaviors that accompany alcohol dependence. The behaviors need not always be observed in an individual, nor do they need to be observable to the same degree in everyone who is alcohol dependent. Edwards and his colleagues modified several of Jellinek's concepts, including the notion that alcoholics experience loss of control. Rather, the alcohol dependency syndrome holds that those who are alcohol dependent have *impaired control*, suggesting that people drink heavily because, at certain times and for a variety of reasons, they do not exercise control over their drinking.

Edwards and Milton Gross (1976) described seven essential elements of the alcohol dependency syndrome. First is a *narrowing of drinking repertoire*, suggesting that a person tends to drink the same beverage the same time of day and the same day of the week. Second is a *salience of drink-seeking behavior*, meaning that drinking begins to take priority over all other aspects of life. A third element of the alcohol dependency syndrome is *increased tolerance*. As noted earlier, alcohol does not produce as much

tolerance as do some other drugs, but some drinkers gradually become accustomed to going about their daily routine "at blood alcohol levels that would incapacitate the non-tolerant drinker" (Edwards & Gross, 1976, p. 1059).

A fourth element of the alcohol dependency syndrome is *withdrawal symptoms*. As previously mentioned, the severity of withdrawal depends on length and amount of use. Those who are alcohol dependent *avoid withdrawal symptoms by further drinking*, the fifth characteristic of the alcohol dependency syndrome. A mildly dependent person might relieve the morning "blues" by having a drink with lunch, but some drinkers use the strategy of avoiding withdrawal symptoms by maintaining a steady alcohol level.

The sixth element is the *subjective awareness of the compulsion to drink*. The final element of the alcohol dependency syndrome is *reinstatement of dependence after abstinence*. Edwards and Gross believe that time of reinstatement is inversely related to the degree of dependence. Moderately dependent people may not reinstate drinking for months, whereas severely dependent patients may resume full dependence in as little as 3 days.

Evaluation of the Disease Model Despite the continuing popularity of the disease model of alcoholism, only limited empirical evidence supports the concept. Moreover, this model fails to address our first two questions: "Why do people begin to drink?" and "Why do some people continue to drink at a moderate level?" One key concept in the disease model is loss of control or impaired control—the inability to stop or moderate alcohol intake once drinking begins. Research has not supported this key concept. G. Alan Marlatt and his colleagues (Marlatt, Demming, & Reid, 1973; Marlatt & Rohsenow, 1980) conducted experiments suggesting that many effects of alcohol, including impaired control, are due more to expectancy than to any pharmacological effect of alcohol. Their experimental design, called the *balanced placebo design*, included four groups, two of which expected to be given alcohol and two of

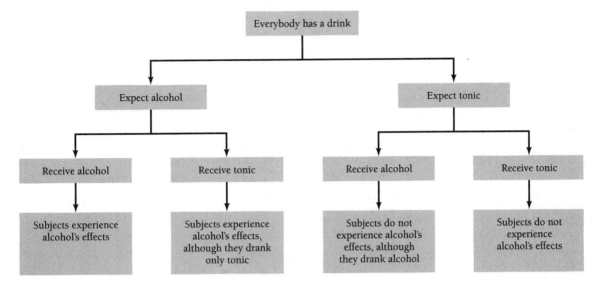

Figure 14.3 Balanced placebo design.

which did not. Two groups actually received alcohol, and two did not. Figure 14.3 shows all four combinations.

Using the balanced placebo design, several studies (Marlatt et al., 1973; Marlatt & Rohsenow, 1980) showed that people who think they have received alcohol behave as though they have (whether they have or not). Even for those who had been in treatment for problem drinking, expectancy appeared to be the controlling factor in the craving for alcohol and in the amount consumed. These findings suggest that loss of control and craving for alcohol result from expectancy rather than from some physical property of alcohol. This well-controlled study did not provide support for the disease model of alcoholism.

Some investigators (Marlatt, 1987; McMurran, 1994) have criticized the disease model of alcohol, arguing that it does not adequately consider environmental, cognitive, and affective determinants of abusive drinking; that is, in its emphasis on the physical properties of alcohol, the disease model neglects the cognitive and social learning aspects of drinking.

Cognitive-Physiological Theories

Several alternatives to the disease model emphasize the combination of physiological and cognitive changes that occur with alcohol use. Rather than hypothesizing that alcohol use and misuse are based only on the chemical properties of alcohol, these models contend that alcohol use also depends on the cognitive changes experienced by drinkers.

The Tension Reduction Hypothesis   As the name suggests, the tension reduction hypothesis (Conger, 1956) holds that people drink alcohol because of its tension-reducing effects. This hypothesis has much intuitive appeal because alcohol is a sedative drug that leads to relaxation and slowed reactions.

However, alcohol's effects on physiological processes are not simple (Levenson, Sher, Grossman, Newman, & Newlin, 1980). Moderate doses of alcohol stimulate some responses (such as heart rate); other responses (such as pulse wave velocity, a measurement that relates to the heart muscle's ability to contract) become slower, and yet other responses (such as skeletal muscle tension) remain unaffected. Such a complex pattern of physiological responses does not support a simple version of the tension reduction hypothesis.

Studies that have manipulated tension or anxiety to observe their effects on participants' readiness to consume alcohol have yielded contradictory results. No relationship appeared in one study (Higgins & Marlatt, 1973) that measured the relationship between the threat of a painful shock and subsequent amount of alcohol consumed, but a later study (Higgins & Marlatt, 1975) found that male participants who expected to be evaluated by a woman on the basis of their looks (and thus were considered to be anxious) drank more than those participants who expected no such evaluation.

A longitudinal study (Rohsenow, 1982) of men who were heavy social drinkers found social anxiety to be negatively related to drinking; that is, the *less* socially anxious the participants were, the more they drank. This study also found that men who had social support for their drinking were the ones who tended to drink most heavily. Thus, men may drink to attain a positive mood rather than to avoid a negative state of tension.

A review of some of these same studies found no support for the tension reduction hypothesis (Wilson, 1987). These studies showed that alcohol may increase, decrease, or have no effect on tension in both social drinkers and problem drinkers. In addition, situational variables other than the alcohol itself may reduce tension. For example, in the social setting of a familiar bar, some men may feel less shy about approaching women. In the same setting, some women experience increased tension and react defensively to sexual advances. Social learning history may determine the degree of relaxation in many social situations.

Although the original version of the tension reduction hypothesis has found little support, a reformulation of this view seems to be more viable. A group of researchers at Indiana University (Levenson et al., 1980; Sher, 1987; Sher & Levenson, 1982) discovered that high levels of alcohol consumption decrease the strength of responses to stress. They labeled this decrease the **stress-response-dampening (SRD)** effect. People who had been drinking did not respond as strongly as nondrinking participants to either physiological or psychological stressors. Interestingly, people whose personality profile suggested a high risk of developing problem drinking showed the strongest SRD effect, and those whose profile indicated a low risk showed a weaker effect (Sher & Levenson, 1982). These results suggest that rather than reducing tension, alcohol may cause some people to avoid tension.

The Self-Awareness Model A second approach, proposed by Jay Hull, is based on social psychological theories of self-awareness (Hull, 1981, 1987; Hull & Bond, 1986). Hull built a model of drinking behavior on the observation that alcohol consumption indirectly affects behavior through changes in cognitive processes. He then hypothesized that alcohol can interfere with cognition to make thought more superficial and to decrease negative self-feedback. Negative self-feedback consists of statements such as "I can't do anything very well" or "I shouldn't be such a coward." By making cognitions more superficial, alcohol enables people either to reduce or to avoid these kinds of tension-producing self-statements and thus to think better of themselves than when they are not drinking.

Hull's explanation of drinking is therefore based on changes in self-awareness. By inhibiting the use of normal, complex information-processing strategies, such as memory and information acquisition, drinking makes people less self-aware. Decreased self-awareness leads to decreased monitoring of behavior, resulting in the disinhibition that commonly occurs among drinkers.

The self-awareness model also proposes the idea that drinkers become less self-critical as they become less self-aware because they fail to process information that reflects badly on them. Hull (1987) hypothesized that this effect may be the reason why some people consume alcohol—to avoid self-awareness. Reduced self-awareness might also be rewarding through decreased self-censure for inappropriate (but personally attractive) social behavior. Therefore, loss of self-awareness can offer some rewards, which explains why people drink and why some people drink unwisely. What this model fails to elaborate is who will fall into each category.

Alcohol Myopia Claude Steele and his colleagues (Steele & Josephs, 1990) have developed a model of alcohol use and abuse based on alcohol's psychological and physical properties. This model hypothesizes that alcohol use creates effects on social behaviors that produce *alcohol myopia*, a type of shortsightedness in which alcohol blocks out insightful cognitive processing and alters thoughts related to the self, stress, and social anxiety. That is, "Alcohol makes us the captive of an impoverished version of reality in which the breadth, depth, and time line of our understanding is constrained" (Steele & Josephs, 1990, p. 923).

Part of alcohol myopia is drunken excess, the tendency for those who drink to behave more excessively. This tendency appears as increased aggression, friendliness, sexiness, and many other exaggerated behaviors. Tendencies to behave in such extreme ways are usually inhibited, but when people drink, they experience less inhibition, and their behavior becomes more extreme.

Another aspect of alcohol myopia is self-inflation, a tendency to inflate self-evaluations. When asked to rate the importance of 35 trait dimensions for their real and ideal selves, drunk participants rated themselves higher on traits that were important to them and on which they had rated themselves low when sober (Banaji & Steele. 1989). Thus, drinking allowed participants to see themselves in a better light than they did when they were not drinking, confirming the ability of alcohol to inflate a person's self evaluation.

A third aspect of alcohol myopia is "drunken relief" (Steele & Josephs, 1990, p. 928); that is, people who drink tend to worry less and pay less attention to their worries. When consumed in large quantities, alcohol alone may produce drunken relief, but in smaller quantities and combined with distracting activity, it can also produce a powerful stress reduction effect. People who combine the effects of alcohol with a pleasant distraction can experience a significant relief from anxiety, but neither alcohol by itself nor a pleasant distraction by itself appears to bring about the same level of anxiety relief (Steele, Southwick, & Pagano, 1986). Therefore, drunken relief is not entirely an effect of alcohol but of alcohol in combination with other factors in the social environment that provide distraction.

The Social Learning Model

Many psychologists accept the social learning model as the most useful explanation for why people begin to drink, why they continue to drink in moderation, and why some people drink in a harmful manner (Abrams & Niaura, 1987). Social learning theory conceives of drinking as learned behavior, acquired in the same manner as other behaviors.

According to social learning theory, people begin to drink for at least three reasons. First, the taste of alcohol and its immediate effects may bring pleasure (positive reinforcement); second, a person may have decided earlier that drinking alcohol is consistent with personal standards (cognitive mediation); and third, the person may learn to drink by observing others (modeling). Any one or a combination of these factors is sufficient to initiate and guide drinking behavior. Social learning was a prominent feature of drinking for Chad. He began to drink with his friends and continued to drink in the company of fraternity brothers who also drank. Now that he is not around his fraternity friends so much, he drinks less.

The social learning model also offers three explanations for why people drink too much. First, excessive drinking may serve as a coping response; that is, the initial effect of small doses may be interpreted by drinkers as enhancement of their ability to cope. This response can give drinkers a sense of power and also a feeling of avoiding responsibility or minimizing stress. People then continue to drink as long as they perceive that alcohol has desirable effects.

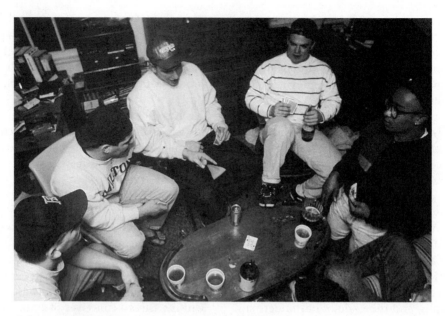

College social gatherings may encourage binge drinking.

Second, drinkers tend to adjust their level of alcohol according to the amounts they see others consuming. Evidence indicates that people who observe a heavy-drinking model will consume more alcohol than those who observe a light-drinking model or no model at all (Caudill & Marlatt, 1975), Thus, modeling can explain both the initiation of drinking and the tendency of some people to drink to excess.

A fourth explanation for excessive drinking offered by the social learning model is based on the principles of negative reinforcement. Most heavy drinkers have learned that they can avoid or reduce the painful effects of withdrawal symptoms by maintaining blood alcohol concentrations at a particular level. As this level begins to drop, the alcohol addict feels the discomfort of withdrawal. These symptoms can be avoided by ingesting more alcohol; thus, negative reinforcement increases the probability that heavy drinking will continue.

Social learning theory provides an explanation for why people start drinking, why some continue to drink in moderation, and why others become problem drinkers. In addition, social learning the-

ory also suggests a variety of treatment techniques to help people overcome excessive drinking habits. Because drinking behavior is learned, it can be unlearned or relearned, with either abstinence or moderation as a goal of therapy.

In Summary

The question of why people drink has three components: (1) Why do people begin drinking? (2) Why do some people drink in moderation? (3) Why do others drink to excess? Theories of drinking behavior should be able to offer explanations for each of these questions. This section discussed three theories or models, each of which offers a partial explanation. The *disease model* assumes that people drink excessively because they have the disease of alcoholism. One variation of the disease model—the alcohol dependency syndrome—assumes that alcohol dependent people have impaired control and drink heavily for a variety of reasons. Cognitive-physiological models, including the *tension reduction hypothesis,* the *self-awareness model,* and *alcohol myopia,* propose that people drink because alcohol produces alterations in cognitive function that allow people to escape tension and negative self-evaluations. *Social learning theory* assumes that people acquire drinking behavior in the same manner in which they learn other behaviors—that is, through positive or negative reinforcement, modeling, and cognitive mediation. All three models offer some explanation of why some people continue to drink, but none of them has a satisfactory explanation for why some people can drink in moderation and others abuse alcohol.

Changing Problem Drinking

Despite a recent and steady decline in the percentage of drinkers in the United States, an increasing number of people seek help for problem drinking, with nearly a million people receiving treatment on any given day (Rouse, 1998). People between ages 25 and 44 are the most likely to seek treatment, and men outnumber women by a ratio of 3 to 1 (USDHHS, 1997). However, the disproportion may be partially a result of women's greater tendency to seek help in non-alcohol-specific settings, such as mental health-treatment services (Weisner & Schmidt, 1992). Five out of six people who receive treatment do so on an outpatient rather than inpatient basis (USDHHS, 1997). Although private, for-profit facilities emphasize inpatient treatment, these programs are eight times more costly than outpatient treatment (Hayashida et al., 1989). In addition to the various treatment settings, a majority of alcoholics are able to quit drinking without formal treatment (McMurran, 1994; Sobell, Cunningham, & Sobell, 1996).

Change without Therapy

Some problems (and even some diseases) disappear without formal treatment, and problem drinking is no exception. When a disease disappears without treatment, the term spontaneous remission is used to describe the cure. Many authorities in the field of problem drinking do not accept the term *spontaneous remission;* they prefer the term *unassisted change* to describe a switch from problem to non-problem drinking (McMurran, 1994). Even the term *unassisted change* may be misleading because people who change their drinking patterns may have the help and support of many people, including family members, employers, and friends. Many people are able to change from problem to non-problem drinking without formal treatment (Sobell et al., 1996); others fluctuate among problem drinking, light drinking, and abstinence (Clark & Cahalan, 1976).

Although many problem drinkers are able to quit on their own or to moderate their drinking, others seek professional help or the assistance of traditional groups such as Alcoholics Anonymous. Presently, nearly all treatment programs in the United States are oriented toward abstinence; a few in other countries allow for the possibility that some problem drinkers can control their alcohol intake.

Treatments Oriented toward Abstinence

All formal treatments—even those that permit the possibility of resuming drinking—seek immediate abstinence as their goal. This section examines several treatment programs aimed at total and permanent abstinence.

Alcoholics Anonymous   Alcoholics Anonymous (AA) is one of the most widely used alcohol treatment programs, and it is often a component of other treatment programs. Founded in 1935 by two former alcoholics, AA has become the best known of all approaches to problem drinking. The organization follows a very strict version of the disease model and combines it with quasi-religious meetings that are designed to bring the problem drinker into the group. To adhere to the AA doctrine, a person must maintain total abstinence from alcohol. Part of the AA philosophy is that those who are in need of joining AA can never drink again and that problem drinkers are addicted to alcohol and have no power to resist it. According to AA, alcoholics never recover but are always in the process of recovering. They will be alcoholics for a lifetime, even if they never take another drink.

AA and other 12-step programs have become increasingly popular, attracting large numbers of people. A survey of U.S. adults (Room & Greenfield, 1993) revealed that nearly 5% of adults had sought help at some time during their lives for drinking problems, and for those who had sought help, 60% of the men and 80% of the women had attended AA meetings (Weisner, Greenfield & Room, 1995).

The anonymity offered to those who attend AA meetings presents serious barriers to researchers wishing to conduct controlled experimental follow-up studies of members. One of the few controlled studies (Brandsma, Maultsby, & Welsh, 1980) found a high dropout rate for AA members. The AA group showed the highest dropout rate: 68% versus 57% for the other treatment groups in the study. In addition, the AA participants were most likely to binge drink during the 3 months of the study. Thus, AA is no more effective than alternative treatments and is possibly less so.

Other research on AA has indicated that it may be more effective for some problem drinkers than for others. Men with lower educational levels who have high needs for authoritarianism, dependence, and sociability may be good candidates (Miller & Hester, 1980). AA also seems to work better for people who need to give as well as to receive help (Maton, 1988).

Psychotherapy Nearly as many psychotherapeutic techniques have been used to treat alcohol abuse as there are psychotherapies. This variety should not be surprising because a variety of psychiatric and behavioral problems often accompany alcohol abuse. Whether these disorders are the cause or the effect of heavy drinking, the immediate goal of all treatment approaches is sobriety, because no psychotherapy is successful with intoxicated patients. For this reason, psychotherapeutic approaches are often combined with detox-

ification, AA, or some form of chemical treatment aimed at stopping drinking.

In terms of setting, treatment may be centered in Veterans Administration hospitals, care units in other hospitals, private treatment clinics, offices of psychiatrists and psychologists, halfway houses, or one of a variety of other treatment facilities. In terms of form, psychotherapeutic treatment can be divided into group procedures and individual therapy, with patients frequently participating in both within a single treatment regimen.

Group therapy for alcoholics has both advantages and disadvantages. Observing others who have successfully stopped drinking can raise expectancies for achieving the same goal, and patients within a group setting are more likely to receive praise and recognition from other group members for staying away from problem drinking. Another advantage of group treatment is the opportunity that groups provide to allow the patient to give help. The experience of being helpful is, itself, often therapeutic, and AA members who reach the final step of their program often sponsor a new member. This type of responsibility can be beneficial to both persons (Maton, 1988).

However, group therapy is sometimes rather superficial in dealing with individual problems, so individual psychotherapy may be preferable. How effective are the various individual therapy programs for alcohol abuse? Unfortunately, reports of success are frequently exaggerated, with some private treatment centers claiming a greater than 90% recovery rate (Hunter, 1982). Well-controlled studies, however, usually yield somewhat lower success rates, depending on the type of treatment (multimodal programs typically report higher rates than single-approach treatments); the sample composition (healthy, middle-social class, married, employed alcoholics have the highest improvement rates); the definition of success (abstinence versus improved); and the interval before follow-up (longer periods before follow-up report lower success rates) (Emrick & Hansen, 1983). The percentage of successes ranges from 4% to 42%, with perhaps 19% to 20% being the median. Even these rates are subject to decline as a result of relapse in the months and years following treatment (Armor, Polich, & Stambul, 1976; Wiens & Menustik, 1983).

Chemical Treatments Many treatment programs for problem drinking include administering drugs that interact with alcohol to produce a range of unpleasant effects. The most commonly used of these drugs is **disulfiram** (Antabuse). The unpleasant effects include flushing of the face, chest pains, a pounding heart, nausea and vomiting, sweating, headache, dizziness, weakness, difficulty in breathing, and a rapid decrease in blood pressure. These effects do not occur unless disulfiram and alcohol are both ingested. Disulfiram does have side effects of its own, including skin eruptions, fatigue, drowsiness, headache, and impotence. As with all side effects to drugs, these vary from person to person, and some individuals have few or none.

A major problem with disulfiram therapy is patient compliance (Fuller et al., 1986). People are not eager to take a drug that will make them sick if they drink. Because disulfiram must be taken at least twice weekly, patients are frequently hospitalized to ensure compliance, but this strategy is not practical for long-term treatment. Noncompliance, of course, lowers the effectiveness of this treatment because low levels of the drug may not cause the unpleasant effects after a person drinks alcohol. Despite the extremely unpleasant effects of drinking while on disulfiram, research does not show it alone to be any more effective than other treatments (Fuller et al., 1986; Miller & Hester, 1980).

Aversion Therapy Drugs like disulfiram, which produce nausea when combined with alcohol, are intended to produce an aversion to drinking or to act as a punishment for drinking. Thus they would technically be considered aversion therapies. However, the term **aversion therapy** is more commonly applied to the classical conditioning technique of using an electric shock, an emetic drug, or some other aversive stimulus to countercondition the patient's response to alcohol. In the classical conditioning paradigm, the unconditioned stimulus (shock or the emetic drug) is paired one or more times with the conditioned stimulus (sight, smell, taste, or image of alcohol) so that it will elicit the unconditioned response (aversion or withdrawal from alcohol). Through this process, drinking should come to be associated with an aversive condition and thus be avoided. When the unconditioned stimulus is a high level of shock, aversive therapy programs do not work well: Their success rates are low and their dropout rates high (Miller & Hester, 1980).

Rather than relying on electric shock, many alcohol treatment programs use **emetine**, a drug that induces vomiting, as the aversive stimulus. This aversive therapy procedure pairs emetine with the sight, smell, taste, and thought of alcohol. One evaluation of the effectiveness of emetine treatment (Wiens & Menustik, 1983) found that 63% of patients were not drinking at the end of 1 year, but only 31% were abstinent after 3 years. This relapse rate indicates that emetine aversion therapy, like many other treatment programs for alcohol and drug abuse, loses much of its effectiveness after a moderately long time.

Aversion conditioning has also been used in programs oriented toward moderation in drinking. Indeed, aversion therapy may be more useful in bringing about controlled drinking among problem drinkers than in inducing abstinence, even when abstinence is the goal (Miller & Hester, 1980).

Controlled Drinking

Until the late 1960s, all alcohol cessation treatments were aimed at total abstinence. Then something quite unexpected happened. In 1962 in London, D. L. Davies found that 7 of the 93 recovered alcoholics whom he studied were able to drink "normally" (defined as consumption of up to three pints of beer or its equivalent per day) for at least a 7-year period following treatment. These moderate drinkers represented less than 8% of those Davies studied, but this finding was still remarkable because it opened up the possibility that diagnosed alcoholics could successfully return to nonproblem drinking. All seven of the controlled drinkers had been completely abstinent for at least a few months following treatment, yet all had been able to resume "normal" drinking without relapsing into a heavy, harmful pattern of drinking.

Prompted by Davies's results, a study in the United States (Armor, Polich, & Stambul, 1976) showed that controlled drinking occurred in 3% to 20% of patients who received treatment oriented toward abstinence. Publicity about this study produced a wave of criticism from those holding the position that alcoholics can never drink again. A more extensive study (Polich, Armor, Braiker, 1980) replicated the earlier results and led to an interest in treatments with controlled drinking as the goal.

Abstinence-oriented programs usually teach that the urge to drink will always be present and that if it is indulged even for a single drink, total relapse is inevitable. In contrast, controlled drinking programs do not have such a self-fulfilling prophecy built into them. Instead, they emphasize moderating patients' behavior and finding environmental supports that will reinforce moderation. They teach patients to monitor their intake, set weekly goals for total consumption, intersperse nonalcoholic drinks with alcoholic ones, and dilute drinks. In addition, behaviorally oriented controlled drinking programs train patients in a variety of human relations skills so they can modify all their self-destructive behaviors (Alden, 1988).

More recent evidence suggests that problem drinkers can moderate their drinking without the assistance of formal cessation programs. A survey of former drinkers (Sobell, Cunningham, & Sobell, 1996) showed that more than half of former heavy drinkers were able to drink moderately after resolving their problems with alcohol. Of those who became controlled drinkers, most did so on their own. This survey confirms some earlier evidence (Pukish & Tucker, 1994) that controlled drinking is a more likely outcome for problem drinkers who quit on their own than for those who enter treatment.

Despite potential advantages of controlled drinking, most treatment centers in the United States have resisted the possibility that former problem drinkers can learn to moderate their use of alcohol. In Great Britain, nearly all treatment centers accept the principle of controlled drinking treatment (McMurran, 1994). Some therapists and treatment centers in the United States are beginning to realize that traditional treatments work for less than half of alcoholics and that matching patient to treatment can offer a higher success rate (Neimark, Conway, & Doskoch, 1994).

What factors predict success in controlled drinking? Several characteristics relate to positive outcomes, including low severity of dependence and belief in the possibility of controlled drinking (Rosenberg, 1993). The best candidates for controlled drinking are people under age 40 who have not had long histories of problem drinking and serious alcohol-related physiological damage. In addition, married people do better than unmarried people, and people who attribute their drinking to situational factors are better candidates than those who believe they are physically dependent on alcohol. Also, people with regular employment are more likely to succeed than those who are frequently out of work. Finally, people who quit on their own have a better chance of becoming controlled drinkers than those who seek treatment for their drinking problems. All these factors suggest that controlled drinking can be successful for some problem drinkers.

However, none of the findings in favor of controlled drinking programs should be interpreted as evidence that moderate drinking is indicated for *all* alcohol abusers. No responsible proponent of controlled drinking would advocate such a course of action. One cannot state too strongly that *controlled drinking is not for everyone*. Some former alcohol addicts must abstain completely, and even those drinkers who are candidates for controlled drinking must apparently undergo at least 1 month of complete abstinence to allow the toxic effects of excessive drinking to diminish. In addition, former alcohol abusers who initially learn control may gradually or even abruptly escalate their consumption until they reach complete relapse.

The Problem of Relapse

Problem drinkers who successfully complete either an abstinence-oriented or a moderation-oriented treatment program do not necessarily maintain their goals. As we saw with smoking, people who complete a treatment program usually improve quite a bit, but the problem of relapse is often substantial. Interestingly, the time course and rate of relapse is similar for those who complete treatment programs for smoking, alcohol abuse, or opiate abuse (Hunt, Barnett, & Branch, 1971). Most relapses occur within 90 days after the end of the program. At 12 months after the end of treatment, only about 35% of those completing the programs are still abstinent.

Since the early 1970s, treatment programs have improved, and relapse rates have declined. Studies obviously vary in success rate, depending on such factors as severity and duration of the drinking problem, age of the drinker, type of treatment, and definition of success. Amid this diversity of contributing factors, generalizations are difficult. However, a reasonable estimate is that with some relapse or "booster" training, roughly two-thirds of those treated for alcohol abuse show some improvement after 1 year; about a third are still improved (either abstinent or drinking in a controlled manner) after 3 years; and about a sixth are still improved after 5 years. These figures, of course, are rough estimates. Furthermore, some studies, especially those using abstinence as the criterion for success, show much lower success rates. The Rand Report (Polich et al., 1980), for example, found that only 7% of treated alcoholics did not drink at all in the 4 years following treatment. One long-term study (Vaillant, 1983) reported that after a 40-year follow-up, only 5% remained abstinent. Although complete abstinence may be too strict a standard to impose, relapse following treatment for alcohol abuse remains a serious problem.

Most behavior-based treatment regimens include training for relapse prevention (Marlatt & Gordon, 1980). As discussed in Chapter 13, relapse prevention training is aimed at changing cognitions so that the addict comes to believe that one slip does *not* equal total relapse. Programs that incorporate relapse prevention into their regimen, train participants in the use of coping skills, and attempt to enhance self-efficacy tend to have the highest rates of success (Annis & Davis, 1988).

In Summary

Despite a decline in the percentage of drinkers in the United States, the number of people seeking help for their drinking problems has continued to grow. In addition to formal treatment programs, many problem drinkers are able to quit without therapy. Traditional alcohol treatment programs have been oriented toward abstinence, but most have had only moderate success. The effectiveness of the AA programs are difficult to assess because members are anonymous. Psychotherapeutic approaches to changing problem drinking usually deal with a wide range of personal problems and are not limited to the problem of drinking. People most likely to be helped by psychotherapy are healthy, middle-class, married and employed. The drug disulfiram has been used for some time to curb alcohol consumption, but its drastic effects hinder its usefulness. Electric shock and emetine have been used with limited success as aversive stimuli.

Controlled drinking might be a reasonable goal for a substantial minority of all problem drinkers. Although many medically oriented therapists do not consider controlled drinking a viable alternative to abstinence, attitudes toward alcohol treatment are undergoing changes, and controlled drinking may become a more accepted goal.

With all alcohol treatment approaches, relapse has been a persistent problem. Most relapses occur within 3 months after the end of treatment, and after 12 months, only about one third of those who complete the program are still abstinent. Relapse depends on severity and duration of the drinking problem, age of the drinker, type of treatment, and definition of success. Relapse training, especially programs teaching that one slip does not equal complete relapse, can help people to stop abusing alcohol, but complete abstinence probably occurs in a very small percentage of problem drinkers.

Other Drugs

Illicit drugs have created many serious problems in the United States, but these problems are mainly social and not related to physical health. Compared with the effects of smoking cigarettes, drinking alcohol, eating unwisely, and failing to exercise, relatively few people die from the effects of illegal drugs. For example, cocaine, the deadliest of the illicit drugs, kills only one person for every 1,000 killed by tobacco products (Rouse, 1998). Even one death from illicit drugs, of course, is too many, and this section addresses some of the negative health consequences of both legal and illegal drugs. Table 14.1 shows the rates of use of various drugs, including alcohol and nicotine.

Health Effects

Both legal and illegal drugs pose potential health hazards. However, illegal drugs present certain risks not found with legal drugs, regardless of pharmacological effects. Illegal drugs may be sold as one drug when they are actually another; buyers have no insurance as to dosage; and illegally manufactured drugs may have impurities that are dangerous chemicals themselves. In addition, the sources of illegal drugs can be dangerous people. Legal drugs are free from these risks, but they are not always safe or harmless. For any drug to have an effect, it must intervene in biological processes. For example, psychoactive drugs produce their effects by crossing the blood-brain barrier and changing the brain's chemistry. Such actions are not without risks.

All drugs have potential hazards, but drugs termed *safe* are tested by the federal Food and Drug Administration (FDA) and defined as safe. The FDA considers a drug safe if its potential benefits outweigh its potential hazards. Many drugs, such as antibiotics, have been approved even though they produce severe side effects in some people. The more potentially beneficial a drug, the more likely it is to be labeled safe despite unpleasant side effects.

The FDA classifies drugs into five categories, based on their potential for abuse and their potential medical benefits. Schedule I includes drugs judged to be high in abuse potential and with no accepted medical use. Included in this category are heroin, LSD, and marijuana. Schedule II includes drugs that have high abuse potential, capable of causing severe psychological or physical dependence but having some medical use. In this category are most opiates, some barbiturates, amphetamines, and cocaine. Schedule III consists of drugs judged to produce moderate or low physical dependence or high psychological dependence but with accepted medical uses, such as some opiates and some tranquilizers. Schedule IV drugs, such as phenobarbital and most tranquilizers, are judged to have low abuse potential, limited dependence properties, and accepted medical uses. Schedule V contains drugs with less abuse potential than those in Schedule IV.

Drugs in Schedule V do not require a prescription and are available over the counter in drug stores; drugs in Schedule I are not legally available; and those in Schedules II, III, and IV are available only by prescription. This classification has evolved somewhat haphazardly over the past 100 years and represents legislative and social convention rather than scientific findings.

Sedatives Sedatives are drugs that induce relaxation and sometimes intoxication by lowering the activity of the brain, the neurons, the muscles, and the heart, and even by slowing the metabolic rate. In low doses, these drugs tend to make people feel relaxed and even euphoric. In high doses,

Table 14.1 Lifetime, past year, and past month use of various drugs, including nonmedical use of legal drugs, persons aged 12 years and older, United States, 1997

Drug	Lifetime use	Use during past year	Use during past month
Sedatives	2.0%	0.3%	0.1%
Tranquilizers	3.3	1.0	0.4
Heroin	1.0	0.2	0.1
Alcohol	86.4	67.3	54.3
Stimulants	5.0	0.7	0.3
Cocaine	11.3	0.6	0.2
Crack cocaine	2.1	0.2	0.1
Marijuana	34.8	8.1	4.6
LSD	8.3	0.7	0.2
Analgesics	4.8	1.8	0.7
Cigarettes	73.9	33.1	30.4
Smokeless tobacco	18.1	4.8	3.5

Source: Preliminary Results from the 1997 National Household Survey on Drug Abuse (p. 122), by U.S. Department of Health and Human Services (DHHS publication No. SMA 98-3251), 1998, Washington, DC: U.S. Government Printing Office.

they cause loss of consciousness and can result in coma and death due to their inhibitory effect on the brain center that controls respiration. Sedatives include barbiturates, tranquilizers, opiates, and methadone, but the most commonly used drug in this category is alcohol.

Depressant effects are a major problem with sedative drugs, and these effects are additive when sedatives are taken in combination. The effect of mixing two or more of these drugs can be depression of the respiratory system to a dangerously low level. Some people mix alcohol with tranquilizers or other depressants, providing a potentially lethal combination. Furthermore, sedatives and stimulants have opposite effects, but these effects do not cancel each other; instead, both sets of effects occur. For example, caffeine (the stimulant drug in coffee) will not sober a person intoxicated on alcohol (a sedative). Rather, caffeine merely makes a drunken person more alert and less sleepy—not less drunk.

Barbiturates are synthetic drugs used medically to induce sleep. Taken recreationally, barbi-turates produce effects similar to alcohol: relaxation and intoxication in small doses, drunkenness and unconsciousness in larger doses. Because they are ingested in pill form, barbiturate overdoses are more common than alcohol overdoses. Barbiturates produce both tolerance and dependence, although the tolerance properties are difficult to assess. Many people can take barbiturates in the form of sleeping pills over an extended time without increasing the dose, whereas others rapidly escalate their dosage to dangerous levels. People who use barbiturates as sleeping pills on a regular basis are not able to sleep without them, and they manifest withdrawal symptoms when they stop taking them—two definite indications of dependence. Withdrawal is similar to that from alcohol, lasting up to a week and including tremor, nausea, vomiting, sweating, and sleep disturbances, and sometimes hallucinations and deliriums.

Tranquilizers are relatively recent, dating only to the 1960s. The most prominent variety of these chemical compositions are those of the *benzodiazepine* group. Like barbiturates, tranquilizers induce

BECOMING HEALTHIER

1. Avoid drinking 5 or more drinks on any one occasion. This level of drinking confers more risks than benefits.

2. Avoiding alcohol may not be the healthiest choice, and light to moderate drinkers have health advantages over those who abstain as well as over those who drink unwisely.

3. One or two drinks per day can confer health benefits, but impaired judgment and coordination can present dangers for even low levels of alcohol consumption.

4. Occasional light drinking presents some risks but does not convey as many benefits as more regular drinking.

5. Do not drive, operate machinery, or swim after drinking.

6. Do not escalate your drinking; keep to one or two drinks per day.

7. Even light drinking can be a risk for pregnant women.

8. If one or both of your parents experienced drinking problems, you may be at elevated risk. Manage this risk by moderating your drinking.

9. If you have an extremely pleasant experience with any drug (including alcohol) the first time you try it, be aware that this drug may present problems for you with future use.

10. Drugs that produce dependence are more dangerous than those that do not. Be aware and cautious about using such drugs, which include alcohol and nicotine as well as opiates, barbiturates, and amphetamines.

11. Illegal drugs without tolerance or dependence potential can be dangerous simply because they are illegal.

depression, but they are less likely to produce sleep and more likely to suppress anxiety. Recognition of the dangers of this class of drug has led to a decreased in prescriptions and fewer health problems.

Benzodiazepines produce both tolerance and dependence, but only over an extended period. Neither tolerance nor dependence is particularly severe if the drug is taken in small or even moderate amounts. In large amounts, however, these drugs not only produce tolerance and dependence but also cause disorientation, confusion, and even rage, a paradoxical effect for a tranquilizer.

Another category of depressants is the **opiates**, drugs derived from the opium poppy. Opium can also be refined into *morphine,* which can be further chemically treated to produce *heroin.* Synthetic compounds, including *meperidine* and *methadone,* are chemically similar to the opiates and produce similar effects.

Opium has been used for centuries for both medical and recreational purposes. It can be in-

gested by swallowing, sniffing, smoking, or injecting under the skin, into a muscle, or intravenously, making it one of the most versatile drugs for transmission into the body. In the 19th century in the United States, physicians prescribed opiates frequently and for a variety of conditions. Today, the principal medical use of opiates is to relieve pain. Because they act on the central nervous system and the digestive system, opiate drugs are also prescribed for cough and for diarrhea. Opiates cross the blood-brain barrier and attach to receptors in the brain, altering the interpretation of pain messages. The physical condition responsible for the pain is not halted, of course, but the person's subjective experience of pain diminishes. Opiate drugs, therefore, have important medical uses.

Opiates produce both tolerance and dependence after only a brief time, sometimes as little as 24 hours, thus making opiates like heroin easily abused. However, heroin use is not common in the United States (see Table 14.1). Johnston,

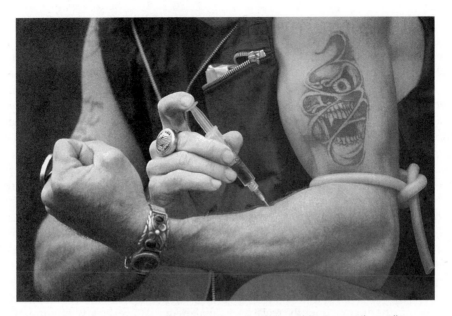

Injection drug use can pose health hazards from the drug and from unsterile needles.

O'Malley, and Bachman (1997; 1998) reported significant increases in the annual use of heroin and other opiates among young adults and high school seniors from 1979 to 1995, with most of the increase occurring between 1994 and 1995.

Stimulants Stimulant drugs tend to make some people feel more alert and energetic, more able to concentrate, and more able to work long hours. They make other users feel jittery, anxious, and unable to sit still. More specifically, stimulants tend to produce alertness, reduce feelings of fatigue, elevate mood, and decrease appetite. They are synthetic but are similar in chemical structure to norepinephrine, the neurotransmitter identified as the brain's main excitatory chemical. After a decline in the nonmedical use of stimulants from 1975 to the early 1990s, there has been a slight increase in the use of illegal stimulants in the United States by high school seniors, college students, and young adults from 1991 to 1995 (Johnston et al., 1997; 1998).

Amphetamines are stimulant drugs that are often abused due to their mood altering effects. In addition, amphetamines produce such physical symptoms as increased blood pressure, slower heart rate, increased respiration, relaxation of bronchial muscles, dilation of pupils, increased EEG activity, and increased blood supply to the muscles. These effects can be dangerous to the cardiovascular system, especially for people who have heart problems or other cardiovascular diseases. Amphetamines can also produce psychological effects, including hallucinations and paranoid delusions. High energy levels combined with paranoid delusions can make amphetamine users dangerous to society. In addition to these physical, psychological, and social effects, amphetamines produce both tolerance and dependence. Thus, they are undesirable as diet pills, despite their appetite suppressant effects.

Another stimulant drug, **cocaine**, is extracted from the coca plant, which grows in the Andes Mountains in South America. In the 1880s, several European physicians, including Sigmund Freud, discovered that cocaine was capable of blocking neural transmission at the site of application and therefore was useful for **anesthesia**. For a time, cocaine was used as an anesthetic for surgery, especially eye surgery. In the 1890s, it became a popular drug in

America and was widely available in tonics, wines, and soft drinks. Soon, however, people began to recognize the dangers of cocaine, and the passage of U.S. federal drug laws restricted its use. Today the medical uses of cocaine are quite limited because more effective anesthetics have been developed.

Cocaine acts as a stimulant to the nervous system, and the strength and duration of its action depend not only on dose but also on mode of administration. Although South American Indians take cocaine orally by chewing the coca leaves, this method is seldom used elsewhere. Instead, cocaine is snorted through the nasal passages, smoked or "freebased," or injected intravenously. The stimulant effects of cocaine are short, lasting only 15 to 30 minutes. During this time, the user often feels a powerful euphoria, a strong sense of well-being, and heightened attention. But when the effects wear off, the user frequently feels fatigued, sluggish, and anxious and is left with a strong craving to repeat the experience. Frequently the user increases the dose in a futile effort to make the euphoria last longer the next time. The stimulant effects of increased doses of cocaine can endanger the cardiovascular system.

The tolerance and dependence properties of cocaine are still debated, but people who use cocaine repeatedly eventually stop getting the "high" they initially felt. With heavy use, many people experience frequent anxiety, insomnia, depression, and irritation of the nose. Even heavy users suffer few withdrawal symptoms, the main criterion for determining physical dependence. However, most heavy users who quit suffer serious depression, coupled with a strong desire to continue taking the drug. The term *psychological dependence* may seem appropriate, but this term is a problem because it can be applied to many habitual behaviors, both drug and nondrug, good and bad. Cocaine can become an important part of the lives of users, and these people tend to have problems as a result of their cocaine use.

The health effects of prolonged, heavy use of cocaine are still not clearly understood. A study of lifetime cocaine use among young adults (Braun, Murray, & Sidney, 1997) investigated whether it was related to such cardiovascular risk factors as elevated blood pressure, rapid heart rate, or lack of physical activity. Participants included African American and European American men and women 18 to 32 years old. Heavy cocaine use was associated with being White, older, and less educated, and having a higher use of other legal and illegal drugs. No relationship appeared between prolonged, heavy use of cocaine and various cardiovascular risk factors, but longitudinal studies are required to determine if continued use of cocaine might be related to cardiovascular risk factors later in life.

During the early 1990s, a group of neuropharmacology researchers (Hearn et al., 1991) discovered that cocaine and alcohol interact in the body to form a third chemical, *cocaethylene,* which produces or enhances the euphoria that cocaine users experience. However, the mixture of cocaine and alcohol is potentially lethal and accounts for a higher death rate and a greater rate of emergency room admissions than either drug alone.

Crack cocaine has become a serious social problem in the United States, partially because this form of cocaine is cheap and widely available. Crack, a form of freebase cocaine, is ingested by smoking. The use of crack among high school seniors, college students, and young adults declined between the mid-1980s and the early 1990s, but it has begun to increase in recent years. For example, from 1986 to 1991 yearly crack use declined for high school seniors from 4.1% to 1.5%, but since 1991 the annual prevalence has risen from 1.5% to 2.4% in 1997 (Johnston et al., 1998). The annual use of both cocaine and crack cocaine is quite low in the general population (see Table 14.1).

Marijuana The most commonly used illegal drug in the United States is *marijuana* (see Table 14.1). Its potential for serious health consequences is still debated, but few authorities regard it as a major health risk. In fact, Stephen Sidney and his associates (Sidney, Beck, Tekawa, Quesenberry, & Friedman, 1997) found no increased death rates for marijuana users, except for men who died of

AIDS. Although this study does not determine cause and effect, if seems safe to assume that marijuana did not cause death from AIDS, but rather that men receiving a diagnosis of AIDS may have subsequently increased their use of marijuana.

Marijuana is composed of the leaves, flowers, and small branches of *Cannabis sativa,* a plant that flourishes in almost every climate in the world. The intoxicating ingredient in marijuana, delta-9-tetrahydrocannabinol (THC), comes from the resin of the male plants and especially the female plants. The most reliable physiological effect of THC is increased heart rate, which occurs with the consumption of heavy doses. Although a rapid heartbeat may present health hazards to users with coronary problems, no evidence exists that marijuana in small or moderate doses causes any organic damage. Nevertheless, any drug used chronically and in heavy doses poses a danger to health. Thus, marijuana, like nicotine, alcohol, or aspirin, has some potential to impair health, and, if smoked as frequently as cigarettes, it would be at least as harmful to the respiratory system as tobacco.

Marijuana has been used medically to treat glaucoma and to prevent the vomiting and nausea associated with chemotherapy. During the 1970s, controlled studies (Sallan, Zinberg, & Frei, 1975) demonstrated that orally administered THC in gelatin capsules was capable of reducing nausea and vomiting in cancer patients treated with chemotherapy. At about the same time, researchers noticed that healthy young marijuana smokers experienced a lessening of pressure within their eyes, decreasing glaucoma (Hepler & Frank, 1971). In 1992, however, the Drug Enforcement Administration rejected all pleas for reclassifying marijuana to Schedule II. Nevertheless, marijuana continues to be used illegally for nausea, glaucoma, muscle relaxation, and as an appetite stimulant for AIDS patients (Grinspoon & Bakalar, 1995).

The desired psychological effects of marijuana are euphoria, a sense of well-being, feelings of relaxation, and heightened sexual responsiveness; these are usually attained by experienced smokers who expect to attain them. On the negative side, marijuana also has an effect on short-term memory, judgment, and time perception. Although the effects of marijuana on memory and cognition are usually slight (Ferraro, 1980), even small deficits may be hazardous when a person is operating an automobile or engaging in any other potentially dangerous activity.

Marijuana does not seem to produce physiological dependence, and no withdrawal symptoms accompany the cessation of marijuana use. One study (Miller & Cisin, 1983) reported that nearly 75% of adults ages 26 and older who had been marijuana users stopped taking the drug. Also, marijuana does not seem to create tolerance; regular users are not ordinarily compelled to escalate dosage in order to achieve the same effect. The psychological effects of marijuana, like those of alcohol and other drugs, seem to depend partially on setting and expectation.

Recreational use of marijuana in the United States is a relatively recent phenomenon. Only 2% of people born between 1930 and 1940 used marijuana before age 21, but more than half the people born during the 1970s used this drug before their 21st birthday (Johnson & Gerstein, 1998). Unlike the use of most other illicit drugs, marijuana use among young people has recently increased in the United States. Johnston et al. (1998) reported a steep rise in marijuana use among 8th-graders, 10th-graders, and 12th-graders from 1991 to 1997 after more than a decade of slow decline. From 1991 to 1997, annual use of marijuana among 12th-grade students nearly doubled from 22% to 39%, while monthly use doubled from 12% to 24% (Johnston et al., 1998). Lifetime use among college students and young adults is more than 50%, but that number has not changed much since 1991. During the early 1990s, monthly use among college students and young adults remained relatively constant—at around 14% to 15%, but during 1995, that rate jumped to nearly 19% for college students, a possible result of increased marijuana smoking among high school students during the early 1990s (Johnston, O'Malley, & Bachman, 1997).

Anabolic Steroids   In recent years, many athletes have used **anabolic steroids** (AS) to increase their muscle bulk and to decrease body fat. Is this practice a potential health hazard? Before addressing this question, we briefly describe anabolic steroids and discuss their positive effects.

Steroids can be either endogenous (manufactured by the body) or synthetic. Endogenous steroids are produced by the adrenal glands, which secrete cortisone, and by the ovaries and testes, which secrete estrogen and testosterone. The effects of anabolic steroids include thickening of vocal cords, enlargement of the larynx, increased muscle bulk, and decreased body fat. These last two properties make AS attractive to athletes, bodybuilders, and people who wish to alter their appearance. Anabolic steroids have some medical uses, including reduction of inflammation and control of some allergic reactions.

On the other hand, anabolic steroids are potentially dangerous. They can upset the chemical balance in the body, produce toxicity, and shut off the body's production of its own steroids, leaving the person more susceptible to stress and infection and altering reproductive functioning. Other hazards include increased coronary risk factors, heart attack, abnormal liver function, stunted height, and severe mood and psychotic disorders (Goldberg et al., 1996).

Anabolic steroids do not seem to produce tolerance or dependence. However, some authorities (Shroyer, 1990) have argued that the use of steroids often leads to psychological dependence. This argument is based on the observation that the effects of steroid use—bulky muscle development and increased athletic performance—are secondary reinforcers. Thus, some people have a strong motivation to maintain steroid use and may suffer loss of self-esteem when the drugs are discontinued.

Some young people use anabolic steroids to prevent injuries—despite a lack of medical evidence that steroids can protect against injuries. If anything, anabolic steroids are more likely to produce injuries, both to the person taking them and to others coming into physical contact with that person. However, increased muscle mass and aggression may not be an inevitable consequence of steroid use. A study of monkeys (Rejeski, Brubaker, Herb, Kaplan, & Koritnik, 1988) suggested that steroid use can increase both aggression and submission. Dominant subjects fought with each other and with the most submissive subjects. Animals that lost fights became more submissive, displaying behaviors much like those that Martin Seligman (1975) described as learned helplessness. These submissive subjects thus became vulnerable to injuries, in part because of their increased levels of steroids. The authors found similarities between the increased aggression of their monkeys and anecdotal reports of human athletes' behaviors.

Monthly use of steroids is less than 1% for high school students, college students, and young adults (Johnston et al., 1997). Although rates of steroid use are low, this drug presents more direct health hazards than other illicit drugs, and indirect health effects are also a potential risk.

Drug Misuse and Abuse

Most people believe that some drugs are acceptable and even desirable because of the medical benefits they confer. But all *psychoactive* drugs—drugs that cross the blood-brain barrier and alter mental functioning—are potentially harmful to health. Most have the capacity for tolerance or dependence (see Table 14.2). Even drugs that are not psychoactive have the potential for unpleasant side effects. For example, penicillin can cause nausea, vomiting, diarrhea, swelling, and skin eruptions. In addition, people who have allergies to penicillin can die from ingesting it. Caffeine, a drug found in coffee and cola drinks, can produce effects that meet the DSM-IV criteria of substance dependence. For example, one study (Strain, Mumford, Silverman, & Griffiths, 1994) found that a high percentage of people who believed that they were dependent on caffeine had been unsuccessful in quitting or cutting down, showed withdrawal symptoms when denied caffeine, and continue to use the drug despite knowledge that

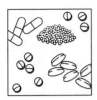

Table 14.2 Summary of the characteristics of psychoactive drugs

Name	Source	Medical use	Mode of ingestion	Effects	Duration of effects	Tolerance	Dependence
Stimulants							
Caffeine	Natural (tea, coffee, etc.)	Anti-depressant	Swallowed	Increases alertness, reduced fatigue	1–2 hrs.	Yes	No
Cocaine	Natural (coca plant)	Local anesthetic	Swallowed, injected, sniffed	Produces euphoria, suppresses appetite	15–30 mins.	?	?
Amphetamines	Synthetic	Appetite suppressant	Swallowed, injected	Produces alertness, reduces fatigue	4 hrs.	Yes	Yes
Nicotine	Natural (tobacco plant)	None	Smoked, sniffed, chewed	Elevates blood pressure	30 mins.	Yes	Yes
Depressants							
Barbiturates	Synthetic	Sedative	Swallowed	Relaxes, intoxicates	Varies depending on type	Yes	Yes
Tranquilizers	Synthetic	Anxiety reducer	Swallowed	Relaxes, intoxicates	3–4 hrs.	Yes	Yes
Opiates	Natural (opium poppy) semi-synthetic	Analgesic	Swallowed, sniffed, smoked, injected	Produces euphoria, sedates	4–6 hrs.	Yes	Yes
Methadone	Synthetic	Treatment for heroin addiction	Swallowed	Prevents heroin withdrawal	12–24 hrs.	Yes	Yes
Alcohol	Natural (fruits, grains)	External antiseptic	Swallowed	Relaxes, intoxicates	1–2 hrs.	Yes	Yes
Marijuana	Natural (cannabis)	Treatment for glaucoma, antiemetic	Smoked	Relaxes, intoxicates	2–3 hrs.	?	No
Steroids	Natural, synthetic	Agent for reducing inflammation and rashes	Swallowed, injected, applied to skin	Builds muscles, increases blood pressure, reduces immune system functioning	7–14 days	Yes	No

its use may cause persistent or recurrent physiological and psychological problems. Therefore, even a drug that is safe for most people is not without substantial risks for some.

Almost all drugs that have potential medical or health benefits also have the potential for misuse and abuse. The moderate use of alcohol, for instance, is related to decreased cardiovascular mortality. The *misuse* of alcohol—defined as inappropriate but not health-threatening levels of consumption—can result in social embarrassment, violent acts, and injury. And *abuse* of alcohol—defined as frequent, heavy consumption to the point of addiction—can lead to cirrhosis, brain damage, heart attack, and fetal alcohol syndrome.

Treatment for Drug Abuse

Treatment for the use and abuse of illegal drugs is similar to treatment of alcohol abuse, both in the philosophy and the administration of treatment. The goal of treatment for all types of illegal drug use is total abstinence. In many cases, the programs that treat drug abusers often coexist physically with treatment programs for alcohol abuse, and patients who are receiving treatment for their drug problems participate in the same therapy as those who are receiving therapy for their alcohol problems. The philosophy that guides Alcoholics Anonymous led to the development of Narcotics Anonymous, an organization devoted to helping drug users abstain from using drugs.

The reasons for entering drug abuse treatment programs are often similar to those for entering treatment for alcohol abuse. These reasons are primarily social. The abuse of illegal drugs leads to legal, financial, and interpersonal problems, as does alcohol abuse. Like alcohol, most illegal drugs produce impairments of judgment that lead to accidents, making accidental injury the leading health risk for drug abuse. Unlike alcohol abuse, the abuse of illegal drugs does not often directly damage health. However, when health problems occur, they are likely to be major and life threatening. Such crises may precipitate a person's decision to seek treatment or lead family members to enforce treatment.

Inpatient treatment programs for drug abuse are strikingly similar to those designed to treat alcohol abuse, but they do differ from programs for alcohol abuse in several minor ways. The detoxification phase of inpatient hospitalization is typically shorter and less severe for most types of drug use than it is for alcohol, for which withdrawal can be life threatening. Alcohol is a depressant drug, as are barbiturates, tranquilizers, and opiates. Therefore, all these drugs have similar symptoms during withdrawal, including agitation, tremor, gastric distress, and possibly perceptual distortions. Stimulants such as amphetamines and cocaine produce different withdrawal symptoms, namely lethargy and depression. These differences necessitate different medical care during detoxification.

One similarity between drug and alcohol abuse treatment is the high rate of relapse. As noted earlier, alcohol, smoking, and opiate treatment all share a high rate of relapse (Hunt et al., 1971), and the first 6 months after treatment are critical. To ameliorate this problem, drug treatment programs, like alcohol treatment interventions, typically include some aftercare or "booster" sessions. Frequently, this continued care comes from joining a support group such as Narcotics Anonymous. However, evidence exists that more comprehensive psychosocial services can boost the effectiveness of drug treatment (McLellan, Arndt, Metzger, Woody, & O'Brien, 1993).

Preventing and Controlling Drug Use

Chapter 13 presented information on attempts to decrease smoking in children and adolescents by various interventions aimed at discouraging their experimentation with cigarettes and smokeless tobacco. Similar efforts have been applied to decrease the use of other drugs (Goldberg et al., 1996), but programs aimed at children and adolescents are not the only approach to controlling drug use.

A more common control technique is the limitation of availability. This strategy is common in all Western countries through the existence of laws that limit the legal access to drugs. However, legal restriction of drugs has a number of side effects, some of which create other social problems (Robins, 1995). For example, when the United States legally prohibited the manufacture and sale of alcohol, illegal manufacture and distribution flourished, creating a large criminal enterprise, huge profits, loss of tax revenue, and corruption among law enforcement agencies. Therefore, the limitation of availability has negative as well as positive consequences.

The prevention attempts aimed at keeping children and adolescents from experimenting with drugs are intended to inhibit initiation, with the goal of eliminating the use of drugs completely (McMurran, 1994). As with the efforts at preventing smoking (see Chapter 13), those aimed at preventing drug use do not have an impressive success rate. Some programs have been counterproductive, increasing drug use or increasing adolescents' beliefs that drug use is more prevalent than it is (Donaldson, Graham, Piccinin, & Hansen, 1995). As with smoking prevention programs, drug prevention programs that rely on scare tactics, moral training, factual information about drug risks, and boosting self-esteem generally are ineffective (Donaldson et al., 1995). Indeed, a meta-analysis of the effectiveness of Project DARE (Drug Abuse Resistance Education), a widely used school-based drug education program, showed that this popular intervention is not very effective, even in the short term (Ennett, Tobler, Ringwalt, & Flewelling, 1994).

Some types of prevention programs are more effective than others. Peer programs that involve adolescents rather than adults as counselors are usually quite effective (Tobler, 1986). These programs typically involve developing social skills necessary to resist social pressure to use drugs. In addition, research (Chilcoat, Deshion, & Anthony, 1995) has demonstrated that parental monitoring of children's activities and whereabouts decreased the risk for drug involvement among children of elementary school age.

Another strategy is the control of the harm of drug use. This strategy involves the assumption that people will use psychoactive drugs, sometimes unwisely, but that reduction of the health consequences of drug use should be the first priority (McMurran, 1994). Rather than taking a moralistic stand on drug use, this strategy takes a practical approach to minimizing the dangers of drug use. An example of the harm reduction strategy is to help injection drug users exchange used needles for sterile ones and thus slow the spread of HIV infection. The controversy surrounding such programs is representative of the debate over the harm reduction strategy.

In Summary

Abuse of alcohol is a serious health problem in most developed nations, but other drugs—including depressants, stimulants, cocaine, marijuana, and anabolic steroids—are also potentially harmful to health. At one time, many of these drugs have been available over the counter or through a physician's prescription. Although the abuse of these drugs often leads to a number of social problems, their health risks are much less than those associated with nicotine or alcohol. Treatments for drug abuse are similar to those for alcohol abuse, and programs aimed at prevention are similar to those aimed at preventing smoking. A new strategy called harm reduction aims at decreasing the social and health risks of taking drugs by changing drug policies.

Answers

This chapter addressed six basic questions.

1. **What are the major trends in alcohol consumption?**

   People have consumed alcohol worldwide and before recorded history. Alcohol consumption in the United States reached a peak during the first 3 decades of the 19th century, dropped sharply during the mid-1800s as a result of the "temperance" movement, and continued at a steady rate until it declined even more during Prohibition. Currently, rates of alcohol consumption in the United States are going down, with only a little more than half the adults classified as current drinkers, 15% as binge drinkers, and 5% as heavy drinkers. Adult European Americans have higher rates of drinking than members of other ethnic groups.

2. **What are the health effects of drinking alcohol?**

Drinking has both positive and negative health effects. Prolonged, heavy drinking of alcohol often leads to cirrhosis of the liver and other serious health problems, such as heart disease and brain dysfunction. Moderate drinking may have certain long-range health benefits in reducing heart disease, probably due to its ability to increase HDL.

3. **Why do people drink?**

Models for drinking behavior should be able to explain why people begin drinking, why some can drink in moderation, and why others drink to excess. The *disease model* assumes that people drink excessively because they have the disease of alcoholism. Cognitive-physiological models, including the *tension reduction hypothesis,* the *self-awareness model,* and *alcohol myopia,* propose that people drink because alcohol allows people to escape tension and negative self-evaluations. *Social learning theory* assumes that people acquire drinking behavior through positive or negative reinforcement, modeling, and cognitive mediation.

4. **How can people change problem drinking?**

About one person in five problem drinkers may be able to quit without therapy. Treatment programs in the United States are oriented toward abstinence. Alcoholics Anonymous is the most popular treatment program, but despite its prominence, its effectiveness has not been established. The drug disulfiram has been used for some time to curb alcohol consumption, but its drastic effects hinder its usefulness. Controlled drinking might be a reasonable goal for a substantial minority of all problem drinkers, but candidates must be carefully selected.

5. **What problems are associated with relapse?**

Relapse is common among heavy drinkers who have quit, although many are able to maintain abstinence or to drink in a controlled manner. Most relapses occur during the first 3 months. After a year, about 65% of all successful quitters have resumed drinking in a harmful manner. Relapse rates are reduced in programs that include "booster" sessions.

6. **What are the health effects of other drugs?**

Other drugs—including depressants, stimulants, cocaine, marijuana, and anabolic steroids—have had some medical use, but they also are potentially harmful to health. The principal problems from most of these drugs are social, not physical. Treatments for drug abuse are similar to those for alcohol abuse, and programs aimed at prevention are similar to those aimed at preventing smoking.

Glossary

addiction Dependence on a drug such that stopping results in withdrawal symptoms.

alcohol dehydrogenase A liver enzyme that metabolizes alcohol into aldehyde.

aldehyde dehydrogenase An enzyme that converts aldehyde to acetic acid.

amphetamines One type of stimulant drug.

anabolic steroids Steroid drugs that increase muscle bulk and decrease body fat but also have toxic effects.

anesthesia Loss of sensations of temperature, touch, or pain.

aversion therapy A type of behavioral therapy based on classical conditioning technique and using some aversive stimulus to countercondition the patient's response.

barbiturates Synthetic sedative drug used medically to induce sleep.

cirrhosis A liver disease resulting in the production of nonfunctional scar tissue.

cocaine A stimulant drug extracted from the coca plant.

delirium tremens A condition induced by alcohol withdrawal and characterized by excessive trembling, sweating, anxiety, and hallucinations.

delta alcoholism A drinking pattern characterized by an inability to abstain from alcohol.

dependence A condition that occurs when a drug becomes incorporated into the functioning of the body's cells so that it is needed for "normal" functioning.

disulfiram A drug that causes an aversive reaction when taken with alcohol; used to treat alcoholism; Antabuse.

emetine A drug that induces vomiting.

ethanol The variety of alcohol used in alcoholic beverages.

fetal alcohol syndrome (FAS) A pattern of physical and psychological symptoms found in infants whose mothers drank heavily during pregnancy.

gamma alcoholism A drinking pattern characterized by loss of control.

Korsakoff syndrome A brain dysfunction found in some long-term heavy users of alcohol and resulting in both physiological and psychological impairment.

sedatives Drugs that induce relaxation and sometimes intoxication by lowering the activity of the brain, the neurons, the muscles, and the heart, and even by slowing the metabolic rate.

spontaneous remission Disappearance of problem behavior or illness without treatment.

stress response-dampening (SRD) Decrease in strength of responses to stress, caused by consumption of alcohol.

tolerance The condition of requiring increasing levels of a drug in order to produce a constant level of effect.

tranquilizers A type of sedative drug that reduces anxiety.

withdrawal Adverse physiological reactions exhibited when a drug-dependent person stops using that drug; the withdrawal symptoms are typically unpleasant and opposite from the drug's effects.

Suggested Readings

Heather, N., & Robertson, I. (1990). *Problem drinking* (2nd ed). Oxford, England: Oxford University Press.

The authors present evidence that problem drinking is not a disease but a learned behavior disorder and should be treated as such. This edition is directed at both the general public and professionals in the field of alcohol treatment.

McMurran, M. (1994). *The psychology of addiction.* London: Taylor & Francis.

Mary McMurran is a British psychologist whose background is in treatment of drug and alcohol problems. Her book is an interesting review of the history, legislation, theory, treatment, and prevention of drug use. Writing in Great Britain, she offers a different view of substance abuse from that of most U.S. therapists and theorists.

 Neimark, J., Conway, C., & Doskoch, P. (1994, September–October). Back from the drink. *Psychology Today, 27,* 46–49.

This article in a popular magazine offers a short, readable review of current statistics and trends on alcohol use and abuse. The review highlights the critical factors for successful quitting and includes tips for moderating your own drinking. Available through InfoTrac College Edition by Wadsworth Publishing Company.

 Nestle, M. (1997). Alcohol guidelines for chronic disease prevention: From Prohibition to moderation. *Nutrition Today, 32*(2), 86–92.

Marion Nestle tells about the experience of being a member of the panel that recommended moderate alcohol consumption in the most recent Dietary Guidelines for Americans. That advice for moderation is a departure from the Prohibitionist sentiment that has ruled official pronouncements concerning drinking.

CHAPTER 15

Eating to Control Weight

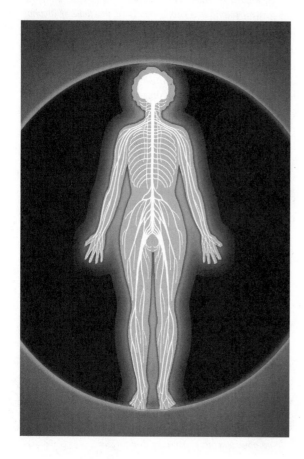

QUESTIONS

This chapter focuses on six basic questions:

1. How does the digestive system function?

2. What factors are involved in weight maintenance?

3. What is obesity and how does it affect health?

4. Is dieting a good way to lose weight?

5. What is anorexia nervosa and how can it be treated?

6. What is bulimia and how can it be treated?

JESSICA AND ELISE: DIETING GONE WRONG

Jessica, a 20-year-old college junior majoring in psychology, was a model student. She worked hard, earned excellent grades, and had high ambitions for a future career. Like many young college women, Jessica wanted to lose a few pounds—8 or 10. However, unlike most other college women, she was already dangerously thin—five feet four inches tall and weighing 81 pounds. Jessica had **anorexia nervosa,** an eating disorder that includes intentional starvation and a distorted body image.

At age 15, Jessica weighed 130 pounds, ate well, and was a normal teenager. In 4 years all this had changed. When she was 16, Jessica took a job as a dance instructor. Her employer suggested that she lose a few pounds, so Jessica began a conscientious program to lose weight. When her weight dropped to 110 pounds, her parents, boyfriend, and girlfriends all complemented her on how good she looked. However, Jessica continued to diet, and her eating habits became stranger as her concern with weight intensified. She would skip breakfast but drink five or six cups of coffee every morning. Her only food of the day was lunch, which consisted of a slice of low-calorie cheese on a half piece of diet bread. She would pick at her lunch for 20 to 30 minutes and eventually consume about half of it. After eating, she would go to the dance studio, where she exercised strenuously for 6 or 7 hours. After work, if daylight permitted, she would ride her bike for several miles or play a couple of sets of tennis. In addition to her morning coffee, she would drink one or two cups of hot tea and three or four diet drinks a day.

As her weight continued to drop, Jessica began to hide her weight loss beneath large, loose-fitting clothing. She weighed herself several times a day and spent a good deal of time looking at herself in a mirror. Where others saw an emaciated body, Jessica always saw a figure that seemed too fat. She also worried that her parents or doctor would put her in a hospital and force her to gain weight.

When her weight dropped below 90 pounds, Jessica began noticing soft black hair growing on parts of her body. At the same time, she began to feel cold all the time, even on hot summer days. Despite constantly feeling sick, Jessica was neither concerned nor displeased about her loss of weight. Except for believing that she was a little too fat, she liked her body as it was and had no desire to reverse the downward spiral of weight loss. On the contrary, she became even more determined to lose additional weight and began to fast completely for 4 or 5 days at a time.

Elise was a senior in high school who had always been an excellent student. She made good grades and was involved in many school-related activities, but like Jessica and many other young women, she was unhappy with her weight. Elise wanted to weigh less than 100 pounds, a weight she felt was reasonable for her 5'2" frame, but she weighed over 120 pounds. She began eating less—not eating at all during the day, missing dinner due to school-related activities, and fooling her family into thinking that she was eating. Like Jessica, she tended to wear baggy clothing, so at first her family and friends did not notice her weight loss. Unlike Jessica, Elise found fasting difficult and did not feel like exercising to lose weight, so she began to vomit as a way to compensate for eating. Soon she added laxatives as an additional technique. She kept both practices secret from her family, who she believed would have tried to stop her.

It was not her disordered eating that resulted in her receiving treatment, but rather it was signs of depression—she cried easily, was always tired, and didn't seem to enjoy anything. Elise's family insisted that she go to a psychiatrist, who recognized her eating problems and tried to get Elise to recognize them, too. Elise listened to her psychiatrist and trusted her, forming a positive relationship, but she resisted the notion that she had an eating problem.

Not only did Elise deny her eating problems, but she also continued to vomit and abuse laxatives as ways to lose weight. By the time she graduated from high school, she had lost more than 15 pounds (but still weighed 104 pounds, 5 pounds away from her goal). Her weight began to be an issue with her family and friends, who told her that she was too thin and that she looked terrible. Despite the amount of weight she had lost, she did not meet the criteria to be diagnosed as anorexic according to the *Diagnostic and Statistical Manual of Mental Disorders* (American Psychiatric Association, 1987, 1994). Those criteria include weight loss to the point that the person is 15% below ideal weight, which Elise was not. However, she exhibited the distorted body image, fear of gaining weight, and **amenorrhea** (cessation of menstrual periods) that are symptoms of anorexia.

Elise's diagnosis was **bulimia,** an eating disorder consisting of binge eating followed by some method to compensate for the binge, such as fasting, excessive exercising, or purging through either vomiting or using laxatives. Elise exhibited these symptoms, forcing herself to vomit and abusing laxatives, even when the amount of food she had eaten was not excessive.

Elise's eating problems got worse when she began college. She purged by both vomiting and using laxatives. But the more laxatives she consumed, the less effective they became. So she increased the dosage to the point of once taking 45 tablets in less than 2 days. This precipitated a medical crisis, resulting in her being hospitalized and receiving psychotherapy. Her therapist tried to convince Elise to accept a reasonable body image, to eat reasonably, and to stop purging.

Elise tried hard to get better over the next 5 years, but her distorted body image continued. She is still

unhappy with her weight, but she continues to work on her recovery. She purged for years but says that the urge to do so has decreased.

Like millions of Americans, Jessica and Elise suffer from some form of **eating disorder.** An eating disorder is any serious and habitual disturbance in eating behavior that produces unhealthy consequences. This definition excludes both starvation resulting from the inability to find enough food and unhealthy eating resulting from inadequate information about nutrition. Also excluded are disturbances in eating behavior such as pica, or the eating of nonnutritive substances such as plastic and wood, and the rumination disorder of infancy—that is, regurgitation of food without nausea or gastrointestinal illness. Neither of these latter disorders presents serious health problems to adults, and they are of relatively minor importance in health psychology. This chapter examines in detail the three major problems of eating—overeating and dieting, anorexia nervosa, and bulimia—each related to difficulties in weight maintenance. To put these in context, we first consider the organs and functions of the digestive system.

The Digestive System

The human body can digest a wide variety of plant and animal tissues, converting these foods into usable proteins, fats, carbohydrates, vitamins, and minerals. The digestive system takes in food, processes it into particles that can be absorbed, and excretes the undigested wastes. The particles that are absorbed through the digestive system are transported through the bloodstream so as to be available to all body cells. These molecules nourish the body by providing the energy for activity as well as the materials for body growth, maintenance, and repair.

The digestive tract is a modified tube, consisting of a number of specialized structures. Also included in the digestive system are several accessory structures connected to the digestive tract by ducts. These ducted glands produce substances that are es-

sential for digestion, and the ducts provide a way for these substances to enter the digestive system. Figure 15.1 shows the digestive system.

In humans and other mammals, some digestion begins in the mouth. The teeth tear and grind food, mixing it with saliva. Several **salivary glands** furnish the moisture that allows the food to be tasted. Without such moisture, the taste buds on the tongue would not function. Saliva also contains an enzyme that digests starch, and so some digestion begins before food particles leave the mouth.

Swallowing is a voluntary action, but once food is swallowed, its progress through the **pharynx** and **esophagus** is largely involuntary. **Peristalsis** propels food through the digestive system, beginning with the esophagus. Peristaltic movement is the rhythmic contraction and relaxation of the circular muscles of structures in the digestive system. In the stomach, rhythmic contrac-

CHECK YOUR HEALTH RISKS

Check the items that apply to you.

❑ 1. My weight concerns me a great deal.

❑ 2. Food is a danger that can be managed by careful thought and mental preparation in order not to eat too much.

❑ 3. I have lost 10 pounds or more over the past two years.

❑ 4. I have gained 10 pounds or more over the past two years.

❑ 5. I am more than 30 pounds overweight.

❑ 6. My waist is as big as or bigger than my hips.

❑ 7. I have been on at least 10 different diet programs in my life.

❑ 8. I have fasted, used laxatives, or used diet drugs to lose weight.

❑ 9. My family has been concerned that I am too thin, but I disagree.

❑ 10. My coach or instructor has suggested that weighing less could improve my athletic performance.

❑ 11. I often feel guilty about eating.

❑ 12. I sometimes lose control over eating and eat far more than I had planned.

❑ 13. I would like to have liposuction surgery to remove fat from my body.

❑ 14. I have vomited after eating as a way to control my weight.

Each of these items represents a health risk from improper eating or unhealthy attitudes about eating. Unhealthy eating contributes to the development of several diseases, and preoccupation with weight and frequent dieting can also be unhealthy. Count your check marks to evaluate your risks. As you read this chapter, you will learn that some of these items are riskier than others.

---

tions mix the food with **gastric juices** secreted by the stomach and the glands that empty into the stomach. The major digestive activity of the stomach is proteins digestion, initiated by the action of the enzyme **pepsin**. Little absorption of nutrients occurs in the stomach; only alcohol, aspirin, and some fat-soluble drugs are absorbed through the stomach lining. The major function of the stomach is to mix food particles with gastric juices, preparing the mixture for absorption in the small intestine.

The mixture of food particles and gastric juices moves into the small intestine a little at a time. The high acidity of the gastric juices results in a very acidic mixture, and the small intestine cannot function in high acidity. To reduce the level of acidity, the pancreas secretes several acid-reducing

enzymes into the small intestine. These **pancreatic juices** are also essential for digesting carbohydrates and fats.

The digestion of starch that begins in the mouth is completed in the small intestine. The upper third of the small intestine absorbs starch and other carbohydrates. Protein digestion, initiated in the stomach, is also completed when proteins are absorbed in the upper portion of the small intestine. Fats, however, enter the small intestine almost entirely undigested. **Bile salts** produced in the **liver** and stored in the **gall bladder** break down fat molecules into a form that is acted on by a pancreatic enzyme. Absorption of fats occurs in the middle one-third of the small intestine. The bile salts that aid the process are reabsorbed later in the lower third of the small intestine.

Associated
structures:

parotids
tongue
teeth
salivary
glands

liver

gallbladder

pancreas

Major
components:

mouth
(oral cavity)

pharynx

esophagus

stomach

small
intestine

large
intestine
(colon)

rectum

anus

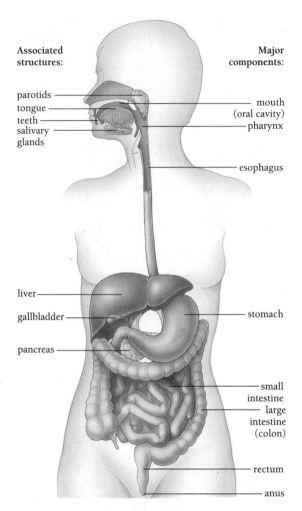

Figure 15.1   The digestive system.   *Source: Introduction to Microbiology* (p. 556), by J. L. Ingraham & C. A. Ingraham, 1995, Belmont, CA: Wadsworth. Copyright © 1995 by Wadsworth Publishing Company. Reprinted by permission.

Large quantities of water pass through the small intestine. In addition to the water that people drink, digestive juices increase the fluid volume. Of all the water that passes into the small intestine, 90% is absorbed. This absorption process also causes vitamins and electrolytes to pass into the body at this point in digestion.

From the small intestine, digestion proceeds to the large intestine. As with other portions of the digestive system, movement through the large intestine occurs through peristalsis. However, the peristaltic movement in the large intestine is more sluggish and irregular than in the small intestine. Bacteria inhabit the large intestine and manufacture several vitamins. Although the large intestine has absorptive capabilities, it typically absorbs only water, a few minerals, and the vitamins manufactured by its bacteria.

Feces consist of the materials left after digestion has taken place. Feces are composed of undigested fiber, inorganic material, undigested nutrients, water, and bacteria. Peristalsis carries the feces through the large intestine, through the **rectum**, and finally through the **anus**, where they are eliminated.

In addition to the structures of the digestive system, several brain structures and hormones are important for eating and digestion. The **hypothalamus** (see Figure 15.2) contains centers that are involved in eating. Damage to the lateral hypothalamus decreases eating, possibly due to decreased responsiveness to taste (Pinel, 1997). Damage to the ventromedial hypothalamus is associated with substantial weight gain due to increased stomach motility and increases in insulin production (Kalat, 1998). Rapid emptying of the stomach prompts eating, which furnishes the materials for weight gain. Insulin is a hormone that allows body cells to take in glucose for their use. High insulin production leads to the intake of more glucose than cells can use, and the excess is converted into fat. Thus, high insulin production results in obesity.

Two additional hormones are related to eating and weight control. **Cholecystokinin (CCK)** is a peptide hormone produced by the intestines and is also a neurotransmitter in the brain. Its production is related to feelings of satiation. **Leptin** is a protein hormone discovered in 1994 (Auwerx & Staels, 1998). Genetically obese mice (Pelleymounter et al., 1995) and overfed mice (Campfield, Smith, Guisez, Devos, & Burn, 1995) lost weight when injected with leptin. The weight loss occurred because the mice decreased their food intake and increased their activity level. Although leptin would

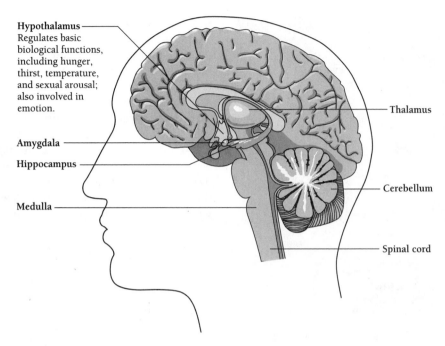

Hypothalamus
Regulates basic
biological functions,
including hunger,
thirst, temperature,
and sexual arousal;
also involved in
emotion.

Thalamus

Amygdala

Hippocampus

Cerebellum

Medulla

Spinal cord

Figure 15.2 Hypothalamus and other brain structures.

seem to be a miracle cure for obesity, a review of the extensive research (Auwerx & Staels, 1998) on its use indicated that leptin is involved in weight maintenance in complex ways but is no cure for obesity.

In summary, the digestive system turns food into nutrients by a process that begins in the mouth with the breakdown of food into smaller particles. Digestive juices continue to act on food particles in the stomach, but digestion of most types of nutrients occurs in the small intestine. Digestion is completed with the elimination of the undigested residue. In addition to the digestive system structures, brain structures and several hormones are involved in eating and weight maintenance. The digestive system is plagued by more diseases and disorders than any other body system. Many digestive disorders are not of active concern to health psychology, but several, such as obesity, anorexia nervosa, and bulimia have important behavioral components.

Factors in Weight Maintenance

A stable weight is maintained when the calories absorbed from food equal those expended for body metabolism plus physical activity. However, this balance is not a simple calculation. Caloric content varies with foods, with fat having more calories per volume than carbohydrates or proteins. The degree of absorption depends on how rapidly food passes through the digestive system and the composition of the foods. The body turns dietary fat into body fat more easily than it does other types of fuels (Rodin, 1992), putting those who eat a high-fat diet at higher risk for obesity than those whose diet is lower in fat (Tremblay, Plourde, Després, & Bouchard, 1989).

Furthermore, large differences exist in people's metabolic rates, and an individual's metabolism can vary from time to time. Activity level is another source of variability, with greater activity requiring greater caloric expenditures. To understand the

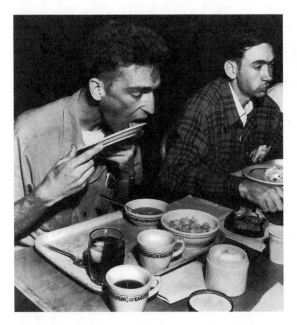

Experimental starvation produced an obsession with food and a variety of negative changes in the behavior of these volunteers.

complexities of weight loss through reduction of food intake, consider an extreme example, an experiment in which participants were systematically starved.

Experimental Starvation

More than 50 years ago, Ancel Keys and his colleagues (Keys, Brozek, Henschel, Mickelsen, & Taylor, 1950) developed an interest in the physical effects of starvation. They had an opportunity to study conscientious objectors during World War II, men who volunteered to be part of a study on starvation as an alternative to military service.

For the first 3 months of the project, the 36 volunteers ate regularly and participated in various tests. In most ways the participants were quite normal young men; their weights were normal, their IQs were in the normal to bright range, and they were emotionally stable. All held religious convictions that forbade fighting, and they volunteered for this project as a substitute for military

service. After the 3 months of normal eating and establishing caloric requirements, the men were put on half their previous rations, with the goal of reducing their body weight to 75% of previous levels. Although the researchers cut the participants' caloric intake in half, they were careful to give them adequate nutrients so that the men were never in any danger of actually starving.

At first these men lost weight rapidly. They were constantly hungry, but the initial pace of weight loss did not last. To continue losing weight, the men had to consume even fewer calories, which led to a few dropping out of the experiment. Nevertheless, most stayed with the project through the whole 6 months, and most met their goal of losing 25% of their body weight.

The behaviors that accompanied the semistarvation were quite surprising to Keys and his colleagues. At the beginning the men were optimistic and cheerful, but these feelings soon vanished. The men became irritable and aggressive and began to fight among themselves, behavior that was completely out of character. Although the men continued this bellicose behavior throughout the 6 months of starvation, they also became apathetic and avoided physical activity as much as they could. They became neglectful of their dormitory, their own physical appearance, and their girlfriends.

The men were, of course, hungry, and they became increasingly obsessed with thoughts of food. Mealtimes became the center of their lives, and they tended to eat very slowly and to be very sensitive to the taste of their food. At the beginning of the period of caloric reduction, no physical restrictions had been imposed to prevent the men from cheating on their diets. But about 3 months into the starvation, the men felt that they would be tempted to cheat if they left the dormitory alone. As a result, they were allowed to go out only in pairs or in larger groups. These dedicated, polite, normal, stable young men had become abnormal and unpleasant under conditions of semistarvation.

Obsession with food and continued negative outlook also characterized the refeeding phase of the project. During refeeding, the plan was for the men to regain the weight they had lost. This phase was to have lasted 3 months, with food introduced at gradually increasing levels, but the men objected so strongly that the pace of refeeding was accelerated. As a result, the men ate as much and as often as they could, some as many as five large meals a day. By the end of the refeeding period, most men had regained their preexperimental weight. In fact, many were even slightly heavier. About one-half were still preoccupied with food, and for many, their prestarvation optimism and cheerfulness had not completely returned.

Experimental Overeating

A study in experimental starvation does not seem attractive to volunteers, but an experiment on overeating might sound like fun to many people. Ethan Allen Sims and his associates (Sims, 1974, 1976; Sims et al., 1973; Sims & Horton, 1968) found a group of people who should have been especially interested and appreciative—prisoners. Inmates at the Vermont State Prison volunteered to gain 20 to 30 pounds as part of an experiment on overeating. Sims's interest was analogous to Keys's—an understanding of the physical and psychological components of overeating. Special living arrangements were made for these prisoners, including plentiful and delicious food. In addition, the experiment included a restriction of physical activity to make weight gain easier.

Did these men gain weight? With an increase in calories and a decrease in physical activity, weight gain was nearly assured. At first they gained fairly easily. But soon the rate of weight gain slowed, and the participants had to eat more and more to continue gaining. As with the men in the starvation study, these men needed about 3,500 calories to maintain their weight at normal levels, but many had to double that amount to continue gaining. Not all the men were able to attain their weight goals, regardless of how much they ate. One man did not reach his goal even though he ate over 10,000 calories per day.

Were the overeating prisoners as miserable as the starving conscientious objectors? No, but they did find overeating unpleasant. Food became repulsive to them, despite the excellent quality and preparation. They had to force themselves to eat, and many considered dropping out of the study.

When the weight-gain phase of the study was over, the prisoners cut down their food intake dramatically and lost weight. Not all lost as quickly as others, and two had some trouble returning to their original weight. An examination of these two men's medical backgrounds revealed some family histories of obesity, although the men themselves had never been overweight. These results indicate that normal-weight people have trouble increasing their weight substantially and that, even if they do, the increased weight is difficult to maintain.

In Summary

Weight maintenance depends largely on two factors: the number of calories absorbed through food intake and the number expended through body metabolism and physical activity. Weight gain occurs when more nutrients are present than are required for maintenance of body metabolism and physical activity. Weight loss occurs when insufficient nutrients are present to furnish the necessary energy for body metabolism and activity. An experiment in starvation showed that loss of too much weight leads to irritability, aggression, apathy, lack of interest in sex, and preoccupation with food. Another experiment in overeating showed that gaining weight can be almost as difficult as losing it for some people.

Overeating and Obesity

Many people assume that overeating is the sole cause of obesity, but the weight maintenance equation is quite complex. Not all obese people eat a great deal; many overweight people eat less than normal-weight people and even less than some thin people. As the studies on experimental starvation and overeating show, metabolic level changes with food intake as well as with energy output to alter the efficiency of nutrient use by the body.

In addition, individual variations in body metabolism allow some people to burn calories faster than others. Thus, two people who eat the same amount may have different weights. Certainly, these findings are not true of all people; some obese people are fat because they eat a lot, do too little physical activity, or some combination of the two (Bray, 1992). Before examining the health consequences of obesity, we look at the meaning of obesity and consider the question of why some people are overweight.

What Is Obesity?

What is obesity? Answers to this question vary by personal and social standards. Should obesity be defined in terms of health? Appearance? Body mass? Percentage of body fat? Weight charts? Total weight? No definition of obesity would consider only body weight, because some individuals have a small skeletal frame and others are more muscular. Muscle tissue and bone weigh more than fat, so some people can be heavier yet leaner than normal, as athletes often are. Therefore, an accurate measure of percentage of body fat is a better index of obesity than total weight.

Determining percentage and distribution of body fat is not as easy as consulting a chart, and several different methods exist to assess body fat. Many new technologies for imaging the body—computer tomography, ultrasound, and magnetic resonance imaging—can be applied to assessing fat content, but these methods have the drawbacks of being very expensive and relatively inaccessible. Simpler methods are less accurate but more accessible. The skinfold technique involves measuring the thickness of a pinch of skin. Although this method is relatively easy and inexpensive, it is not very accurate (Bray, 1992). The water immersion technique is awkward, requiring a person to be lowered into water to determine the amount of displacement. Although this technique accurately records the percentage of body fat, it does not measure the distribution of body fat, and it is moderately expensive. However, the waist-to-hip ratio method does measure distribution, making this measurement preferable to most other methods when estimating body fat and its distribution.

Another method is the **body mass index (BMI)**, defined as body weight in kilograms (kg) divided by height in meters squared (m²), that is, $BMI = kg / m^2$. George Bray (1992) has suggested that the BMI is the preferred estimate of obesity, and most recent investigators have chosen this definition. Although BMI does not consider a person's age, gender, or body build, David Williamson (1993) argued that this index can provide a standard for measuring obesity, which he defined as a BMI of 27.8 or more for men and 27.3 or more for women. (A 5'10" man with a BMI of 27.8 would weigh 194 pounds, and a 5'4" woman with a BMI of 27.3 would weigh 159.) These numbers are approximately 20% above the weights in the 1983 Metropolitan Life Insurance Company's height-weight charts for people with a medium frame. Table 15.1 shows a sample of BMI levels and their corresponding heights and weights.

Most people (and many researchers) continue to rely on the charts that provide normal weight ranges for various heights and body frame sizes. The charts published by the Metropolitan Life Insurance Company are based on statistics from the Society of Actuaries and thus reflect weight ranges with the lowest mortality. Table 15.2 shows both the 1959 and the 1983 charts, and a comparison shows that being overweight has been redefined in an upward direction.

Overweight is often defined in terms of social standards, and such definitions usually have little to do with health. The criteria for ideal weight have changed during human history (Beller, 1978; Bennett & Gurin, 1982). During the times when food supply was uncertain (the most frequent situation throughout history), carrying some supply of fat on the body was a type of insurance and was thus considered attractive. Fat could also be considered a mark of prosperity; fat advertised to the world that a person could afford an ample supply of food. Only in very recent history has this standard changed. Before 1920, thinness was considered unattractive, possibly due to the association between thinness and diseases or perhaps its association with poverty (Bennett & Gurin, 1982).

Thinness is no longer considered unattractive. In fact, today it is as highly desirable as plumpness was in the previous centuries, especially for women. An early study (Garner, Garfinkel, Schwartz, & Thompson, 1980) examined changes in the body weight of *Playboy* centerfolds and also Miss America candidates from 1959 to 1978 and found that weights for both groups had decreased relative to average weight of the general population. A follow-up study (Wiseman, Gray, Mosimann, &

Ahrens, 1992) examined the same relationship from 1979 to 1988. During that time, Miss America contestants became significantly thinner, indicating that the socially ideal weight for women dropped during both decades. Clearly, obesity, like beauty, is in the eye of the beholder.

Despite the nearly constant attempts of many people to achieve thinness, obesity in the United States has increased by one-third during the past 2 decades (Katan, Grundy, & Willett, 1997). During this time, many women have become both more conscious of and more dissatisfied with their weight, even when their weight is normal. A

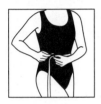

Table 15.1 Body mass index scores and their corresponding heights and weights

Height in inches	Body mass index, kg / m2							
	17.5*	21	23	25	27	30	35	40**
	Weight in pounds							
60	90	107	118	128	138	153	179	204
61	93	111	122	132	143	158	185	211
62	96	115	126	136	147	164	191	218
63	99	118	130	141	142	169	197	225
64	102	122	134	145	157	174	202	232
65	105	126	138	150	162	180	210	240
66	109	130	142	155	167	186	216	247
67	112	134	146	159	172	191	223	255
68	115	138	155	164	177	197	230	262
69	118	142	155	169	182	203	236	270
70	122	146	160	174	188	207	243	278
71	125	150	165	179	193	215	250	286
72	129	154	169	184	199	221	258	294
73	132	159	174	189	204	227	265	302
74	136	163	179	194	210	233	272	311
75	140	168	184	200	216	240	279	319
76	144	172	189	205	221	246	287	328

*BMI of 17.5 after intentional starvation meets one DSM-IV definition of anorexia nervosa.
**BMI of 40 is considered morbid obesity by Bender, Trautner, Spraul, & Berger, 1998.

national survey (Biener & Heaton, 1995) revealed that many women of normal weight are unwisely concerned that they weigh too much. In this survey, nearly half of European American women and one-fourth of African American women with a body mass index under 25 (see Table 15.1) were currently trying to lose weight. Interestingly, these dieters stated that their primary motive was to improve their health. However, the dieters in this survey had a history of 50% more weight fluctuation than the nondieters, which may be a health risk. This survey estimated that 2 million women in the United States (13% of all women) were using unhealthy strategies to lose weight, such as fasting, vomiting, using diet pills, and taking laxatives. A later study (Jeffery & French, 1996) showed that low-income women were more likely than high-income women to engage in most of these unhealthy practices and also to exercise less, eat fewer fruits and vegetables, and consume more sweets and "junk" foods. Therefore, concern about weight and health does not translate into healthy eating.

Why Are Some People Obese?

Just as there are several definitions of obesity, there are several models that attempt to explain why some people are obese. These models, which should be able to explain both the development and the maintenance of obesity, include the setpoint model and the positive incentive model.

The Setpoint Model   The setpoint model holds that weight is regulated around a **setpoint**, a type of internal thermostat. When fat levels rise above or fall below a certain level, physiological and psychological mechanisms are activated that encourage a return to setpoint. The findings from the study on experimental starvation and the studies on experimental overeating are consistent with the concept of a setpoint, which predicts that deviations from normal weight in either direction are achieved only with difficulty. When fat levels fall below setpoint, the body takes action to pre-

serve fat levels. Part of that action includes slowing the metabolic process to require fewer calories, thus making the body more conservative in its energy expenditures. People on diets have difficulty in continuing to lose weight because their bodies fight against depletion of fat stores. With conditions of prolonged and serious starvation, this slowed metabolism is expressed behaviorally as listlessness and apathy—both of which were exhibited by Keys's starving volunteers.

Increased hunger is the body's other corrective action when fat supplies fall below setpoint. Again, this mechanism seems to be consistent with the results of the Keys et al. (1950) study on starvation. The men who dieted to 75% of their normal body weight became miserable and hungry, and they stayed that way until they were back to their original weight. During the entire time they were below their normal weight (which would be below setpoint), they were obsessed with food. When they were allowed to eat, they preferred the high-calorie foods that tended to increase their fat stores most rapidly, a situation that is consistent with setpoint theory.

The experiment on overeating also fits with setpoint theory (Bennett & Gurin, 1982). The prisoners who tried to gain more than their normal weight were fighting their natural setpoint. According to the setpoint concept, the bodies of the overfed prisoners should have sent messages that they had enough fat stored already and did not need more. This message should have translated into something like "Stop eating," which seems to have happened because the prisoners found eating unpleasant.

The setpoint hypothesis also received support from a study of how people adjust to weight loss and weight gain (Leibel, Rosenbaum, & Hirsch, 1995). This study involved underfeeding obese men and women until they lost 10% to 20% of their baseline body weight and overfeeding normal weight men and women until they gained 10% of their baseline body weight. Participants who lost weight also lost energy, expending 15% less than before they were underfed; participants

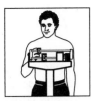

Table 15.2
Metropolitan Life Insurance Company's desirable weights for the years 1959 and 1983

Height		Small frame		Medium frame		Large frame	
		1959	1983	1959	1983	1959	1983
Women							
4 ft. 10 in.		92–98 lb.	102–111 lb.	96–107 lb.	109–121 lb.	104–119 lb.	118–131 lb.
4	11	94–101	103–113	98–110	111–123	106–122	120–134
5	0	96–104	104–115	101–113	113–126	109–125	122–137
5	1	99–107	106–118	104–116	115–129	112–128	125–140
5	2	102–110	108–121	107–119	118–132	115–131	128–143
5	3	105–113	111–124	110–122	121–135	118–134	131–147
5	4	108–116	114–127	113–126	124–138	121–138	134–151
5	5	111–119	117–130	116–130	127–141	125–142	137–155
5	6	114–123	120–133	120–135	130–144	129–146	140–159
5	7	118–127	123–136	124–139	133–147	133–150	143–163
5	8	122–131	126–139	128–143	136–150	137–154	146–167
5	9	126–135	129–142	132–147	139–153	141–158	149–170
5	10	130–140	132–145	136–151	142–156	145–163	152–173
5	11	134–144	135–148	140–155	145–159	149–168	155–176
6	0	138–148	138–151	144–159	148–162	153–173	158–179
Men							
5 ft. 2 in.		112–120 lb.	128–134 lb.	118–129 lb.	131–141 lb.	126–141 lb.	138–150 lb.
5	3	115–123	130–136	121–133	133–143	129–144	140–153
5	4	118–126	132–138	124–136	135–145	132–148	142–156
5	5	121–129	134–140	127–139	137–148	125–152	144–160
5	6	124–133	136–142	130–143	139–151	138–156	146–164
5	7	128–137	138–145	134–147	142–154	142–161	149–168
5	8	132–141	140–148	138–152	145–157	147–166	152–172
5	9	136–145	142–151	142–156	148–160	151–170	155–176
5	10	140–150	144–154	146–160	151–163	155–174	158–180
5	11	144–154	146–157	150–165	154–166	159–179	161–184
6	0	148–158	149–160	154–170	157–170	164–184	164–188
6	1	152–162	152–164	158–175	160–174	168–189	168–192
6	2	156–167	155–168	162–180	164–178	173–194	172–197
6	3	160–171	158–172	167–185	167–182	178–199	176–202
6	4	164–175	162–176	172–190	171–187	182–204	181–207

Source: From "New Weight Standards for Men and Women," by Metropolitan Life Insurance Company, 1959, *Statistical Bulletin,* 40, p. 1. Copyright © 1959, 1983 by The Metropolitan Life Insurance Company. Adapted by permission.

who gained weight increased their total expenditure of energy. Like Keys's conscientious objectors, the people who lost weight became increasingly hungry, and this hunger along with decreased energy made it very difficult for them to maintain weight loss. In contrast, the increased energy and decreased hunger of the overfed participants hampered their ability to maintain weight gain.

Questions remain concerning the usefulness of the setpoint model, including why some people's setpoint is set at obese. One answer may be that the setpoint has a hereditary component. Evidence from studies of adopted children (Stunkard et al., 1986) and of identical twins reared together or apart (Stunkard, Harris, Pedersen, & McClean, 1990) have suggested a role for heredity in weight. A close relationship existed between the weight of adopted children and that of their biological parents, but there was no relationship between their weight and that of their adoptive parents. The study of identical twins indicated that the correlations between weights of twin pairs were high, even when the twins were not reared together. The heritability of obesity may also vary by gender (Allison, Heshka, Neale, Lykken, & Heymsfield, 1994; Stunkard, 1989), with obesity more heritable in women than in men. Concluding that weight has a genetic component is not the same as saying that weight is genetically determined; genes influence fat only indirectly through effects on eating and metabolism. This relationship between biology and behavior means that both must be understood in order to solve the puzzle of obesity.

Most advocates of the setpoint model (Bennett & Gurin, 1982, Nisbett, 1972; Polivy & Herman, 1983) do not believe that it explains all cases of weight deviation and concede that variations from setpoint are possible. People can become obese by overeating, or they can keep their weight lower than setpoint through constant efforts to restrain their eating.

Although the setpoint concept is consistent with many of the findings about weight maintenance, some pieces of information do not fit with this model (Pinel, 1997). From an evolutionary point of view, humans (and other animals) should have a tendency to store fat, because an unreliable food supply makes stored fat a buffer against famine and thus a survival advantage. Those humans with the tendency not only to store fat but also to metabolically protect those fat stores would be at a substantial advantage in most situations in human history (Beller, 1978). This evolutionary view predicts a tendency to gain and difficulty in losing weight, but it does not suggest a setpoint around which weight is regulated.

Why would the setpoint be set at the level of obesity for some people but not others? A setpoint that dictates obesity for some and thinness for others makes very little sense. For example, variations in setpoint should not occur disproportionately in the United States. That is, setpoints should not differ from decade to decade or country to country. However, obesity is much more common in the United States than in other industrialized nations and has increased in the past 2 decades (Katan et al., 1997), suggesting some social influence as well as biological factors in obesity.

The Positive Incentive Model   The failure of setpoint theory to explain some factors related to eating and weight maintenance has led to the formulation of the positive incentive model. This model holds that the positive reinforcers of eating have important consequences for weight maintenance. This view suggests that people have several types of motivation to eat, including personal pleasure, social context, and biological factors (Pinel, 1997). The personal pleasure factors concentrate on the pleasures of eating, including the taste of food and how pleasurable eating is at any given time. The social context of eating includes the cultural background of the person eating, as well as what people are present and whether or not they are eating. Biological factors involved in eating include the length of time since eating and blood glucose levels. This model, then, includes biological factors in eating but holds that people learn to regulate their eating rather than having a setpoint that controls food intake (Ramsay, Seeley, Bolles, & Woods, 1996).

The setpoint model ignores the factors of taste, learning, and social context in eating, factors that are unquestionably important (Rozin, 1996). For each person in each instance, the act of choosing something to eat has a long history of personal experience and cultural learning. A preferred food is not equally appealing under all circumstances. For example, some foods do not seem to go together, even if each food is individually tasty. Various cultures have restrictions (and requirements) on what to eat and when. People tend to get hungry on a schedule that corresponds to mealtimes, but people in the United States are much more likely to eat cereal for breakfast than for dinner. Such cultural and learned factors also affect the caloric value of chosen foods and how much a person eats, and these choices influence body weight. For example, a women who is dieting might desire a brownie but choose a diet soda instead.

The positive incentive view predicts a variety of body weights, depending on food availability, individual experience with food, cultural encouragement to eat various foods, and the cultural ideal for body weight. The availability of an abundant food supply is necessary but not sufficient to produce obesity. People must overeat to become obese, and the quantity of food a person eats is related to how palatable the food is. Some tastes, such as sweet, are innately determined through the action of taste buds, but preference for flavor combinations seems to be the result of learning (Capaldi, 1996). In industrialized countries, a huge food industry promotes food products as desirable through massive advertising campaigns, and many of these foods are high in fat and sugar. This situation influences individual food choices that promote population-wide obesity.

Another factor that promotes overeating in industrialized countries is the availability of a variety of foods. Eating a very desirable food leads to decreased pleasure in eating it. (Hetherington & Rolls, 1996); that is, people become satiated for any particular food. When food supplies are limited in variety (but not in quantity), this factor can lead to lower levels of food consumption; but a new taste can tempt someone who is full to eat

more. Indeed, if eating a sufficient amount terminated a meal, dessert would not be so popular (Pinel, 1997).

Variety is important in boosting eating, even in rats. One study (Sclafani & Springer, 1976) showed that a "supermarket" diet produced weight gains of 269% in laboratory rats. The diet consisted of a changing variety of foods chosen from the supermarket, including chocolate chip cookies, salami, cheese, bananas, marshmallows, chocolate, peanut butter, and sweetened condensed milk. The combination of high fat and high sugar plus the changing variety led to enormous weight gain. Are humans very different? The availability of a wide variety of tasty food should produce widespread obesity, which is exactly the situation that exists in the United States today. This wide variety of foods allows people to always have some foods that furnish a new taste, and people in such situations never become satiated for all available foods.

How, then, do some people escape obesity? The answer lies in culture and learning: The ideal body type is thin, especially for women, so dieting and food restriction have become a way of life for many people. These people are able to avoid overeating through conscious effort to restrict food intake. Such efforts should create different eating patterns in these individuals, and a series of experiments (Polivy & Herman, 1983) indicated that restrained eaters differ from others in their taste sensitivity, constant awareness of eating, and the problem of lapsing and eating too much.

In summary, some evidence not consistent with the setpoint model fits better with the positive incentive theory of eating and weight maintenance, including individual food preferences, cultural influences in eating, cultural influences on body composition, and the relationship between food availability and obesity. Both the setpoint and positive incentive models suggest that some people will be obese, and this situation is disturbing to those who want to adhere to fashion and those who believe that obesity constitutes a serious health problem.

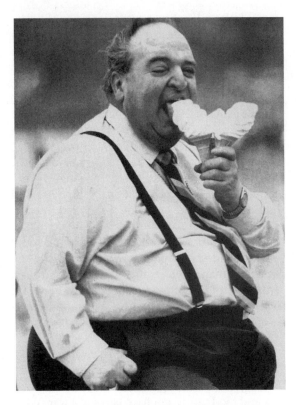

The weight maintenance equation is complex, but overeating is a cause of obesity.

Is Obesity Unhealthy?

The question of obesity's effect on health is complicated. The answer depends on one's degree of obesity, history of weight cycling, and distribution of weight. Although being moderately overweight is probably not an independent risk factor for heart disease or for all-cause mortality, being severely obese, having a history of weight losses and gains, and having a high waist-to-hip ratio place a person at an elevated health risk.

In general, a U-shaped relationship seems to exist between weight and poor health; that is, the very thinnest and the very heaviest people are at greatest risk for all-cause mortality. Such a relationship appeared in a study that followed a group of women for 26 years (Lindsted & Singh, 1997). A

positive relationship between body mass and mortality appeared after 8 years for middle-aged women, but a U-shaped relationship emerged after 26 years. This U-shaped curve does not apply to individual causes, such as heart disease (Manson et al., 1995; Rimm et al., 1995) or ischemic stroke (Rexrode et al., 1997). Instead, it appears when considering death from all causes.

Extreme obesity is a risk. A recent large-scale study from Germany (Bender, Trautner, Spraul, & Berger, 1998) showed no relationship between obesity and all-cause mortality for men with BMI scores up to 32, and only a very weak relationship for women in this range. Moderate obesity (up to a BMI of 36) produced a relatively weak risk for all-cause mortality. Only when BMI scores rose above 40 did both men and women more than double their risk for all-cause mortality. (A BMI of 40—defined as morbid obesity—is equivalent to 278 pounds for a man 5 feet 10 or 232 pounds for a woman 5 feet 4. See Table 15.1 for other weights and heights.) In terms of attributable risk, 67% of deaths among morbidly obese men and 57% among morbidly obese women were due to their excess weight. A summary of these levels of risk appears in Table 15.3.

Both age and ethnicity complicate the interpretation of risk from obesity. For young and middle-aged adults, being overweight is a risk for all-cause mortality and especially for death due to cardiovascular disease (Stevens et al., 1998). After age 65, the relationship no longer exists, and losing weight after age 50 increases risk (Diehr et al., 1998). Also, very thin people do not have the lowest mortality rates (Durazo-Arvizu, McGee, Cooper, Liao, & Luke, 1998). For African American men and women, the healthiest BMI levels were around 27. For European Americans, the lowest mortality rates were associated with BMI levels of 24 to 25.

Besides gross and morbid obesity, weight cycling (yo-yo dieting) presents a health risk. One study (Borkan, Sparrow, Wisniewski, & Vokonas, 1986) found that weight changes alone were associated with the risk factors for coronary heart

Table 15.3   Categories of obesity and risks for all-cause mortality based on body mass index (BMI)

Degree of RR obesity	BMI range	Risk for men	Relative Risk	Risk for women	Relative Risk
Moderate	25 to 32	None	1.0	Very low	1.1
Obese	32 to 36	Low	1.3	Low	1.2
Gross	36 to 40	High	1.9	Low	1.3
Morbid	40+	Very high	3.1	Very high	2.3

Information based on Bender et al. (1998)

disease. A report from the Framingham study (Lissner et al., 1991) indicated that people with a history of weight cycling had a significant increase in risk for all-cause mortality, heart disease, and cancer. This study also found that fluctuation in weight carried more of a risk than obesity itself.

A study of Harvard alumni (Lee & Paffenbarger, 1992) found that men who either lost or gained weight had a higher death rate from all causes and from coronary heart disease than men with stable weight, and a study of middle-aged and older men (Yaari & Goldbourt, 1998) found that weight loss was associated with increased mortality risks, even if the men had lost weight intentionally. In a review of the research on weight cycling, Kelly Brownell and Judith Rodin (1994b) concluded that this pattern of weight loss and gain is associated with increased cardiovascular disease and all-cause mortality, and research since this review (Rexrode et al., 1997) confirms this conclusion.

A third weight-related factor associated with morbidity and mortality is a person's distribution of weight. During the past 2 decades, evidence has suggested that people who accumulate excess weight around their abdomen are at greater risk than people who carry their excess weight on their hips and thighs. As part of the Health Professionals Follow-up Study, middle aged and older male physicians were examined (Walker, et al., 1996), but no relationship appeared between body mass index and risk of stroke. However, when considering the ratio of waist size to hip size, a substantial relationship appeared. Men whose waists were about the same size as their hips were 2.3 times more likely to have stroke than a comparison group of men whose waist-to-hip ratio was 0.89 or less. Other studies too have found that the waist-to-hip ratio is a good predictor of a variety of health problems (see the Would You Believe . . . ? box).

In conclusion, obese people have heightened risks of developing certain health problems, especially diabetes and cardiovascular disease. Table 15.4 summarizes studies showing that gross obesity, changes in weight, and fat distributed around the waist all relate to increased mortality rates, especially from heart disease.

In Summary

Obesity can be defined in terms of health or social standards, and the two are not always the same. The ideal weight for health can be seen in the Metropolitan Insurance Company weight charts or reflected in the body mass index (BMI). Social standards, however, have dictated a standard of thinness with a lower body weight than is ideal for health.

Obesity can be accounted for by the setpoint model and by the positive incentive model. Setpoint theory explains obesity in terms of a high setpoint for body weight, whereas positive incentive theory holds that people gain weight when they have an abundant supply of tasty food.

WOULD YOU BELIEVE...?

A Big Butt Is Healthier Than a Fat Gut

Would you believe that a big butt is better than a fat gut, at least in terms of health risks? All fat is not equal: Abdominal fat creates more of a health risk than fat in the thighs and hips. In recent years, researchers have begun looking at the waist-to-hip ratio as a predictor of disease, especially heart disease. Women generally have lower waist-to-hip ratios than men and they also have lower rates of heart disease. A woman with a waist of 28 inches and a hip measurement of 36 would have a ratio of 0.78, while a man with 36 inch waist and a 41 inch hip measurement would have a ratio of 0.88. Each of these ratios is considered to be in the healthy range for women and men respectively. A ratio of 1.0 or higher could be dangerous, especially for women.

One early study (Hartz, Rupley, & Rimm, 1984) examined obese women and found that those whose waist measurements were large compared with their hip measurements had an elevated risk of diabetes, hypertension, and gallbladder disease. Later studies (Sjöström, 1992a; 1992b) found that the dangers of a high waist-to-hip ratio apply to men as well as to women. For both genders, the location of fat on the body is related to the risk of heart disease. The amount of fat is not as important as its distribution. Men are more likely to show the pattern of central fat distribution with accumulated fat around the middle, whereas women are more prone to develop large hips and thighs. Thus, men not only have a higher waist-to-hip ratio than women, but they also have a greater likelihood of developing heart disease.

The accumulation of fat around the middle is related to risk factors for heart disease, even during adolescence and early adulthood (van Lenthe, van Mechelen, Kemper, & Twisk, 1998). Weight around one's middle may be a better predictor of all-cause mortality than body mass index. A study on a large group of Iowa women (Folsom et al., 1993) showed that the larger the waist-to-hip ratio, the higher the death rate. This dose-response relationship remained after controlling for BMI, smoking, educational level, marital status, estrogen use, and alcohol consumption. Folsom et al. concluded that waist-to-hip ratio is a better predictor of death in older women than body mass index. Similarly, the Nurses' Health Study (Rexrode et al., 1998), after adjusting for body mass index, found that women with a waist-to-hip ratio of 0.88 or higher had more than a three-fold risk for coronary heart disease compared with women with a ratio less than 0.72. Authors of this study concluded that a high waist-to-hip ratio is an independent risk factor for heart disease in women.

However, the health risk of a big gut may not be equal for all people. Examining the distribution of body fat and its relationship to heart disease in African American and European American men and women revealed differences (Freedman, Williamson, Croft, Ballew, and Byers, 1995). The relationship between fat around one's middle and ischemic heart disease appeared, but this risk did not extend to African American women. The relative risk for African American men and European American men was essentially identical, and the risk for European American women was highest of all. However, African American women with weight distributed around the middle had no extra risk of heart disease. Some evidence (Biener & Heaton, 1995) indicates that African American women are less concerned about losing weight than European American women, and this reduced concern may be justified. For other subgroups, however, a fat gut is more dangerous to health than a big butt.

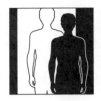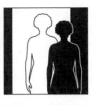

Table 15.4
The relationship between weight and disease or death

Study	Sample	Results
	Effects of obesity	
Lindsted & Singh, 1997	Seventh-Day Adventist women	A U-shaped relationship exists between BMI and all-cause mortality so that obese older women may not be at risk.
Manson et al., 1995	middle-aged women	Heaviest women have a fourfold risk for cardiovascular disease.
Rexrode et al., 1997	middle-aged women	BMI of 32+ doubles risk of ischemic stroke.
Rimm et al., 1995	men 65 and older	BMI of 33+ is a strong predictor of heart disease.
Bender et al., 1998	obese men	No increase in all-cause mortality up to BMI of 32. Morbid obesity (BMI of 40+) carries a threefold risk for men and more than a double risk for women.
	Effects of weight cycling	
Borkan et al., 1986	men with history of weight cycling	Weight cycling is associated with hypertension and high cholesterol levels.
Lissner et al., 1991	Framingham men and women	Weight change is more risky than obesity.
Lee & Paffenbarger, 1992	middle-aged men	Weight gain and weight loss are each related to all-cause mortality and CHD death.
	Effects of abdominal fat	
Walker, et al., 1996	middle-aged men and older men	High waist/hip ratio is related to a double risk for stroke.
Hartz et. al., 1984	middle-aged and older men	Large waist is a risk for diabetes, hypertension, and gallbladder disease.
Sjöström, 1992	men and women	High waist/hip ratio increases the risk for heart disease.
Folsom et al., 1993	middle-aged men	Waist/hip ratio is a better predictor than BMI of all-cause mortality.
Freedman et al., 1995	African American women	Central fat does not predict heart disease.
Freedman et al., 1995	All other groups	Central fat predicts heart disease.

Obesity is associated with increased mortality, heart disease, adult-onset diabetes, and digestive tract diseases, but the relationship between weight and all-cause mortality is a U-shaped one; that is, the very thinnest and the very heaviest people are at the greatest risk for death. Most people who are moderately overweight and who have no coronary risk factors are not at an increased risk for heart disease or all-cause mortality. Nevertheless, severe obesity, a history of weight cycling, and carrying excess weight around the waist rather than the hips are all risks of death from several causes, especially heart disease.

Dieting

Many people in the United States have some knowledge of the risks of obesity, weight cycling, and an unfavorable waist-to-hip ratio, and a large number of these people are trying to maintain a healthy weight. Nevertheless, obesity in the United States has risen sharply during the past 10 years (Jeffery & French, 1998). Why are people gaining weight, and what are they doing to try to lose weight?

Researchers have proposed several reasons for the steady increase in obesity over the past 2 decades. Robert Jeffery and Simone French (1998) cited evidence that Americans are eating more of their meals in fast food restaurants and are viewing more television, including video tapes and cable TV. They also demonstrated that both behaviors are related to a larger body mass index and to weight gain—at least in some people. Another possible explanation for increases in weight during the past 2 decades is a rise in consumption of sweets. People in the United States have reduced dietary fat from about 40% of energy intake to 33%, they have increased their intake of sugar from 120 pounds person to about 150 pounds (Connor & Connor, 1997). The exchange of fat for sugar is not a healthy one. A low-fat, high-carbohydrate diet may be able to reduce total cholesterol, but it does so largely by lowering HDL

cholesterol (Katan et al., 1997). Although most people believe that by reducing fat they automatically benefit with a leaner body and a longer life, they are mistaken. This finding demonstrates that people lack the information to make wise dietary choices.

The trend toward dieting has become more severe in the past few decades. During the mid-1960s, only 10% of overweight adults were dieting (Wyden, 1965), but during subsequent years those percentages steadily increased, so that currently nearly 70% of high school girls and more than 20% of high school boys have dieted at some time (French, Story, Downes, Resnick, & Blum, 1995). Adults too are increasingly likely to diet. A survey of adolescents and adults (Serdula et al., 1993) showed that two-thirds of the women and more than half of the men were trying either to lose or to not gain weight, making weight concerns a common experience to a majority of people in the United States. However, many of these dieters do not have sufficient excess weight to put them at risk for disease or death.

Approaches to Losing Weight

To lose weight or keep from gaining weight, people have several choices. They can (1) restrict the types of food they eat, (2) change their eating behaviors, (3) increase their level of exercise, (4) rely on drastic medical procedures, or use a combination of these approaches.

Restricting Types of Food Maintaining a diet consisting of a variety of foods with smaller portions is a reasonable and healthy strategy, but many people find it difficult simply to eat less. The approach of restricting types of foods has been a popular dieting strategy, but because a variety of foods is necessary for adequate nutrition, severely restricting or eliminating a food category may be nutritionally unwise.

Restricting carbohydrates has been a popular approach, possibly because low-carbohydrate diets often allow dieters to eat high-fat foods, which most

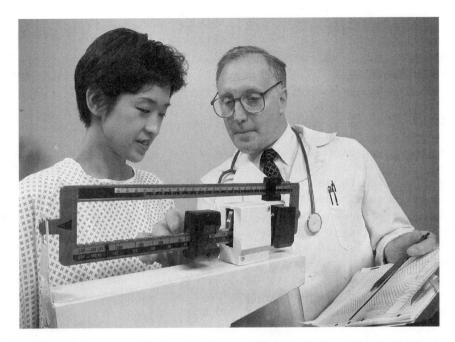

Dieting is increasingly common among those who do not need to lose weight for health reasons.

people find tasty. However, low-carbohydrate diets are open to severe criticism for being both ineffective and potentially dangerous. Evidence of ineffectiveness comes from research indicating that eating fat tends to increase fat intake rather than induce satiety (Tremblay et al., 1989). Thus, high-fat diets tend to be counterproductive in helping people lose weight. Such diets also produce fatigue and depression as frequent side effects, which some people develop after a few days on such diets. The primary danger of a high-fat diet is the increase in serum cholesterol. People who lose weight on such diets do so for the same reason that people on any diet lose weight: They consume fewer calories.

High-carbohydrate, low-fat diets have also had their advocates (Ornish, 1993). These diets strive to increase the amount of foods with "complex" carbohydrates while lowering fat intake. Fruits, vegetables, and whole-grain cereals contain complex carbohydrates, but sugar does not. Fats come

from animal and vegetable fats such as oils and butter, but many meats contain a high proportion of fats. Therefore, low-fat, high-carbohydrate diets are often vegetarian or modified vegetarian diets. Some dieters find these programs easy to follow, because they allow a greater volume of food (carbohydrates are lower in calories per volume, so a person can eat more). However, for some dieters, the food choices are not their favorites, and the feeling of constantly being deprived of preferred foods often leads to "cheating" and failure. Nutritionally, high-carbohydrate diets are safe and effective programs for controlling weight, especially if the carbohydrates are consumed in the form of fruits and vegetables.

Some diets are more extreme, restricting the dieter to a limited group of foods or even a single food. All-fruit diets, egg diets, and even the pound cake diet fall into this category. Of course, such diets are nutritional disasters. They produce weight loss by restricting calories; dieters get tired of the monotony of one food and eat less than they would if they were eating a variety. "All the hard-boiled eggs you want" turns out to be not many!

Taking monotony a step further are the liquid diets, which exist in a variety of forms and under various brand names. Liquid diets have the advantage of being nutritionally more balanced than most restricted food diets. Still, liquid diets and their equivalent meals in the form of puddings or bars have the disadvantage of being monotonous and repetitive, and they tend to be low in fiber. These diets, like all others, work by restricting calorie intake. Although current researchers may disagree on the advantages of low-fat or low-carbohydrate diets, they are likely to agree that diets high in fiber from fruits and vegetables are good choices (Connor & Connor, 1997; Katan et al, 1997).

In conclusion, any diet must be viewed as a lifelong eating pattern. Diets low in animal fats and high in fruits, vegetables, and whole grain cereals will generally produce weight loss and promote health. To be effective, however, any diet must be one that a person will be able to maintain throughout life.

Behavior Modification Programs

Although dieting should be seen as a permanent modification in one's eating habits, such a change is a difficult task. People who advocate a behavior modification approach to eating behaviors tend to treat eating problems directly rather than viewing overeating as a symptom of some other problem.

The behavior modification approach toward treating obesity was originated by Richard Stuart (1967), who reported a much higher success rate than with previous approaches. Most behavior modification programs use a broad assortment of techniques and focus on eating in a particular situation, at a particular time, and in association with particular feelings. Clients often keep eating diaries to focus their awareness on the types of foods they eat and under what circumstances as well as to provide data the therapist can use to devise a personal plan for changing unhealthy eating habits.

Because weight loss is not a behavior, these programs tend to reinforce good eating habits rather than the numbers of pounds lost. In other words, the behaviors, not the consequences, are rewarded. Behavior modification programs can affect weight by altering behavior and thus can be successful with some obese patients. However, not all obese people profit from these programs (White & White, 1988).

Exercise

The importance of exercise in weight loss has become increasingly apparent. Because metabolic rate slows down when food intake decreases, some form of physical activity is necessary to speed up metabolism. Exercise is known to counteract metabolic slowdown and thus may be an indispensable part of weight-reduction programs. Indeed, exercise alone is sufficient to cause some weight loss, and exercise can alter fitness and the distribution of fat (Blair, 1993). We have seen that fat distribution is a greater risk for heart disease than the percentage of body fat. Exercise can also decrease body mass index (Kahn et al., 1997). (The role of exercise is more fully discussed in Chapter 16.)

Drastic Methods of Losing Weight

People sometimes take drastic measures to lose weight, and physicians sometimes recommend drastic measures for severely obese patients. Even with medical supervision, some weight reduction programs present risks, sometimes to the point of being life threatening.

One approach that turned out to be more dangerous than initially believed was taking drugs to reduce appetite. In the 1950s and 1960s, diet pills were widely prescribed. These drugs were amphetamines, stimulant drugs that increase the activity of the nervous system, speed up metabolism, and suppress appetite. Unfortunately, these drugs lose their appetite-suppressing effect within a few weeks, so the dosage must be increased to maintain the desired effect. These diet pills can be effective for a short time, but for people who need to lose a considerable amount of weight and who therefore must continue taking amphetamines, dependence may become a more serious problem than obesity.

Increasing evidence of the dangers of amphetamines led to the development of other diet drugs. Most were chemically similar to amphetamines and shared their disadvantages, including the possibility of abuse. Two of these alternatives, fenfluramine and phenylpropylalamine were once believed to be safe and effective. However, in the Fall of 1997, the Food and Drug Administration warned people to stop taking these two drugs—known collectively as fen-phen—because their combination may contribute to heart valve damage. Other diet pills continue to be developed and will be available as long as people desire an easy solution to weight loss.

Fasting is another weight-loss measure that can be dangerous. Under conditions of food restriction, the body metabolizes fat and muscle tissue about equally, and some muscle tissue is present in essential organs. Thus, severe fasting can lead to the metabolism of internal organs. However, the *protein-sparing modified fast* averts this problem. In this type of program, patients eat high-protein food in very limited amounts. The protein-sparing modified fast spread in popularity in the form of the liquid-protein diet, which used a product high in protein but low in calories. A person on this type of diet would ingest only this preparation and no food. Although the regimen seemed safe under close medical supervision, a number of deaths were reported for people on liquid-protein diets without supervision. The title of the book advocating this approach, *The Last Chance Diet* (Linn, 1976), was more prophetic than the author had intended.

Other drastic measures to control obesity include several types of surgery. One procedure consists of wiring the person's jaws so that she or he is unable to chew. Caloric intake can thus be severely restricted, but such body functions as coughing can be very painful, and vomiting could be deadly. For good reason, this approach is rare.

Surgery has also been performed to remove part of the intestines, preventing food from being absorbed and cutting down on the calories metabolized (Kral, 1992). Because nutrients can no longer be fully absorbed, the person has perma-

nent diarrhea and the potential for vitamin and mineral deficiency, but the procedure usually produces weight loss and is sometimes recommended for severely obese people who have medical conditions that are aggravated by obesity.

Surgical techniques that reduce the size of the stomach may either implant mesh that wraps around the stomach or staple part of the stomach. Both variations assume that not being able to fill the stomach will result in weight loss, and this has been true in some cases (Kral, 1992). In others, the obese people simply eat more frequently.

Another surgical approach to weight loss is to remove adipose tissue through a fat-suctioning technique called liposuction. People who undergo this procedure may gain the weight back, but the technique allows for a recontouring of the body rather than an overall weight loss. This procedure is not useful in controlling obesity (Kral, 1992); rather, it is a cosmetic procedure to change body shape. Despite the discomfort and expense of the surgery, liposuction has become a very popular type of plastic surgery (Brownell & Rodin, 1994a).

Diets that severely restrict calories—that is, allow fewer than 1,000 calories per day—tend to be nutritional risks because of the small amount of food allowed. Most nutrition and diet experts recommend against very low calorie diets, contending that the rapid weight loss they promote is less likely to be maintained than steady, slower weight loss. Nevertheless, some people attempt such diets on their own, a potentially dangerous choice.

Indeed, all these drastic means of losing weight can be dangerous. Although anyone can attempt a very low calorie diet or a fast without a physician's guidance, these programs are recommended only for those who are severely obese and whose obesity is an immediate health threat. For those who participate under such circumstances as well as for those who attempt a drastic diet on their own, keeping weight off is a major problem. Indeed, regardless of weight loss method, maintaining weight loss is a challenge.

Maintaining Weight Loss In Chapters 13 and 14 we saw that about two-thirds of the people who initially quit smoking or stop drinking will eventually relapse. For people who successfully lose weight, maintaining that loss is equally difficult. A large number of studies have confirmed the difficulty of maintaining weight loss (NIH Technology Assessment Conference Panel, 1993). However, most of these studies looked at highly selected dieters, including those who were extremely obese and those who sought professional help in losing weight. For those people, weight control should probably be treated as a chronic illness, with continued professional assistance in maintaining weight loss (Wing, 1992). Obviously, information on the long-term success of people dieting on their own is very sparse (Tinker & Tucker, 1994), yet this approach is the one that most people use.

Effective formal weight reduction interventions typically include posttreatment programs to help dieters maintain weight loss. These programs are usually more successful than those that lack a posttreatment phase. For example, a posttreatment program that included social support, aerobic exercise, and continued contact with the therapist was more successful 18 months later than one that included only a weight-loss phase (Perri et al., 1988). Dieters who participated in the posttreatment programs had regained only 17% of their lost weight compared to the 67% gained by those involved in only the diet phase of the program. This study demonstrated that weight loss can be maintained and that several posttreatment techniques can help dieters keep off most of their lost weight.

The social environment may be a factor in maintaining weight loss. Formerly obese people who lost weight and maintained a normal weight experienced an increase in positive relationships and social events, which may have reinforced their efforts to lose weight (Tinker & Tucker, 1994). Thus, successful weight loss seems to be enhanced by an environment that rewards these efforts. People's motivation for dieting may also play a role in maintaining weight loss. The motivation to go on the diet was a significant predictor

of success for dieters in both losing weight and maintaining weight loss 2 years after their weight loss (Williams, Grow, Freedman, Ryan, & Deci, 1996). People who decided for themselves to begin dieting were more successful than those who began dieting as a response to pressure from family, friends, or physicians.

In contrast to the difficulty that adults have in keeping off lost weight, obese children who lose weight are more likely to maintain that loss. A 10-year follow-up of formerly obese children who had participated in a weight-loss program (Epstein, Valoski, Wing, & McCurley, 1994) demonstrated that more than one-third of the children decreased the degree of obesity, and another 30% were no longer obese. Children who adopted a more active lifestyle were the most successful in maintaining weight loss.

Is Dieting a Good Choice?

Although dieting can produce weight loss, it may not be a good choice. Dieting has psychological costs and may not be effective in improving health. Dieters often behave like starving people: They are irritable, obsessed with food, finicky about taste, easily distractible, and hungry. These behavioral abnormalities make dieting foolish, especially for dieters who are close to the best weight for their health (Polivy & Herman, 1995). Dieters can be divided into two groups: those who are obese and those who are of normal weight (Brownell & Rodin, 1994a). Dieting may be a good choice for those who are sufficiently overweight to endanger their health, but as we have discussed, most dieters are not. For those who are of normal weight or even underweight, dieting is not a wise choice. Instead, developing reasonably healthy eating patterns is a better choice.

Ironically, weight loss may be a health risk for some people. Several studies (Pamuk, Williamson, Serdula, Madans, & Byers, 1993; Williamson & Pamuk, 1993) explored the mortality risks of weight loss and found an increased risk for those who lost weight. Another study (Andres, Muller, & Sorkin,

1993) found that the pattern with the lowest mortality risk was one of modest weight gain during adulthood. Indeed, Reubin Andres (1995) is critical of all weight charts that do not consider age as a factor. He acknowledges the existence of a U-shaped relationship between weight and mortality, but he insists that the nadir of the U-shaped curve increases with age. After looking at the research, he stated that many people would be healthier if they gained some weight as they age—up to seven pounds a decade.

Of course, some people who lose weight voluntarily benefit from their weight loss. Overweight European American women who had obesity-related illnesses decreased their mortality risk by losing weight, especially if they lost 20 pounds or more (Williamson et al., 1995), but thin women who lose weight tend to increase their risk for cardiovascular disease (Harris, Ballard-Barbasch, Madans, Makuc, & Feldman, 1993). Middle-aged and elderly men who lose weight slightly increase their mortality risk (Yaari & Goldbourt, 1998).

In Summary

The near obsession with thinness in our culture has led to a plethora of diets, many of which are neither safe nor permanently effective. Most diets produce some initial weight loss in response to the restriction of caloric intake, but maintaining the reduced weight levels is a matter of lifelong changes in basic eating habits. In addition, people who wish to lose weight should incorporate some sort of exercise routine into their daily schedule. Despite a recent decline in fat consumption, people in the United States are now heavier than ever, because they have increased the number of calories consumed.

Losing weight is easier than maintaining weight loss, but programs that include posttreatment and frequent follow-up can be successful in helping people maintain a healthy weight. Behavior modification programs are generally more successful than other types of programs, and people whose lives change in positive ways after weight loss may be motivated to maintain their weight loss. In addition, behavior modification programs with obese children have greater success in promoting permanent weight loss than similar programs with adults.

Dieting is a good choice for some people but not for others. Morbidly obese people and those with a high waist-to-hip ratio should try to lose weight and keep it off. However, most people who diet for cosmetic reasons would be healthier if they did not lose weight, and people who lose and then regain weight have a higher risk for mortality than those who are slightly obese but who are able to maintain a stable weight. Thus, weight maintenance, especially for people who are not severely obese, is a healthier pattern than weight fluctuation.

Eating Disorders

Besides overeating, two other eating disorders have received considerable attention both in the popular media and in the scientific literature. These unhealthy eating habits are anorexia nervosa and bulimia.

The term *anorexia nervosa* literally means lack of appetite due to a nervous or physiological condition; *bulimia* means continuous, morbid hunger. Neither meaning, however, is quite accurate. The patterns of eating behavior to which these labels apply are only marginally related to the literal meaning of the two terms. People with anorexia nervosa have not lost their appetite. Ordinarily, they are perpetually hungry, but they insist that they do not wish to eat. Like Jessica, our first case study, these people become preoccupied with losing weight, and their self-induced starvation often results in a life-threatening condition. Similarly, bulimia has come to mean more than continuous morbid hunger. The chief identifying mark of this eating disorder is repeated bingeing and purging, the purge usually coming after eating huge quantities of food, usually high in calories and loaded with carbohydrates, fat, or both. Like Elise, our second case study, people with bulimia ordinarily purge by vomiting, but fasting and using laxatives and diuretics are also frequently part of the purging process.

These two eating disorders obviously have much in common, and Elise experienced symptoms of both. In fact, many authorities regard them as two dimensions of the same illness. Others see them as two separate but related illnesses. We regard neither of them as an illness; they are both unhealthy eating patterns that, along with overeating, may eventually produce physical illness. Although a person may show symptoms of both, in this section we discuss anorexia nervosa and bulimia separately, as each has a somewhat different set of behaviors and each produces its own complex of physiological disorders.

Anorexia Nervosa

Anorexia nervosa is an eating disorder characterized by intentional self-starvation or semistarvation, sometimes to the point of death. People with anorexia are extremely afraid of gaining weight and have a distorted body image, seeing themselves as being too heavy, even though they are exceedingly thin. The *Diagnostic and Statistical Manual of Mental Disorders (DSM-IV)* of the American Psychiatric Association (1994) defined anorexia nervosa as intentional weight loss to a point that a person weighs less than 85% of weight considered normal by the Metropolitan Life Insurance tables or has a body mass index of 17.5 or less.

Despite recent publicity on anorexia, neither the disorder nor the term is new. The first two authentic, documented cases of intentional self-starvation were reported by Richard Morton in 1689 (Sours, 1980). Morton wrote about an 18-year-old English girl who had died of the effects of anorexia some 25 years earlier and about an 18-year-old boy who had survived. Both had shown a remarkable indifference to starvation, and both had been described as sad and anxious. Over the next 2 centuries, several other cases were reported, but often these were not clearly distinguished from tuberculosis or consumption.

In London, Sir William Gull (1874) studied several cases of intentional self-starvation during the 1860s. He regarded the condition as a psychological disorder and coined the term anorexia nervosa to indicate loss of appetite due to "nervous" causes—that is, psychological factors. From that time until about 1910, Gull's psychopathological conception pervaded the psychological and psychiatric literature. From about 1910 until the late 1930s, some medical authorities tried to link anorexia nervosa with atrophy of the anterior lobe of the pituitary gland, but this medical view soon lost favor.

During the 1940s and 1950s, speculation proliferated concerning the causes and cures of anorexia nervosa. Some psychiatrists hypothesized that the ailment was a denial of femininity and a fear of motherhood. Other theorists suggested that it represented an attempt on the part of the young woman to reestablish unity with her mother. Unfortunately, none of these hypotheses proved fruitful in expanding the scientific understanding of anorexia nervosa. The last 3 decades have seen a shift away from this sort of speculation and a turn toward the view that anorexia is a learned syndrome of behavior (Darby, Garfinkel, Garner, & Coscina, 1983). Recent emphasis has been on describing the disorder in terms of behaviors and physiological effects, demographic correlates, and effective treatment procedures.

Description of Anorexia   This chapter opened with a description of Jessica, a college junior who showed classical symptoms of anorexia. When first interviewed, her weight had dropped from 130 to 81 pounds, but Jessica's story was far from over. In this section, we continue with the case of Jessica, pointing out how it matches or deviates from a composite model of hundreds of cases of anorexia nervosa.

Like Jessica, most anorexics are young, White women who are outwardly compliant and high achievers in school. They are preoccupied with food, usually like to cook for others (Jessica didn't), insist that others eat their food, but eat almost nothing themselves. They lose from 15% to 50%

of their body weight, yet continue to see themselves as overweight. Like Jessica, they are ambitious, perfectionistic, and come from high-achieving families. Their preoccupation with body fat usually leads to a strenuous program of exercise—dancing, jogging, calisthenics, or playing tennis. Excessively active and energetic behavior continues until their weight loss reaches a level that produces fatigue and weakness, making further activity impossible.

Whether the characteristics connected with anorexia precede the weight loss or are a consequence of starvation is sometimes a difficult question. For example, anorexic women often display some hostility toward their mothers. But whereas many anorexics exhibit an increase in hostility before their excessive dieting, for others the mother-daughter friction seems to revolve around the daughter's lack of concern over weight loss that the mother considers alarming.

A second characteristic that may either precede or follow dieting is *amenorrhea,* cessation of the menses. Because the attainment of a given percentage of body fat is necessary for menstruation, postpubescent women develop amenorrhea if they lose enough weight. However, cessation of the menstrual cycle often precedes dieting (Neuman & Halvorson, 1983). This somewhat puzzling event reinforces the view that simple explanations of anorexia nervosa are inadequate and that complex factors are related to both the causes and the course of the disorder.

After substantial weight loss has occurred, individual differences tend to disappear, and accounts of the disorder itself are remarkably similar. Interestingly, most of the descriptions are also consistent with the sketch of starving conscientious objectors drawn by Keys et al. (1950). Thus, these conditions are probably an effect of starvation and not its cause. As weight loss becomes more than 25% of one's previous normal weight, the person constantly feels chilled, grows a soft, downy covering of body hair, loses scalp hair, loses interest in sex, and develops an unusual preoccupation with food. As starvation nears a perilous level, the anorexic becomes more hostile

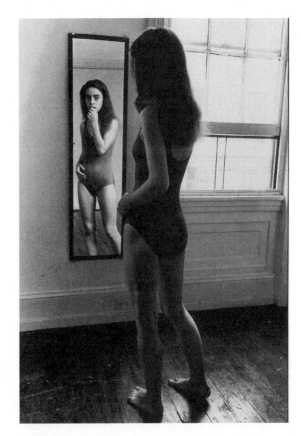

No matter how thin they get, anorexics continue to see themselves as too fat.

toward family and friends who try to reverse the weight loss.

Many authorities, including Hilde Bruch (1973, 1978, 1982), have regarded anorexia nervosa as a means of gaining control. Bruch, who spent more than 40 years studying eating disorders and the effects of starvation, reported that prior to dieting, anorexics typically are troubled girls who feel incapable of changing their lives. These young women often see their parents as overdemanding and in absolute control of their life, yet they remain too compliant to rebel openly. They try to seize control of their life in the most personal manner possible: by changing the shape of their body. Short of force-feeding, no one can stop these young women from controlling their own body size and shape. They take great pleasure and pride in doing something that is difficult and often compare their superior willpower with that of others who are overweight or who shun exercise. Bruch (1978) stated that anorexics enjoy being hungry and eventually regard any food in the stomach as dirty or damaging.

Becky Thompson (1994) has taken a somewhat different view, holding that women often use eating as a way to cope with problems in their lives. Thompson proposed that explaining anorexia as an extension of fashion-consciousness is demeaning to women, trivializing the problems that prompt eating disorders. In interviewing and treating a variety of women from many ethnic backgrounds, Thompson concluded that physical, psychological, and sexual assaults on women are among the factors contributing to eating problems.

Who Is Anorexic? Anorexia nervosa cuts across cultural boundaries (Steinhausen, Winkler, & Meier, 1997), but it remains somewhat more prevalent among upper-middle-class and upper-class White women in North America and Europe. In terms of incidence, most clinicians and researchers believe that anorexia has become more common in the United States than it was 40 years ago, but anorexia nervosa is still a very rare disorder. One estimate (Hoek, 1993) placed the incidence of anorexia at about 8 for every 100,000 people per year. However, among some populations the incidence rates are much higher. Young women between the ages of 15 and 19 are at elevated risk (Lucas, Beard, O'Fallon, & Kurland, 1991; Steinhausen et al., 1997), and young women who attend ballet classes or modeling academies are at especially high risk. The competitive, weight-conscious atmosphere of professional schools for dance and modeling prompt the development of anorexia, and 6.5% of dance students and 7% of modeling students met the diagnostic criteria for anorexia nervosa (Garner & Garfinkel, 1980). Athletic competition is also a risk for anorexia, and athletes with eating disorders can be found in programs for all sports, even those that do not emphasize appearance or an overly thin body (Thompson & Sherman, 1993). In addition, women who decline to participate in studies about eating disorders may be more likely to have such disorders, and their absence lowers the frequency estimates below the actual number (Beglin & Fairburn, 1992). Analyzing a number of studies that used different methodologies led to the conclusion (Hsu, 1990) that the prevalence of anorexia nervosa in all women in the United States and Western Europe is between 0.7% and 2.1%.

Over the years anorexics have tended overwhelmingly to be women, and research and treatment have focused on women. Men make up about 5% to 10% of all anorexics (Garfinkel & Garner, 1982). This estimate—that 90% to 95% of all anorexics are women—has remained constant over a period of years, but it is based mostly on clinical impressions and incomplete empirical data.

Male anorexics are quite similar to female anorexics in social class and family configuration, symptoms, treatment, and prognosis as well as in the behaviors and personality characteristics before the onset of anorexia (Crisp & Burns, 1990), but men are less likely than women to receive a diagnosis. In addition, gay men are slightly overrepresented among the anorexics, but sexual orientation is probably not an important factor in anorexia among men. Indeed, one recent study (Carlat, Camargo, & Herzog, 1997) found that more than half of male anorexics identified themselves as asexual, a finding consistent with loss of sexual interest among female anorexics.

Treatment for Anorexia Anorexia has a much higher mortality than bulimia, making successful treatment a matter of life or death for some anorexics. Nearly 6% of all anorexics die from their disorder (Neumarker, 1997). Most die of cardiac arrhythmia, but suicide is also a frequent cause of death. Despite the very real possibility of death, anorexia nervosa remains one of the most difficult behavior disorders to treat because most anorexics see nothing wrong with their eating behavior, resent suggestions that they are too thin, and resist any attempt to change their eating. Therefore, parents and friends have great difficulty motivating anorexics to seek treatment. Threats, pleas, and criticisms are likely to have a negative effect (Szmukler, Eisler, Russell, & Dare, 1985). Short of force, family and friends have few options. The one aspect of the environment that anorexics can control is their own body. As long as they refuse to eat, their control remains sovereign.

As starvation continues, anorexics eventually reach the point of fatigue, exhaustion, and possible physical collapse. At that point some sort of treatment is usually forced on them. After 2 years of self-imposed starvation and weighing only 52 pounds, Jessica was forced by her parents to seek treatment. She was then hospitalized and fed intravenously.

The immediate aim of almost any treatment program for anorexia is medical stabilization of any danger due to physical symptoms of starvation (Goldner & Birmingham, 1994). After that, anorexics need to work toward restoration of normal weight, healthy eating, and good body image. Recommendations concerning the methods of achieving these goals are not universally accepted. Some believe that hospitalization is required, especially for medical stabilization and restoration of weight, but others have found little evidence to support the need for inpatient treatment (Hsu, 1990). Weight restoration is an important step in the treatment of anorexia, but anorexics resist attempts to get them to eat. Tube feeding and intravenous feeding can provide methods of forcing nutrient intake, but force-feeding may be undesirable because it deprives the patient of control and may impede the growth of a trusting relationship between therapist and patient.

Weight restoration is a step in therapy but is not a cure for anorexia nervosa, and anorexics need to change their body image as well as their eating habits. As Elliot Goldner and C. Laird Birmingham (1994, p. 139) put it:

> In order to recover, anorexic individuals will have to confront those things they fear most and will have to surrender the feelings of accomplishment gained by

weight control. A therapeutic alliance is needed to catalyze and nurture the anorexic individual's motivation for recovery.

Most therapists recommend that both family therapy and individual therapy accompany weight-gain programs (Bloom, Kogel, & Zaphiropoulos, 1994; Goldner & Birmingham, 1994). These recommendations for family therapy seem sound, because both psychopathology (Kog & Vandereycken, 1985) and sexual abuse (Thompson, 1994; Wonderlich, Brewerton, Jocic, Dansky, & Abbott, 1997) are common in the family experiences of anorexics. For these reasons, most treatment programs are designed to change the anorexic's social environment, her attitude toward herself, and her distorted view of her body.

Behavior modification has sometimes been used to promote weight gain (Hsu, 1990), but this procedure is not often oriented toward changing the maladaptive cognitions that accompany anorexia. Since the mid-1970s, cognitive behavior therapy has become increasingly popular as a treatment for anorexia nervosa, and it has shown some success in both changing eating behavior and changing cognitions. Practitioners of cognitive behavior therapy recognize that the pleasure and gratification derived from the effects of self-starvation act as potent reinforcers for anorexic eating habits (Garner, Garfinkel, & Bemis, 1982). They attempt to change anorexics' faulty thinking patterns and their erroneous beliefs, which extend beyond matters of weight and body image. Cognitive behavior therapists attack these irrational beliefs while maintaining a warm and accepting attitude toward patients. Anorexics are taught to discard the absolutist, all-or-none thinking pattern expressed in such self-statements as "If I gain one pound, I'll go on to gain a hundred." Patients are also encouraged to stop centering all attention on themselves and to realize that others do not have the same high standards for their behavior that they do. Finally, therapists need to point out the errors in superstitious food beliefs such as "Any sweet is instantly converted into fat" or

BECOMING HEALTHIER

1. Get good information about nutrition and use that information to help you choose a healthy diet.

2. Be more concerned with eating a healthy diet than with what you weigh.

3. Consult a chart that contains height-weight recommendations or body mass index, rather than a fashion magazine, to determine what is the correct weight for you.

4. Give up dieting. Instead, consider any dietary change as a permanent change in the way you eat.

5. Concentrate less on food restriction and more on exercise as a way to change your body shape.

6. Do not lose weight unless you have made a realistic plan that would allow you to keep the weight off. Weight cycling is more dangerous to health than being somewhat overweight.

7. If you lose weight, know when to stop. Listen to people who tell you that you have lost enough.

8. Do not hide how little you weigh from friends or family by wearing baggy clothing.

9. Find ways to make eating a pleasurable experience. Feelings of deprivation and going without favorite foods can make you too miserable to care about eating correctly.

9. Do not use diet drugs, fast, or go on a very low calorie diet to lose weight, even if you are very obese.

10. Do not vomit as a way to keep from gaining weight.

11. Learn how to see someone who is normal weight or slightly overweight as attractive. Look for such people in the news and in the media.

"Laxatives prevent the absorption of calories" (Thompson & Sherman, 1993). When patients understand the superstitious nature of these beliefs, they can become more realistic about the effects of food on body composition.

In general, cognitive behavior therapy has been more successful with anorexia nervosa than psychoanalytic approaches. Indeed, therapists who use a psychoanalytic framework need to be careful to avoid the sexist bias that often accompanies this approach (Bloom, Kogel, & Zaphiropoulos, 1994). However, no treatment offers a high rate of success. A number of studies (Eckert, 1983; Garfinkel, Moldofsky, & Garner, 1977) have found some long-term benefits of cognitive behavior therapy, especially when benefit is defined in terms of weight gain.

Relapse always remains a possibility. Some patients gain weight while hospitalized but have no intention of retaining it subsequent to release. Anorexics who have attained normal weight may not have attained normal attitudes toward food and eating (Hsu, 1990). Many hospitalized patients gain weight because they know that doing so is a prerequisite for hospital discharge. After leaving the hospital, few anorexics learn to eat normally. Some slip back to self-starvation, others attempt suicide, some become depressed, and some develop bulimia (Goldner & Birmingham, 1994; Hsu, 1990). Similarly, a review of the outcomes for male and female anorexics (Burns & Crisp, 1990) showed that anorexics often gain enough weight during treatment to be in the normal weight range, but about 50% relapse or develop other psychological or eating-related problems. About 20% remain underweight despite extensive treatment. Also, this review found that about 5% of anorexics die and that death becomes even more likely when eating disorders persist for 4 years or longer.

After being hospitalized, Jessica became convinced that continuing self-starvation threatened her life. With almost no psychological or psychiatric intervention, she gradually began a weight-restoration program, and within 6 months her weight was up to 110 pounds. Her appearance was normal, but she had suffered severe and permanent physical damage. She continued to see herself as overweight, a view typical of anorexics.

Bulimia

Bulimia is often regarded as a companion disorder to anorexia nervosa. Like anorexia, bulimia affects mostly women and often centers around maladaptive attempts at weight control. Unlike anorexics, who rely mostly on strict fasts to lose more and more weight, bulimics engage in binge eating; that is, they consume huge quantities of food in an uncontrolled manner. As defined by the fourth edition of the *Diagnostic and Statistical Manual of Mental Disorders (DSM-IV)* of the American Psychiatric Association (1994) bulimia nervosa involves recurrent episodes of binge eating, a sense of lack of control over eating, and inappropriate, drastic measures to compensate for bingeing. Some bulimics fast or exercise excessively, but most use self-induced vomiting to maintain a relatively normal weight. Binge eating may occur without any attempts to purge, but this pattern does not meet the DSM-IV criteria for bulimia.

The seemingly bizarre practice of binge eating followed by purging is not new. The ancient Romans sometimes indulged in very similar eating rituals. After they had feasted on great quantities of rich food, these Romans would retire to the vomitorium, empty their stomachs, and then return to eat some more (Friedländer, 1968). The ancient Romans were neither the first nor the last to binge and purge, but theirs was perhaps the only society to have elevated this practice to such a refined state. Today, millions of women (and a smaller

number of men) continue this custom of bingeing and purging as a means of controlling weight.

Description of Bulimia   In many ways, Elise, our second case study, was not typical of people with bulimia, but in other ways she was. Like most other bulimics, she began purging as part of a diet. The common pattern for bulimia involves binge eating compensated by fasting, with this pattern developing into one of vomiting or laxative abuse or both as methods of purging. Unlike most bulimics, Elise's binges were never a central part of her eating problem, but her purging behavior was. Like most bulimics, Elise felt guilty about her bingeing and purging and after several years, managed to end this cycle.

Depression is a frequent correlate of bulimia, but some authorities question whether it is a cause or an effect. One study (Pope & Hudson, 1984) reported that half the bulimic women had been depressed for a year or more before the onset of bulimia. Whether depression causes bulimia or bulimia causes depression is still unknown, but the majority of bulimics experience depression.

A second correlate of bulimia is a history of alcohol or drug abuse. Research suggest that bulimics are two to five times more likely than other people to have serious problems with alcohol (Cauwells, 1983; Garfinkel & Garner, 1982; Pope & Hudson, 1984). In addition, binge eaters have higher rates of substance abuse, drunkenness, marijuana use, and cigarette use than the population at large (Holderness, Brooks-Gunn, & Warren, 1994). Like many college students, Elise's alcohol use was not always wise, but her drinking never got her into serious trouble, and, except for laxatives, she did not misuse drugs.

Another behavior more common among bulimics than among the general population is **kleptomania**, the compulsive stealing of unneeded items. Although most kleptomania bulimics steal food and laxatives—items related to their bingeing and purging—they may also pilfer such items as alcohol, clothing, cosmetics, and jewelry. In other words, although bulimia is an expensive habit and some bulimics steal to obtain food, a disproportionate number seem to take items that have no relationship to food or to their bingeing (Pyle, Mitchell, & Eckert, 1981).

Childhood experiences with sexual abuse, physical abuse, and posttraumatic stress are additional correlates of bulimia (Dansky, Brewerton, Kilpatrick, & O'Neil, 1997; Welch, Doll, & Fairburn, 1997). A disproportionate number of female bulimics have been victims of sexual abuse during childhood. Stephen Wonderlich's team of researchers (Wonderlich, Wilsnack, Wilsnack, & Harris, 1996) surveyed a nationally representative sample of bulimic women and reported that nearly one-fourth of all female victims of childhood sexual abuse displayed bulimic behaviors later on. Wonderlich et al. called childhood sexual abuse a significant risk factor for bulimia and estimated that a substantial fraction (one-sixth to one-third) of bulimic behavior in women is attributable to childhood sexual abuse. A later review of more than 50 studies (Wonderlich et al., 1997) showed that childhood sexual abuse is more closely associated with bulimia than it is with anorexia. Although not all victims of childhood sexual abuse become bulimic and not all bulimics are victims of childhood abuse, there is a relationship between the two.

Perhaps as a result of depression, a substantial number of bulimics attempt suicide. Two studies (Garfinkel & Garner, 1984; Pope & Hudson, 1984) found that between 20% and 33% of bulimics in treatment had made at least one serious suicide attempt. Because many suicide attempts are not successful, one might guess that bulimic women are not deadly serious. However, bulimia remains a largely hidden disorder, and the possibility exists that many young women who kill themselves were secretly suffering from bulimia.

Another characteristic of bulimics is a close relationship with food. One study (Lehman & Rodin, 1989) revealed that bulimics derive a greater percentage of their self-nurturance from food than from any other source. However, while treating themselves with food, bulimics frequently criticize themselves harshly. In addition, they tend to react more strongly to negative events and to experience sustained negative reactions that interfere with effective coping. These findings painted a picture of bulimics as people who use food for comfort. Because bulimics experience many negative feelings and have difficulty coping with the negative experiences in their lives, they have a great need for comfort.

Elise felt a lot of stress in her life when she started purging, and her life centered around controlling her eating. When she ate more than she thought she should (and her criteria were very strict), she would vomit or take laxatives. Indeed, she often took laxatives in anticipation of eating and feared her stomach being full for long. Unlike most bulimics, Elise did not plan eating sprees in advance or collect special types of food for her binges. Also unlike most bulimics, she was not completely secretive about vomiting or laxative abuse. On the other hand, Elise was like many other bulimics in her continued belief that she was too heavy. She thought that if she could weigh less than 100 pounds, she would be happier. This continued dissatisfaction of one's body reflects the distorted thinking that is even more typical of bulimics than of anorexics (Cash & Deagle, 1997).

Who Is Bulimic?   In at least one way the population of bulimics is quite similar to that of anorexics. Both eating disorders occur far more often in women than in men, with about 90% to 95% of both groups being women (DSM-IV, American Psychiatric Association, 1994). In other ways, however, the two populations differ. Although anorexia nervosa is spreading to all social classes and ethnic groups, upper-middle- and upper-class Whites are still overrepresented. Bulimia, however, is a more democratic disorder. Its prevalence seems to be about equally spread throughout the various social classes, although firm evidence for this assumption is still lacking.

How prevalent is bulimia? Is its incidence increasing or decreasing? Early surveys generally found high prevalence rates, much higher than the rates for anorexia. Two investigations of college students in the 1980s (Halmi, Falk, & Schwartz, 1981; Pyle et al., 1983) found that between 8% and 13% of women met the DSM-III criteria for bulimia and that 1.4% of the men were bulimic. Similarly, a survey conducted in a shopping mall (Pope, Hudson, & Yurgelun-Todd, 1984) yielded an estimate of 10.3% of women with binge eating and a fear of loss of control over eating.

However, the definition of bulimia has changed in later editions of the American Psychiatric Association's *Diagnostic and Statistical Manual of Mental Disorders (DSM)*. The 1980 edition of the DSM (DSM-III)—which yielded prevalence rates around 10% for women—failed to include purging as an essential feature of bulimia, defining it only in terms of bingeing. Although bingeing may be fairly common, bulimia is not widespread according to the definitions in DSM-III-R (1987) and DSM-IV (1994). These stricter definitions, which include fasting, excessive exercising, or purging as methods of compensating for bingeing, have generally led to decreased estimates of the prevalence of the disorder. More recent studies (Hoek, 1993; Pemberton, Vernon, & Lee, 1996) reflect these more stringent criteria, yielding low estimates of bulimia. Around 1% of women and about 0.2% of men meet the current definition of bulimia.

Is prevalence of bulimia on the increase? One review (Fairburn, Hay, & Welch, 1993) noted not only higher rates of bulimia in younger women but also a higher lifetime occurrence. That is, women born after 1960 were at higher risk to have ever been bulimic than women born before 1950, indicating that the prevalence of bulimia is increasing. This estimate held that between 0.5% and 1.0% of young adult women are bulimic, but this may be an underestimate. Perhaps as many as 10% to 15% of college-age women have engaged in binge eating on a regular basis, but with the revised criteria of the DSM-IV, the rate for young women has dropped to about 1% to 3%.

Is Bulimia Harmful? To many people, bingeing and purging may seem to be an acceptable means of controlling weight. To others, comfort derived from eating helps them cope with stress and anxiety, making bingeing and purging a difficult pattern to relinquish (Rodin, 1992; Thompson, 1994). Although guilt is a nearly inevitable part of bulimia and some mental health problems accompany bulimia, the question remains: Is bulimia harmful to physical health? Unlike anorexia nervosa, which has a mortality rate of 2% to 15% (Sours, 1980), bulimia is very seldom fatal. Nevertheless, there are serious detrimental consequences to both bingeing and purging.

Binge eating is harmful in several ways. First, the intake of large quantities of sweets can result in **hypoglycemia**, or a deficiency of sugar in the blood. This may seem paradoxical because the typical binge eater consumes huge amounts of sugar. High intake of sugar, however, activates the pancreas to release excessive amounts of insulin, and insulin drives down blood sugar levels. Low blood sugar results in dizziness, fatigue, and depression. The low blood sugar level frequently produces cravings for more sugar, which in turn prompt the person to eat more cake, candy, ice cream, and other sweets. Second, binge eaters seldom eat a balanced diet. They usually lack sufficient fatty acids, a major energy source, and consequently they may experience lethargy and depression. Third, binge eating is expensive. Bulimics can spend more than $100 a day on food; this leads to other problems, such as financial difficulties or stealing. Also, binge eaters are almost invariably preoccupied with food. They think almost constantly of the next binge and have little time or energy for other activities. This obsession sometimes leads to the loss of a job and more frequently to disinterest in sex and other social activities (Cauwells, 1983).

Purging also leads to several physical problems. One of the most common consequences of frequent vomiting is damaged teeth; hydrochloric acid from the stomach erodes the enamel that protects the teeth. Many long-time bulimics need extensive dental work; thus dentists are sometimes the first health care professionals to suspect bulimia. Hydrochloric acid is also implicated in damage to other parts of the digestive system, particularly the mouth and esophagus. Unlike the stomach, they are not naturally protected against hydrochloric acid. Bleeding and tearing of the esophagus are not uncommon among bulimics, and many longtime sufferers report reverse peristalsis, a spontaneous regurgitation of food, often after eating quite moderately (Boskind-White & White, 1983) .

Besides damage to teeth, mouth, and esophagus, other potential dangers of frequent purging include anemia, electrolyte imbalance, and alkalosis. **Anemia,** a reduction in the number of red blood cells, leads to generalized weakness and a lack of vitality. **Electrolyte imbalance** is caused by the loss of such body minerals such as sodium, potassium, magnesium, and calcium and leads to muscle cramps and weakness. **Alkalosis,** an abnormally high level of alkaline in the body tissues due to the loss of hydrochloric acid, results in generalized fatigue and frequent headaches. In addition, purging through excessive use of laxatives and diuretics may lead to kidney damage, dehydration, and a spastic colon, or the loss of voluntary control over excretory functions. In summary, bulimia is not a benign eating practice but a serious disorder with a multitude of harmful consequences.

Treatment for Bulimia   In one important respect, the treatment of bulimia has a critical advantage over therapy programs for anorexia nervosa. Anorexics cling to their dangerous eating behaviors, but bulimics usually do not approve of their own eating habits, and many of them would like to change. Unfortunately, this motivation does not guarantee that bulimics will seek therapy. A perception that their eating is far from normal can keep bulimics from treatment. One study (Furnham & Kramers, 1989) found that both anorexics and bulimics judged the eating patterns of normal people to be at great variance from their own eating, but they were mistaken. The eating patterns of normal people deviate greatly from the standards that anorexics and bulimics perceive as normal, and this unrealistic perception of the eating pattern they must achieve to be normal may be one factor that prevents people with eating disorders from seeking treatment.

The immediate aim of treatment for bulimics is a change in eating patterns, but other long-term goals must also be included. For example, one therapy (Boskind-White & White, 1983) aims to change clients' attitudes toward themselves and their eating habits. This therapy relies heavily on intensive group therapy, with the emphasis on helping clients gain control over their whole life, not just their eating habits. In addition, clients are encouraged to set reasonable rather than idealistic goals. Most bulimics set a goal of "never again," but this goal is a near guarantee of failure because slips are likely to occur. Total bingeing often follows one lapse, especially for perfectionists who set an unrealistic goal of complete abstinence.

In addition to group therapy, cognitive behavior therapy is common in the treatment of bulimia (Agras, 1993). Cognitive behavior therapists can suggest a variety of techniques to their clients, such as keeping a diary on the factors related to bingeing and on their feelings after purging; monitoring their caloric intake and purging; eating slowly; eating regular meals; clarifying their distorted views of eating and weight control; and undergoing a procedure called *exposure plus response prevention.* In exposure plus response prevention, therapists require bulimics to eat a great deal but then prevent them from vomiting. Some researchers (Hsu, 1990; Wilson, 1989) advocate the use of exposure plus response prevention, but others believe this technique may not significantly increase the effectiveness of cognitive behavioral programs (Compas, Haaga, Keefe, Leitenberg, & Williams, 1998). A review on the effectiveness of cognitive behavioral treatment for bulimia (Compas et al., 1998) found that the average reduction in the frequency of binge eating was 80%, an unusually high percentage of success for any type of therapy.

Interpersonal psychotherapy has also been used successfully in treating bulimics (Agras, 1993). Interpersonal psychotherapy is a nonintrospective, short-term therapy that was originally applied to depression. It focuses on present interpersonal problems and not on eating, taking the approach that eating problems tend to appear in late adolescence when interpersonal issues present major developmental challenges. In this view, eating problems represent maladaptive attempts to cope. The success rate of interpersonal therapy is comparable to cognitive behavioral therapy (Agras, 1993), but it may not provide additional help for people with a binge eating disorder who failed to respond to cognitive behavioral therapy (Agras et al., 1995),

Drugs, especially antidepressants, have been used for some time in the treatment of bulimia. Controlled studies using these drugs tend to show decreases in the frequency of binges, but drugs are not a substitute for psychotherapy for most patients (Mitchell & de Zwaan, 1993). Indeed, cognitive behavioral therapy is more effective than antidepressant drugs in managing bulimia, and drugs alone are not as good a choice as this type of psychotherapy (Compas et al., 1998).

A combination of educational and cognitive psychology approaches can be effective in treating at risk women who have not yet developed bulimia (Kaminski & McNamara, 1996). The risks include low self-esteem, poor body image, a strong need for perfectionism, a history of repeated dieting, and other dysfunctional eating behaviors or attitudes. College women with such attitudes and behaviors were randomly assigned to receive no treatment or a 7-week treatment consisting of educational information about realistic weights and healthy eating habits as well as cognitive strategies for enhancing self-esteem, challenging negative thinking styles, improving body image, and combating social pressures for thinness. The treatment group showed significantly greater improvement in self-esteem and body satisfaction than those in the control group and manifested fewer destructive dieting practices and less need for perfectionism. Results of this study are encouraging, suggesting that intervention can change the attitudes and risky behaviors that are symptomatic of bulimia before the appearance of the disorder.

In Summary

Some people begin a weight-loss program that seemingly gets out of control and turns into an almost total fasting regimen. This eating disorder, called *anorexia nervosa,* is uncommon but most prevalent among young, high-achieving, compliant women. Anorexia is very difficult to treat successfully because people with this disorder continue to see themselves as too fat and thus lack any motivation to change their eating habits.

Bulimia is an eating disorder characterized by uncontrolled binge eating, usually accompanied by guilt and followed by vomiting or other purgative methods. Although people with bulimia differ from one another in some ways, many of them share certain personal characteristics. In general terms, bulimics, compared with other people, are more likely to be depressed, abuse alcohol and other drugs, and steal items they do not intend to use. In addition, they are more likely to have been victims of childhood sexual abuse, to be dissatisfied with their bodies, and to use food for self-nurturance.

Treatment for bulimia has generally been more successful than treatment for anorexia, partly because of bulimics' greater motivation to change. Antidepressant drugs have been used with limited success to treat bulimia, but the more successful programs for eating disorders are those that include cognitive behavioral techniques, which seek to change not only eating patterns but also the pathological concerns about weight and eating that characterize both anorexia nervosa and bulimia.

Answers

This chapter addressed six basic questions.

1. **How does the digestive system function?**

   The digestive system turns food into nutrients by breaking down food into particles that can be absorbed. The process of breaking down food begins in the mouth and continues in the stomach, but absorption of most nutrients occurs in the small intestines. Hormones such as cholecystokinin (CCK), insulin, and leptin affect eating, and the hypothalamus and other brain structures are involved in eating in complex ways.

2. **What factors are involved in weight maintenance?**

Weight maintenance depends largely on two factors: the number of calories absorbed through food intake and the number expended through body metabolism and physical activity. Experimental starvation has demonstrated that losing weight leads to irritability, aggression, apathy, lack of interest in sex, and preoccupation with food. Initial weight loss may be easy, but the slowing of metabolic rate makes drastic weight loss difficult. Experimental overeating has demonstrated that gaining weight can be almost as difficult and unpleasant as losing it.

3. **What is obesity and how does it affect health?**

Obesity can be defined in terms of percent body fat, Body Mass Index, or social standards; each criterion yields different estimates for the prevalence of obesity. Over the past 20 years, obesity has become more common in the United States whereas the ideal body has become thinner, leading to questions about the causes for obesity.

The difficulty of either losing or gaining weight has led several investigators to adopt the notion of a natural setpoint for weight maintenance, but an alternative view holds that positive aspects of eating lead people to overeat when a variety of tasty foods is available.

Obesity is associated with increased mortality, heart disease, adult-onset diabetes, and digestive tract diseases, with the very thinnest and the very heaviest people at the greatest risk for death. Severe obesity, a history of weight cycling, and carrying excess weight around the waist rather than the hips are all risks of death from several causes, especially heart disease.

4. **Is dieting a good way to lose weight?**

A cultural obsession with thinness has led to a plethora of diets, many of which are neither safe nor permanently effective. Changing to healthier eating patterns and incorporating exercise are wise choices for weight change, whereas surgery, diet drugs, fasting, and very low calorie diets are not.

5. **What is anorexia nervosa and how can it be treated?**

Anorexia nervosa is an eating disorder characterized by self-starvation. This disorder is most prevalent among young, high-achieving, compliant women but is uncommon, affecting only about 1% of the population. Anorexics are very difficult to treat successfully because they continue to see themselves as too fat and thus they lack any motivation to change their eating habits.

6. **What is bulimia and how can it be treated?**

Bulimia is an eating disorder characterized by uncontrolled binge eating, usually accompanied by guilt and followed by vomiting or other purgative methods. Bulimia is more common than anorexia, affecting between 1% and 2% of the population. Their motivation to change eating patterns make bulimics better therapy candidates than anorexics. Treatment for bulimia, especially cognitive behavioral therapy, has generally been successful in treating bulimics.

Glossary

alkalosis   An abnormally high level of alkaline in the body.

amenorrhea   Cessation of the menses.

anemia   A low level of red blood cells, leading to generalized weakness and lack of vitality.

anorexia nervosa   An eating disorder characterized by intentional starvation, distorted body image, excessive amounts of energy, and an intense fear of gaining weight.

anus   Opening through which feces are eliminated.

bile salts   Salts produced in the liver and stored in the gall bladder that aid in digestion of fats.

body mass index (BMI)   An estimate of obesity determined by body weight and height.

bulimia   An eating disorder characterized by periodic bingeing and purging, the latter usually taking the form of self-induced vomiting or laxative abuse.

cholecystokinin (CCK)   A peptide hormone released by the intestines that may be involved in feelings of satiation after eating.

eating disorder   Any serious and habitual disturbance in eating behavior that produces unhealthy consequences.

electrolyte imbalance   A condition caused by loss of body minerals.

esophagus   The tube leading from the pharynx to the stomach.

feces   Any materials left over after digestion.

fenfluramine   A prescription diet drug.

gall bladder   A sac on the liver in which bile is stored.

gastric juices   Stomach secretions that aid in digestion.

hypoglycemia   Deficiency of sugar in the blood.

hypothalamus   A small structure beneath the thalamus, involved in the control of eating, drinking, and emotional behavior.

kleptomaniacs   People who compulsively steal items they neither need nor intend to use.

leptin   A protein hormone produced by fat cells in the body and related to eating and weight control.

liver   The largest gland in the body; it aids digestion by producing bile, regulates organic components of the blood, and acts as a detoxifier of blood.

pancreatic juices   Acid-reducing enzymes secreted by the pancreas into the small intestine.

pepsin   An enzyme produced by gastric mucosa that initiates digestive activity.

peristalsis   Contractions that propel food through the digestive tract.

pharynx   Part of the digestive tract between the mouth and the esophagus.

phenylpropylalamine   A nonprescription diet drug.

rectum   The end of the digestive tract leading to the anus.

salivary glands   Glands in the mouth that furnish moisture that helps in tasting and digesting food.

setpoint   A hypothetical ratio of fat to lean tissue at which a person's weight tends to stabilize.

Suggested Readings

Bennett, W., & Gurin, J. (1982). *The dieter's dilemma: Eating less and weighing more.* New York: Basic Books.

This book presents the setpoint hypothesis and evidence that supports it, along with a review of approaches to dieting. The authors combine a presentation of evidence with advice to those interested in losing weight, for a readable and often entertaining book.

Bruch, H. (1978). *The golden cage: The enigma of anorexia nervosa.* Cambridge, MA: Harvard University Press.

Written by one of the leading authorities on anorexia nervosa, this nontechnical book describes anorexia and suggests methods of treating this eating disorder.

 Polivy, J. (1996). Psychological consequences of food restriction. *Journal of the American Dietetic Association, 96,* 589–594.

Janet Polivy reviews the research on food restriction, including Keys's experiment on starvation, to show the psychological consequences of restricting food intake. She argues that the costs of dieting may be too high and that eating a healthy diet is a better choice for physical and mental health. Available through InfoTrac College Edition from Wadsworth Publishing Company.

Rodin, J. (1992). *Body traps.* New York: William Morrow.

Judith Rodin is one of the leading researchers in the field of eating, obesity, and eating disorders. In this popular book, she summarizes her work and that of other researchers and analyzes the ways that people can become trapped by body concerns, food, and dieting.

CHAPTER 16

Exercising

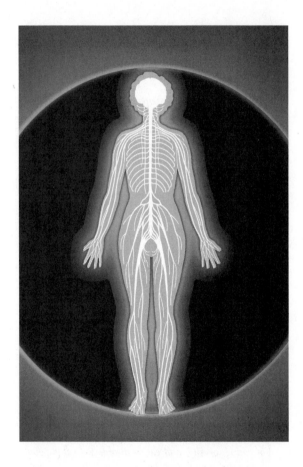

QUESTIONS

This chapter focuses on seven basic questions:

1. What are the different types of physical activity?

2. What are the health-related reasons to exercise?

3. Does physical activity benefit the cardio-vascular system?

4. What are some other health benefits of physical activity?

5. Can physical activity be hazardous?

6. How much is enough but not too much?

7. What are some problems in maintaining an exercise program?

JIM FIXX: CAN EXERCISE EXTEND YOUR LIFE?

When Jim Fixx was 35 years old, he was 50 pounds overweight, smoked two packs of cigarettes a day, and except for an occasional game of tennis or touch football, generally lived a sedentary existence as a magazine editor. But at that point, his life changed dramatically. By his account, the impetus for this transformation was a pulled leg muscle he incurred while playing tennis (Fixx, 1977). To rehabilitate his leg and avoid another muscle pull, Fixx began a modest running program. Painfully he jogged half a mile or so three or four times a week. Gradually he increased both his distance and his speed, and running began to play an increasingly important role in his life. This exercise slowly altered both his physical appearance and his attitude toward his health. He lost weight, stopped smoking, felt physically rejuvenated, and came to believe strongly in the preventive and curative powers of running. Perhaps too much so. On a warm July day in 1984, Jim Fixx died while returning from his afternoon run. The cause of death was listed as sudden **cardiac arrhythmia** due to coronary artery disease.

Because Jim Fixx, like some other runners, died during or immediately after exercising, some contro-versy arose over the potential hazards of strenuous physical activity. However, Fixx had a family history of heart problems; his father suffered a heart attack at age 35 and died of another one at 43. Fixx, then, out-lived his father by 9 years—so perhaps his 17 years of long-distance running produced more benefits than risks. Some people may conclude that exercise is hazardous to health. Others, however, might argue that Fixx would have died earlier if he had not become a runner (Pietschmann, 1984).

The death of Jim Fixx spotlighted several questions that had long been asked about the benefits and dangers of vigorous physical activity. Does exercise reduce heart disease? Does it contribute to longevity? Can physical activity protect against cancer? Does it enhance personal well-being and psychological health? How much is necessary to maintain good health? How much is too much? Can it be a health hazard? This chapter examines the available evidence on these issues and attempts to reach some conclusions about the health effects of both moderate and strenuous physical activity.

Types of Physical Activity

Depending on definition, only about 5% to 25% of adults in the United States engage in regular, vigorous exercise (Kirschenbaum, 1997), and more than one-fourth do not engage in any leisure-time physical activity (USDHHS, 1996). Although exercise can include hundreds of different kinds of physical activity, physiologically there are only five different types of exercise: isometric, isotonic, isokinetic, anaerobic, and aerobic. Each has different goals, different activities, and different advocates. Each can contribute to some aspect of fitness or health, but only aerobic exercise benefits cardiorespiratory health.

Isometric exercise is performed by contracting muscles against an immovable object. Although the body does not move in isometric exercise, muscles push hard against each other or against an immovable object and thus gain strength. Pushing hard against a solid wall is an example of isometric exercise. Because joints do not move, it may not be apparent that exercise is occurring, but the contraction of muscles produces gains in strength—and little else. This type of physical activity can improve muscle strength, which can be especially important for older people in preserving independent living (Tanji, 1997).

Isotonic exercise requires the contraction of muscles and the movement of joints. Weight lifting and many forms of calisthenics fit into this category. Programs based on isotonic exercise can improve muscle strength and muscle endurance if the program is sufficiently lengthy. Again, older people can profit from this isotonic exercise, but most people in a weight-lifting program are body-builders interested in improving the appearance of their body rather than improving health.

Check the items that apply to you.

☐ 1. Whenever the urge to exercise comes over me, I sit down until the urge goes away.

☐ 2. My family history of heart disease means that I am going to have a heart attack whether I exercise or not.

☐ 3. When it comes to exercise, I definitely subscribe to the motto "No pain, no gain."

☐ 4. I have changed jobs in order to have more time to train for races.

☐ 5. I feel anxious and depressed whenever I don't run at least 10 miles a day.

☐ 6. My doctor has advised me to start an exercise program, but I just never quite get around to it.

☐ 7. One of the reasons I exercise is that I believe that a person can't be too thin and

that exercise will help me continue to lose weight.

☐ 8. I may begin an exercise program when I'm older, but now I'm young and in good shape.

☐ 9. I'm too old and out of shape to begin exercising.

☐ 10. I'd probably have a heart attack if I started to jog or run.

☐ 11. I'd like to exercise, but I can't run and walking doesn't help.

☐ 12. I try not to let injuries interfere with my regular exercise.

Each of these items represents a health risk from either too little or too much exercise. Count your check marks to evaluate your risks. As you read this chapter, you will learn that some of these items are riskier than others.

In **isokinetic exercise**, exertion is required for lifting, and additional effort is required to return to the starting position. This type of exercise requires specialized equipment that adjusts the amount of resistance according to the amount of force applied. Isokinetic exercise is superior to both isometrics and isotonics in promoting muscle strength and muscle endurance, but it is inconvenient for many people and requires expensive and elaborate equipment. Its most important use is in physical rehabilitation, helping injured people to regain strength and flexibility with more safety than other types of exercise.

Anaerobic exercises include short-distance running, some calisthenics, softball, and other exercises that require short, intensive bursts of energy but do not require an increased amount of oxygen use. Such short, strenuous exercises improve speed and endurance, but they may be dangerous for people with coronary heart disease.

Aerobic exercise is any exercise that requires dramatically increased oxygen consumption over an extended period of time. One of the most common forms of aerobic exercise is jogging, although many other physical activities can be performed aerobically, including walking, cross-country skiing, dancing, rope skipping, swimming, and cycling.

The important characteristics of aerobic exercise are intensity and duration. Exercise must be intense enough to elevate the heart rate into a certain range, which is computed from a formula based on age and the maximum possible heart rate. In general, the heart rate should stay at this elevated level for 12 to 20 minutes for the aerobic benefits to accrue. This type of program requires elevated oxygen use and provides a workout for both the respiratory system, which furnishes the oxygen, and the coronary system, which pumps the blood. Of the various approaches to fitness, aerobic activity is superior to other types of exercise in developing cardiorespiratory fitness, provided a person engages in some aerobic exercise at least three times a week.

One of the early advocates of aerobic exercise was Kenneth Cooper. However, Cooper (1968, 1982, 1985) is cautious in recommending an aerobic exercise program. First, he recommends a medical examination before beginning a program of aerobic exercise, because potentially dangerous coronary abnormalities can exist without any apparent symptoms. Second, he advocates the use of an exercise electrocardiogram, known as a *stress test,* to detect any abnormal cardiac activity during exercise. Any abnormality in heartbeat or insufficiency in blood supply signals some coronary problem, which may indicate a need for further testing to pinpoint the source. If no problem is indicated, exercise can probably be done with safety. Third, Cooper has been more conservative than others with respect to the distance and frequency of exercise that is necessary to produce health benefits. Many exercise adherents, including Jim Fixx, advocated running long distances 6 or 7 days a week. However, Cooper maintains that jogging or running three miles a day for 5 days a week confers an optimum level of cardiovascular fitness. He believes that more frequent exercise or more distance does not confer much additional benefit and may increase the chances for injuries. In a later section of this chapter, we examine the question of how much exercise is enough and how much is too much.

Reasons for Exercising

People who exercise regularly report a variety of reasons for exercising. Surveys (Carmach & Martens, 1979; Koplan, Powell, Sikes, Shirley, & Campbell, 1982) have revealed answers such as "Exercise helps people become physically fit," "I want to lose weight," "It strengthens my heart," "Exercise helps people live longer," "I don't feel so depressed when I exercise," "I just feel better," "I'm addicted to it." This chapter looks at evidence relating to each of these reasons as well as to the benefits and potential hazards of physical activity.

Physical Fitness

First, does physical activity help people become physically fit? The effects of exercise on fitness depend both on the duration and intensity of the exercise and on the definition of fitness. To most exercise physiologists, fitness is a complex condition consisting of muscle strength, muscle endurance, flexibility, and cardiorespiratory (aerobic) fitness. Each of the five types of exercise can contribute to these four different aspects of fitness, but no one type fulfills all the requirements.

In addition, fitness can be considered in terms of both organic and dynamic fitness. *Organic fitness* is the capacity for action and movement that is determined by inherent characteristics of the body. These organic factors include genetic endowment, age, and health limitations. *Dynamic fitness,* which is determined by experience, is probably what most people think of in connection with the term *fitness.* Dynamic fitness is affected by exercise, whereas organic fitness is not. A person can have a good level of organic fitness and yet be "out of shape" and perform poorly. Another person may train and improve dynamic fitness but still be unable to win races because of relatively poor organic fitness. Athletes who want to be champions need to have been very selective about choosing their biological parents in order to have inherited a high level of organic fitness. Aspiring champions also need to train to gain the dynamic fitness necessary for optimal athletic performance. The following discussion is concerned almost exclusively with dynamic fitness and its components, because this type of fitness can be modified through exercise.

Muscle Strength and Endurance   Two components of physical fitness are muscle strength and muscle endurance. Muscle strength is a measure of how strongly a muscle can contract. This type of fitness can be achieved through isometric, isotonic, isokinetic, and to a lesser extent, anaerobic exercise. All these types of exercise have the capability to increase muscle strength, because they contract muscles.

Muscle endurance differs from muscle strength in that it requires continued performance. Some strength is necessary for muscle endurance, but the opposite is not true: A muscle may be strong but not have the endurance to continue its performance. Exercises that improve strength require greater exertion for limited repetitions; exercises that improve endurance require less exertion but are performed many times. Both muscle strength and muscle endurance are improved by similar types of exercises, including isometric, isotonic, and isokinetic.

Flexibility   Flexibility is the range of motion capacity of a joint. The types of exercises that develop muscle strength and muscle endurance generally do not improve flexibility. Moreover, flexibility is specific to each joint, so that exercises designed to develop flexibility tend to be quite varied. In addition to being a component of fitness, flexibility also decreases the likelihood of injury in other types of physical activity, especially aerobic and anaerobic exercise.

Flexibility is best attained through slow, sustained stretching exercises. Fast, jerky, bouncing movements are not recommended, because they can cause soreness and injury. Also, flexibility training should not be as intense as strength and endurance training.

Aerobic Fitness   Of all the types of physical activity, aerobic exercise contributes most to cardiorespiratory fitness. Aerobic exercise greatly increases the body's requirement for oxygen, thereby causing the respiratory system to work harder and the heart to pump blood at a higher rate.

Research strongly suggests that exercise increases aerobic fitness and protects against death from heart disease. A 5-year follow-up of healthy middle-aged men (Lakka et al., 1994) revealed that those with high aerobic fitness, compared to those with low fitness, were only about one-fourth as likely to have heart attacks.

Interestingly, aerobic fitness also protects men against death from all causes. Steven Blair et al. (1995) administered a treadmill test to middle-aged men from Cooper's clinic in Dallas at two different times, nearly 5 years apart. He then tracked them for an additional 5 years. At the end of the follow-up, men who were high in cardiorespiratory fitness at both the first and the second treadmill examinations were only one-third as likely to have died as men who were unfit at both tests. A more important finding, however, was that men who increased their cardiorespiratory fitness from the first testing to the second reduced their all-cause mortality risk by 44%. This latter finding demonstrates that *changes* in cardiorespiratory fitness affect mortality risk.

When people acquire aerobic fitness, they improve cardiorespiratory health in several ways. First, they increase the amount of oxygen that can be used during strenuous exercise, and second, they increase the amount of blood pumped with each heartbeat. These changes result in a lowering of both resting heart rate and resting blood pressure and increase the efficiency of the cardiovascular system (Pollock, Wilmore, & Fox, 1978). Thus, aerobic fitness is an important contributor to physical health and well-being.

Weight Control

Does physical activity contribute to weight control? Many people exercise to lose weight or to sculpt a more ideal body by improving their body composition—that is, the percentage of fat tissue on the body or the ratio of fat to muscle. Exercise increases muscle tissue and can therefore change this ratio.

Increased physical activity is recommended for people who wish to stop smoking but who are concerned about gaining too much weight (Fiore et al., 1996; Tsoh et al., 1997). Research confirms this recommendation. One study (Kawachi, Troist, Robnitzky, Coakley, & Colditz, 1996) found that

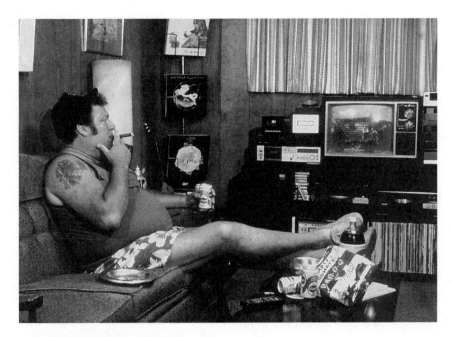

Sedentary lifestyle is a risk for several chronic illnesses.

women who increased their level of physical activity after quitting smoking gained less weight than those who quit but did not become more physically active. Women who quit smoking but moderately increased their level of physical activity gained only about four pounds. This study suggests that women who use weight concerns as an excuse to continue smoking will be much healthier if they stop smoking and initiate a moderate exercise program.

Whether one quits smoking or not, physical activity is recommended for weight control. Indeed, exercise is at least equal to dieting in controlling weight and much better than dieting in changing the ratio of fat to muscle tissue. In one study (Wood et al., 1988), sedentary obese men were randomly assigned to one of three groups: dieters, runners, or controls. The dieters did not exercise, the runners did not diet, and the controls did neither. After a year, the running group and the dieting group had both lost weight, whereas people in the control group had not. However, some important differences emerged in comparing the dieters and the runners. Although both groups had lost an equal amount of weight, the dieters lost both fat and lean tissue, whereas the runners lost only fat tissue and retained more lean muscle tissue.

Exercise does not produce much weight loss through burning calories; for example, more than 30 minutes of tennis is required to work off the calories in two doughnuts. However, sitting and eating doughnuts is a risk for obesity in two ways—the sitting and the eating. Sedentary people are much more likely than active ones to be overweight. One group of researchers (Ching et al., 1996) found that the number of hours spent watching television was related to risk of obesity; men who watched a lot of TV were much more likely to be overweight than those who watched little TV. Another group (Andersen, Crespo, Bartlett, Cheskin, & Pratt, 1998) found much the same results when they examined television watching and its relationship to weight and body mass in a nationally representative sample of 8- to 16-year old children. These studies suggest that the weight loss associated with exercise may come not only from spending time on activities that burn calories but also from avoiding sedentary activities that may lead to consuming calories—such as watching TV while eating snacks.

Most of the weight loss associated with exercise, however, comes from the elevation of metabolic rate, the rate at which the body metabolizes calories. William Bennett and Joel Gurin (1982) suggested another possibility for the role of physical activity, speculating that physical activity may lower a person's *setpoint*. As Chapter 15 explained, the setpoint model holds that the body works to keep fat levels relatively fixed, so dieters cannot lose (or gain) much weight unless the setpoint is adjusted. Moderate levels of physical activity seem to be capable of producing such adjustments. Thus, exercise may be capable of increasing metabolic rate and adjusting setpoint, both of which would produce changes in weight that exceed the number of calories spent in any activity.

How much exercise is enough to bring about weight loss? Recent evidence (Kahn et al., 1997) indicates that moderate physical activity is sufficient to help control weight. Women who walk as little as 4 hours a week decrease their body mass index as well as improve their waist-to-hip ratio. Men who jog or run 1 to 3 hours a week are able to control their weight and improve body composition. Thus, although strenuous exercise will also bring about loss of weight, even moderate physical activity can be a helpful ingredient in weight-loss programs

Is exercise helpful for people who are already thin, or will it make them too thin? A review (Forbes, 1992) concluded that if people have a low body mass index at the beginning of an exercise program, they may have a tendency to lose some lean body weight. However, thin exercisers can maintain lean body mass through proper diet. The review also found that moderate-weight exercisers who do not decrease total weight often increase lean body weight, suggesting that even when exercisers fail to lose weight, they increase lean body mass and decrease body fat.

In Summary

All physical activity can be subsumed under one or more of five basic categories: isometric, isotonic, isokinetic, anaerobic, and aerobic. Each of these five exercise types has advantages and disadvantages for improving physical fitness, but only aerobic exercise benefits cardiorespiratory health.

People have a variety of reasons for maintaining an exercise regimen, including physical fitness, aerobic health, and weight control. The various types of exercise can increase dynamic fitness, strengthen muscles, improve endurance, and add flexibility. Aerobic fitness reduces death not only from cardiovascular disease but from all causes. Smokers who fear weight gain if they stop smoking should adopt a regular exercise program to help prevent unwanted weight. Overweight people can lose weight through moderate physical activity, highly active thin people can maintain lean body mass through proper diet, and people of moderate weight can increase lean body weight without an overall weight gain.

Cardiovascular Benefits of Physical Activity

More important than physical fitness or weight control is the issue of exercise and cardiovascular health. Does regular exercise reduce the chances of heart disease? During the earlier years of the 20th century, physicians often advised patients with heart disease to avoid strenuous physical activity, based on the belief that too much physical activity could damage the heart and threaten a person's life. In more recent years, however, evidence has suggested that exercise can protect against heart disease.

Early Studies

The history of the positive cardiovascular effects of physical activity began in England during the early 1950s and involved London's famous double-decker buses. Jeremy Morris and his colleagues

(Morris, Heady, Raffle, Roberts, & Parks, 1953) discovered that physically active male conductors differed from less active bus drivers in incidence of heart disease. This study, of course, did not prove that physical activity decreases the chances of coronary heart disease (CHD), because workers may have been selected for jobs on the basis of body type, personality, or some other factor associated with a high or low risk of CHD.

Ten years later, another study (Kahn, 1963) gave a little more support to the notion that physical activity can protect against heart disease. Comparing the death rates among sedentary versus active men showed differences in deaths from CHD. More important, the potential benefits from past activity disappeared after a few years. When former mail carriers switched to more sedentary clerical jobs, their rates of CHD changed. After more than 5 years of working as a clerk, former carriers had an incidence of death from CHD equal to that of men who had always been clerks. This finding suggests that exercise should be incorporated into one's lifestyle on a continuing basis.

These studies seemed to suggest that workers who are physically active have a reduced risk of coronary heart disease. However, the studies did not address the problem of self-selection that clouds any conclusion about exercise benefits. Furthermore, none of the early studies measured the workers' activity levels off the job. Most of these issues have been addressed in more recent studies, including a series of investigations by Ralph Paffenbarger, a professor of epidemiology at the Stanford University School of Medicine. Paffenbarger investigated the relationship between physical activity and health in two large populations of participants: San Francisco longshoremen and Harvard alumni.

In the early 1970s, Paffenbarger and his associates (Paffenbarger, Gima, Laughlin, & Black, 1971; Paffenbarger, Laughlin, Gima, & Black, 1970) published several reports of a study involving a large number of San Francisco longshoremen whom they had followed since 1951. In general, they found that CHD death rates were much higher

for workers with low versus high activity. In these studies, the problem of initial self-selection was not a major factor, because all workers in both the high- and low-activity groups had begun their employment with at least 5 years of strenuous cargo handling. From these and other studies, Paffenbarger concluded that high-intensity exercise produces a training effect that protects against coronary heart disease.

In the late 1970s, Paffenbarger and his associates (Paffenbarger, Wing, & Hyde, 1978) published a landmark epidemiological investigation that avoided most of the flaws found in earlier studies. Paffenbarger et al. found extensive medical records of former Harvard University students dating back to 1916 and sent detailed questionnaires to the men who were still living.

To measure the weekly total energy expenditure of these men, the investigators used a composite physical activity index that took into account all activity, both on and off the job. By asking these men such questions as how many flights of stairs they climbed, how far they walked, and what sports they played and for how long, the investigators were able to arrive at an estimate of energy expenditure per week, measured in kilocalories (kcal). For example, walking up one flight of 10 stairs per day was equated to 28 kcal per week, light sports such as golf or softball were rated at 5 kcal per minute, and strenuous sports such as running, skiing, or swimming were rated at 10 kcal per minute.

Paffenbarger et al. then divided the Harvard alumni into high- and low-activity groups. Of those men whose energy levels could be determined, about 60% expended fewer than 2,000 kcal per week and were thus placed in the low-activity group; the 40% who expended more than 2,000 kcal made up the high-activity group. (Note that 2,000 kcal of energy is approximately that expended in 20 miles of jogging or its equivalent.)

Paffenbarger et al. (1978) reported that the least active Harvard alumni had an increased risk of heart attack over their more physically active classmates, with 2,000 kcal per week as the breaking point. Beyond this level, increased exercise paid no dividends in terms of reduced risk of fatal or nonfatal heart attacks. Figure 16.1 shows this relationship. In addition, exercise benefited men who smoked or had a history of hypertension.

During the 1980s and 1990s, Paffenbarger and his associates published reports on these same male Harvard alumni that addressed the question of longevity and exercise. One study (Paffenbarger, Hyde, Wing, & Hsieh, 1986) found an inverse relationship between the amount of exercise and all-cause mortality up to 3,500 kcal per week. In 1993, Paffenbarger et al. reported that men who initiated a moderately vigorous physical activity program during middle age or older had a lower risk of death from all causes than men who did not begin such a program. In addition, both total expenditure of energy and expenditure from vigorous exercise were inversely related to all-cause mortality (Lee, Hsieh, & Paffenbarger, 1995).

Later Studies

All studies on the cardiovascular effects of exercise discussed to this point have one important limitation: They focus exclusively on men. To complete the picture of the health benefits of exercise, research must be extended to women.

One of the first studies to include women was the Framingham Heart Study (Dawber, 1980). Even though both men and women participated in this investigation, the study was limited because nearly all participants reported relatively similar levels of activity. As a result, when the investigators looked at the coronary benefits of activity for all participants, they found very few. However, when they compared extremely inactive participants with the maximally active, they found that inactive men and women were about three times more likely to develop coronary heart disease. The Alameda County Study also found that both men and women can decrease cardiovascular disease and increase life span through leisure-time physical activity (Kaplan, Strawbridge, Cohen, & Hungerford, 1996). In addition a study of post-menopausal women in Iowa (Kushi, et al., 1997) found that

older women who exercised moderately at least four times a week had much lower rates of all-cause mortality than women who were sedentary. Even moderate physical activity once a week significantly reduced the chances of death from CVD. In this study, vigorous activity also reduced death rates but was not superior to moderate physical activity.

Can women reduce their risk of CVD by doing ordinary housework? Unfortunately, one study that addressed this question (Pols, Peeters, Twisk, Kemper, & Grobbee, 1997) found that neither housework nor job-related activity lowered women's cardiovascular risk factors. Although this study of middle-aged and older Dutch women found that such leisure-time activities as sports, cycling, and gardening tended to lower blood pressure, reduce body mass index, improve waist-to-hip ratio, and decrease waist circumference, work activity and housework did not contribute to a favorable cardiovascular profile. Because some women performed heavy work on the job and others spent a lot of time doing housework, the authors were somewhat perplexed by this finding and suggested additional research on the benefits of all types of physical activity for women's cardiovascular health.

Could these differences in longevity be the result of genetic differences rather than differences in physical activity? A study from Finland (Kujala, Kaprio, Sarna, & Koskenvuo, 1998) strongly suggests that heredity is *not* the answer. This study followed healthy men and women from the Finnish Twin Cohort and looked at differences in level of physical activity between pairs of twins—one of whom had died and one of whom had survived. Results showed that people who walked briskly for 30 minutes as little as six times a month reduced their death rate by 44%, indicating that light to moderate leisure-time physical activity reduces all-cause death rate, even after genetic factors are taken into account.

People who engage in regular, moderately intense physical activity can expect an average increase in longevity of about 2 years (USDHHS, 1996). A cynic might criticize this finding by

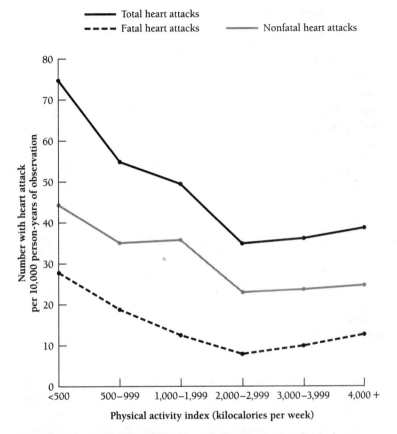

Figure 16.1 **Age-adjusted first heart attack rates by physical activity index in a 6- to 10-year follow-up of male Harvard alumni.**
Source: Adapted from "Physical Activity as an Index of Heart Attack Risk in College Alumni," by R. S. Paffenbarger, Jr., A. L. Wing, and R. T. Hyde, 1978, *American Journal of Epidemiology, 108,* p. 166. Copyright © 1978 by The Johns Hopkins University School of Hygiene and Public Health. Adapted by permission of the publisher and Dr. Paffenbarger.

pointing out that a person would need to jog a total of about 2 years between the ages of 20 and 80 to increase longevity by 2 years. Why live another 2 years if one spends that time exercising? Paffenbarger et al. (1986) contended that physical activity does not merely extend the life span 2 years at the end, but it adds quality years throughout a person's life. They concluded that exercise not only protects against disease and death but contributes to enhanced health in all age groups. This contention was confirmed by research (Vita, Terry, Hubert, & Fries, 1998) showing that women and

men who exercised regularly, had a favorable body mass index, and did not smoke had much lower levels of disability during the later years of life.

Exercise and Stroke

Although physical activity is a strong protector against cardiovascular disease generally, it is somewhat less protective against stroke, or at least the evidence is less clear. One study, for example, (Gillum, Mussolino, & Ingram, 1996) followed African American and European American men and women and found only a slight relationship between exercise and fatal and nonfatal stroke for both groups of men and for African American women. However, sedentary European American women nearly doubled their risk for stroke over their more active counterparts. The authors concluded that more than a fourth of strokes in European American women could be prevented by a more active lifestyle.

In contrast, a 32-year follow-up of the Framingham study (Kiely, Wolf, Cupples, Beiser, & Kannel, 1994) looked at mostly White men and women and found no protective effect of physical activity against stroke among women. However, men who exercised moderately or vigorously significantly reduced their risk for stroke. A study of middle-aged British men (Wannamethee & Shaper 1992) found that physical activity offered some protection against stroke, and the Honolulu Heart Program (Abbott, Rodriguez, Burchfiel, & Curb, 1994) found similar results. This latter study found inactive middle-aged men to have a slightly greater risk for stroke than active men of the same age, but older sedentary men were three to four times more likely to have a stroke than older physically active men.

Thus, physical activity seems to offer some protection against stroke for middle-aged and older men and women. Because stroke is far less common than coronary heart disease among middle-aged people, exercise does not have as dramatic an impact on stroke as it does on heart disease. However, as people become older and more prone to stroke, the benefits of physical activity become more dramatic: Older people, especially men, who exercise regularly greatly reduce their chances of stroke.

Exercise and Cholesterol Levels

How does exercise protect against cardiovascular disease? Some evidence, from both human and animal studies, suggests that exercise may increase high-density lipoprotein (HDL), the so-called "good" cholesterol. In addition, a program of reg-ular physical activity may actually lower LDL, the "bad" cholesterol. If both processes occurred, total cholesterol might remain the same, but the ratio of total cholesterol to HDL would become more favorable and the risk for heart disease would decrease.

Studies with humans have generally found that even moderate levels of exercise, with or without dietary changes, can bring about a favorable ratio of total cholesterol to HDL. An early study (Laporte, Brenes, & Dearwarter, 1983) found a dose-response relationship between amount of physical activity and HDL, with marathon runners having very high rates of good cholesterol and thus very low ratios of total cholesterol to HDL. Another early study (Wood et al., 1988) assigned overweight, sedentary men to a diet group, an aerobic exercise group, or a control group. After 1 year, both the exercisers and the dieters raised HDL levels without changing LDL, but the controls did not. By raising HDL while keeping LDL constant, the aerobic exercisers (as well as the dieters) improved their ratio of total cholesterol to HDL.

Later studies found that moderate exercise, such as walking and gardening, is associated with increased HDL and decreased total cholesterol for men (Caspersen, Bloemberg, Saris, Merritt, & Kromhout, 1991) and that leisure-time activity reduces both *triglycerides* and LDL (Lakka & Salonen, 1992). Again, these findings support the notion that some level of exercise raises HDL without increasing LDL and thus leads to a favorable ratio of total cholesterol to HDL for physically active men.

Women, too, can improve their total cholesterol to HDL ratio by beginning a regular physical activity program. The Stanford Five-City Project (Young, Haskell, Jalulis, & Fortmann, 1993) investigated coronary risk factors for both men and women who had changed their levels of physical activity. Physically active men increased their HDL, lowered their body mass, and decreased their coronary heart disease risk score. Physically active women also increased their HDL while lowering their resting pulse rate. Although the association between physical activity and HDL was not quite as high for women as for men, a later study (Siscovick et al., 1997) found that physically active women had a more favorable cholesterol profile than physically active men. In addition, a dose-response relationship appeared between intensity of regular exercise and favorable cardiovascular risk factors. Similarly, a national sample of women who were serious recreational runners (P. T. Williams, 1996) revealed that the more these premenopausal women ran, the higher their HDL levels. For every mile run per week, there was an increase in high density lipoprotein and a more favorable lipid profile. These findings suggest that both men and women who begin a regular exercise program can increase their HDL and lower their risk for heart disease.

Children and young adults can also benefit from an active lifestyle. A study of male and female 12-, 15-, and 18-year olds (Raitakari et al., 1994) found differences in lipid profiles of the physically active and the physically inactive. Physically active young men had lower triglycerides, higher HDL, and a lower total cholesterol to HDL ratio, and physically active young women had lower triglycerides and lower body fat than their inactive peers. These studies suggest that regular aerobic exercise may protect against heart disease by increasing HDL and by improving the ratio of total cholesterol to HDL.

Humans are not alone in their ability to raise HDL with physical activity. Some investigators have conducted experiments on animals to determine the effects of exercise on cholesterol and atherosclerosis. For example, one study (Kramsch, Aspen, Abramowitz, Kreimendahl, & Hood, 1981) demonstrated that exercise can have a beneficial effect on the cardiovascular system of monkeys fed a diet high in cholesterol. Compared with sedentary monkeys, physically active monkeys had significantly higher HDL levels, lower LDL levels, less narrowing of arteries, and fewer sudden deaths. These results, of course, do not mean that people can eat high-fat diets and then rely on exercise to protect them against coronary heart disease, but they do suggest that regular physical activity may raise HDL without raising total cholesterol and may provide some protection against cardiovascular disease.

In Summary

For nearly 50 years evidence has accumulated suggesting a positive relationship between physical activity and reduced incidence of coronary heart disease. The early studies had many flaws and tended to include only men. However, later research has confirmed a strong association between a regimen of moderate to brisk physical activity and coronary health. Regular activity also protects both women and men against stroke, but this protection is not as strong as it is for heart disease. In addition, physical activity can control high blood pressure, lower body mass index, improve the waist-to-hip ratio, and raise HDL, thereby improving the ratio of total cholesterol to high-density lipoprotein. In addition, regular activity can add as much as 2 years to one's life while decreasing disability, especially in later years.

Other Health Benefits of Physical Activity

Besides contributing to physical fitness, weight control, and cardiovascular health, regular exercise confers several other health benefits, including protection against some kinds of cancer, prevention of bone density loss, control of diabetes, and improved sleep. In addition, regular physical activity appears to offer several psychological benefits, including a defense against depression, a reduction of anxiety, a buffer against stress, and enhanced self-esteem.

Protection against Cancer

Although most people who exercise do so for physical fitness, weight control, or cardiovascular health, several studies have associated physical activity with reduced chances of some cancers. For example, a prospective study (Vena et al., 1985) compared the lifetime occupational physical activity of three different groups: men with colon cancer, men with rectal cancer, and men who had neither a digestive disease nor any type of cancer. Interestingly, no relationship of any kind appeared between physical activity and rectal cancer, whereas the risk of colon cancer increased as occupational physical activity decreased. This study showed that the more sedentary the job and the longer the time spent with such a job, the greater the risk for colon cancer. Other research (Slattery, Schumacher, Smith, West, & Abd-Elghany, 1990; White, Jacobs, & Daling, 1996) has confirmed that high intensity activity corresponds to a reduction in colon cancer in both men and women. These results provide some promise that exercise may protect against colon cancer, one of the leading causes of cancer death for both women and men.

Can physical activity protect women against breast cancer? Evidence on this question is still somewhat inconsistent, but a majority of research studies is beginning to suggest that many women can help protect themselves against breast cancer through regular exercise. A recent review of studies on breast cancer and physical activity (Gammon, John, & Britton, 1998) reported that most (but not all) studies found that occupational physical activity as well as recreational exercise reduced breast cancer rates by 12% to 60%, and that high levels of intense activity were not necessary to achieve these results. One of these studies (Bernstein, Henderson, Hanisch, Sullivan-Halley, & Ross, 1994) found that women who had exercised at least 4 hours per week since early adolescence had a 50% reduction in incidence of breast cancer compared with less active women. The greatest protection appeared in women who had given birth, but physically active childless women also showed some benefit. A second study (Thune, Brenn, Lund, & Gaard, 1997) found that increased leisure-time activity was related to reduced risk of breast cancer in Norwegian women and that the relationship was most pronounced in young, lean premenopausal women who exercised at least 4 hours a week.

Can exercise protect men against prostate cancer? Research on this question has produced somewhat contradictory findings. Some evidence (Le Marchand, Kolonel, & Yoshizawa, 1991) suggests that older men who spent most of their working life in sedentary or relatively inactive jobs had a somewhat *lower* chance of developing prostate cancer. However, this study did not assess leisure-time activity. In a study that did account for total physical activity (Lee, Paffenbarger, & Hsieh, 1992), physically active Harvard alumni were much less likely to develop prostate cancer than their more sedentary cohorts.

Finally, can men lower their risk of cancer deaths in general through exercise? Exercise protected middle-aged British men from cancer in general, but especially from lung cancer and cancers of the digestive tract (Wannamethee, Shaper, & Macfarlane, 1993). This study looked at such activities as walking, cycling, playing golf, swimming, playing tennis, and running, and found an inverse relationship between level of physical activity and cancer deaths as well as between physical activity and all noncardiovascular diseases. Although researchers have largely found that physical activity can lessen men's risk of several kinds of cancer, they have not addressed the question of exercise and cancer in women.

Prevention of Bone Density Loss

Exercise has also been recommended as a protection against **osteoporosis**, a disorder characterized by a reduction in bone density due to calcium loss and resulting in brittle bones. Is this recommendation valid? An early review of research (Harris, Caspersen, DeFriese, & Estes, 1989) concluded that physical activity offers strong protection against osteoporosis in postmenopausal women but is less effective in preventing this disorder in premenopausal women. Since this review, evidence has accrued suggesting that physical activity can protect women both during and after menopause and may even help prevent loss of bone mineral density in older men.

For example, a retrospective study (Greendale, Barrett-Connor, Edelstein, Ingles, & Halle, 1995) asked a group of older men and women to recall their level of physical activity as teenagers, at age 30, and at age 50. They found that both men and women with a history of physical activity had more bone mineral density than the more sedentary people but about the same number of bone fractures. Another retrospective study (Zhang, Feldblum, & Fortney, 1992) asked menopausal women about their level of physical activity during high school. The authors found a dose-response relationship between high school physical activity and current levels of bone mineral density, suggesting that perimenopausal women who exercised regularly continued to be protected against loss of bone mineral density. A similar study (Jagal, Kreiger, & Darlington, 1993) asked two groups of postmenopausal women to recall their levels of physical activity at ages 16, 30, and 50. One group consisted of women who had suffered a hip fracture and the other was a group of controls who had not suffered any recent bone fractures. When the researchers looked at both past and present levels of activity, they noted some interesting findings. Past physical activity—both moderate and vigorous—protected women ages 55 to 84 from hip fracture, and present moderate activity was also protective. However, present vigorous physical activity showed a slightly positive relationship to hip fractures. The message from this research is that older women should continue with moderate activity, but highly active older women should perhaps slow down a little.

Starting an exercise program may help older women retain bone mineral density. An experimental study (M. E. Nelson et al., 1994) of previously sedentary women ages 50 to 70 divided participants into a control group that remained sedentary and an exercise group that began moderate physical activity. Women in the exercise group preserved their bone mineral content while those in the sedentary control group experienced a decrease in bone mineral density. Moreover, the exercise group increased muscle mass and muscle

strength. This body of research suggests that both men and women should start exercising while young and continue into old age as a possible protection against a variety of disorders, including loss of bone mineral density and osteoporosis.

Control of Diabetes

Physical activity may also be a useful weapon in the control of diabetes. A study that followed male University of Pennsylvania alumni over a 15-year period (Helmrich, Ragland, Leung, & Paffenbarger, 1991) showed a direct relationship between leisure-time physical activity and incidence of diabetes; that is, men who were the most physically active had the lowest rates of adult-onset diabetes. This relationship remained when the investigators controlled for obesity, blood pressure, and parental history of diabetes. In fact, men at greatest risk for diabetes—those with high body mass index, parental history of the disease, and hypertension—received the greatest protective effect.

A prospective study (Manson et al., 1992) also found that physical activity offers some protection against the development of adult-onset diabetes. This large-scale investigation of male physicians reported an inverse dose-response relationship between amount of exercise and incidence of diabetes; that is, the more days per week these men exercised, the less likely they were to develop noninsulin-dependent diabetes. After the investigators controlled for smoking, hypertension, and other coronary risk factors, the negative relationship between amount of exercise and incidence of diabetes persisted. Another study (Moy et al., 1993) followed insulin-dependent mostly European American male and female children and adolescents and found that sedentary male diabetics were three times more likely to die than more active male diabetics. However, the trend for female diabetics was not as pronounced.

Although these studies reported a modest protective benefit for physical activity, they do not suggest that exercise is a panacea for the control of diabetes. Nevertheless, they do indicate that physical activity can be a useful adjunct in the treatment of insulin-dependent diabetes and can offer some protection against the development of noninsulin-dependent diabetes.

Aid to Sleep

Can physical activity help people sleep better? Although evidence on this question is still sparse, at least one study (King, Oman, Brassington, Bliwise, & Haskell, 1997) found that moderate exercise can help at least some people improve their sleep. Participants in this investigation were sedentary men and women, 50 to 76 years of age with moderate sleep complaints; that is, they took at least 25 minutes to fall asleep and then slept for only about 6 hours.

The researchers divided participants into an experimental (exercise) group and a wait-list (control) group. Participants in the experimental group engaged in 30 to 40 minutes of brisk walking four times a week, while those in the control group remained sedentary. After 16 weeks, people in the exercise group showed significant improvements in sleep; they decreased sleep onset by 15 minutes and increased sleep duration by 45 minutes. The authors concluded that 8 weeks of moderate, regular exercise may be needed to obtain these benefits. Although this study shows promise, more research is clearly needed before physical activity can be prescribed as treatment for sleep disorders.

Psychological Benefits of Physical Activity

The physiological benefits of physical activity are well established, but what about the psychological benefits? Can exercise lessen depression, reduce anxiety, lower stress levels, or increase self-esteem? People who exercise list psychological reasons nearly as often as physiological ones when asked about the benefits they receive from exercise (Harris, 1981). Does the evidence support these claims?

William P. Morgan, one of the leading authorities in this area, believes that physical activity has great potential for treating and preventing some psychological disorders. Nevertheless, Morgan (1997a) insists that most of the current research on this topic has serious methodological problems and that some enthusiastic conclusions are based more on wishful thinking than on scientific evidence. In general, the link between physical activity and psychological functioning is less clearly established than the one between physical activity and physiological health. In addition, any evaluation of the therapeutic effects of exercise on psychological disorders must consider the problems raised by the placebo effect. Few studies on the psychological benefits of physical activity have sufficiently controlled for the 35% to 38% improvement that might be excepted from a placebo effect alone. Although a causal relationship between physical activity and improved psychological health has not yet been firmly established, some correlational evidence suggests that a regular exercise regimen can decrease depression, reduce anxiety, buffer stress, and increase self-esteem.

Decreased Depression   At any point in time, 5% to 9% of women and 2% to 3% of men in the United States are suffering from major depression (Morgan, 1997b). The *Diagnostic and Statistical Manual of Mental Disorders (DSM-IV)* of the American Psychiatric Association (1994) defines a major depressive episode as "a period of at least 2 weeks during which there is either depressed mood or the loss of interest or pleasure in nearly all activities" (p. 320). During a lifetime, as many as 25% of women and 12% of men may suffer from major depression (DSM-IV). If physical activity can relieve major depression, then millions of people can be helped by a therapy that is easily available to nearly everyone.

People who exercise regularly are generally less depressed than sedentary people. When groups of exercisers are compared to groups of sedentary people on different measures of depression, highly active people are usually less depressed, but such data do not reveal the direction of causation. Depressed people may simply be less motivated to exercise. This section examines the effects of exercise as a preventive measure for depression in normal people and also as a therapeutic intervention for clinically depressed individuals.

Does exercise reduce depression in normal, nonclinical individuals? A brief look at the research reveals some evidence supporting the view that physical activity can, indeed, lower depressive moods in a variety of people, including pregnant women from ethnically diverse backgrounds (Koniak-Griffin, 1994), elderly male and female nursing home residents (Ruuskanen & Parkatti, 1994), college students (Stein & Motta, 1992), law enforcement personnel (Norvell & Belles, 1993), and a representative sample of people in the Alameda County study (Camacho, Roberts, Lazarus, Kaplan, & Cohen, 1991). These studies seem to indicate that various types of physical activity can lessen depression in individuals with nonclinical depression.

Can physical activity be an effective technique for helping clinically depressed patients? Either alone or as an adjunct to drug therapy and psychotherapy, aerobic exercise may be a useful tool for the clinician. One pioneer in running therapy is John Greist, who along with his associates (Greist, 1984; Greist, Eischens, Klein, & Linn, 1981; Greist & Greist, 1979; Greist et al., 1978, 1979), has found tentative evidence supporting the use of running as a treatment for depression. In a pilot study, Greist et al. (1978) assigned moderately depressed men and women patients either to a running group or to one of two kinds of individual psychotherapy—time-limited or time-unlimited. Patients in the running group received no conventional psychotherapy and were not permitted to talk about their depression during running therapy. Initially, they ran with a running leader in small groups for an hour three or four times a week. Later they ran less with the leader and more on their own, but they were encouraged to run at least three times a week. As a whole, patients who received the running treatment were somewhat less depressed after treatment than those in either the time-limited or the time-unlimited therapy group.

Since this early study, several other investigators have examined the usefulness of running as a psychotherapeutic tool. One well-controlled study (Rueter & Harris, 1980) randomly assigned clinically depressed college students to either a running and counseling group or to a counseling-only group and found that patients in the running and counseling group became significantly less depressed than those who received only counseling. Also, Greist (1984) randomly assigned depressed patients to one of three treatment groups: aerobic exercise, Benson's (1975) relaxation training, or group psychotherapy. At the end of a 3-month follow-up, only the exercise and relaxation groups showed improvement. Patients who had received group therapy showed some regression toward original levels of depression. A later study (Bosscher, 1993) randomly assigned depressed inpatients to either a short-term running program or to a treatment-as-usual program, which included both physical and relaxation exercises. Patients in the running program increased their self-esteem and lowered their depressive symptoms, whereas patients in the treatment-as-usual group showed no significant improvements.

A review of research on the effectiveness of physical activity as treatment for clinical depression (Martinsen & Morgan, 1997) led to the conclusions that: (1) aerobic exercise is more effective than no treatment; (2) physical activity is at least as effective as psychotherapy; (3) aerobic and nonaerobic exercise seem to be equally effective in treating depression, (4) no dose-response relationship exists between aerobic exercise and decreased amounts of depression; that is, depressed patients do not continue to benefit from ever-increasing levels of physical activity; (5) to date, no evidence exists showing the therapeutic value of exercise for severe forms of major depression, and (6) evidence does not yet exist that exercise can prevent relapse into a major depression. In addition, there are no well-controlled studies comparing the effectiveness of physical activity and drug therapy for depressed patients.

Martinsen and Morgan (1997, p. 105) concluded that "physical exercise may be an alternate or adjunct to traditional forms of treatment in mild to moderate forms of unipolar depression."

Despite this therapeutic potential, few health psychologists possess the training in exercise physiology and cardiovascular medicine to supervise exercise programs without the aid of physicians, athletic trainers, or others trained in this area.

Reduced Anxiety   Many people report that they exercise to feel more relaxed and less anxious. Does exercise play a role in anxiety reduction? The answer may depend on the type of anxiety. **Trait anxiety** is a general personality characteristic or trait that manifests itself as a more or less constant feeling of dread or uneasiness. **State anxiety** is a temporary, affective condition that stems from a specific situation. Feelings of worry or concern over a final examination or a job interview are examples of state anxiety. This type of anxiety is usually accompanied by physiological changes, such as increased perspiration and rapid heart rate.

Research on the effects of physical activity on trait and state anxiety suffers from many of the same methodological limitations as research on physical activity and depression: that is, only a few of the studies have had an adequate number of participants and have used random assignment to experimental, placebo, or control groups. Nevertheless, sufficient evidence suggests that a moderate program of physical activity can reduce both trait and state anxiety, at least in some people (Raglin, 1997). Moreover, exercise need not be aerobic or vigorous to be effective. As one would expect, highly anxious people experience a greater decrease in anxiety than do people with lower levels, but both groups can profit from moderate physical activity.

How does physical activity help reduce anxiety? William P. Morgan (1973) has been interested in this question for many years. One hypothesis is that exercise simply provides a change of pace—a chance to relax and forget one's troubles. In support of this change of pace hypothesis, exercise demonstrated no stronger therapeutic effect than meditation (Bahrke & Morgan, 1978). Studies that have shown that other techniques to reduce anxiety, including biofeedback, transcendental meditation, "time out" therapy, and even beer drinking in a pub atmosphere, can also be effective (Morgan, 1981). Each of these interventions provides a change of pace and all have been demonstrated to be associated with reduced levels of state anxiety.

Change of pace may not be the only avenue through which physical activity alleviates anxiety. Research suggests that exercise can increase self-esteem (Bosscher, 1993), improve body composition (Norvell & Belles, 1993), enhance social interaction (USDHHS, 1996), alleviate fatigue and anger (Pierce & Pate, 1994), and increase feelings of self-mastery (USDHHS, 1996). Each of these positive results may lead to enhanced self-efficacy and decreases in anxiety.

Although any one of a variety of interventions that break into a stressful daily routine may help relieve anxiety, physical activity seems particularly suitable. From a practical standpoint, walking and jogging have several advantages over most other forms of treatment: They can be done by almost anyone, nearly anywhere, and with very little expense.

Buffer against Stress   Can exercise reduce stress? More importantly, can it protect people against the harmful effects of stress? Research on the first question has generally produced an affirmative answer. For example, many people view exercise as the most effective strategy for reducing tension and eliminating a bad mood (Thayer, Newman, & McClain, 1994).

Answers to the second question are more difficult, because a direct causal link between stress and subsequent illness has not yet been firmly established. Thus, no conclusive evidence exists for exercise's buffering effects. For example, some research (Sinyor, Golden, Steinert, & Seraganian, 1986) failed to find much stress-buffering benefit for exercise in healthy young men who began an aerobic exercise program or a weight-lifting intervention.

Other researchers have found some support for the hypothesis that exercise produces a buffering effect against stress-related effects. Exercise can moderate the effects of laboratory stressors—such as video games or mental arithmetic tasks—on cardiovascular reactivity in mildly hypertensive people (Perkins, Dubbert, Martin, Faulstich, & Harris, 1986). Under conditions of high stress, adolescents who exercise regularly have fewer physical illnesses than those who rarely exercised (Brown & Lawton, 1986). In addition, physically fit people report fewer stress-related health problems and also fewer depressive symptoms than less active people (Roth & Holmes, 1985).

Finally, some research indicates that physically active adolescent girls are more resistant than sedentary girls to stress-related illnesses such as sore throat and diabetes (Brown & Siegel, 1988) and also that physically active college women experience fewer stress-related illnesses than their less active school mates (Brown, 1991). Also, exercise can also buffer European American and African American women against stress-related increases in blood pressure and heart rate (Rejeski, Thompson, Brubaker, & Miller, 1992).

These studies suggest that exercise is at least as powerful as personal hardiness (see Chapter 6) in buffering the negative effects of stress. Although evidence does not overwhelmingly favor the idea that exercise has protective effects, no study has shown that physical activity lowers one's resistance to stress or places one in greater jeopardy of developing physical symptoms. Figure 16.2 shows some of the positive effects of exercise.

Increased Self-Esteem Do people who exercise regularly increase their self-esteem? Do they have more self-confidence and improved feelings of self-worth? In the previous sections, we saw that exercise is associated with decreases in both depression and anxiety and that it may have some ability to buffer stress. This section considers the possibility that exercise might be related to increases in self-esteem.

Reviews of the literature dealing with the relationship between exercise and self-esteem (Sonstroem, 1984, 1997) revealed that the majority of studies showed a significant positive relationship between self-esteem and exercise. Although

these studies suggested that exercise raises self-esteem, their methodological limitations prevent this conclusion. Few of the studies employed an experimental design, with random assignment to experimental, placebo, or control groups. Also, no single definition of self-esteem was used. Many studies adopted a global definition, defining self-esteem as having a positive feeling about oneself. Such broad definitions confound any relationship between exercise and self-esteem. That is, adherence to a regular exercise program may improve physical health, enhance body image, raise physical fitness, boost feelings of self-mastery, increase social support, bolster feelings of self-control, or improve physical self-efficacy. Any one or combination of these factors can lead to better feelings about oneself. Despite attempts to identify a more precise pathway through which physical activity relates to self-esteem (Sonstroem, 1997), it may not be necessary to know the exact variables responsible for improved self-esteem as long as increased feelings of self-worth and self-confidence are associated with an exercise program.

We have seen that people who regularly exercise decrease their risk of cardiovascular disease, cancer, and diabetes; improve their cholesterol ratio; sleep better and longer; have lower levels of depression; decrease anxiety; and have fewer stress-related illnesses. Exercise may not be the direct cause of enhanced feelings of self-esteem (Sonstroem, 1984), but it may contribute indirectly through each of these factors, in addition to achieving weight loss, improved appearance, increased levels of physical energy, and greater self-discipline. Participation in an exercise program is strongly associated with feeling good about oneself.

In Summary

During the past 35 years, research has accumulated to support the hypothesis that physical activity is associated with both cardiovascular health and improved psychological functioning. The first Surgeon General's report on physical activity and health (USDHHS, 1996) examined much of that

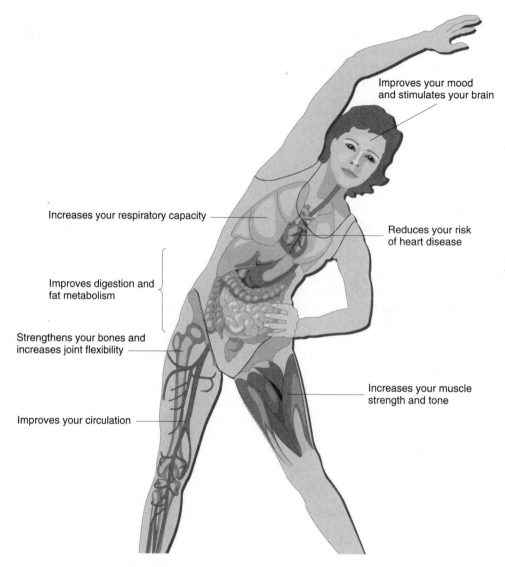

Improves your mood
and stimulates your brain

Increases your respiratory capacity

Reduces your risk
of heart disease

Improves digestion and
fat metabolism

Strengthens your bones and
increases joint flexibility

Increases your muscle
strength and tone

Improves your circulation

Figure 16.2   Some of the physical and psychological benefits of exercise.   *Source: An Invitation to Health* (7th ed., p. 493), by D. Hales, 1997, Pacific Grove, CA: Brooks/Cole. Copyright © 1997 by Brooks/Cole Publishing Company. Reprinted by permission of Wadsworth Publishing Co.

research and found that regular moderate physical activity can reduce the incidence of cardiovascular disease, diabetes, colon cancer, and high blood pressure. Moreover, physical activity can reduce symptoms of depression and anxiety, increase feelings of well-being, and enhance ability to perform daily tasks. The International Society of Sport Psychology (1992) issued a position statement delineating the benefits of physical activity on both short-term and long-term personal well-being and

Table 16.1 Reasons for exercising and research supporting these reasons

Reasons for exercising	Findings	Principle source(s)
"Exercise helps people become physically fit."	Exercise improves several kinds of physical fitness, including cardiovascular fitness	Lakka et al. (1994); Blair et al. (1995)
"I want to lose weight."	Exercise is a slow way to burn calories, but it may change setpoint.	Fiore et al. (1996); Tsoh (1997)
"It strengthens my heart"	Both the heart and the cardiovascular system benefit from exercise.	Kramsch et al. (1981); USDHHS (1996)
"Exercise helps people live longer."	Exercise may increase longevity by 2 years or more.	Lee et al. (1995); Kujala et al. (1998); Vita et al. (1998)
"I don't feel so depressed when I exercise." and "I just feel better."	Exercise can reduce anxiety, stress, and depression, as well as increase self-esteem.	International Society of Sports Psychology (1992); Sonstroem (1997); Martinsen & Morgan (1997)
"I'm addicted to it."	Exercise is not physiologically addictive, but some people become dependent on it.	McMurray et al. (1984); Hoffmann (1997)

self-esteem. The society also suggested that physical activity can reduce anxiety and stress and have a positive effect on hypertension, osteoporosis, and adult-onset diabetes. Moreover, regular exercise is as effective as any form of psychotherapy in lessening depression.

An earlier section of this chapter examined several reasons why people exercise. Table 16.1 lists some of these reasons, summarizes research evidence, and cites at least one study pertaining to each reason.

No strong causal relationship has been established between physical activity and health, because people who exercise regularly generally engage in other health-related activities, such as eating more fruits and vegetables, wearing seat belts, and not smoking (Pate, Heath, Dowda, & Trost, 1996). Nevertheless, sufficient correlational evidence exists to suggest that regular physical activity can be an effective adjunct in the treatment or prevention of cardiovascular disease, some types of cancer, diabetes, osteoporosis, insomnia, depression, anxiety, and stress. In addition, moderate exercise is related to enhanced feelings of well-being, self-esteem, and improved body image.

Hazards of Physical Activity

Although physical activity can enhance physical functioning; reduce anxiety, stress, and depression; and increase feelings of self-esteem, it also poses hazards to one's physical and psychological health. Some athletes overtrain to the point of **staleness** and, as a consequence, suffer from negative mood, fatigue, and depression (O'Connor, 1997). In addition, some highly active people suffer exercise-related injuries and others allow exercise to assume an almost addictive importance. In this section, we look at some of these hazards of too much physical activity.

Exercise Addiction

Some people become so dependent on exercise that it interferes with other parts of their lives, but the evidence is not clear concerning the underlying physiological mechanisms for exercise addiction. In Chapter 14, we saw that addictions produce tolerance, dependence, and physiological withdrawal symptoms. For exercise to produce physical addiction, some neurochemical must be

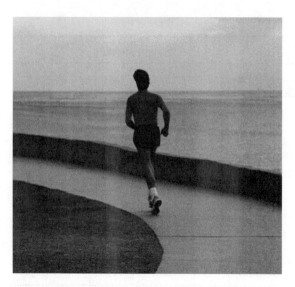

Exercise poses hazards as well as benefits for those who exercise vigorously.

involved. Although some researchers have speculated that vigorous and prolonged aerobic exercise can increase endorphins, the evidence is not clear. Research (Hoffmann, 1997; McMurray, Sheps, & Guinan, 1984) raises doubts that endorphin levels increase in response to exercise.

Exercise can result in what some people call *psychological addiction;* that is, it can become a habitual behavior and extremely resistant to extinction. Although the term *psychological addiction* is not universally accepted, William Glasser (1976) used this concept to describe several positive habits, including running and meditation. Glasser termed these habits *positive addictions* and argued that running and meditation are opposites of those habits usually considered negative addictions, such as taking drugs. Like negative addictions, positive addictions involve regular, compulsive use and withdrawal symptoms on cessation. Indeed, runners can become so psychologically dependent on running that they experience withdrawal symptoms on days when they do not run (Conboy, 1994). However, these withdrawal symptoms, which include anxiety, guilt, restlessness, tension,

and irritability, may be more psychological than physical (Sachs, 1982).

Running addiction becomes a negative habit when the athlete develops either staleness or injuries and yet refuses to stop vigorous physical activity. Morgan (1979) compared the process of overuse to the development of other negative addictions. Initially, the tolerance for running is low, and it has many unpleasant side effects. But persistence eases the unpleasant aspects, and the pleasure of meeting goals becomes a powerful reinforcer. Like most social drinkers who have a casual, nonobsessive relationship with alcohol, most runners are able to incorporate running into their lives without drastic changes in lifestyle. Other runners, however, cannot. Those who continue to increase their running must make changes in their lives to accommodate the time required to exercise. Morgan called these runners *negatively addicted.*

One aspect of this addiction is increased neglect of family and job responsibilities due to the time and commitment required for running. A second facet of running addiction is a progressive self-absorption, with a great deal of concentration on internal experiences. A third aspect of running addiction is the continuation of running after medical orders to stop. In this respect, the addicted runner behaves very much like the anorexic or the alcoholic, continuing a behavior that is harmful or even self-destructive. Addicted runners, in fact, have often been compared to anorexics. Thinness is the most obvious characteristic common to the two groups, but it is by no means the only one. Anorexic women and addicted male runners are alike in the need for mastery of the body, unusually high expectations of self, tolerance or denial of physical discomfort and pain, a single-minded commitment to endurance, and preoccupation with exercise and body image (Yates, Leehey, & Shisslak, 1983).

In addition, serious runners—both male and female—are often preoccupied with weight and frequently show symptoms of eating disorder (Kiernan, Rodin, Brownell, Wilmore, & Crandall, 1992). Indeed, physical activity may play an

WOULD YOU BELIEVE...?

Misunderstandings about Exercise

Would you believe that exercise does not increase appetite? Although some people believe that exercise makes them hungry, such a belief—like several others regarding exercise—is not based on scientific evidence.

Because exercise requires energy and energy is obtained through food, exercise should logically increase one's appetite for food. In fact, only very light, brief exercise and very heavy exercise increase appetite. Moderate, sustained exercise *decreases* appetite. Decrease of appetite is associated with most aerobics programs and tends to last for about as long as the exercise lasted. For this reason, Kenneth Cooper (1982) advised people wishing to lose weight to do their aerobic exercise in the late afternoon so their appetite for dinner would be decreased.

Very heavy, sustained exercise, such as long-distance running, does increase appetite but not immediately after the exercise. Because such exercise uses many calories, this increase in appetite is part of the body's regulation system. But this system apparently works imperfectly. Many marathon runners must force themselves to eat adequate calories.

Some evidence suggests that exercise affects obese people and thin people differently. One review study (Hill, Drougas, & Peters, 1994) reported that obese people tend to eat less during exercise periods, whereas thin people eat more. Even when the taste of food was greatly enhanced, obese women did not increase their food intake. Nor is this finding limited to humans. Hill et al. also reported on a study showing that animals almost never take in more calories than they expend through exercise. These findings suggest that fat people should not avoid exercise out of fear of increasing their appetite and adding unwanted extra pounds.

Would you believe that exercise is not an effective method of spot reduction? Despite some exercise promoters' claims, a particular calisthenic exercise will not reduce fat in a particular part of the body. Such a belief is one of the most appealing and enduring of all exercise myths. Unfortunately, it is not true. Muscle and fat have little to do with one another, and it is possible to have both in the same spot. Long-time tennis players, for example, typically have more muscle in the playing arm than in the nonplaying arm, but the fat content of the two arms is about equal (Gwinup, Chelvam, & Steinberg, 1971). This evidence that the playing arm of a tennis player can be exercised vigorously with no loss of fat refutes the concept of spot reduction.

Reduction of fat happens more in some spots than in others. When weight is lost, both fat and muscle tissue are depleted. If a person exercises during weight reduction, muscle tissue is built up while fat is being lost. Spot reduction appears to be the result, because fat tends to be lost from the places where it was most abundant. Therefore, the hips, thighs, or stomach may reduce more quickly than other spots during a program of diet and exercise, but this is not due to the effect of spot reducing exercises. Most exercise physiologists believe that fat distribution on the body is under strong genetic control, so some spots may never look like the ideal.

A person's belief in spot reducing can be hazardous, both physically and financially. Certain calisthenics that have been promoted as spot-reducing aids can cause injury. These include straight-leg sit-ups, deep knee bends, and any exercise involving bouncing stretches. Such exercises should be avoided for spot reducing or any other purpose. The financial hazards come from the purchase of exercise equipment and enrollment in expensive health clubs that promise spot reduction. No exercise can cause a loss of fat in a particular spot, so equipment advertisements that promise to do so are deceptive.

Would you believe that pain and injury during exercise is nature's way of telling you to quit? Although some people believe that exercise should

(continued)

WOULD YOU BELIEVE...?

Misunderstandings about Exercise *(continued)*

hurt and that injury is no reason to stop or even slow down, this belief can be dangerous and may lead to further injuries and even to permanent disability.

Pain is a message from the body that there is something wrong. Ignoring pain messages often results in more pain and even further injury. Those who exercise regularly face a dilemma. Minor injuries often occur in people who exercise for fitness or for training. Unfortunately, their desire to retain the effects of fitness training creates a strong temptation to ignore the pain and continue to exercise. Although the wise exerciser would seek professional advice about pain, few people do, probably because they do not want to be told to stop exercising. Nevertheless, prudent advice would be to stop exercising if the pain gets worse during exercise.

---

intimate part in the development of eating disorders. One study (Davis, Kennedy, Ravelski, & Dionne, 1994) looked at women hospitalized for eating disorders and found that more than three-fourths of the patients had engaged in excessive exercise, with 60% involved in competitive athletics.

Additional support for the relationship between high intensity exercising and problem behaviors came from Caroline Davis, Howard Brewer, and Dorothy Ratusny (1993), who developed the Commitment to Exercise Scale, which yields an Obligatory factor and a Pathological factor. Obligatory exercisers engage in activity because they believe their well-being is dependent on their exercising, whereas Pathological exercisers continue to exercise in the face of adverse circumstances, such as injuries, or permit their activity to take precedence over other aspects of their lives. Research by Davis et al. found that both male and female committed exercisers tend to be preoccupied with weight control and to have an excess of eating disorders. In addition, the men in this study tended to be perfectionistic, obsessive, and compulsive. Other research (Slay, Hayaki, Napolitano, & Brownell, 1998) has confirmed the close association between being an obligatory runner and having unhealthy concerns about weight control and body image.

Like a drug addict, the obligatory exerciser is willing to endure discomfort and social neglect for the sensations obtained from the exercise experience. Perhaps this fanaticism can be best expressed in the words of one fanatic runner:

> One day last spring I was having an exceptionally good run. I was running about 10 miles a day at that time and on this particular day I had decided to extend my workout. I was around the 14-mile point and I was preparing to cross a one-lane bridge when all of a sudden a large cement mixer turned the corner and began to cross the bridge. I never thought for a second about stopping and letting the truck pass. I simply continued and said to myself, "Come on you son-of-a-bitch and I'll split you right down the middle—there will be concrete all over the road!" The driver slammed on the brakes and swerved to the side as I sailed by. That was really scary afterward, but at the time I really felt good. I have felt equally strong and indestructible many times since, but never have taken on a cement truck again. (Morgan, 1979, pp. 63, 67)

Injuries from Physical Activity

Excluding head-to-head challenges with cement trucks, what are the chances of experiencing injuries from exercise? Many people with a regular exercise program accept minor injuries and soreness as an almost inevitable component of their program. However, irregular exercise produces even more injuries and more discomfort, with "weekend athletes" accounting for a disproportional number of injuries.

Several factors can decrease the probability of injury. One of these is appropriate equipment. For example, proper running shoes are a necessity for running, jogging, or even exercise walking (Cooper, 1982). Another factor, supervised training, can decrease the chances of injury by preventing improperly performed exercise or an overly ambitious program. Strenuous exercise, especially for people who have been sedentary, can be a danger. For such people and for those who have been diagnosed as being at risk for coronary heart disease, supervised exercise is a wise precaution.

However, musculoskeletal injuries are not uncommon, especially among runners, and the greater the distance and greater the frequency of running, the more likely it is that people will injure themselves. The Surgeon General's report (USDHHS, 1996) found that about half of runners had experienced an injury during the past year. This review also found, as expected, that the injury rate was lower for walkers than for joggers and that previous injury is a risk factor for subsequent injury. To reduce chances of musculoskeletal injuries, previously inactive people wishing to begin exercising should warm up with slow, easy stretching exercises, begin their activity slowly, and gradually increase their pace toward a reasonable goal.

Other Health Risks of Physical Activity

Besides muscular and skeletal injuries, avid exercisers encounter a number of other health hazards. Heat, cold, dogs, and drivers can all be sources of danger. During exercise, body temperature rises. It can be maintained at 104°F with no danger (Pollock et al., 1978). Fluid intake before, after, and even during exercise can protect against overheating by allowing the exerciser to cool off by sweating. However, conditions of extremely high air temperature, high humidity, and sunlight can combine to raise body temperature and prevent sweat from evaporating from the skin surface. If the body is prevented from cooling itself, dangerous overheating may occur.

Cold temperatures can also be dangerous for outdoor exercising, but proper clothing can provide protection. Layered clothing for the body and gloves, hat, and even a face mask can protect against temperatures of 20°F and below (Pollock et al., 1978). Temperatures below zero, especially when combined with wind, can be dangerous even to people who are not exercising.

Death during Exercise

Many patients who have had heart attacks are put into an exercise program, and such programs generally include close supervision. Although these coronary patients are at an elevated risk during exercise, the cardiovascular benefit they receive from exercising ordinarily outweighs the risk (USDHHS, 1996). Nevertheless, exercise programs for those who have been diagnosed as having coronary heart disease should be undertaken only with a physician's permission and under the supervision of specialists in cardiac rehabilitation.

What about people who have no known disease? Is it possible for a person who looks and feels well to die unexpectedly during exercise? Yes—but it is also possible to die unexpectedly while watching TV or sleeping. One study (Thompson, Funk, Carleton, & Sturner, 1982) examined the causes and frequency of sudden death during jogging as well as during nonvigorous activities and found that the probability of sudden death increased during exercise. The risk of dying during jogging was seven times greater than the risk of dying during nonvigorous activities. In other words, although conditioned athletes like Jim Fixx may experience cardiac arrest at any time, they are much more likely to die during exercise. This statistic seems to be an indictment of exercise, but the causes of sudden death during exercise should first be examined.

A review of studies on sudden death during exercise (Thompson, 1982) found that the majority of these deaths were due to atherosclerotic cardiovascular disease. In many cases, the people who died had known of their disease. However, the coronary arteries may narrow substantially with no apparent symptoms of cardiovascular disease. This condition would likely be diagnosed during an exercise stress test, but not all people who begin and continue an exercise program have had such tests. Testing is highly recommended for people over 40 years old who plan to start an exercise program, especially if they are overweight, smoke, or have a family history of coronary disease.

In contrast to physically fit people, those with low levels of habitual exercise are much more likely to have a fatal or nonfatal heart attack during vigorous activity. People who do not exercise regularly are far more likely to die during exercise than physically fit men. One study (Mittleman et al., 1993) interviewed patients who had very recently suffered myocardial infarction and found that those who had a history of exercising less than once a week were more than 40 times as likely to have a heart attack during exercise than patients who exercised five or more times a week. In a similar study (Willich et al., 1993), researchers interviewed male and female patients who had recently suffered a myocardial infarction and asked about their physical exertion at the time of their heart attack. They found that people who did not exercise regularly were much more likely than frequent exercisers to experience a heart attack while engaging in physical exertion. By themselves, these findings reveal little about the benefits or hazards of regular, habitual exercise. They merely indicate that heart attacks are more likely to occur during periods of exertion than during times of inactivity.

Is exercise beneficial or hazardous to coronary health? Physician Gregory Curfman (1993) believes that it may be both, but he commented that "exercise performed at frequent intervals over a long time span provides protection against both the development of coronary artery disease and the triggering of myocardial infarction by strenuous exertion" (p. 1731). Curfman warned that sudden, heavy exertion may put sedentary people at risk of sudden heart attack. However, the overall cardiac risk for active people is much less than it is for sedentary individuals (USDHHS, 1996), which suggests that regular exercise protects against death from heart attack.

In Summary

Exercise has hazards as well as benefits. Potential hazards include exercise addiction—that is, a pathological and compulsive need to devote long periods of time to strenuous physical activity. Also, exercise may lead to injuries, but appropriate preparation, such as stretching before jogging or running, using suitable shoes, and stopping when injuries first occur, can reduce these injuries. Joggers should also avoid working out in extreme temperatures, and they should know how to avoid dogs, drivers, and darkness. Death during exercise is a possibility, and people with heart disease are more likely to die while exercising than at other times. Nevertheless, people who exercise regularly are much less likely than sporadic exercisers to die of a heart attack during intense physical exertion.

How Much Is Enough but Not Too Much?

Research has indicated that some amount of exercise is inversely related to a variety of disorders and diseases and also that some amount of exercise may be hazardous. These disparate findings raise the question, How much is enough but not too much?

During the 1980s, many people, perhaps led by devoted runner/writers such as Jim Fixx, believed that they had to achieve aerobic fitness through

BECOMING HEALTHIER

1. If you don't exercise, make plans to start a program of regular physical activity.

2. Don't start too fast. If you are overweight or over 40, consult a physician before beginning.

3. Once you have determined that you are ready to begin an exercise program, start slowly. The first day you may feel as though you can run a mile. Don't give in to that temptation.

4. Exercising too vigorously on the fist day will result in injuries or at least sore muscles. If you are stiff and sore the next day, you overdid it, and you won't feel like exercising on the second day.

5. If you are exercising for weight control, don't weigh yourself every day, and try not to become preoccupied with your weight or body shape.

6. If you are in the process of quitting smoking, use exercise as a way to prevent weight gain.

7. Choose and use correct equipment when you exercise.

8. If you exercise in a location unfamiliar to you, check out your surroundings before you begin. Several types of potential dangers may be in your path.

9. Remember that in order to receive maximum health benefits from your exercise program, you must stick to it. About 70% of those who begin drop out after a couple of years.

10. To acquire muscle tone as well as aerobic fitness, include a combination of types of exercise such as working out with weights or other isotonic exercise as well as aerobics.

---

vigorous exercise if they were to enhance their health. At the same time, Ralph Paffenbarger and his colleagues (1986) were reporting that high levels of physical activity were more beneficial than moderate levels. Based on research at that time, health professionals were advising people to structure their exercise program around at least 20 minutes of sustained activity at an intensity level of 50% to 85% of their maximum heart rate for 4 or 5 days a week. Although this level of exercise confers cardiovascular fitness, some have questioned the necessity of such a highly structured program.

In recent years, some experts have seen exercise as a subset of physical activity and have emphasized the value of moderate physical activity, including walking, gardening, bicycling, climbing stairs, and swimming (Pratt, 1999). Recent evidence suggests that moderate walking is sufficient to produce the desired health benefits. For example, one study (Duncan, Gordon, & Scott, 1991) found that previously sedentary young women

showed a reduction in their coronary risk factors with 45 minutes of walking 5 days a week.

In 1995, a 20-member panel of experts reviewed this and other evidence on frequency and intensity of physical activity (Pate et al., 1995) and recommended that every adult should accumulate 30 minutes of moderate physical activity a day, or at least on most days. These experts also suggested that sedentary people should begin a program of moderate, regular physical activity.

> If Americans who lead sedentary lives would adopt a more active lifestyle, there would be enormous benefit to the public's health and to individual well-being. An active lifestyle does not require a regimented, vigorous exercise program. Instead, small changes that increase daily physical activity will enable individuals to reduce their risk of chronic disease and may contribute to enhanced quality of life. (Pate et al., 1995, p. 406)

Subsequent research has supported this advice. For example, one report from the Honolulu Heart Program (Hakim et al., 1998) found that older

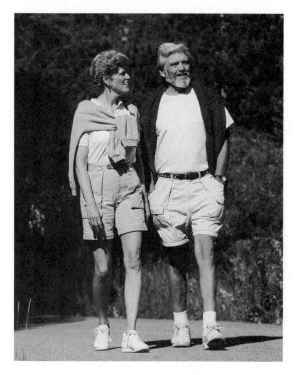

Walking is one form of physical activity that offers more advantages than hazards for most people.

of maximum aerobic capacity for 20 to 60 minutes 5 days a week. After 2 years, participants in both groups increased their physical activity and their cardiorespiratory fitness, showing that lifestyle changes were as least as beneficial as a more intensive exercise program. The second study (Andersen et al., 1999) introduced similar interventions to obese women and also included a low-fat diet for both groups. Both groups lost weight, reduced triglycerides, and decreased their total cholesterol. The authors concluded that diet plus moderate physical activity is a suitable alternative to diet plus structured aerobic exercise. These studies suggest that moderate levels of physical activity can confer cardiovascular health as effectively as vigorous exercise.

Maintaining a Physical Activity Program

Adherence to nearly all medical regimens is a serious problem (see Chapter 4), and exercise is no exception. Only 30% of people who begin an exercise program continue for an average of 3.5 years (Rodin & Salovey, 1989), and about half the participants in therapeutic exercise programs drop out within 6 months (Martin & Dubbert, 1985). Dropout rates in prescribed exercise regimens are about the same as those found in other compliance studies, and they closely parallel the relapse rates reported in smoking and alcohol cessation programs.

Predicting Dropouts

The first step toward maintaining a physical activity program is to identify the personal, social-environmental, and exercise program variables related to noncompliance. In a review of research, Rod Dishman and Janet Buckworth (1997) identified several personal attributes that predict adherence to physical activity. In general, those most likely to stick to an exercise plan are men, people with a past history of physical activity, those with higher levels of education and income, and

men who included a daily walk of two or more miles cut their risks for sudden cardiac death in half. Another study from the Cooper Clinic in Dallas (Stofan, DiPietro, Davis, Kohl, & Blair, 1998) found much the same results when both women and men were included.

In addition, two groups of researchers have shown that relatively small lifetime changes in levels of physical activity are at least as beneficial as traditional structured programs. The first study (Dunn et al., 1999) compared the effects of a lifestyle intervention with a traditional structured program of fitness, body composition, and other cardiovascular risk factors. The lifestyle intervention used Bandura's (1986) cognitive social theory and Prochaska's (1994) transtheoretical model to train slightly overweight men and women to gradually increase their level of moderate physical activity. The traditional intervention called for participants to exercise vigorously at 50% to 85%

younger people. Smokers, blue-collar workers, and people with low self-efficacy for maintaining an exercising program are most likely to drop out. Also, people who see themselves as having poor health either are reluctant to enter a physical activity program or have a high rate of quitting if they do.

Two frequently reported social-environmental factors for nonadherence are lack of access to exercise facilities and perceived lack of time (Dishman & Buckworth, 1997), but both are probably excuses rather than legitimate reasons for quitting. Health clubs and gymnasiums are not necessary for a walking program, and most people could find time if they reordered their priorities. A third social-environmental variable is social support. Individuals who receive encouragement from spouse and friends are less likely to drop out than people without this support. Also, group exercise programs usually have lower dropout rates than in-dividual programs. However, evidence for social support as a strong predictor is still sparse (Dishman & Buckworth, 1997).

Among the exercise program variables, the most common reason for stopping is injury. Of the people who engage in high-intensity physical activity, as many as 50% per year develop injuries serious enough to force them to stop (Dishman & Buckworth, 1997; USDHHS, 1996). As noted earlier, the more frequent and more intense the activity, the greater the chance that an injury will lead to temporary or permanent dropout. Thus, intense, frequent physical activity is one of the best predictors of noncompliance.

Increasing Maintenance

The second step in increasing adherence to physical activity is establishing an intervention strategy for all patients, with special attention for those at greatest risk of dropping out. Behavior modification and cognitive behavioral methods have had some success in reducing the dropout rate of exercisers. These programs ordinarily use a multimodal approach that relies on reinforcement for healthy behaviors, contracting, self-monitoring,

instruction, modeling, goal setting, increased self-efficacy, relapse prevention, and a variety of other strategies. Most of these have been discussed in earlier chapters and need no additional elaboration here. In general, psychological interventions have improved adherence to physical activity programs by about 15% to 20% (Dishman & Buckworth, 1997). In other words, if a program without an intervention has a 40% compliance rate, adding a psychological intervention may increase compliance to about 55% to 60%.

An important part of relapse prevention is protection against slips leading to full relapse. G. Alan Marlatt and Judith Gordon (1980) called this phenomenon the *abstinence violation effect* (see Chapter 13). With physical activity, people don't violate their abstinence, but rather they go a few days without any exercise behavior. Injury, illness, travel, or other breaks in daily routine can lead to an abstinence violation effect if people use four or five days of inactivity as an excuse to give up their physical activity regimen. Relapse prevention programs attempt to warn participants that they may be tempted to permanently quit exercising after a period of inactivity. As with smoking, drinking, or dieting, one slip does not equal complete relapse, and exercisers can be taught that the sooner they resume physical activity, the easier it will be. Although behavioral and cognitive behavioral strategies have demonstrated some success, especially when used in combination, maintenance remains a serious problem in most health-related exercise programs.

In Summary

The health benefits of physical activity can be gleaned from relatively low levels of exercise. Experts now say that if every person would accumulate 30 minutes of moderate physical activity five or six times a week, they would reduce their risk of chronic disease and probably enhance their quality of life.

Dropout rates in prescribed exercise regimens are about the same as those found in other compliance studies; that is, after about 3 years, only

30% of the people who began an exercise program maintained that program. This rate closely parallels the relapse rates reported in smoking and alcohol cessation programs. The two most common reasons (excuses) given for dropping out of an exercise program are lack of access to exercise facilities and lack of time. Programs designed to improve adherence to physical activity programs are able to boost maintenance by about 15% to 20%.

Answers

This chapter addressed seven basic questions.

1. **What are the different types of physical activity?**

   All physical activity can be subsumed under one or more of five basic categories: isometric, isotonic, isokinetic, anaerobic, and aerobic. Each of these five exercise types has advantages and disadvantages for improving physical fitness.

2. **What are the health-related reasons to exercise?**

   Most people who exercise do so for muscle strength, muscle endurance, flexibility, cardiorespiratory or aerobic fitness, and weight control. One or another of the five types of physical activity can help people achieve these goals, but no one type of exercise promotes all types of fitness. Physical activity is at least as effective as diet in a weight-control program and much better than dieting in changing the ratio of fat to muscle.

3. **Does physical activity benefit the cardiovascular system?**

   Most results on the health benefits of exercise have confirmed a positive relationship between regular physical activity and enhanced cardiovascular health. This relationship suggests that a regimen of moderate, brisk physical activity should be prescribed as one of several components in a program of coronary health.

4. **What are some other health benefits of physical activity?**

   In addition to improving cardiovascular health, regular physical activity may protect against some kinds of cancer, especially colon cancer; help prevent bone density loss, thus lowering one's risk of osteoporosis; control adult-onset diabetes, especially in those men most at risk; and help people sleep better and longer.

   Besides improving physical fitness and health, regular exercise can confer certain psychological benefits. Specifically, research has demonstrated that aerobic and nonaerobic exercises can decrease depression, reduce anxiety, a buffer against the harmful effects of stress, and enhance feelings of self-esteem.

5. **Can physical activity be hazardous?**

   Several hazards accompany both regular and sporadic exercise. Some runners appear to be addicted to exercise, becoming obsessed with body image and fearful of being prevented from following their exercise regimen. Injuries are frequent among veteran runners, but the most serious hazard is sudden death while exercising. However, people who exercise regularly are much less likely than sporadic exercisers to die of heart attack during heavy physical exertion.

6. **How much is enough but not too much?**

   During the past 20 years, "experts" have gradually decreased their estimation of the amount of physical activity necessary to benefit cardiovascular health. The latest recommendation was provided by a 20-member panel of experts who recommended that every adult should accumulate 30 minutes of moderate physical activity a day, or at least on most days.

7. **What are some problems in maintaining an exercise program?**

   Exercise is frequently prescribed as therapy, especially for coronary heart disease. Unfortunately, dropout rates are about as high for this medical recommendation as they are for others. Behavioral interventions have had some limited success in improving compliance with health-related exercise programs.

Glossary

aerobic exercise Exercise that requires an increased amount of oxygen consumption over an extended period of time.

anaerobic exercise Exercise that does not require an increased amount of oxygen.

cardiac arrhythmia Irregularity in the heartbeat rhythm.

isokinetic exercise Exercise requiring exertion for lifting and additional effort for returning weight to the starting position.

isometric exercise Exercise in which muscles are contracted against an immovable object.

isotonic exercise Exercise that requires the contraction of muscles and the movement of joints, as in weight lifting.

osteoporosis A disease characterized by a reduction in bone density, brittleness of bones, and a loss of calcium from the bones.

staleness Negative mood, fatigue, and depression as a result of overtraining in athletes.

state anxiety A temporary condition of dread or uneasiness stemming from a specific situation.

trait anxiety A personality characteristic that manifests itself as a more or less constant feeling of dread or uneasiness.

Suggested Readings

Blair, S. N. (1994). Physical activity, fitness, and coronary heart disease. In C. Bouchard, R. J. Shephard, & T. Stephens (Eds.), *Physical activity, fitness, and health: International proceedings and consensus statement* (pp. 579–590). Champaign, IL: Human Kinetics.

Steven Blair reviews the literature on the effects of physical activity on heart disease and concludes that a seden- tary lifestyle and poor physical fitness are important risk factors for heart disease.

Fixx, J. F. (1980). *Jim Fixx's second book of running.* New York: Random House.

This is a well-written book by one of the people who helped popularize running and jogging. This book supplements Fixx's first book, which turned out not to be the complete book of running.

McAuley, E. (1994). Physical activity and psychosocial outcomes. In C. Bouchard, R. J. Shephard, & T. Stephens (Eds.), *Physical activity, fitness, and health: International proceedings and consensus statement* (pp. 551–568). Champaign, IL: Human Kinetics.

An authority on the psychosocial outcomes of exercise, Edward McAuley reviews the literature and concludes that the area still suffers from methodologically weak designs, imprecise outcome measures, lack of sufficient follow-up, and confusion between physical fitness and physical activity.

 Rosellini, L. (1997, November 10). How far should you go to stay fit? The battle between tough and tame. *U.S. News & World Report, 123,* 95–96.

This brief article presents the clash between two philosophies of exercise: the older approach that encourages people to "tough it out" to attain fitness and the newer view that says any exercise is good. The article also covers research and policy on fitness and health. Available through InfoTrac College Edition from Wadsworth Publishing Company.

U. S. Department of Health and Human Services (USDHHS). (1996). *Physical activity and health: A report of the Surgeon General.* Atlanta, GA: Centers for Disease Control and Prevention.

With this first Surgeon General's report on physical activity, the U. S. Government officially recognized the health-related benefits of exercise. This volume discusses the effects of physical activity on cardiovascular disease, cancer, diabetes, arthritis, osteoporosis, and psychological health.

CHAPTER 17

Future Challenges

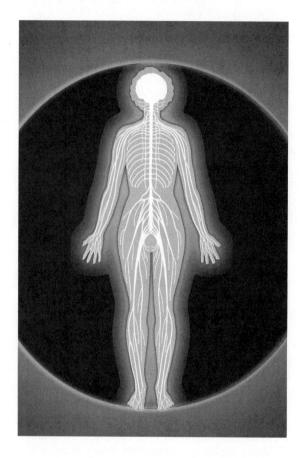

QUESTIONS

This chapter focuses on three basic questions:

1. What role does health psychology play in contributing to the goals of *Healthy People 2000*?

2. What training do health psychologists receive and what kinds of work do they do?

3. What is the outlook for the future of health psychology?

At the beginning of the third millennium, health psychology faces myriad challenges as it strives to become an important contributor to people's health. No longer a nascent science, health psychology has become established as an important profession within the discipline of psychology—a science capable of making significant contributions to the health of the nation.

As Americans have become increasingly health conscious, they have come to realize that their physical well-being is not solely in the hands of medical professionals and that they have an important share of the responsibility in maintaining their own health. They are aware of the dangers of smoking, abusing alcohol, eating improperly, and not exercising regularly. They know that they should learn to cope better with stress, make and keep regular medical and dental appointments, and follow the advice of their health care professionals. This knowledge does not always translate into action, and people have difficulty changing their behavior and lifestyle. But over the past 30 years, U.S. residents have managed to make some healthy changes in their behavior. The percentage of smokers has fallen, the amount of alcohol consumed has decreased, and the use of seatbelts and other safety measures has increased. People have started to become more conscious of what they eat and to consume more fruit and vegetables and less red meat and other saturated fats.

These positive changes are reflected in declining mortality for heart disease, stroke, cancer, homicide, and unintentional injuries (USBC, 1998), but unhealthy and risky behaviors continue to contribute to an increasing rate of chronic obstructive pulmonary disease. This chapter looks at the nation's health goals and at the role and status of health psychology in confronting the principal challenges facing the field.

Healthier People

An example of the influence of health consciousness on a national policy level is *Healthy People 2000* (USDHHS, 1991), a report that detailed 3 broad goals, 22 priority areas, and 300 main objectives for improving the health of people in the United States. The broad goals included increasing the span of healthy life, reducing health disparities among Americans, and achieving access to preventive services for all people in the United States. This report was followed by *Healthy People 2010: Draft for public comment* (USDHHS, 1998b), which called for public comment on these goals, priority areas, and objectives.

Increasing the Span of Healthy Life

The first goal—to increase the span of healthy life—is different from that of increasing life expectancy. Rather than striving for longer lives, many people are now trying to increase their number of well-years. A **well-year** is "the equivalent of a year of completely well life, or a year of life free of dysfunction, symptoms, and health-related problems" (Kaplan & Bush (1982, p. 64). This concept has grown in acceptability since 1946, when the World Health Organization charter defined health in terms of positive states of mental and physical well-being.

In addition to striving to increase well-years, health psychologists advocate the concept of **health expectancy**, defined as that period of life a person spends free from disability (Robine & Ritchie, 1991). For example, the life expectancy at age 65 is about 14 additional years for men and 19 years for women, but health expectancy is only 8 more years for men and 10 years for women, leaving both men and women with a discrepancy that represents years of disability (Robine & Ritchie, 1991). The differences between life expectancy and health expectancy are even larger when comparing the richest and poorest segments of the population. Wealthy people not only live longer but also having more years of healthy life. In addition, the disorders that shorten life are not necessarily the same as those that compromise health. For example, circulatory disorders head both lists, but disorders producing restricted movement and respiratory disorders are responsible for producing lost health expectancy, whereas cancer and accidents are major sources of lost life expectancy. Therefore, interventions aimed at increasing life expectancy do not necessarily improve health expectancy.

The need to increase the health of older people is important not only to improve their quality of life but also to help manage health care costs. Due to their tendency to have chronic illnesses, older people use health care services more heavily than younger people, with a rate of physician contacts twice as high for those over 75 as for those between ages 15 and 44 (USDHHS, 1998a). In an editorial in the *New England Journal of Medicine,* Andrew Kramer (1995) advocated a change in emphasis for health care for older people. Rather than concentrating on acute care delivered in hospitals, Kramer argued for the promotion of primary care and long-term care, strategies that might help improve quality of life for older people.

In addition, life expectancy may not continue to increase in the next century as it has in the past century. Although life expectancy has increased steadily over the past 100 years, without some breakthrough that changes the process of aging, it is not likely to increase much beyond 85 years (Olshansky, Carnes, & Cassel, 1993). Nevertheless, people's later years can include better health *and* a better quality of life, a situation that would benefit both the individual and the health care system.

Reducing Health Disparities

The United States has made much progress toward achieving the objectives of *Healthy People 2000,* but most of those gains have been by higher socioeconomic groups. Huge discrepancies in health status continue among various socioeconomic and ethnic groups (USDHHS, 1998b). When *Healthy People 2000* was published in 1991, the plan for reducing ethnic and socioeconomic disparities was to target minority groups separate from the general population. However, with

Healthy People 2010 (USDHHS, 1998b), the emphases shifted away from targeting special groups and toward high standards of improved health for everyone. With such a plan, the Department of Health and Human Services hopes to eliminate disparities in infant mortality, cancer screening, cardiovascular disease, diabetes, HIV/AIDS, sedentary lifestyle, obesity, and other health areas that now show large discrepancies between the general population and at least one minority group.

Currently, the United States does a poorer job of dispensing health care to its citizens than any other industrialized country, and this problem is reflected in many health statistics. For example, the United States ranks 21st in the world in infant mortality, 17th in life expectancy for men, and 16th in life expectancy for women (Consumers Union, 1992).

Social and economic factors contribute to these low rankings, but the underlying reasons for the relationship between socioeconomic factors and health are complex (Anderson & Armstead, 1995) and include education, income, occupational status, and ethnic background. In the United States, these factors are not separate: African Americans, Hispanic Americans, and Native Americans have lower average educational levels and incomes than European Americans and Asian Americans. Thus, the factor of ethnicity is difficult to separate from income and education, complicating the interpretation of the underlying reasons for health disparities among people of different ethnic backgrounds.

For example, African Americans, compared with European Americans, have a shorter life expectancy as well as a higher infant mortality rate, more homicide deaths, increased cardiovascular disease rates, higher cancer mortality, and more tuberculosis and diabetes (USBC, 1998). Inadequate medical treatment and lack of health education may be responsible for much of this disparity, but discrimination in health care provision is also a factor. For example, African Americans receive less aggressive treatment for symptoms of coro-

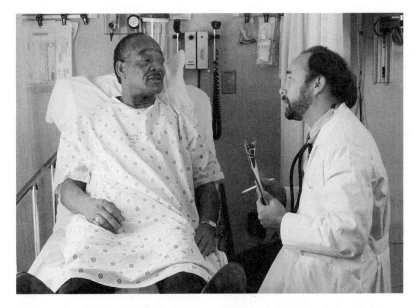

Reducing health disparities is one of the goals included in Healthy People 2010.

nary heart disease and are less likely to be referred to a cardiologist than European Americans (Crawford, McGraw, Smith, McKinlay, & Pierson, 1994) even though both groups are equally likely to seek health care.

Health discrepancies also exist when poor African Americans and poor European Americans are compared. Place of residence may partially explain the disadvantage of poor African Americans—poor Blacks and poor Whites tend to live in different circumstances. A majority of poor European Americans live in areas that are not classified as poverty areas, whereas only a small minority of poor African Americans lived outside poverty areas. Such residential isolation results in extreme segregation and concentration of African Americans in substandard housing and in neighborhoods with violence and without social ties—circumstances that relate to a variety of health risks (Anderson & Armstead, 1995).

Low economic status and the lack of access to medical care affect Native Americans at least as strongly as they effect African Americans. The In-

dian Health Service supports health care for Native Americans, but the level of funding is only half that spent on other Americans (Japsen, 1994). This situation may be a factor in the shorter life expectancy, higher mortality rate, higher infant mortality, and higher rates of infectious illness for Native Americans compared with European Americans (Grossman, Krieger, Sugarman, & Forquera, 1994).

Socioeconomic status, however, is not the only answer to the question of discrepancy between Native Americans and European Americans. One study (Cheadle et al., 1994) showed that even with socioeconomic status adjusted, Native Americans had a higher prevalence of risk-taking behaviors and poorer health status than people who were not Native Americans. Native Americans, then, are one of the groups poorly served by the current system of health care and health education in the United States.

Many Hispanic Americans also experience low socioeconomic status and poor education but not all groups of Hispanic Americans are equally affected, and their health and longevity tend to vary accordingly. Cuban Americans generally have higher education and economic levels than Mexican Americans or Puerto Ricans; thus, Cuban Americans are more likely to have jobs that include health insurance as a benefit, making them more likely to have access to regular health care and physician visits (Treviño, Moyer, Valdez, & Stroup-Benham, 1991).

For Hispanic Americans without insurance coverage, their ethnic background and geographic location may affect the health care they receive. Compared with Mexican Americans living near the U.S.-Mexican border, Puerto Ricans are more likely to live in places that offer better accessibility to Medicaid and thus more opportunity for frequent visits to physicians (Apodaca, Woodruff, Candelaria, Elder, & Zlot, 1997). Puerto Ricans, however, are poorer than other Hispanic Americans and have higher levels of health problems (USDHHS, 1995).

Hispanic Americans fare about the same as or better than European Americans on health and mortality measures. Hispanic Americans have a lower death rate than European Americans (USDHHS, 1997), including death from heart disease, stroke, and lung cancer. These low death rates are puzzling, given the high rates of smoking, obesity, and hypertension among Hispanic Americans. The poor health habits of Hispanic Americans, combined with their low disease prevalence, may reflect a transition in which immigrants are adopting European American lifestyles but have not yet developed the chronic diseases typical of the United States.

This same trend applies to all immigrant groups—those who adopt the lifestyle of the U.S. soon have the patterns of disease and death characteristic of the United States. Asian Americans who have adopted Western habits increase their risks, but Asian Americans still have more favorable health status and life expectancy than other ethnic groups (USDHHS, 1997). Asian Americans have lower infant mortality, longer life expectancy, lower lung and breast cancer deaths, and lower cardiovascular death rates.

Low income has an obvious connection to lower standards of health care, and people without health insurance and access to a physician are at increased risk. However, universal access to health care does not remove the disparities among socioeconomic groups (Anderson & Armstead, 1995). Even in countries that have universal access to health care, health disparities between poor and wealthy people continue to exist, suggesting that factors other than receiving health care are involved in maintaining health.

Education and socioeconomic level are two factors that may influence health status—independent of access to health care. Across ethnic groups, people who have higher education and income also have better health and longevity than those with lower education and income. As we saw in Chapter 13, education is significantly related to cigarette smoking, the leading cause of death in the United States (CDC, 1998d). People with fewer than 12 years of education are much more likely to smoke than those with college degrees. In addition, people with low education and low socioeconomic status are more likely to eat a high-fat diet and less likely to engage in leisure-time physical activity than people with high education and socioeconomic levels (Anderson & Armstead, 1995; USDHHS, 1991). These behaviors are related to a variety of disorders, explaining at least part of the relationship between poor health and low education and socioeconomic status. Improved access to health care will probably eliminate some of the disparities among ethnic groups, but changes in health-related behaviors and improved living conditions will also be necessary.

Increasing Access to Preventive Services

The third goal of *Healthy People 2000* is to achieve access to preventive services for all people living in the United States. In general, preventing disease and disability would seem to be more cost effective than curing these disorders after people become sick or disabled. However, whether prevention saves money or not depends on the type of prevention and the target audience. *Primary prevention* consists of immunizations and programs that encourage lifestyle changes; this type of prevention is usually a good bargain. Programs that encourage people to quit smoking, eat properly, exercise, and moderate their drinking generally have low cost and little potential to do harm (Leutwyler, 1995). In addition, some of these behaviors, such as smoking and inactivity, are risks for many health problems, and efforts oriented toward changing these behaviors can pay off by decreasing risks for several disorders (Winett, 1995). Although immunizations have some potential for harm, they remain good choices unless the risks from side effects of the immunization are comparable to the risk of catching the disease. Thus, primary prevention efforts tend to pose few risks and have many benefits.

Secondary prevention consists of screening people at risk for developing a disease in order to find problems in their early and more treatable stages. However, such efforts can be costly because the number of people at risk may be much larger than the number who have developed the disease. Based on the economic considerations of cost-benefit analysis—that is, how much money is spent and how much is saved—secondary prevention may not be the solution to the problem of rising health care costs. Cost-benefit analyses (Leutwyler, 1995) have revealed that some prevention efforts, such as control of hypertension, are no more cost effective than curative interventions, such as coronary bypass operations, because many people who receive preventive care would never have developed heart disease.

However, if a program adds well-years to life, then cost-efficiency analysis can determine the cost per well-year. Such information can help individuals and policy makers decide which health programs offer the best outcomes (in terms of well-years) for the least cost. In these terms, the interventions that health psychologists provide can justify their costs (Sobel, 1995).

The *Healthy People 2000* goals that are oriented toward prevention incorporate both primary and secondary prevention efforts. The primary prevention goals include increasing physical activity, improving nutrition, decreasing tobacco use, decreasing alcohol and illegal drug use, increasing health education in schools and communities, increasing dental care, and increasing immunizations for a variety of childhood and adult diseases. Secondary prevention goals include testing homes for radon and lead as well as screening for a variety of other conditions. These screenings include testing newborns for genetic disorders, assessing adults (especially men) for hypertension, measuring adults for high serum cholesterol, testing women over age 40 for breast cancer, testing at-risk individuals for HIV, and assessing children and older people for vision and hearing problems.

A review of progress toward each of the 300 main objectives listed in *Healthy People 2000* is included in *Healthy People 2010* (USDHHS, 1998b). A variety of health care professionals, including psychologists, have a role in helping the nation achieve the goals and objectives of *Healthy People 2000*.

In Summary

People in the United States and other industrialized countries are becoming more health conscious, and both government policy and individual behavior reflect this concern. *Healthy People 2000* stated three broad goals for the U.S. population: (1) increasing healthy years of life, (2) decreasing disparities among specialized groups in health care delivery, and (3) increasing access to preventive services for everyone. The first goal includes increasing the number of *well-years*—that is, years free of dysfunction, disease symptoms, and health-related problems. The goal also includes the concept of *health expectancy*—that is, the period of life a person spends free from disability. The second goal—decreasing disparities in health care—is far from being met, in part because people in the upper socioeconomic level continue to make greater gains in health status than do those in the lower levels. Finally, the United States has made some small strides toward increasing access to preventive services for everyone. Primary prevention consists of programs that encourage lifestyle changes such as quitting smoking, eating properly, exercising, and drinking alcohol in a healthy manner. Secondary prevention consists of looking at people who are at risk for developing a disease so that potential problems can be avoided or controlled in their early stages. Primary prevention programs are usually cost efficient, whereas secondary prevention interventions sometimes are not.

The Profession of Health Psychology

One important goal of health psychology is to help translate knowledge into action. The field of health psychology rests on the premise that psychology can contribute to health in four major ways: (1) accumulating more information on behaviors and lifestyles as they relate to health and illness, (2) helping to promote and maintain health, (3) contributing to the prevention and treatment of disease, and (4) helping to formulate health policy and promote the health care system (Matarazzo, 1982).

The first contribution—accumulating more information on behaviors and lifestyles as they relate to health and illness—is a necessary but not sufficient condition for improving health. Although psychology has made substantial contributions toward the body of health knowledge, much of this information is being gathered by other disciplines, such as epidemiology, immunology, dietetics, sociology, and medical anthropology. Psychology's historical involvement in changing human behavior places it in a position to: (1) help people eliminate unhealthy practices and (2) support their attempts to incorporate healthy behaviors into an ongoing lifestyle.

The prevalence of such chronic disorders as asthma, arthritis, Alzheimer's disease, AIDS, cancer, cardiovascular disease, diabetes, headaches, and stress is a challenge for psychology—and specifically, health psychology—in the field of

health. How successfully has health psychology progressed toward meeting this challenge?

Progress in Health Psychology

Since the founding of health psychology, the field has grown rapidly, and this growth has been apparent both in the amount of research published by psychologists on health-related topics and in the growing number of psychologists who work in health care settings.

In 1969, William Schofield published an article in the *American Psychologist* that gave a major impetus to health psychology. Analyzing the research publications in psychology that dealt with health, he found that only 19% of the research articles dealt with topics other than the traditional mental health concerns of psychology. This finding brought about a call for a wider scope of psychological services and research. The American Psychological Association (APA) appointed a task force to perform a further analysis; this task force concluded that health was not a common area of research for psychologists (APA Task Force on Health Research, 1976). During the past 2 decades, psychology research on health issues has accelerated to the point where health psychology has changed the field of psychology, making health-related issues common topics in psychology journals.

Employment opportunities have also increased for health psychologists since the early 1980s. A survey of job announcements in the *APA Monitor* from mid-1982 to mid-1983 (Altman & Cahn, 1987) found an average of about 27 job announcements per month seeking psychologists for health-related positions. Our examination of the December, 1998 *APA Monitor* found nearly 100 advertisements for psychologists to work in health-related fields. Several of these descriptions specifically included the term *health psychologist,* and the others included a description of the setting or the work that suggested a health-related job. These advertisements represented a wide variety of positions, including faculty appointments in universities and medical schools, postdoctoral research fellowships, predoctoral internships, and employment in hospitals, clinics, private practices, health maintenance organizations, and pain clinics.

The 1998 job advertisements were divided between clinical psychologist and teaching/research psychologist positions. The clinical skills sought included assessment, therapy, biofeedback, stress management, and experience working with eating disordered and chronic pain patients. Many job descriptions, especially for jobs in hospitals and medical schools, stipulated that the person hired be part of an interdisciplinary team. Our analysis also discovered that openings for psychologists in health-related fields were spread throughout the United States and Canada. Thus, employment opportunities exist for psychologists trained to work in health-related areas.

The Training of Health Psychologists

The training of health psychologists includes a grounding in psychological principles and substantial preparation in neurology, endocrinology, immunology, public health, epidemiology, and other medical subspecialties. Standards for the preparation of health psychologists follow the Boulder model of 1949, which views psychologists as both scientists and practitioners. These standards are also consistent with those established by the National Working Conference on Education and Training in Health Psychology of 1983, which defined the core program in psychology to which health psychologists should be exposed. Health psychologists now receive a solid core of graduate training in such areas as (1) the biological bases of behavior, health, and disease; (2) the cognitive and affective bases of behavior, health, and disease; (3) the social bases of health and disease, including knowledge of health organizations and health policy; (4) the psychological bases of health and disease, with emphasis on individual differences; (5) advanced research, methodology, and statistics; (6) psychological and health measurement; (7) interdisciplinary collaboration; and (8) ethics and professional issues (Belar, 1997). In addition to this core, many health psychologists have recommended postdoctoral training, with at least 2 years of specialized training in health psychology to follow a Ph.D. or Psy.D. in psychology (Belar, 1997; Matarazzo, 1987a). This training might include some combination of internships and residencies in which health psychologists would learn to provide treatment in hospitals and other traditional health care settings.

Cynthia Belar (1997) has called for continuing education for psychologists so that they can develop new competencies and specializations to provide new types of services. The growing market for psychologists in health care and the shrinking, competitive market for psychologists providing traditional mental health care make practice in health psychology attractive to both new and continuing practitioners. Belar maintained that training psychologists for new specializations in health care should be a priority for the profession and warned that psychologists should be thoroughly trained before taking jobs in the health care system. She also stressed the importance of training practitioners to be both researchers and clinicians, echoing the traditional emphasis on the combination of scientific knowledge and practical skills.

The Work of Health Psychologists

Health psychologists work in a variety of settings and perform many different functions. They work in universities, hospitals, clinics, health maintenance organizations (HMOs), and private practice. In addition, many work for federal agencies such as the Centers for Disease Control and Prevention and the National Institutes of Health. They teach, conduct research, and provide a medley of services to individual patients as well as to private and public agencies. Much of their work is collaborative in nature; that is, health psychologists frequently work with a team of health professionals, including physicians, nurses, physical therapists, and counselors.

The services provided by health psychologists working in clinics and hospitals fit into several categories. One type of service provides alternatives to pharmacological treatment; for example, biofeedback might be an alternative to analgesic

WOULD YOU BELIEVE...?

Your Doctor May Be a Psychologist

Would you believe that health psychologists may become primary providers of health care? When you make an appointment at your HMO, the provider you see may be a psychologist. The growth of health psychology has put health psychologists in a variety of settings to provide care, but they typically act as consultants rather than as primary providers. That situation may change. Kaiser Permanente of Northern California has designated psychologists as primary health care providers in its health maintenance facilities (Bruns, 1998). These psychologists are designated Behavioral Medicine Specialists and serve as part of teams that implement an integrated care approach to health care services.

Including psychologists as primary providers has advantages. Many patients come to health care fa-cilities with complaints or problems that are psychological but are reluctant to accept referrals for psychiatric help. Psychologists as primary providers can manage many problems in the initial consul-tation rather than after many referrals and consulta-tions. Therefore, psychologists as primary providers can save health care dollars by avoiding unnecessary services.

This innovation was not initiated by psychologists seeking additional roles but by the HMO seeking savings in providing care. Behavioral Medicine Specialists can decrease the number of medical visits and help to keep patients well. Because these goals are important in controlling health care costs and in promoting wellness, health psychology may play a more prominent role than in the past.

---

drugs for headache patients. Another type of service is the primary treatment of physical disorders that respond favorably to behavioral interventions, such as chronic pain and some gastrointestinal problems. Several other types of services that psychologists might provide are related to traditional clinical psychology and include ancillary psychological treatment for patients who are hospitalized, such as cardiac or cancer patients. Health psychologists employed in hospitals and clinics also help improve the rate of patient compliance with their medical regimens and provide some assessments using psychological and neuropsychological tests. Those who concentrate on prevention and behavior changes are more likely to be employed in health maintenance organizations, school-based prevention programs, or worksite wellness programs. All these organizations use services that trained health psychologists can perform.

The Centers for Disease Control and Prevention have entered into a partnership with psychologists to expand behaviorally based programs (Cavaliere, 1995; Herring, 1997). In this partnership, psychologists are involved in designing and conducting prevention programs on a national level, a focus consistent with a mandate from the U.S. Congress to increase support for behavioral and social sciences. Involvement of health psychologists in governmental agencies and expansion of behavior research in health would not only create additional jobs; it would also expand health psychology's influence in health research and public health.

Most health psychologists engage in several activities. The combination of teaching and research is common among those in educational settings. Health psychologists who work in medical centers may teach medical students, conduct research, perform clinical services, or carry out some combination of these activities. Those who work in service delivery settings are much less likely to teach and do research and are more likely to spend most of their time providing diagnosis and therapy.

In Summary

Health psychology can contribute to health in four ways: (1) by accumulating information on behaviors and lifestyles that relate to health and illness, (2) by helping to promote and maintain health, (3) by contributing to the prevention and treatment of illness, and (4) by helping to formulate health policy and promote the health care system. To maximize their contributions to health care, health psychologists must be both broadly trained in the science of psychology and specifically trained in the knowledge and skills of such areas as neurology, endocrinology, immunology, epidemiology, and other medical subspecialties. Health psychologists with a solid background in generic psychology and specialized knowledge in medical fields are currently employed in a variety of settings, including universities, hospitals, clinics, private practice, and health maintenance organizations. They typically collaborate with other health care professionals in providing services for people with physical disorders rather than for traditional areas of mental health care. Research in health psychology is also likely to be a collaborative effort that includes the professions of medicine, epidemiology, nursing, pharmacology, nutrition, and exercise physiology.

Outlook for Health Psychology

Despite the growth of health psychology and its ability to contribute to health care, the field faces several challenges. One major challenge is acceptance by other health care practitioners, an acceptance that continues to grow. As they become involved in health care, psychologists will be forced to attend to such problems as the escalating cost of medical care, which will include a justification of their own salary. Although the diagnostic and therapeutic techniques used by health psychologists have demonstrated effectiveness, these procedures also have substantial financial costs. Health psychology must meet the challenges of justifying its costs by offering needed services in the chang-

ing health care system and in a changing society. In addition, it must be cautious in the claims it makes.

Future Challenges for Health Care

Health care in the United States faces several future challenges. Two of the more crucial ones are the changing patterns of illness and the escalating cost of health care. These two challenges are only partially interrelated. The increase in chronic illness has probably not contributed as much to rising health care costs as has the increased use of technology, the building of new hospital rooms, and the growth of specialization among physicians.

Changing Profile of Disease Chapter 1 identified several important changes in the pattern of illness that have contributed to the development of health psychology. One change was a shift in the leading causes of death and disability from infectious diseases to chronic illnesses, such as cardiovascular disease (CVD) and cancer. We saw that cardiovascular disease—including heart disease and stroke—currently accounts for nearly 40% of deaths in the United States, nearly 75% more than the deaths from cancer. Research in health psychology has reflected this discrepancy; considerably more attention is paid to heart disease than to cancer. Psychologists, for example, have devoted much work to the increased risk of cardiovascular disease related to the Type A (coronary prone) behavior pattern and have intensively investigated behavioral interventions for reducing serum cholesterol, lowering blood pressure, encouraging exercise, and promoting a heart-healthy diet. As Margaret Chesney (1993) has suggested, this emphasis on heart disease may be misplaced.

During the 1980s and early 1990s, CVD decreased while cancer increased; since the mid-1990s both are declining. Figure 17.1 shows the trends for these two causes of death since 1900. If deaths from CVD continue to decrease more sharply than deaths from cancer, the proportion

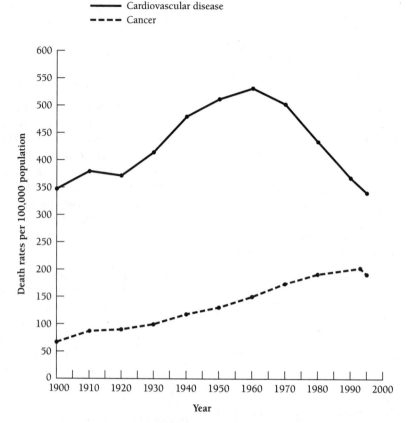

Figure 17.1   Death rates for cardiovascular disease and cancer per 100,000 population, United States, 1900–1991.   *Source:* Data from *Historical Statistics of the United States: Colonial Times to 1970* (p. 38), by U.S. Bureau of the Census, 1975, Washington, DC: U.S. Government Printing Office; and from *Statistical Abstracts of the United States: 1998* (p. 104), by U.S. Bureau of the Census, 1998, Washington, DC: U.S. Government Printing Office.

of total deaths due to cancer will increase, and this increase may boost interest in cancer prevention during the early years of the 21st century. Thus, in the coming decades, the behavioral aspects of cancer should receive more attention.

A second reason for an increased attention to cancer is its prominence as a cause of death among young and middle-aged adults. Figure 17.2 shows the death rates from CVD and cancer for various age groups and the greater tendency for children and adults from age 50 to 65 to die of

cancer. Cancer accounts for more premature death than CVD, and thus efforts to prevent cancer, and especially childhood cancer, would add years of life expectancy in the United States.

The third reason why cancer may attract more research is because it is easily the leading cause of death in young and middle-aged women. In 1995, cancer accounted for 37% of the deaths in women between the ages of 15 and 64. Coronary heart disease and stroke combined accounted for only 22% of their deaths (USBC, 1998). Like other

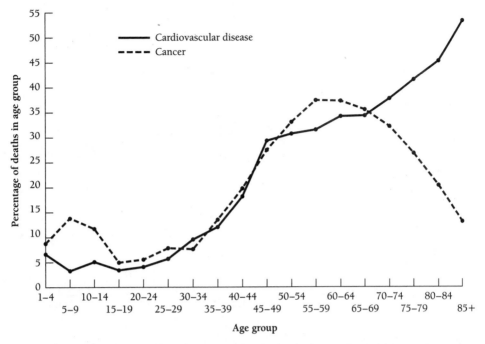

Figure 17.2 **Death rates from cardiovascular disease (CVD) and cancer by age, United States, 1995.** *Source:* Data from *Statistical Abstracts of the United States, 1998* (p. 102), by U.S. Bureau of the Census, 1998, Washington DC: U.S. Government Printing Office.

health research, health psychology has in the past not only emphasized heart disease over cancer but has also been slanted much more toward men than women. The founding of the Office of Research on Women's Health within the National Institutes of Health (Matthews et al., 1997) has been a force in changing this situation. With an increasing emphasis on research dealing with women's health, cancer should receive increased attention, and future research on disorders that affect both women and men should include as many women as men.

Because cancer is the leading cause of death in people under 65, future health psychologists must become increasingly involved in identifying the personality and behavioral correlates of cancer and in helping people change the behaviors and lifestyles associated with this disease. In addition,

they should expand their current practices of helping cancer patients manage pain and helping those patients and their families cope with the illness.

Reducing unintentional injuries is a goal to which psychologists can also contribute, and such injuries are the leading cause of death for young people between the ages of 15 and 24. Motor vehicle crashes, intentional violence, and suicide are the leading killers of young people, and the behavioral bases of these causes of death are obvious. Violent injury and death are declining in the United States, but this society is still more violent than other industrialized nations. As discussed in Chapter 12, psychologists have recently become involved in exploring the causes of unintentional injuries and strategies for preventing them.

The aging of the U.S. population presents an additional challenge to health psychologists. After

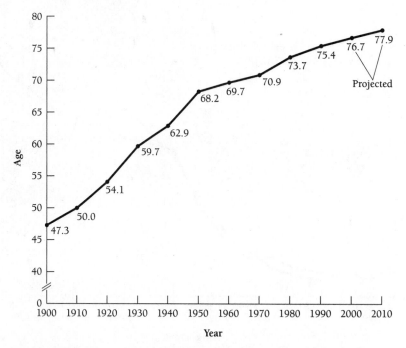

Figure 17.3   Actual and projected life expectancy, United States, 1900–2010.   *Source:* Data from *Historical Statistics of the United States: Colonial Times to 1970* (p. 55), by U.S. Bureau of the Census, 1975, Washington, DC: U.S. Government Printing Office; and from *Statistical Abstracts of the United States: 1998* (p. 25), by U.S. Bureau of the Census, 1998, Washington, DC: U.S. Government Printing Office.

age 65, many people develop chronic illnesses and suffer from chronic pain. As we have seen, health psychology has a role in preventing illness, promoting health, and helping people cope with pain. In old age, lifestyles can still be changed to help prevent illness, but health psychology's alliance with gerontology will more likely produce an emphasis on promoting and maintaining health, managing pain, promoting the health care system, and formulating health care policy.

Since 1900, the number of people in the United States 65 years old or older has increased from about 3 million to more than 30 million. In 1900, only 4% of the population was over 65, whereas in 1997, nearly 13% of U.S. citizens had reached that age. During this same period, life expectancy increased from 47 years to more than 76 years. By the year 2010, life expectancy is pro-

jected to be more than 77 years (see Figure 17.3), with more than 18 million people, or 6.2% of the total population, over age 75 (USBC, 1998). In contrast, in 1900 only 5.6 million, or 3.1% of the population, were over 75.

During its early years, health psychology was only moderately involved in issues of concern to older people. That situation changed, with health psychologists becoming more involved in issues of aging, and a committee of Division 38 is devoted to these problems. Health-related articles appear frequently in psychology journals concerned with aging, and a journal specifically oriented to issues of health in the aging, *Behavior, Health, and Aging,* began publication in 1990. During the next few decades, as the population continues to age, psychology will play an important role in helping older people achieve and maintain healthy and productive lifestyles and adjust to the problems of chronic illness.

What will be the profile of illness and death in the 21st century? Will the trends of the 20th century continue, or will some other pattern emerge? Cardiovascular disease and cancer are likely to continue for some time as the two leading causes of death in the United States. However, infectious illness has made something of a comeback (Weitz, 1996). AIDS and tuberculosis are two examples of the re-emergence of infectious diseases. Twenty-five years ago, AIDS was unknown, and now it is considered a major, worldwide health threat and ranks among the leading causes of death in the United States. Tuberculosis was the second leading cause of death in 1900 but fell off the list as the century progressed. During the 1980s, the incidence of tuberculosis began to increase. Furthermore, the current cases of tuberculosis are more resistant to antibiotics and thus more difficult to treat. Thus we see that new infectious diseases can emerge and old ones can re-emerge in more resistant forms. As chronic diseases continue and infectious diseases persist, health psychologists will likely contribute to preventing and managing these disorders.

Controlling Health Care Costs Health care costs in the United States have escalated at a higher rate than inflation and other costs of living. This escalation has left many people in the United States unable to afford health care and others in the position of fearing that they will not be able to do so in the future. A number of factors have contributed to the high costs, including the proliferation of hospitals, the growth of technology, a large proportion of physicians who are specialists, and growing administrative costs. Figure 17.4 shows where health care dollars go, with hospitals receiving 35% and physicians 20% of the dollars spent. The high cost of hospitalization is partly due to technology; when hospitals buy the latest technology, costs rise for all patients, even those who do not use the equipment. Another reason for the high cost of hospitalization is overbuilding by

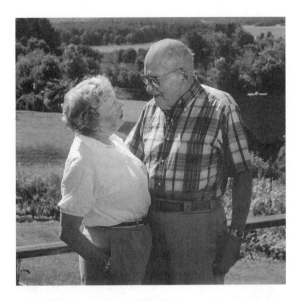

Increasing the span of healthy life is a goal for health psychologists.

hospitals, resulting in the need to pay for these hospital beds by filling them. Indeed, areas of the country with more hospital beds available have higher rates of hospitalization than areas with fewer beds (Consumers Union, 1992).

Although physicians receive little more than half the health care dollars that hospitals get, the number of specialists adds to the cost of medical care; the scarcity of family practitioners (and the lack of incentive for going into family practice) also plays a role in escalating health care costs. Hospitals with expensive technology and specialist physicians who use this technology both contribute to the increasing (and increasingly expensive) role of technology in medicine.

Administrative costs are a substantial factor in high health care costs in the United States (Weitz, 1996). The complex system of insurance, private physicians, private and public hospitals, and government-supported medical programs such as Medicare has produced different procedures, forms, payment plans, allowed expenses, maximum payments, and deductibles for medical services. Thus, payment is a complex matter of

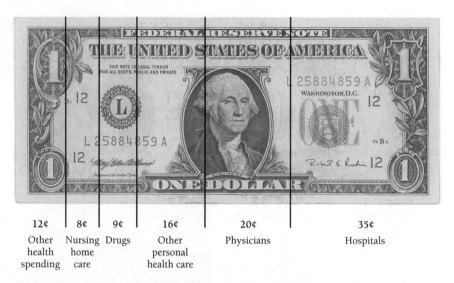

Figure 17.4 **Where health care dollars go.**   *Source: Health, United States, 1998* (p. 346), by U.S. Department of Health and Human Services, 1998, (DHHS publication No. PHS 98-1232), Washington, DC: U.S. Government Printing Office.

filling out and filing forms, not only by patients but also by health care providers. At least 20% of the costs of health care goes to administrative expenses (Consumers Union, 1992).

Health care reform has been recognized as an urgent priority for the United States, but containing costs has proven difficult. The traditional fee-for-service system allowed physicians to charge whatever fees their patients and the insurance companies would pay. This system was partially responsible for some of the increases in health care costs. During the 1980s, health maintenance organizations (HMOs) proliferated (Weitz, 1996). Although HMOs were originally established to provide preventive care as well as treatment, corporations entered the HMO market and profit became a motive. Thus, the growth of HMOs did not contain rising health care costs.

Examining other countries that are faced with similar health problems and their solutions can give direction about ways to provide health care. Other industrialized countries such as Canada, Japan, Australia, the countries of Western Europe, and Scandinavia also have high rates of cardiovascular disease and cancer as well as aging popula-

tions, presenting similar problems for their health care systems (Caragata, 1995; Ikegami, 1992). Many of these countries do a better job of providing health care to a larger percentage of their residents at lower costs than does the U.S. system.

Germany, Canada, and Great Britain all have found ways to control the factors that spin health care costs out of control in the United States (Weitz, 1996). The history of health care costs for these countries and the United States appears in Figure 17.5. These countries have managed to contain health care expenditures by controlling all of the factors that account for the rise in medical costs for the United States: growth of hospitals, availability of medical technology, abundance of specialists, and complex administrative requirements.

All these countries limit hospital proliferation by making the government responsible for giving money for capital expenditures to hospitals rather than allowing hospitals to overbuild. This same process limits purchases of expensive technology. The limits on technology also decrease patients' access to this technology and technological medicine, which may be a drawback in some cases. In other cases, patients in the United States are over-

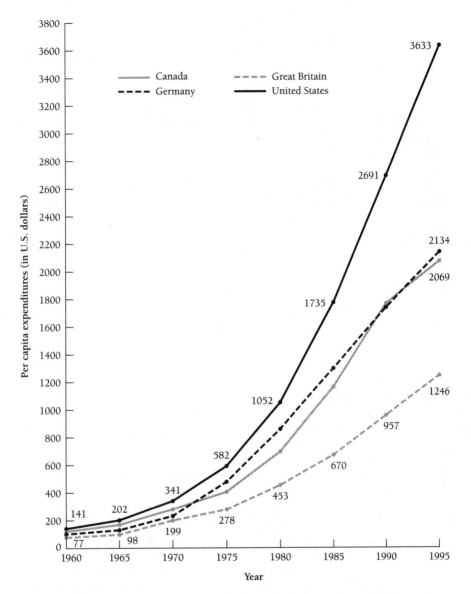

Figure 17.5 Health care expenditures in Canada, Germany, Great Britain, and United States, 1960 to 1995. *Source: Health, United States, 1998 (p. 342), by U.S. Department of Health and Human Services, 1998, (DHHS publication No. PHS 98-1232), Washington, DC: U.S. Government Printing Office.*

treated, and limiting access could actually boost health and life expectancy.

By devising systems in which all people have access to health care, Germany, Canada, and Great Britain have eliminated the competitive health in-

surance business and its costs. These three countries have different systems for paying for health care, but each has universal coverage. Without advertising to attract customers and the without multitude of different filing procedures, forms, allowed procedures, deductibles, and other differences among insurers, administrative costs are much lower than in the United States (Weitz, 1996).

Some restrictions of costs in the United States are similar to those in Canada, Germany, and Great Britain (Weitz, 1996). For example, many physicians in the United States now have restrictions on their fees. In Canada, fees are set as a result of negotiations between government and physicians' groups, and these negotiated fees represent the limit of what physicians can charge for their services. Great Britain has limited the number of specialists trained and the access to those specialists. Medicine has traditionally been a highly paid career, but U.S. physicians feel that they need high salaries because the average physician finishes medical training with almost $80,000 of debt. Specialty practice offers the opportunity for higher salaries. In the other countries, medical education is subsidized so that young physicians do not have such debts, and medical practice is a highly paid career in these societies. Despite limitations on training and practice, physicians in the other countries are more satisfied with their practices than are U.S. physicians (Weitz, 1996).

Another approach to controlling health care costs is to reduce the need and the demand for services (Fries, 1998). Health psychologists have a role in both approaches. As we have seen in discussions of chronic diseases such as cardiovascular disease, cancer, and chronic obstructive pulmonary disease, behavior plays a major role in the development of these conditions; people with a healthy lifestyle are much less likely to develop these disorders. Those with good health habits have lifetime medical costs of about half of costs for people with poor health habits. Promotion of good health habits is an important way to decrease the need for medical services.

Reducing the demand for medical services is another approach to controlling health care costs. Although limiting access to medical care has achieved reductions of the use of medical services, this strategy does not affect demand and leaves patients dissatisfied with their level of care. An alternative approach is reduction of demand for medical services that have only marginal benefits. The availability of a wide range of medical technology has led to the widespread belief that modern medicine can cure any disease; this belief has fostered an overreliance on medicine to heal rather than a reliance on good health habits to avoid disease. Building feelings of personal efficacy for health can help reduce the demand for medical services (Fries, 1998), but boosting efficacy requires training. Several pilot programs have indicated that such training is less expensive than providing health care, making such programs a good buy. Additional research may reveal that this approach can be a good strategy for containing health care costs.

Controlling health care costs will probably require substantial changes in the U.S. health care system. Insurance companies, hospitals, and physicians will all be affected, and no system can provide a good quality of medical care for low costs. Some countries, however, do a better job than the United States, serving a larger proportion of the population and achieving better health and longer life.

A Note of Cautious Optimism

Health psychology has contributed to the field of health by developing a research base, assessments, and treatment techniques. Although health psychologists face exciting prospects, both researchers and practitioners must not allow their enthusiasm to lead to claims they cannot fulfill. That is, both caution and optimism are appropriate for health psychology at this point.

The caution reflects the limits on what health psychologists know and what treatments they can offer. Practitioners in health psychology must not claim more than they can deliver (Belar, 1997; Kaplan, 1984). To be fully effective, clinical health psychologists must be part of a comprehensive treatment program, with the correct balance of biological and behavioral treatment. Research has identified many behavioral components of disease, but the interaction among biology, social situation, and behavioral factors is complex, and health psychologists cannot ignore the other components in this interaction.

Evan Pattishall (1989) proposed two rules, deduced from a review of the history of behavioral medicine, that health psychology should heed to guard against inappropriate enthusiasm: "Rule 1: Don't propose more than you have data to support, and Rule 2: Don't promise more than you can deliver" (p. 44).

Health psychology has been fairly cautious in its promises of cures, and health psychologists who offer treatment are well acquainted with the difficulties of changing behavior. The temptation to promise changes in behavior is strong, but health psychologists must continue to be conservative.

The optimism in health psychology reflects the growth and maturation of the field and the promise of future contributions. Health psychologists must continue to develop a research base on the interaction among behavior, biology, and social factors (Human Capital Initiative Report, 1996). There is still much to learn about the role of behavior in the development and recovery from disease as well as the psychological factors that affect living with chronic conditions.

Even more important, health psychologists must take a leading role in creating a scientific knowledge of disease prevention. This approach is new to health care, because the dominant model in medicine, the biomedical model, does not emphasize prevention. The biomedical model holds that pathogens cause disease and biochemistry furnishes cures. The alternative model, the biopsychosocial model, allows not only for a more complex view of disease but also for an inclusion of behavioral and social factors that may be important in preventing disease and enhancing health. Promoting the biopsychosocial model is important in changing the emphasis from treatment to prevention (Belar, 1997).

In Summary

The outlook for health psychology includes both caution and optimism. Health psychology has made significant contributions to health care research and practice, but health psychology must meet several challenges to continue to grow. These challenges include making a place for health psychology within a health care field that must deal with changes in the pattern of disease and rising health care costs. The shift from infectious to chronic diseases has made cardiovascular disease and cancer the leading causes of death, with cardiovascular disease receiving greater emphasis; this emphasis may be inappropriate. Although the rates of both these diseases are declining, cancer is responsible for more premature deaths than cardiovascular disease, necessitating a greater effort to prevent cancer and extend life for those with cancer.

Health care costs have risen in the United States more rapidly than in other industrialized countries, yet some of those countries manage to provide health care to a wider segment of their populations and with a better outcome in life expectancy. The United States needs to reform its health care policy, with prevention emphasized to a greater degree. This emphasis would boost the nation's health as well as cut health care costs.

The role of psychology in health care is a reason for optimism, but health psychologists must also be cautious in their claims and continue to build a research base that will furnish information about the interconnections among psychological, social, and biological factors in health.

Answers

This chapter addressed three basic questions.

1. **What role does health psychology play in contributing to the goals of** *Healthy People 2000?*

    Health psychology is one of several disciplines that have a role in helping the nation achieve the goals and objectives of *Healthy People 2000*. The three broad goals of this document are (1) increasing the span of healthy life, (2) reducing health disparities among various ethnic groups, and (3) increasing access to preventive services for everyone. Health psychologists advocate healthy years of life, not merely more years. They cooperate with other health professionals in reducing health discrepancies among different income groups, and they have been involved with both primary and secondary prevention of disorder, disease, and disability.

2. **What training do health psychologists receive and what kinds of work do they do?**

Health psychologists receive doctoral-level training in the basic core of psychology, including (1) the biological, cognitive, psychological, and social bases of behavior, health, and disease; (2) advanced research, methodology, and statistics; (3) psychology and health measurement; (4) interdisciplinary collaboration; and (4) ethics and professional issues. In addition, they often receive at least 2 years of postdoctoral work in a specialized area of health psychology.

Health psychologists are employed in a variety of settings, including universities, hospitals, clinics, private practice, and health maintenance organizations. Many work for governmental agencies such as the CDC and the National Institutes of Health.

3. **What is the outlook for the future of health psychology?**

The outlook for the future of health psychology is one of cautious optimism. The optimism reflects psychology's contributions to (1) understanding and treating the chronic diseases that have become the leading causes of death in industrialized countries; and (2) helping people make behavior changes that lead to better prevention and thus help control health care costs. The caution reflects the knowledge that behavior change is difficult and that prevention is not the focus of health care at this point in time. To play an important role in future health care, health psychologists must continue to build a research base and to develop more effective strategies for behavior change.

Glossary

health expectancy   The period of life that a person spends free from disability.

well-year   The equivalent of a year of complete wellness.

Suggested Readings

Belar, C. D. (1997). Clinical health psychology: A specialty for the 21st century. *Health Psychology, 16,* 411–416.

In this presidential address to Division 38 of APA, Cynthia Belar outlines goals for clinical health psychologists for the 21st century, including accumulating a scientific body of knowledge, disseminating this knowledge, using the knowledge in their practice, and providing appropriate training for future health psychologists.

 Smith, R. (1997). The future of healthcare systems: Information technology and consumerism will transform health care worldwide. *British Medical Journal, 314,* 495–496.

This brief editorial reports on the predictions of a panel of invited experts on health care concerning future trends throughout the world. The predictions address six possibilities, and the article presents these possibilities and their relation to current systems in the major industrialized countries. Available through InfoTrac College Edition by Wadsworth Publishing Company.

Sobel, D. S. (1995). Rethinking medicine: Improving health outcomes with cost effective psychosocial interventions. *Psychosomatic Medicine, 57,* 234–244.

David Sobel makes a persuasive argument for the effectiveness and cost-effectiveness of the types of interventions that health psychologists have to offer.

Stone, G. C. (1984). A final word [editorial]. *Health Psychology, 3,* 585–589.

The first editor of Health Psychology looks back over the first three volumes of the journal and outlines some of his ideas for the future direction of the profession of health psychology.

REFERENCES

Abbott, R. D., Rodriguez, B. L., Burchfiel, C. M., & Curb, J. D. (1994). Physical activity in older middle-aged men and reduced risk of stroke: The Honolulu Heart Program. *American Journal of Epidemiology, 139,* 881–893.

Abraham, C., & Sheeran, P. (1994). Modelling and modifying young heterosexuals' HIV-preventive behaviour: A review of theories, findings and educational implications. *Patient Education and Counseling, 23,* 173–186.

Abrams, D. B., & Niaura, R. S. (1987). Social learning theory. In H. T. Blane & K. E. Leonard (Eds.), *Psychological theories of drinking and alcoholism* (pp. 131–178). New York: Guilford Press.

Abramson, L. Y., Garber, J., & Seligman, M. E. P. (1980). Learned helplessness in humans: An attributional analysis. In J. Garber & M. E. P. Seligman (Eds.), *Human helplessness: Theory and applications* (pp. 3–34). New York: Academic Press.

Achterberg, J., Kenner, C., & Lawlis, G. F. (1988). Severe burn injuries: A comparison of relaxation imagery and biofeedback for pain management. *Journal of Mental Imagery, 12,* 71–87.

Achterberg-Lawlis, J. (1982). The psychological dimensions of arthritis. *Journal of Consulting and Clinical Psychology, 50,* 984–992.

Acierno, R., Resnick, H. S., & Kilpatrick, D. G. (1997). Prevalence rates, case identification, and risk factors for sexual assault, physical assault, and domestic violence in men and women, part 1 (Health impact of interpersonal violence). *Behavioral Medicine, 23,* 53–65.

Ader, R., & Cohen, N. (1975). Behaviorally conditioned immunosuppression. *Psychosomatic Medicine, 37,* 333–340.

Ader, R., & Cohen, N. (1982). Behaviorally conditioned immunosuppression and murine systematic lupus erythematosus. *Science, 215,* 1534–1536.

Ader, R., & Cohen, N. (1993). Psychoneuroimmunology: Conditioning stress. *Annual Review of Psychology, 44,* 53–85.

Adler, N., & Matthews, K. (1994). Health psychology: Why do some people get sick and some stay well? *Annual Review of Psychology, 45,* 229–259.

Agras, W. S. (1993). Short-term psychological treatments for binge eating. In C. G. Fairburn & G. T. Wilson (Eds.), *Binge eating: Nature, assessment, and treatment* (pp. 270–286). New York: Guilford Press.

Agras, W. S., Telch, C. F., Arnow, B., Eldredge, K., Detzer, M. J., Henderson, J., & Marnell, M. (1995). Does interpersonal therapy help patients with binge eating disorder who fail to respond to cognitive-behavioral therapy? *Journal of Consulting and Clinical Psychology, 63,* 356–360.

Ahlbom, A., & Norell, S. (1990). *Introduction to modern epidemiology* (2nd ed.). Chestnut Hill, MA: Epidemiology Resources.

Ahluwalia, I. B., Grummer-Strawn, L. & Scanlon, K. S. (1997). Exposure to environmental tobacco smoke and birth outcome: Increased effects on pregnant women aged 30 years or older. *American Journal of Epidemiology, 146,* 42–47.

Aiken, L. S., West, S. G., Woodward, C. K., & Reno, R. R. (1994). Health beliefs and compliance with mammography-screening recommendations in asymptomatic women. *Health Psychology, 13,* 122–129.

Ajzen, I. (1985). From intentions to actions: A theory of planned behavior. In J. Kuhland & J. Beckman (Eds.), *Action-control: From cognitions to behavior* (pp. 11–39) Heidelberg, Germany: Springer.

Ajzen, I. (1988). *Attitudes, personality, and behavior.* Chicago: Dorsey Press.

Ajzen, I. (1991). The theory of planned behavior. *Organizational Behavior and Human Decision Processes, 50,* 179–211.

Ajzen, I., & Fishbein, M. (1980). *Understanding attitudes and predicting social behavior.* Englewood Cliffs, NJ: Prentice-Hall.

Åkerstedt, T. (1988). Sleepiness as a consequence of shiftwork. *Sleep, 11,* 17–34.

Albert, C. M., Hennekens, C. H., O'Donnell, C. J., Ajani, U. A., Carey, V. J., Willett, W. C., Ruskin, J. N., & Manson, J. E. (1998). Fish consumption and risk of sudden cardiac death. *Journal of the American Medical Association, 279,* 23–28.

Alden, L. E. (1988). Behavioral self-management controlled-drinking strategies in a context of secondary prevention. *Journal of Consulting and Clinical Psychology, 56,* 280–286.

Alderman, M. H., Cohen, H., & Madhavan, S. (1998). Dietary sodium intake and mortality: The National Health and Nutrition Examination Survey (NHANES I). *Lancet, 351,* 781–785.

Alexander, F. (1950). *Psychosomatic medicine.* New York: Norton.

Allison, D. B., Heshka, S., Neale, M. C., Lykken, D. T., & Heymsfield, S. B. (1994). A genetic analysis of relative weight among 4,020 twin pairs, with an emphasis on sex effects. *Health Psychology, 13,* 362–365.

Alper, J. (1993). Ulcers as infectious diseases. *Science, 260,* 159–160.

Alterman, T., Shekelle, R. B., Vernon, S. W., & Burau, K. D. (1994). Decision latitude, psychologic demand, job strain, and coronary heart disease in the Western Electric Study. *American Journal of Epidemiology, 139,* 620–627.

Altman, D. G., & Cahn, J. (1987). Employment options for health psychologists. In G. C. Stone, S. M. Weiss, J. D. Matarazzo, N. E. Miller, J. Rodin, C. D. Belar, M. J. Follick, & J. E. Singer (Eds.), *Health psychology: A discipline and a profession* (pp. 232–244). Chicago: University of Chicago Press.

American Cancer Society. (1996). *Cancer facts & figures– 1996.* Atlanta: American Cancer Society.

American Cancer Society. (1998). *Cancer facts & figures– 1998.* Atlanta: American Cancer Society.

American Psychiatric Association. (1980). *Diagnostic and statistical manual of mental disorders* (3rd ed.) (DSM III). Washington, DC: Author.

American Psychiatric Association. (1987). *Diagnostic and statistical manual of mental disorders* (3rd ed., rev.) (DSM III-R). Washington, DC: Author.

American Psychiatric Association. (1994). *Diagnostic and statistical manual of mental disorders* (4th ed.) (DSM IV) . Washington, DC: Author.

American Psychological Association (APA). Task Force on Health Research. (1976). Contributions of psychology to health research: Patterns, problems, and potentials. *American Psychologist, 31,* 263–274.

Anda, R. F., Williamson, D. F., & Remington, P. L. (1988). Alcohol and fatal injuries among US adults: Findings from the NHANES I epidemiologic follow-up study. *Journal of the American Medical Association, 260,* 2529–2532.

Andersen, B. L. (1989). Health psychology's contribution to addressing the cancer problem: Update on accomplishments. *Health Psychology, 8,* 683–703.

Andersen, B. L. (1998). Psychology's science in responding to the challenge of cancer: Biobehavioral perspectives. *Psychological Science Agenda, 11*(1), 14–15.

Andersen, R. E., Crespo, C. J., Bartlett, S. J., Cheskin, L. J., & M. Pratt, (1998). Relationship of physical activity and television watching with body weight and level of fatness among children: Results from the third National Health and Nutrition Examination Survey. *Journal of the American Medical Association, 279,* 938–942.

Andersen, R. E., Walden, T. A., Bartlett, S. J., Zemel, B., Verde, T. J., & Franckowiak, S. C. (1999). Effects of lifestyle activity vs structured aerobic exercise in obese women: A randomized trial. *Journal of the American Medical Association, 281,* 335–340.

Anderson, E. A. (1987). Preoperative preparation for cardiac surgery facilitates recovery, reduces psychological distress, and reduces the incidence of acute postoperative hypertension. *Journal of Consulting and Clinical Psychology, 55,* 513–520.

Anderson, N. B. (1993). Reactivity research on socio-demographic groups: Its value to psychophysiology and health psychology. *Health Psychology, 12,* 3–5.

Anderson, N. B., & Armstead, C. A. (1995). Toward understanding the association of socioeconomic status and health: A new challenge for the biopsychosocial approach. *Psychosomatic Medicine, 57,* 213–225.

Anderson, R. N., Kochanek, K. D., & Murphy, S. L. (1997). Report of final mortality statistics, 1995. *Monthly Vital Statistics Report, 45*(11), supp. 2, 23–33.

Andrasik, F., Blanchard, E. B., Arena, J. G., Saunders, N. L., & Barron, K. D. (1982). Psychophysiology of recurrent headaches: Methodological issues and new empirical findings. *Behavior Therapy, 13,* 407–429.

Andres, R. (1995). Body weight and age. In K. D. Brownell & C. G. Fairburn. *Eating disorders and obesity: A comprehensive handbook* (pp. 65–70). New York: Guilford Press.

Andres, R., Muller, D. C., & Sorkin, J. D. (1993). Long-term effects of change in body weight on all-cause mortality: A review. *Annals of Internal Medicine, 119,* 737–743.

Andrew, J. (1970). Recovery from surgery, with and without preparatory instruction for three coping styles. *Journal of Personality and Social Psychology, 15,* 223–226.

Aneshensel, C. S., & Pearlin, L. I. (1987). Structural contexts of sex differences in stress. In R. C. Barnett, L. Biener, & G. K. Baruch (Eds.), *Gender and stress* (pp. 75–95). New York: Free Press.

Annis, H. M., & Davis, C. S. (1988). Self-efficacy and the prevention of alcoholic relapse: Initial findings from a treatment trial. In T. B. Baker & D. Cannon (Eds.), *Assessment and treatment of addictive disorders* (pp. 88–112). New York: Praeger.

Antoni, M. H. (1993). Stress management: Strategies that work. In D. Goleman & J. Gurin (Eds.), *Mind/body medicine: How to use your mind for better health* (pp. 385–397). Yonkers, NY: Consumer Reports Books.

Antoni, M. H., Baggett, L., Ironson, G., LaPerriere, A., August, S., Klimas, N., Schneiderman, N., & Fletcher, M. A. (1991). Cognitive-behavioral stress management intervention buffers distress responses and immunologic changes following notification of HIV-1 seropositivity. *Journal of Consulting and Clinical Psychology, 59,* 906–915.

Antoni, M. H., Schneiderman, N., Fletcher, M. A., Goldstein, D. A., Ironson, G., & LaPerriere, A. (1990). Psychoneuroimmunology and HIV-I. *Journal of Consulting and Clinical Psychology, 58,* 38–49.

Apodaca, J. X., Woodruff, S. I., Candelaria, J., Elder, J. P. & Zlot, A. (1997). Hispanic health program participant and nonparticipant characteristics. *American Journal of Health Behavior 21,* 356–369.

Argyle, M. (1992). Benefits produced by supportive social relationships. In H. O. E. Veiel & U. Baumann (Eds.), *The meaning and measurement of social support* (pp. 13–32). New York: Hemisphere.

Arluke, A. (1988). The sick-role concept. In D. S. Gochman (Ed.), *Health behavior: Emerging research perspectives* (pp. 169–180). New York: Plenum Press.

Armor, D. J., Polich, J. M., & Stambul, H. B. (1976). *Alcoholism and treatment.* Santa Monica, CA: Rand.

Ary, D. V., & Biglan, A. (1988). Longitudinal changes in adolescent cigarette smoking behavior: Onset and cessation. *Journal of Behavioral Medicine, 11,* 361–382.

Ashmore, J. P., Krewski, D., Zielinksi, J. M., Jiang, H., Semenciw, R., & Band, P. R. (1998). First analysis of mortality and occupational radiation exposure based on the National Dose Registry of Canada. *American Journal of Epidemiology, 148,* 564–574.

Astemborski, J., Vlahov, D., Warren, D., Solomon, L., & Nelson, K. E. (1994). The trading of sex for drugs or money and HIV seropositivity among female intravenous drug users. *American Journal of Public Health, 84,* 382–387.

Astin, J. A. (1997). Stress reduction through mindfulness meditation: Effects on psychological symptomatology, sense of control, and spiritual experiences. *Psychotherapy and Psychosomatics, 66,* 97–106.

Auwerx, H., & Staels, B. (1998). Leptin. *Lancet, 351,* 737–742.

Avins, A. L., Woods, W. J., Lindan, C. P., Hudes, E. S., Clark, W., & Hulley, S. B. (1994). HIV infection and risk behaviors among heterosexuals in alcohol treatment programs. *Journal of the American Medical Association, 271,* 515–518.

Avis, N. E., Smith, K. W., & McKinlay, J. B. (1989). Accuracy of perceptions of heart attack risk: What influences perceptions and can they be changed? *American Journal of Public Health, 79,* 1608–1612.

Ayanian, J. Z., & Cleary, P. D. (1999). Perceived risks of heart disease and cancer among cigarette smokers. *Journal of the American Medical Association, 281,* 1019–1021.

Bagley, C., & King, K. (1990). *Child sexual abuse: The search for healing.* London: Tavistock/Routledge.

Bahrke, M. S., & Morgan, W. P. (1978). Anxiety reduction following exercise and meditation. *Cognitive Therapy and Research, 2,* 323–334.

Bailey, J. E., Kellerman, A. L., Somes, G. W., Banton, J. G., Rivara, F. P., & Rushforth, N. P. (1997). Risk factors for violent death of women in the home. *Archives of Internal Medicine, 157,* 777–782.

Baker, E., Israel, B. A., & Schurman, S. (1996). The Integrated Model: Implications for worksite health promotion and occupational health and safety practice. *Health Education Quarterly, 23,* 175–190.

Ballard, J. E., Koepsell, T. D., & Rivara, F. (1992). Association of smoking and alcohol drinking with residential fire injuries. *American Journal of Epidemiology, 135,* 26–34.

Banaji, M. R., & Steele, C. M. (1989). The social cognition of alcohol use. *Social Cognition, 7,* 137–151.

Bandura, A. (1977). *Social learning theory.* Englewood Cliffs, NJ: Prentice-Hall.

Bandura, A. (1986). *Social foundations of thought and action: A social cognitive theory.* Englewood Cliffs, NJ: Prentice-Hall.

Bandura, A. (1989). Human agency in social cognitive theory. *American Psychologist, 44,* 1175–1184.

Barber, J. (1996). A brief introduction to hypnotic analgesia. In J. Barber (Ed.), *Hypnosis and suggestion in the treatment of pain: A clinical guide.* New York: Norton.

Barber, T. X. (1982). Hypnosuggestive procedures in the treatment of clinical pain: Implications for theories of hypnosis and suggestive therapy. In T. Millon, C. J. Green, & R. B. Meagher, Jr. (Eds.), *Handbook of clinical health psychology.* New York: Plenum.

Barber, T. X. (1984). Hypnosis, deep relaxation, and active relaxation: Data, theory, and clinical applications. In R. L. Woolfolk & P. M. Lehrer (Eds.), *Principles and practice of stress management.* New York: Guilford Press.

Barefoot, J. C., Larsen, S., von der Lieth, L., & Schroll, M. (1995). Hostility, incidence of acute myocardial infarction, and mortality in a sample of older Danish men and women. *American Journal of Epidemiology, 142,* 477–484.

Barrett, J. J., Ford, G. R., Stewart, K. E., & Haley, W. E. (1994, August). *Family caregiver appraisals of stressors in senile dementia: Gender differences?* Paper presented at the American Psychological Association, Los Angeles, CA.

Barrett, K. E., Riggar, T. F., & Flowers, C. R. (1997). Violence in the workplace: Preparing for the age of rage. *Journal of Rehabilitation Administration, 21,* 171–188.

Baum, A., Davidson, L. M., Singer, J. E., & Street, S. W. (1987). Stress as a psychophysiological process. In A. Baum & J. E. Singer (Eds.), *Handbook of psychology and health, Vol. 5. Stress* (pp. 1–24). Hillsdale, NJ: Erlbaum.

Baum, A., Gatchel, R. J., & Schaeffer, M. A. (1983). Emotional, behavioral, and physiological effects of chronic stress at Three Mile Island. *Journal of Consulting and Clinical Psychology, 51,* 565–572.

Bazargan, M. (1994). The effects of health, environmental, and socio-psychological variables on fear of crime and its consequences among urban Black elderly individuals. *International Journal of Aging and Human Development, 38,* 99–115.

Beaglehole, R., Bonita, R., & Kjellström, T. (1993). *Basic epidemiology.* Geneva, Switzerland: World Health Organization.

Beaglehole, R., Stewart, A. W., Jackson, R., Dobson, A. J., McElduff, P., D'Este, K., Heller, R. F., Janrozik, K. D., Hobbs, M. S., Parsons, R., & Broadhurst, R. (1997). Declining rates of coronary heart disease in New Zealand and Australia, 1983–1993. *American Journal of Epidemiology, 145,* 707–713.

Beck, A. T. (1976). *Cognitive therapy and the emotional disorders.* New York: International Universities Press.

Beck, A. T., Ward, C. H., Mendelson, M., Mock, J., & Erbaugh, J. (1961). An inventory for measuring depression. *Archives of General Psychiatry, 4,* 561–571.

Becker, M. H. (1979). Understanding patient compliance: The contributions of attitudes and other psychosocial factors. In S. J. Cohen (Ed.), *New directions in patient compliance* (pp. 1–31). Lexington, MA: Lexington Books.

Becker, M. H., Drachman, R. H., & Kirscht, J. P. (1972). Predicting mothers' compliance with pediatric medical regimens. *Journal of Pediatrics, 81,* 843–854.

Becker, M. H., & Maiman, L. A. (1980). Strategies for enhancing patient compliance. *Journal of Community Health, 6,* 113–135.

Becker, M. H., & Rosenstock, I. M. (1984). Compliance with medical advice. In A. Steptoe & A. Mathews (Eds.), *Health care and human behavior*. London: Academic Press.

Beecher, H. K. (1946). Pain of men wounded in battle. *Annals of Surgery, 123,* 96–105.

Beecher, H. K. (1956). Relationship of significance of wound to pain experience. *Journal of the American Medical Association, 161,* 1609–1613.

Beecher, H. K. (1957). The measurement of pain. *Pharmacological Review, 9,* 59–209.

Begleiter, H. & Kissin, J. (Eds.). (1996). *The pharmacology of alcohol and alcohol dependence. Alcohol and alcoholism* (Vol. 2). New York: Oxford University Press.

Beglin, S. J., & Fairburn, C. G. (1992). Women who choose not to participate in surveys on eating disorders. *International Journal of Eating Disorders, 12,* 113–116.

Behrens, V., Seligman, P., Cameron, L., Mathias, C. G. T., & Fine, L. (1994). The prevalence of back pain, hand discomfort, and dermatitis in the US work population, *American Journal of Public Health, 84,* 1780–1785.

Belar, C. D. (1997). Clinical health psychology: A specialty for the 21st century. *Health Psychology, 16,* 411–416.

Beller, A. S. (1978). *Fat and thin: A natural history of obesity.* New York: Farrar, Straus & Giroux.

Belloc, N. (1973). Relationship of health practices and mortality. *Preventive Medicine, 2,* 67–81.

Benca, R. M., Obermeyer, W. H., Thisted, R. A., & Gillin, J. C. (1992). Sleep and psychiatric disorders: A meta-analysis. *Archives of General Psychiatry, 49,* 651–668.

Bender R., Trautner, C., Spraul, M., & Berger, M. (1998). Assessment of excess mortality in obesity. *American Journal of Epidemiology, 147,* 42–48.

Benedetti, C., & Bonica, J. J. (1984). Cancer pain: Basic considerations. In C. Benedetti, C. R. Chapman, & G. Moricca (Eds.), *Advances in pain research and therapy: Vol. 7. Recent advances in the management of pain.* New York: Raven Press.

Ben-Eliyahu, S., Yirmiya, R., Liebeskind, J. C., Taylor, A. N., & Gale, R. P. (1991). Stress increases metastatic spread of mammary tumor in rats: Evidence for mediation by the immune system. *Brain, Behavior, and Immunity, 5,* 193–205.

Benishek, L. A., (1996). Evaluation of the factor structure underlying two measures of hardiness. *Assessment, 3,* 423–435.

Benishek, L. A., & Lopez, F. G. (1997). Critical evaluation of hardiness theory: Gender differences, perception of life events, and neuroticism. *Work & Stress, 11,* 33–45.

Bennett, H. L., & Disbrow, E. A. (1993). Preparing for surgery and medical procedures. In D. Goleman & J. Gurin (Eds.), *Mind/body medicine: How to use your mind for better health* (pp. 401–427). Yonkers, NY: Consumer Reports Books.

Bennett, W., & Gurin, J. (1982). *The dieter's dilemma: Eating less and weighing more.* New York: Basic Books.

Bennett, W. I., Goldfinger, S. E., & Johnson, G. T. (1987). *Your good health: How to stay well and what to do when you're not.* Cambridge, MA: Harvard University Press.

Ben-Shlomo, Y., Smith, G. D., Shipley, M. S., & Marmot, M. G. (1994). What determines mortality risk in male former cigarette smokers? *American Journal of Public Health, 84,* 1235–1242.

Benson, H. (1974). Your innate asset for combating stress. *Harvard Business Review, 52,* 49–60.

Benson, H. (1975). *The relaxation response.* New York: Morrow.

Benson, H., Beary, J. F., & Carol, M. P. (1974). The relaxation response. *Psychiatry, 37,* 37–46.

Benyamini, Y., Leventhal, E. A., & Leventhal, H. (1997). Attributions and health. In A. Baum, S. Newman, J. Weinman, R. West, & C. McManus (Eds.), *Cambridge handbook of psychology, health and medicine* (pp. 72–77). Cambridge, United Kingdom: Cambridge University Press.

Berger, B. D., & Adesso, V. J. (1991). Gender differences in using alcohol to cope with depression. *Addictive Behaviors, 16,* 315–327.

Berkman, L. F. (1986). Social networks, support, and health: Taking the next step forward. *American Journal of Epidemiology, 123,* 559–562.

Berkman, L. F., & Breslow, L. (1983). *Health and ways of living: The Alameda County Study.* New York: Oxford University Press.

Berkman, L. F., Breslow, L., & Wingard, D. (1983). Health practices and mortality risk. In L. F. Berkman & L. Breslow (Eds.), *Health and ways of living: The Alameda County study.* New York: Oxford University Press.

Berkman, L. F., & Syme, S. L. (1979). Social networks, host resistance, and mortality: A nine-year follow-up study of Alameda County residents. *American Journal of Epidemiology, 109,* 186–204.

Bernstein, L., Henderson, B. E., Hanisch, R., Sullivan-Halley, J., & Ross, R. K. (1994). Physical exercise and reduced risk of breast cancer in young women. *Journal of the National Cancer Institute, 86,* 1403–1408.

Berry, D. S., & Pennebaker, J. W. (1993). Nonverbal and verbal emotional expression and health. *Psychotherapy and Psychosomatics, 59,* 11–19.

Betz, N. (1993). Women's career development. In F. L. Denmark & M. A. Paludi (Eds.), *Psychology of women: A handbook of issues and theories* (pp. 627–684). Westport, CT: Greenwood Press.

Bhopal, R. (1998). Spectre of racism in health and health care: Lessons from history and the United States. *British Medical Journal, 316,* 1970–1973.

Bibace, R., & Walsh, M. E. (1979). Developmental stages in children's conceptions of illness. In G. C. Stone, F. Cohen, & N. E. Adler (Eds.), *Health psychology—A handbook* (pp. 285–301). San Francisco: Jossey-Bass.

Bieliauskas, L. A. (1982). *Stress and its relationship to health and illness.* Boulder, CO: Westview Press.

Biener, L., & Heaton, A. (1995). Women dieters of normal weight: Their motives, goals, and risks. *American Journal of Public Health, 85,* 714–717.

Biglan, A., Metzler, C. W., Wirt, R., Ary, D., Noell, J., Ochs, L., French, C., & Hood, D. (1990). Social and behavioral factors associated with high-risk sexual behavior among adolescents. *Journal of Behavioral Medicine, 13*, 245–262.

Bjornson, W., Rand, C., Connett, J. E., Lundgren, P., Nides, M., Pope, F., Buist, A. S., Hoppe-Ryan, C., & O'Hara, P. (1995). Gender differences in smoking cessation after 3 years in the Lung Health Study. *American Journal of Public Health, 85*, 223–230.

Blackwell, B. (1997). From compliance to alliance: A quarter century of research. In B. Blackwell (Ed.), *Treatment compliance and the therapeutic alliance* (pp. 1–15). Amsterdam: Harwood Academic Publishers.

Blair, S. N. (1993). Evidence for success of exercise in weight loss and control. *Annals of Internal Medicine, 119*, 702–706.

Blair, S. N. (1994). Physical activity, fitness, and coronary heart disease. In C. Bouchard, R. J. Shephard, & T. Stephens (Eds.), *Physical activity, fitness, and health: International proceedings and consensus statement* (pp. 579–590). Champaign, IL: Human Kinetics.

Blair, S. N., Kohl, H. W., Barlow, C. E., Paffenbarger, R. S., Jr., Gibbons, L. W., & Macera, C. A. (1995). Changes in physical fitness and all-cause mortality: A prospective study of healthy and unhealthy men. *Journal of the American Medical Association, 273*, 1093–1098.

Blalock, S. J., DeVellis, R. F., Giorgino, K. B., DeVellis, B. M., Gold, D. T., Dooley, M. A., Anderson, J. J. B., & Smith, S. L. (1996). Osteoporosis prevention in premenopausal women: Using a stage model approach to examine the predictors of behavior. *Health Psychology, 15*, 84–93.

Blanchard, E. B., & Andrasik, F. (1982). Psychological assessment and treatment of headache: Recent development and emerging issues. *Journal of Consulting and Clinical Psychology, 50*, 859–879.

Blanchard, E. B., & Andrasik, F. (1985). *Management of chronic headaches: A psychological approach.* New York: Pergamon Press.

Blanchard, E. B., Appelbaum, K. A., Radniz, C. L., Michultka, D., Morrill, B., Kirsch, C., Hillhouse, J., Evans, D. D., Guarnieri, P., Attanasio, V., Andrasik, F., Jaccard, J., & Dentinger, M. P. (1990a). Placebo-controlled evaluation of abbreviated progressive muscle relaxation and of relaxation combined with cognitive therapy in the treatment of tension headache. *Journal of Consulting and Clinical Psychology, 58*, 210–215.

Blanchard, E. B., Appelbaum, K. A., Radniz, C. L., Morrill, B., Michultka, D., Kirsch, C., Guarnieri, P., Hillhouse, J., Evans, D. D., Jaccard, J., & Barron, K. D. (1990b). A controlled evaluation of thermal biofeedback and thermal biofeedback combined with cognitive therapy in the treatment of vascular headache. *Journal of Consulting and Clinical Psychology, 58*, 216–224.

Bloom, C., Kogel, L., & Zaphiropoulos, L. (1994). Beginning the eating and body work: Stance and tools. In C. Bloom, A. Gitter, S. Gutwill, L. Kogel, & L. Zaphiro-

poulos (Eds.), *Eating problems: A feminist psychoanalytic treatment model* (pp. 67–82). New York: Basic Books.

Blumstein, P., & Schwartz, P. (1983). *American couples.* New York: Pocket Books.

Bodnar, J. C., & Kiecolt-Glaser, J. K. (1994). Caregiver depression after bereavement: Chronic stress isn't over when it's over. *Psychology and Aging, 9*, 372–380.

Bohman, M., Sigvardsson, S., & Cloninger, C. R. (1981). Maternal inheritance of alcohol abuse. *Archives of General Psychiatry, 38*, 965–969.

Bolinder, G., Alfredsson, L., England, A., & de Faire, U. (1994). Smokeless tobacco use and increased cardiovascular mortality among Swedish construction workers. *American Journal of Public Health, 84*, 399–404.

Bond, G. G., Aiken, L. S., & Somerville, S. C. (1992). The health belief model and adolescents with insulin-dependent diabetes mellitus. *Health Psychology, 11*, 190–198.

Boney McCoy, S., Gibbons, F. X., Reis, T. J., Gerrard, M., Luus, C. A. E., & Von Wald Sufka, A. (1992). Perceptions of smoking risk as a function of smoking status. *Journal of Behavior Medicine, 15*, 469–488.

Bonica, J. J. (1980). Cancer pain. In J. J. Bonica (Ed.), *Pain.* New York: Raven Press.

Bonica, J. J. (1990). Definitions and taxonomy of pain. In J. J. Bonica (Ed.), *The management of pain* (2nd ed., pp. 18–27). Malvern, PA: Lea & Febiger.

Bonica, J. J., Ventafridda, V., & Twycross, R. G. (1990). Cancer pain. In J. J. Bonica (Ed.), *The management of pain* (2nd ed., pp. 400–460). Malvern, PA: Lea & Febiger.

Bonneau, R., Sheridan, J. F., Feng, N., & Glaser, R. (1991). Stress-induced suppression of herpes simplex virus (HSV)-specific sytotoxic T lymphocyte and natural killer cell activity and enhancement of acute pathogenesis following local HSV infection. *Brain, Behavior, and Immunity, 5*, 170–192.

Borkan, G. A., Sparrow, D., Wisniewski, C., & Vokonas, P. S. (1986). Body weight and coronary disease risk: Patterns of risk factor change associated with long-term weight change. The Normative Aging Study. *American Journal of Epidemiology, 124*, 410–419.

Borrelli, B., & Mermelstein, R. (1994). Goal setting and behavior change in a smoking cessation program. *Cognitive Therapy and Research, 18*, 69–82.

Boskind-White, M., & White, W. C., Jr. (1983). *Bulimarexia: The binge/purge cycle.* New York: Norton.

Bosscher, R. J. (1993). Running and mixed physical exercises with depressed psychiatric patients. Special Issue: Exercise and psychological well-being. *International Journal of Sport Psychology, 24*, 170–184.

Bovbjerg, V. E., McCann, B. S., Brief, D. J., Follette, W. C., Retzlaff, B. M., Dowdy, A. A., Walden, C. E., & Knopp, R. H. (1995). Spouse support and long-term adherence to lipid-lowering diets. *American Journal of Epidemiology, 141*, 451–460.

Bower, P. J., Rubik, B., Weiss, S. J., & Starr, C. (1997). Manual therapy: Hands-on healing. *Patient Care, 31*, 69–81.

Bradley, L. A., Prokop, C. K., Gentry, W. D., Van der Heide, L. H., & Prieto, E. J. (1981). Assessment of chronic pain. In C. K. Prokop & L. A. Bradley (Eds.), *Medical psychology: Contributions to behavioral medicine.* New York: Academic Press.

Bradley, L. A., & Van der Heide, L. H. (1984). Pain-related correlates of MMPI profile subgroups among back pain patients. *Health Psychology, 3,* 157–174.

Brandsma, J. M., Maultsby, M. C., & Welsh, R. J. (1980). *The outpatient treatment of alcoholism: A review and comparative study.* Baltimore: University Park Press.

Brannon, L. (1999). *Gender: Psychological perspectives* (2nd ed.). Boston: Allyn and Bacon.

Brannon, L., & Papadimitriou, M. (1985, October). *Smokers vs. nonsmokers: Perception of risks.* Paper presented at convention of the Louisiana Psychological Association, Lake Charles, LA.

Braun, A. C. (1977). *The story of cancer.* Reading, MA: Addison-Wesley.

Braun, B. L., Murray, D., & Sidney, S. (1997). Lifetime cocaine use and cardiovascular characteristics among young adults: the CARDIA study. *American Journal of Public Health, 87,* 629–634.

Braver, E. R., Ferguson, S. A., Greene, M. A., & Lund, A. K. (1997). Reductions in deaths in frontal crashes among right front passengers in vehicles equipped with passenger air bags. *Journal of the American Medical Association, 278,* 1437–1439.

Bray, G. A. (1992). Pathophysiology of obesity. *American Journal of Clinical Nutrition, 55,* 488S–494S.

Brecher, E. M. (1972). *Licit and illicit drugs.* Boston: Little, Brown.

Brehm, J. W. (1966). *A theory of psychological reactance.* New York: Academic Press.

Breslau, N., Peterson, E., Schultz, L., Andreski, P., & Chilcoat, H. (1996). Are smokers with alcohol disorders less likely to quit? *American Journal of Public Health, 86,* 985–990.

Breuer, J., & Freud, S. (1955). *Studies on hysteria.* In J. Strachey (Ed. and Trans.), *The standard edition of the complete psychological works of Sigmund Freud* (Vol. 2). London: Hogarth Press. (Original work published 1895).

Brock, D. W., & Wartman, S. A. (1990). When competent patients make irrational choices. *New England Journal of Medicine, 322,* 1595–1599.

Broman, C. L. (1993). Social relationships and health-related behavior. *Journal of Behavioral Medicine, 16,* 335–350.

Brookmeyer, R., Gray, S., & Kawas, C. (1998). Projections of Alzheimer's disease in the United States and the public health impact of delaying disease onset. *American Journal of Public Health, 88,* 1337–1342.

Brown, B. (1970). Recognition of aspects of consciousness through association with EEG alpha activity represented by a light signal. *Psychophysics, 6,* 442–446.

Brown, G. W., & Harris, T. O. (1989). *Life events and illness.* New York: Guilford Press.

Brown, J. D. (1991). Staying fit and staying well: Physical fitness as a moderator of life stress. *Journal of Personality and Social Psychology, 60,* 555–561.

Brown, J. D., & Lawton, M. (1986). Stress and well-being in adolescence: The moderating role of physical exercise. *Journal of Human Stress, 12,* 125–131.

Brown, J. D., & Siegel, J. M. (1988). Exercise as a buffer of life stress: A prospective study of adolescent health. *Health Psychology, 7,* 341–353.

Brown, W. A. (1997, September/October). The best medicine? *Psychology Today, 30,* 56–60, 80, 82.

Brownell, K. D., & Rodin, J. (1994a). The dieting maelstrom: Is it possible and advisable to lose weight? *American Psychologist, 49,* 781–791.

Brownell, K. D., & Rodin, J. (1994b). Medical, metabolic, and psychological effects of weight cycling. *Archives of Internal Medicine, 154,* 1325–1330.

Brownell, P. (1996). Domestic violence in the workplace: An emergent issue. *Crisis Intervention, 3,* 129–141.

Brownlee, S., & Schrof, J. M. (1997). The quality of mercy: Effective pain treatments already exist. Why aren't doctors using them? *U.S. News & World Report, 122*(10), 54–61.

Brownlee-Duffeck, M., Peterson, L., Simonds, J. F., Goldstein, D., Kilo, C., & Hoette, S. (1987). The role of health beliefs in the regimen adherence and metabolic control of adolescents and adults with diabetes mellitus. *Journal of Consulting and Clinical Psychology, 55,* 139–144.

Brownson, R. C., Jackson-Thompson, J., Wilkerson, J. C., Davis, J. R., Owens, N. W., & Fisher, E. B., Jr. (1992). Demographic and socioeconomic differences in beliefs about the health effects of smoking. *American Journal of Public Health, 82,* 99–103.

Bruch, H. (1973). *Eating disorders. Obesity, anorexia nervosa and the person within.* New York: Basic Books.

Bruch, H. (1978). *The golden cage: The enigma of anorexia nervosa.* Cambridge, MA: Harvard University Press.

Bruch, H. (1982). Anorexia nervosa: Therapy and theory. *American Journal of Psychiatry, 139,* 1531–1538.

Brunner, E., White, I., Thorogood, M., Bristow, A., Curle, D., & Marmot, M. (1997). Can dietary interventions change diet and cardiovascular risk factors? A meta-analysis of randomized controlled trials. *American Journal of Public Health, 87,* 1415–1422.

Brunnquell, D., & Hall, M. D. (1984). Issues in the psychological care of pediatric oncology patients. In R. H. Moos (Ed.), *Coping with physical illness 2: New perspectives* (pp. 195–207). New York: Plenum Press.

Bruns, D. (1998). Psychologists as primary care providers: A paradigm shift. *Health Psychologist, 20*(4), 19.

Bryant, R. A. (1993). Beliefs about hypnosis: A survey of acute and chronic pain therapists. *Contemporary Hypnosis, 10,* 89–98.

Burbach, D. J., & Peterson, L. (1986). Children's concepts of physical illness: A review and critique of the cognitive-developmental literature. *Health Psychology, 5,* 307–325.

Bureau of Justice Statistics. (1998a). National Crime Victimization Survey, violent victimization rates by sex, 1973–96. http://www.ojp.usdoj.gov/bjs/glance

Bureau of Justice Statistics. (1998b). Homicide rates by age, 1970–96. http://www.ojp.usdoj.gov/bjs/glance

Burish, T. G., Meyerowitz, B. E., Carey, M. P., & Morrow, G. R. (1987). The stressful effects of cancer in adults. In A. Baum & J. E. Singer (Eds.), *Handbook of psychology and health: Vol. 5. Stress* (pp. 137–173). Hillsdale, NJ: Erlbaum.

Burnette, M. M., Meilahn, E., Wing, R. R., & Kuller, L. H. (1998). Smoking cessation, weight gain, and changes in cardiovascular risk factors during menopause: The Healthy Women Study. *American Journal of Public Health, 88,* 93–96.

Burns, J. W., & Katkin, E. S. (1993). Psychological, situational, and gender predictors of cardiovascular reactivity to stress: A multivariate approach. *Journal of Behavioral Medicine, 16,* 445–465.

Burns, T., & Crisp, A. H. (1990). Outcome of anorexia nervosa in males. In A. E. Andersen (Ed.), *Males with eating disorders* (pp. 163–186). New York: Brunner/Mazel.

Burte, J. M., Burte, W. D., & Araoz, D. L. (1994). Hypnosis in the treatment of back pain. *Australian Journal of Clinical Hypnotherapy and Hypnosis, 15,* 93–115.

Bush, C., Ditto, B., & Feuerstein, M. (1985). A controlled evaluation of paraspinal EMG biofeedback in the treatment of chronic low back pain. *Health Psychology, 4,* 307–321.

Bush, J. P., Melamed, B. G., Sheras, P. L., & Greenbaum, P. E. (1986). Mother-child patterns of coping with anticipatory medical stress. *Health Psychology, 5,* 137–157.

Byrne, J., Fears, T. R., Steinhorn, S. C., Mulvihill, J. J., Connelly, R. R., Austin, D. F., Holmes, G. F., Holmes, F. F., Latourette, H. B., Teta, J., Strong, L. C., & Myers, M. H. (1989). Marriage and divorce after childhood and adolescent cancer. *Journal of the American Medical Association, 262,* 2693–2699.

Bypass Angioplasty Revascularization Investigation. (1997). Five-year clinical and functional outcome comparing bypass surgery and angioplasty in patients with multivessel coronary disease: A multicenter randomized trial. *Journal of the American Medical Association, 277,* 715–721.

Cacioppo, J. T., Poehlmann, K. M., Kiecolt-Glaser, J. K., Malarkey, W. B., Burleson, M. H., Berntson, G. G., & Glaser, R. (1998). Cellular immune responses to acute stress in female caregivers of dementia patients and matched controls. *Health Psychology, 17,* 182–189.

Caggiula, A. W., Christakis, G., Farrand, M., Hulley, S. B., Johnson, R., Lasser, N. L., Stamler, J., & Widdowson, G. (1981). The Multiple Risk Factor Intervention Trial (MRFIT): IV. Intervention on blood lipids. *Preventive Medicine, 10,* 443–475.

Calermajer, D. S., Adams, M. R., Clarkson, P., Robinson, J., McCredie, R., Donald, A., & Deanfield, J. E. (1996). Passive smoking and impaired endothelium-dependent arterial dilation in healthy young adults. *New England Journal of Medicine, 334,* 150–154.

Calhoun, J. B. (1956). A comparative study of the social behavior of two inbred strains of house mice. *Ecological Monogram, 26,* 81.

Calhoun, J. B. (1962, February). Population density and social pathology. *Scientific American, 206,* 139–148.

Calle, E. E., Miracle-McMahill, H. L., Thun, M. J., & Heath, C. W., Jr. (1994). Cigarette smoking and risk of fatal breast cancer. *American Journal of Epidemiology, 139,* 1001–1007.

Camacho, T. C., Roberts, R. E., Lazarus, N. B., Kaplan, G. A., & Cohen, R. D. (1991). Physical activity and depression: Evidence from the Alameda County study. *American Journal of Epidemiology, 134,* 220–231.

Camacho, T. C., & Wiley, J. A. (1983). Health practices, social networks, and change in physical health. In L. F. Berkman & L. Breslow (Eds.), *Health and ways of living: The Alameda County Study.* New York: Oxford University Press.

Cameron, L., Leventhal, E. A., & Leventhal, H. (1993). Symptom representations and affect as determinants of care seeking in a community-dwelling, adult sample population. *Health Psychology, 12,* 171–179.

Cameron, L., Leventhal, E. A., & Leventhal, H. (1995). Seeking medical care in response to symptoms and life stress. *Psychosomatic Medicine, 57,* 37–47.

Campfield, L. A., Smith, F. J., Guisez, Y., Devos, R., & Burn, P. (1995). Recombinant mouse OB protein: Evidence for a peripheral signal linking adiposity and central neural networks. *Science, 269,* 546–549.

Campion, E. W. (1997). Power lines, cancer, and fear. *New England Journal of Medicine, 337,* 44–46.

Cannon, W. (1932). *The wisdom of the body.* New York: Norton.

Capaldi, E. D. (1996). Conditioned food preferences. In E. D. Capaldi (Ed.), *Why we eat what we eat: The psychology of eating* (pp. 53–80). Washington, DC: American Psychological Association.

Caragata, W. (1995, April 3). Medicare wars: Canada's health care cuts. *Maclean's, 108,* 14–15.

Carden, A. D. (1994). Wife abuse and the wife abuser: Review and recommendations. *Counseling Psychologist, 22,* 539–582.

Carlat, D. J., Camargo, C. A., & Herzog, D. B. (1997). Eating disorders in males: A report on 135 patients. *American Journal of Psychiatry, 154,* 1127–1132.

Carlson, C. R., & Hoyle, R. H. (1993). Efficacy of abbreviated progressive muscle relaxation training: A quantitative review of behavioral medicine research. *Journal of Consulting and Clinical Psychology, 61,* 1059–1067.

Carmach, M. A., & Martens, R. (1979). Measuring commitment to running: A survey of runners' attitudes and mental state. *Journal of Sports Psychology, 1,* 25–42.

Carruthers, M. (1983). Instrumental stress tests. In H. Selye (Ed.), *Selye's guide to stress research* (Vol. 2). New York: Scientific and Academic Editions.

Carson, B. S. (1987). Neurologic and neurosurgical approaches to cancer pain. In D. B. McGuire & C. H. Yarbro (Eds.), *Cancer pain management* (pp. 223–243). Philadelphia: Saunders.

Case, R. B., Moss, A. J., Case, N., McDermott, M., & Eberly, S. (1992). Living alone after myocardial infarction. *Journal of the American Medical Association, 267,* 515–519.

Cash, T. F., & Deagle, E. A., III. (1997). The nature and extent of body-image disturbances in anorexia nervosa and bulimia nervosa: A meta-analysis. *International Journal of Eating Disorders, 22,* 107–125.

Caspersen, C. J., Bloemberg, B. P. M., Saris, W. H. M., Merritt, R. K., & Kromhout, D. (1991). The prevalence of selected physical activities and their relation with coronary heart disease risk factors in elderly men: The Zutphen Study, 1985. *American Journal of Epidemiology, 133,* 1078–1092.

Castro, F. G., Coe, K., Gutierres, S., & Saenz, D. (1996). Designing health promotion programs for Latinos. In P. M. Kato & T. Mann (Eds.), *Handbook of diversity issues in health psychology* (pp. 319–345). New York: Plenum Press.

Caudill, B. D., & Marlatt, G. A. (1975). Modeling influences in social drinking: An experimental analogue. *Journal of Consulting and Clinical Psychology, 143,* 405–415.

Caudron, S. (1998). Target: HR. *Workforce, 77*(8), 44–50.

Cauwells, J. M. (1983). *Bulimia: The binge-purge compulsion.* Garden City, NY: Doubleday.

Cavaliere, F. (1995, July). APA and CDC join forces to combat illness. *APA Monitor, 26*(7), 1, 13.

Cecil, H., Evans, R. I., & Stanley, M. (1996). Perceived believability among adolescents of health warning labels on cigarette packs. *Journal of Applied Social Psychology, 26,* 502–519.

Centers for Disease Control and Prevention (CDC). (1992). 1993 revised classification system for HIV infection and expanded surveillance case definition for AIDS among adolescents and adults. *Morbidity and Mortality Weekly Report, 41,* No. RR-17.

Centers for Disease Control and Prevention (CDC). (1993). Cigarette smoking—attributable mortality and years of potential life lost—United States, 1990. *Morbidity and Mortality Weekly Report, 42,* 645–649.

Centers for Disease Control and Prevention (CDC). (1994a). Preventing tobacco use among young people: A report of the Surgeon General. *Morbidity and Mortality Weekly Report, 43,* No. RR-4.

Centers for Disease Control and Prevention (CDC). (1994b). Reasons for tobacco use and symptoms of nicotine withdrawal among adolescent and young adult tobacco users—United States, 1993. *Morbidity and Mortality Weekly Report, 43,* 745–750.

Centers for Disease Control and Prevention (CDC). (1995). Update: Trends in fetal alcohol syndrome—United States, 1979–1993. *Morbidity and Mortality Weekly Report, 44,* 249–251.

Centers for Disease Control and Prevention. (1998a). AIDS among persons aged ≥ 50 years—United States, 1991–1996. *Morbidity and Mortality Weekly Report, 47,* 21–27.

Centers for Disease Control and Prevention (CDC). (1998b). Deaths resulting from residential fires and the prevalence of smoke alarms—United States, 1991–1995. *Morbidity and Mortality Weekly Report. 47,* 803–906.

Centers for Disease Control and Prevention (CDC). (1998c). Incidence of initiation of cigarette smoking—United States, 1965–1996. *Morbidity and Mortality Weekly Report, 47,* 837–840.

Centers for Disease Control and Prevention (CDC). (1998d). Percentage of adults who were current, former, or never smokers, + overall and by race, Hispanic origin, age, and education, National Health Interview Surveys, selected years—United States, 1965–1994. *Tobacco Information and Prevention Source.* http://www.cdc.gov/tobacco

Centers for Disease Control and Prevention (CDC). (1998e). Smoking status of high school seniors—United States, Monitoring the Future Project, 1976–1996. *Tobacco Information and Prevention Source.* http://www.cdc. gov/tobacco

Centers for Disease Control and Prevention (CDC). (1998f). Tobacco use among high school students—United States, 1997. *Morbidity and Mortality Weekly Reports, 47,* 229–233.

Centers for Disease Control and Prevention (CDC). (1998g). Tobacco use prevention program. *Tobacco Information and Prevention Source.* http://www.cdc. gov/tobacco

Chalk, R., & King, P. A. (Eds.). (1998). *Violence in families: Assessing prevention and treatment programs.* Washington, DC: National Academy Press.

Champion, V. L. (1994). Strategies to increase mammography utilization. *Medical Care, 32,* 118–129.

Champion, V. L. & Miller, A. (1997). Adherence to mammography and breast self-examination regimen. In D. S. Gochman Ed., *Handbook of health behavior research II: Provider determinants* (pp. 245–267). New York: Plenum Press.

Chapman, C. R., & Syrjala, K. L. (1990). Measurement of pain. In J. J. Bonica (Ed.), *The management of pain* (2nd ed., pp. 580–594). Malvern, PA: Lea & Febiger.

Chapman, S., Wong, W. L., & Smith, W. (1993). Self-exempting beliefs about smoking and health: Differences between smokers and ex-smokers. *American Journal of Public Health, 83,* 215–219.

Charlee, C., Goldsmith, L. J., Chambers, L., & Haynes, R. B. (1996). Provider-patient communication among elderly and nonelderly patients in Canadian hospitals: A national survey. *Health Communication, 8,* 281–302.

Chaves, J. F., & Brown, J. M. (1987). Spontaneous cognitive strategies for the control of clinical pain and stress. *Journal of Behavioral Medicine, 10,* 263–276.

Cheadle, A., Pearson, D., Wagner, E., Psaty, B. M., Diehr, P., & Koepsell, T. (1994). Relationship between socioeconomic status, health status, and lifestyle practices of American Indians: Evidence from a

Plains reservation population. *Public Health Reports, 109*, 405–413.

Chen, Y., Horne, S. L., & Dosman, J. A. (1993). The influence of smoking cessation on body weight may be temporary. *American Journal of Public Health, 83*, 1330–1332.

Chen, Z., Xu, Z., Collins, R., Li, W., & Peto, R. (1997). Early health effects of the emerging tobacco epidemic in China: A 16-year prospective study. *Journal of the American Medical Association, 278*, 1500–1504.

Cherpitel, C. J. (1994). Cause of casualty and drinking patterns: An emergency room study of unintentional injuries. *Drug and Alcohol Dependence, 35*, 61–67.

Cherpitel, C. J. (1995). Alcohol and casualties: Comparison of county-wide emergency room data with the county general population. *Addiction, 90*, 343–350.

Chesney, M., & Darbes, L. (1998). Social support and heart disease in women: Implications for intervention. In K. Orth-Gomér, M. Chesney, & N. K. Wenger (Eds.), *Women, stress, and heart disease* (pp. 165–182). Mahwah, NJ: Erlbaum.

Chesney, M. A. (1993). Health psychology in the 21st century: Acquired immunodeficiency syndrome as a harbinger of things to come. *Health Psychology, 12*, 259–268.

Chilcoat, H. D., Deshion, T. J., & Anthony, J. C. (1995). Parent monitoring and the incidence of drug sampling in urban elementary school children. *American Journal of Epidemiology, 141*, 25–31.

Chimonczyk, B. A., Salmun, L. M., Megathlin, F. N., Neveux, L. M., Palomadi, G. E., Knight, G. J., Pulkkinen, A. J., & Haddow, J. E. (1993). Association between exposure to environmental tobacco smoke and exacerbations of asthma in children. *New England Journal of Medicine, 328*, 1665–1669.

Ching, P. L. Y. H., Willett, W. C., Rimm, E. B., Colditz, G. A., Gortmaker, S. L., & Stampfer, M. J. (1996). Activity level and risk of overweight in male health professionals. *American Journal of Public Health, 86*, 25–30.

Christ, G. H., Siegel, K., Freund, B., Langosch, D., Hendersen, S., Sperber, D., & Weinstein, L. (1993). Impact of parental terminal cancer on latency-age children. *American Journal of Orthopsychiatry, 63*, 417–425.

Christen, W., Glynn, R. J., Manson, J. E., Ajani, U., & Buring, J. E. (1997). A prospective study of cigarette smoking and risk of age-related macular degeneration in men. *Journal of the American Medical Association, 276*, 1147–1151.

Christensen, A. J., Wiebbe, J. S., & Lawton, W. J. (1997). Cynical hostility, powerful others control expectancies, and patient adherence in hemodialysis. *Psychomotatic Medicine, 59*, 307–312.

Clark, W. B., & Cahalan, D. (1976). Changes in problem drinking over a four-year span. *Addictive Behaviors, 1*, 251–399.

Classen, C., Sephton, S. E., Diamond, S., & Spiegel, D. (1998). Studies of life-extending psychosocial interventions. In J. C. Holland (Ed.), *Psycho-oncology* (pp. 730–742). New York: Oxford University Press.

Clements, L. B., York, R. O., & Rohrer, G. E. (1995). The interaction of parental alcoholism and alcoholism as a predictor of drinking-related locus of control. *Alcoholism Treatment Quarterly, 12*, 97–110.

Cloninger, C. R., Bohman, M., & Sigvardsson, S. (1981). Inheritance of alcohol abuse. *Archives of Psychiatry, 38*, 861–868.

Coambs, R. B., Li, S., & Kozlowski, L. T. (1992). Age interacts with heaviness of smoking in predicting success in cessation of smoking. *American Journal of Epidemiology, 135*, 240–246.

Cochran, S. D. (1984). Preventing medical noncompliance in the outpatient treatment of bipolar affective disorders. *Journal of Consulting and Clinical Psychology, 52*, 873–878.

Cochran, S. D., & Mays, V. M. (1993). Applying social psychological models to predicting HIV-related sexual risk behaviors among African-Americans. Special Issue: Psychosocial aspects of AIDS prevention among African Americans. *Journal of Black Psychology, 19*, 142–154.

Cohen, A., & Colligan, M. J. (1997). Accepting occupational safety and health regimens. In D. S. Gochman (Ed.), *Handbook of health behavior research II: Provider determinants* (pp. 379–394). New York: Plenum Press.

Cohen, S. (1996). Psychological stress, immunity, and upper respiratory infections. *Current Directions in Psychological Science, 5*, 86–90.

Cohen, S., Doyle, W. J., Skoner, D. P., Fireman, P., Gwaltney, J. M., Jr., & Newson, J. T. (1995). State and trait negative affect as predictors of objective and subjective symptoms of respiratory viral infections. *Journal of Personality and Social Psychology, 68*, 159–169.

Cohen, S., Frank, E., Doyle, W. J., Skoner, D. P., Rabin, B. S., & Gwaltney, J. M., Jr. (1998). Types of stressors that increase susceptibility to the common cold in healthy adults. *Health Psychology, 17*, 214–223.

Cohen, S., Glass, D. C., & Phillips, S. (1977). Environment and health. In H. E. Freeman, S. Levine, & L. G. Reeder (Eds.), *Handbook of medical sociology*. Englewood Cliffs, NJ: Prentice-Hall.

Cohen, S., & Herbert, T. B. (1996). Health psychology: Psychological factors and physical disease from the perspective of human psychoneuroimmunology. *Annual Review of Psychology, 47*, 113–132.

Cohen, S., Kamarck, T., & Mermelstein, R. (1983). A global measure of perceived stress. *Journal of Health and Social Behavior, 24*, 385–396.

Cohen, S., Lichtenstein, E., Prochaska, J. O., Rossi, J. S., Gritz, E. R., Carr, C. R., Orleans, C. T., Schoenbach, V. J., Beiner, L., Abrams, D., DiClemente, C., Curry, S., Marlatt, G. A., Cummings, K. M., Emont, S. L., Giovino, G., & Ossip-Klein, D. (1989). Debunking myths about self-quitting: Evidence from 10 prospective studies of persons who attempt to quit smoking by themselves. *American Psychologist, 44*, 1355–1365.

Cohen, S., Tyrrell, D. A. J., Russell, M. A. H., Jarvis, M. J., & Smith, A. P. (1993). Smoking, alcohol consumption, and susceptibility to the common cold. *American Journal of Public Health, 83,* 1277–1283.

Cohen, S., Tyrrell, D. A. J., & Smith, A. P. (1991). Psychological stress and susceptibility to the common cold. *New England Journal of Medicine, 325,* 606–612.

Cohen, S., Tyrrell, D. A. J., & Smith, A. P. (1993). Negative life events, perceived stress, negative affect, and susceptibility to the common cold. *Journal of Personality and Social Psychology, 64,* 131–140.

Cohen, Y., Spirito, A., & Brown, L. K. (1996). Suicide and suicidal behavior. In R. J. Di Clemente, W. B. Hansen, & L. E. Ponton (Eds.), *Handbook of adolescent health risk behavior* (pp. 193–224). New York: Plenum Press.

Cohler, B. J., Groves, L., Borden, W., & Lazarus, L. (1989). Caring for family members with Alzheimer's disease. In E. Light & B. D. Lebowitz (Eds.), *Alzheimer's disease treatment and family stress: Direction for research* (pp. 50–105). (DHHS Publication No. ADM 89–1569). Washington, DC: U.S. Government Printing Office.

Colditz, G. A. (1995). Weight gain as a risk factor for clinical diabetes mellitus in women. *Annals of Internal Medicine, 122,* 481–486.

Colditz, G. A., Bonita, R., Stampfer, M. J., Willett, W. C., Rosner, B., Speizer, F. E., & Hennekens, C. H. (1988). Cigarette smoking and risk of stroke in middle-aged women. *New England Journal of Medicine, 318,* 937–941.

Colditz, G. A., Willett, W. C., Hunter, D. J., Stampfer, M. J., Manson, J. E., Hennekens, C. H., Rosner, B. A., & Speizer, F. E. (1993). Family history, age, and risk of breast cancer. *Journal of the American Medical Association, 270,* 338–343.

Cole, S. W., Kemeny, M. E., & Taylor, S. E. (1997). Social identity and physical health: Accelerated HIV progression in rejection-sensitive gay men. *Journal of Personality and Social Psychology, 72,* 320–335.

Cole, S. W., Kemeny, M. E., Taylor, S. E., Visscher, B. R., & Fahey, J. L. (1996). Accelerated course of human immunodeficiency virus infection in gay men who conceal their homosexual identity. *Psychosomatic Medicine, 58,* 219–231.

Coles, C. D., Smith, I. E., Lancaster, J. S., & Falek, A. (1987). Persistence over the first month of neurobehavioral alternations in infants exposed to alcohol prenatally. *Infant Behavior and Development, 10,* 23–37.

Collis, G. M., & McNicholas, J. (1998). A theoretical basis for health benefits of pet ownership: Attachment versus psychological support. In C. C. Wilson & D. C. Turner (Eds.), *Companion animals in human health* (pp. 105–122). Thousand Oaks, CA: Sage.

Compas, B. E., Haaga, D. A., Keefe, F. J., Leitenberg, H., & Williams, D. A. (1998). Sampling of empirically supported psychological treatments from health psychology: Smoking, chronic pain, cancer, and bulimia nervosa. *Journal of Consulting and Clinical Psychology, 66,* 89–112.

Conboy, J. K. (1994). The effects of exercise withdrawal and mood states in runners. *Journal of Sport Psychology, 17,* 188–203.

Condiotte, M. M., & Lichtenstein, E. (1982). Self-efficacy and relapse in smoking cessation programs. *Journal of Consulting and Clinical Psychology, 49,* 648–658.

Conger, J. (1956). Reinforcement theory and the dynamics of alcoholism. *Quarterly Journal of Studies on Alcohol, 17,* 296–305.

Conn, J. M., Chorba, T. L., Peterson, T. D., Rhodes, P., & Annest, J. L. (1993). Effectiveness of safety-belt use: A study using hospital-based data for nonfatal motor-vehicle crashes. *Journal of Safety Research, 24,* 223–232.

Conn, V. S. (1998). Older women: Social cognitive theory correlates of health behavior. *Women and Health, 26,* 71–85.

Connor, W. E., & Connor, S. L. (1997). The case for a low-fat, high-carbohydrate diet. *New England Journal of Medicine, 337,* 562–563.

Constantini, A., Solano, L., Di-Napoli, R., & Bosco, A. (1997). Relationship between hardiness and risk of burnout in a sample of 92 nurses working in oncology and AIDS wards. *Psychotherapy and Psychosomatics, 66,* 78–82.

Consumers Union. (1992, August). Wasted health care dollars. *Consumer Reports, 57,* 435–448.

Cook, W., & Medley, D. (1954). Proposed hostility and pharisaic-virtue scales for the MMPI. *Journal of Applied Psychology, 38,* 414–418.

Cooper, K. H. (1968). *Aerobics.* New York: Evans.

Cooper, K. H. (1982). *The aerobics program for total well-being.* New York: Evans.

Cooper, K. H. (1985). *Running without fear: How to reduce the risks of heart attack and sudden death during aerobic exercise.* New York: Evans.

Corbitt, G., Bailey, A., & Williams, G. (1990). HIV infection in Manchester, 1959. *Lancet, 336,* 51.

Corcoran, K. J. (1994, August). *Party on? Age, gender, and drinking at a college festival.* Presented at the 102nd convention of the American Psychological Association, Los Angeles, CA.

Cottington, E. M., & House, J. S. (1987). Occupational stress and health: A multivariate relationship. In A. Baum & J. E. Singer (Eds.), *Handbook of psychology and health: Vol. 5. Stress* (pp. 41–62). Hillsdale, NJ: Erlbaum.

Cotton, D. H. G. (1990). *Stress management: An integrated approach to therapy.* New York: Brunner/Mazel.

Cousins, N. (1983). *The healing heart; Antidote to panic and helplessness.* New York: Norton.

Cover, H., & Irwin, M. (1994). Immunity and depression: Insomnia, retardation, and reduction of natural killer cell activity. *Journal of Behavioral Medicine, 17,* 217–223.

Cowley, G. (1998, November 30). Cancer and diet. *Newsweek, 132,* 60–66.

Cowley, G., King, P., Hager, M., & Rosenberg, D. (1995, June 26). Going mainstream. *Newsweek, 125,* 56–57.

Cox, D. J., Freundlich, A., & Meyer, R. G. (1975). Differential effectiveness of electromyographic feedback, verbal relaxation instructions and medication placebo with tension headaches. *Journal of Consulting and Clinical Psychology, 43*, 892–898.

Cox, D. J., & Gonder-Frederick. L. (1992). Major developments in behavioral diabetes research. *Journal of Consulting and Clinical Psychology, 60*, 628–638.

Cramer, J. A., Mattson, R. H., Prevey, M. L., Scheyer, R. D., & Ouellette, V. L. (1989). How often is medication taken as prescribed? *Journal of the American Medical Association, 261*, 3273–3277.

Crawford, S. L., McGraw, S. A., Smith, K. W., McKinlay, J. B., & Pierson, J. E. (1994). Do blacks and whites differ in their use of health care for symptoms of coronary heart disease? *American Journal of Public Health, 84*, 957–964.

Creer, T. L., & Bender, B. G. (1993). Asthma. In R. J. Gatchel & E. B. Blanchard (Eds.), *Psychophysiological disorders: Research and clinical applications* (pp. 151–203). Washington, DC: American Psychological Association.

Crisp, A. H., & Burns, T. (1990). Primary anorexia nervosa in the male and female: A comparison of clinical features and prognosis. In A. E. Andersen (Ed.), *Males with eating disorders* (pp. 77–99). New York: Brunner/Mazel.

Critchlow, B. (1986). The powers of John Barleycorn: Beliefs about the effects of alcohol on social behavior. *American Psychologist, 41*, 751–764.

Cronk, C. E., & Sarvela, P. D. (1997). Alcohol, tobacco, and other drug use among rural/small town and urban youth: A secondary analysis of the monitoring the future data set. *American Journal of Public Health, 87*, 760–764.

Cruickshanks, K. J., Klein, R., Klein, B. E. K., Wiley, T. L., Nondahl, D. M., & Tweed, T. S. (1998). Cigarette smoking and hearing loss: The Epidemiology of Hearing Loss Study. *Journal of the American Medical Association, 279*, 1715–1719.

Cullen, K. J., Knuimon, M. W., & Ward, N. J. (1993). Alcohol and mortality in Busselton, Western Australia. *American Journal of Epidemiology, 137*, 242–248.

Cummings, J. H., & Bingham, S. A. (1998). Fortnightly review: Diet and the prevention of cancer. *British Medical Journal, 317*, 163–167.

Cummings, P., & Psaty, B. M. (1994). The association between cholesterol and death from injury. *Annals of Internal Medicine, 120*, 848–855.

Cunningham, A. J. (1981). Mind, body, and immune response. In R. Ader (Ed.), *Psychoneuroimmunology* (pp. 609–617). New York: Academic Press.

Curfman, G. D. (1993). Is exercise beneficial—or hazardous—to your heart? *New England Journal of Medicine, 329*, 1730–1731.

Cushman, R., James, W., & Waclawik, H. (1991). Physicians promoting bicycle helmets for children: A randomized trial. *American Journal of Public Health, 81*, 1044–1046.

Curtis, A. B., James, S. A., Strogatz, D. S., Raghunathan, T. E., & Harlow, S. (1997). Alcohol consumption and changes in blood pressure among African Americans: The Pitt County Study. *American Journal of Epidemiology, 146*, 727–733.

Czeisler, C. A., Johnson, M. P., Duffy, J. F., Brown, E. N., Ronda, J. M., & Kronauer, R. E. (1990). Exposure to bright light and darkness to treat physiologic maladaptation to night work. *New England Journal of Medicine, 322*, 1253–1259.

D'Agostino, R. B., Belanger, A. S., Kannel, W. B., & Higgins, M. (1995). Role of smoking in the U-shaped relation of cholesterol to mortality in men: The Framingham Study. *American Journal of Epidemiology, 141*, 822–827.

Dahlquist, L. N., Gil, K. M., Armstrong, D., DeLawyer, D. D., Green, P., & Wvori, D. (1986). Preparing children for medical examinations: The importance of previous medical experience. *Health Psychology, 5*, 249–259.

Daly, M. J. (1998). Untangling the genetics of a complex disease. *Journal of the American Medical Association, 280*, 652–653.

Danneberg, A. L., Gielen, A. C., Beilenson, P. L., Wilson, D. H., & Joffe, A. (1993). Bicycle helmet laws and educational campaigns: An evaluation of strategies to increase children's helmet use. *American Journal of Public Health, 83*, 667–674.

Dansky, B. S., Brewerton, T. D., Kilpatrick, D. G., & O'Neil, P. M. (1997). The National Women's Study: Relationship of victimization and posttraumatic stress disorder to bulimia nervosa. *International Journal of Eating Disorders, 21*, 213–228.

Darby, P. L., Garfinkel, P. E., Garner, D. M., & Coscina, D. V. (Eds.). (1983). *Anorexia nervosa: Recent developments in research*. New York: Liss.

Dattore, P. J., Shontz, F. C., & Coyne, L. (1980). Premorbid personality differentiation of cancer and noncancer groups: A list of the hypotheses of cancer proneness. *Journal of Consulting and Clinical Psychology, 48*, 388–394.

Davidson, L. L., Durkin, M. S., Kuhn, L., O'Connor, P., Barlow, B., & Heagarity, M. C. (1994). The impact of the Safe Kids/Healthy Neighborhoods Injury Prevention Program in Harlem, 1988–1991. *American Journal of Public Health, 84*, 580–586.

Davies, D. L. (1962). Normal drinking in recovered alcohol addicts. *Quarterly Journal of Studies on Alcohol, 24*, 321–332.

Daviglus, M. L., Stamler, J., Orencia, A. J., Dyer, A. R., Liu, K., Greenland, P., Walsh, M. K., Morris, D., & Shekelle, R. B. (1997). Fish consumption and the 30-year risk of fatal myocardial infarction. *New England Journal of Medicine, 336*, 1046–1053.

Davis, C., Brewer, H., & Ratusny, D. (1993). Behavioral frequency and psychological commitment: Necessary concepts in the study of excessive exercising. *Journal of Behavioral Medicine, 16*, 611–628.

Davis, C., Kennedy, S. H., Ravelski, E., & Dionne, M. (1994). The role of physical activity in the development and maintenance of eating disorders. *Psychological Medicine, 24*, 957–964.

Davis, C. E., Williams, D. H., Oganov, R. G., Tao, S.-C., Rywiik, S. L., Stein, Y., & Little, J. A., (1996). Sex differences in high density lipoprotein cholesterol in six countries. *American Journal of Epidemiology, 143,* 1100–1106.

Davis, R. C., Smith, B. E., & Nickles, L. B. (1998). The deterrent effect of prosecuting domestic violence misdemeanors. *Crime and Delinquency, 44,* 434–443.

Davison, G. C., Williams, M. E., Nezami. E., Bice, T. L., & DeQuattro, V. L. (1991). Relaxation, reduction in angry articulated thoughts, and improvements in borderline hypertension and heart rate. *Journal of Behavioral Medicine, 14,* 453–468.

Dawber, T. R. (1980). *The Framingham study: The epidemiology of atherosclerotic disease.* Cambridge, MA: Harvard University Press.

Deffenbacher, J. L. (1994). Anger reduction: Issues, assessment, and intervention strategies. In A. W. Siegman & T. W. Smith (Eds.), *Anger, hostility, and the heart* (pp. 239–269). Hillsdale, NJ: Erlbaum.

Deffenbacher, J. L., & Stark, R. S. (1992). Relaxation and cognitive-relaxation treatments of general anger. *Journal of Counseling Psychology, 39,* 158–167.

DeJong, W., & Wallack, L. (1992). The role of designated driver programs in the prevention of alcohol-impaired driving: A critical reassessment. *Health Education Quarterly, 19,* 429–442.

De Leo, D., Carollo, G., Dello Bueno, M. (1995). Lower suicide rates associated with a Tele-Help/Tele-Check service for the elderly at home. *American Journal of Psychiatry, 152,* 632–634.

DeLongis, A., Folkman, S., & Lazarus, R. S. (1988). The impact of daily stress on health and mood: Psychological and social resources as mediators. *Journal of Personality and Social Psychology, 54,* 486–495.

Dembroski, T. M., & MacDougall, J. M. (1985). Beyond global Type A: Relationships of paralinguistic attributes, hostility, and anger-in to coronary heart disease. In T. Field, P. McCabe, & N. Scheiderman (Eds.), *Stress and coping* (pp. 223–241). Hillsdale, NJ: Erlbaum.

Dembroski, T. M., MacDougall, J. M., Williams, R. B., Haney, T. L., & Blumenthal, J. A. (1985). Components of Type A, hostility, and anger-in: Relationship to angiographic findings. *Psychosomatic Medicine, 47,* 219–233.

DeNitto, E. (1993, September 29). 100 leaders monopolize pain relievers. *Advertising Age, 64,* 2.

Derogatis, L. R. (1977). *Manual for the Symptom Checklist-90, Revised.* Baltimore, MD: John Hopkins University School of Medicine.

Derogatis, L. R., Morrow, G. R., Fetting, J., Penman, D., Piasetsky, S., Schmale, A. M., Henrichs, M., & Carnicke, C. L. M. (1983). The prevalence of psychiatric disorders among cancer patients. *Journal of the American Medical Association, 249,* 751–757.

de Vincenzi, I. (1994). A longitudinal study of human immunodeficiency virus transmission by heterosexual partners. *New England Journal of Medicine, 331,* 341–346.

Devins, G. M., Mandin, H., Hons, R. B., Burgess, E. D., Klassen, J., Taub, K., Schorr, S., Letourneau, P. K., & Buckle, S. (1990). Illness intrusiveness and quality of life in end-stage renal disease: Comparison and stability across treatment modalities. *Health Psychology, 9,* 117–142.

Dew, M. A., Bromet, E. J., Brent, D., & Greenhouse, J. B. (1987). A quantitative literature review of the effectiveness of suicide prevention centers. *Journal of Consulting and Clinical Psychology, 55,* 239–244.

Deyo, R. A. (1998, August). Low-back pain. *Scientific American, 279,* 48–53.

DiClemente, C. C. (1981). Self-efficacy and smoking cessation maintenance: A preliminary report. *Cognitive Therapy and Research, 5,* 175–187.

Diehr, P., Bild, D. E., Harris, T. B., Duxbury, A., Siscovick, D., & Rossi, M. (1998). Body mass index and mortality in nonsmoking older adults: The Cardiovascular Health Study. *American Journal of Public Health, 88,* 623–629.

DiMatteo, M. R. (1994). Enhancing patient adherence to medical recommendations. *Journal of the American Medical Association, 271,* 79, 83.

DiMatteo, M. R. (1997). Health behaviors and care decisions: An overview of professional-patient communication. In D. S. Gochman (Ed.), *Handbook of health behavior research II: Provider determinants* (pp. 5–22). New York: Plenum Press.

DiMatteo, M. R., & DiNicola, D. D. (1982). *Achieving patient compliance: The psychology of the medical practitioner's role.* New York: Pergamon Press.

Dinges, D. F., Douglas, S. D., Zaugg, L., Campbell, D. E., McMann, J. M., Whitehouse, W. G., Orme, E. C., Kapoor, S. C., Icaza, E., & Orne, M. T. (1994). Leukocytosis and natural killer cell function parallel neurobehavioral fatigue induced by 64 hours of sleep deprivation. *Journal of Clinical Investigation, 93,* 1930–1939.

Dinges, D. F., Pack, F., Williams, K., Gillen, K. A., Powell, J. W., Ott, G. E., Aptowicz, C., & Pack, A. I. (1997). Cumulative sleepiness, mood disturbance and psychomotor vigilance performance decrements during a week of sleep restricted to 4–5 hours per might. *Sleep, 20,* 267–277.

Dinges, D. F., Whitehouse, W. G., Orne, E. C., Bloom, P. B., Carlin, M. M., Bauer, N. K., Gillen, K. A., Shapiro, B. S., Ohene, F. K., Dampier, C. & Orne, M. T. (1997). Self-hypnosis training as an adjunctive treatment in the management of pain associated with sickle cell disease. *International Journal of Clinical and Experimental Hypnosis, 45,* 417–432.

DiNicola, D. D., & DiMatteo, M. R. (1984). Practitioners, patients, and compliance with medical regimens: A social psychological perspective. In A. Baum, S. E. Taylor, & J. E. Singer (Eds.), *Handbook of psychology and health: Vol. 4. Social psychological aspects of health* (pp. 55–84). Hillsdale, NJ: Erlbaum.

Dishman, R. K., & Buckworth, J. (1997). Adherence to physical activity. In W. P. Morgan (Ed.), *Physical activity and mental health* (pp. 63–80). Washington, DC: Taylor & Francis.

Dolecek, T. A., Milas, N. C., Van Horn, L. V., Farrand, M. E., Gorder, D. D., Duchene, A. G., Dyer, J. R., Stone, P. A., & Randall, B. L. (1986). A long-term nutrition experience: Lipid responses and dietary adherence patterns in the Multiple Risk Factor Intervention Trial. *Journal of the American Dietetic Association, 86,* 752–758.

Doll, R., & Hill, A. B. (1956). Lung cancer and other causes of death in relation to smoking: A second report on the mortality of British doctors. *British Medical Journal,* 1071–1081.

Doll, R., & Peto, R. (1981). *The causes of cancer.* New York: Oxford University Press.

Dollinger, M., Rosenbaum, E. H., & Cable, G. (1991). *Everyone's guide to cancer therapy.* Kansas City: Somerville.

Dolnick, E. (1995). Hot heads and heart attacks. *Health, 9*(4), 58–64.

Donaldson, C. S., Stanger, L. M., Donaldson, M. W., Cram, J., & Skubick, D. L. (1993). A randomized crossover investigation of a back pain and disability prevention program: Possible mechanisms of change. *Journal of Occupational Rehabilitation, 3,* 83–94.

Donaldson, S. I., Graham, J. W., Piccinin, A. M., & Hansen, W. B. (1995). Resistance-skills training and onset of alcohol use: Evidence for beneficial and potentially harmful effects in public schools and in private Catholic schools. *Health Psychology, 14,* 291–300.

Donovan, M. I. (1989). Relieving pain: The current basis for practice. In S. G. Funk, E. M. Tornquist, M. T. Champagne, L. A. Copp, & R. A. Wiese (Eds.), *Key aspects of comfort: Management of pain, fatigue, and nausea* (pp. 25–31). New York: Springer.

Dressler, W. W., & Oths, K. S. (1997). Cultural determinants of health behavior. In D. S. Gochman (Ed.), *Handbook of health behavior research I: Personal and social determinants* (pp. 359–378). New York: Plenum Press.

Driver, H. E., & Swann, P. F. (1987). Alcohol and human cancer [review]. *Anticancer Research, 7,* 309–320.

Dubuisson, D., & Melzack, R. (1976). Classification of clinical pain descriptions by multiple group discriminant analysis. *Experimental Neurology, 51,* 480–487.

Dudgeon, D., Raubertas, R. F., & Rosenthal, S. M. (1993). The Short-Form McGill Pain Questionnaire in chronic cancer pain. *Journal of Pain and Symptom Management, 8,* 191–195.

Dunbar, H. F. (1943). *Psychomatic diagnosis.* New York: Hoeber.

Duncan, J. J., Gordon, N. F., & Scott, C. B. (1991). Women walking for health and fitness: How much is enough. *Journal of the American Medical Association, 266,* 3295–3299.

Dufouil, C. Ducimetiere, P. & Apérovitch, A. (1997). Sex differences in the association between alcohol consumption and cognitive performance. *American Journal of Epidemiology, 146,* 405–412.

Dunkel-Schetter, C., Feinstein, L. G., Taylor, S. E., & Falke, R. L. (1992). Patterns of coping with cancer. *Health Psychology, 11,* 79–87.

Dunkel-Schetter, C., & Lobel, M. (1998). Pregnancy and childbirth. In E. A. Blechman & K. D. Brownell (Eds.), *Behavioral medicine and women: A comprehensive handbook* (pp. 475–482). New York: Guilford.

Dunkel-Schetter, C., & Wortman, C. B. (1982). The interpersonal dynamics of cancer: Problems in social relationships and their impact on the patient. In H. S. Friedman & M. R. DiMatteo (Eds.), *Interpersonal issues in health care.* New York: Academic Press.

Dunn, A. L., Marcus, B. H., Kampert, J. B., Garcia, M. E., Kohl, H. W., III, & Blair, S. N. (1999). Comparison of lifestyle and structured interventions to increase physical activity and cardiorespiratory fitness. *Journal of the American Medical Association, 281,* 327–334.

Duquette, A., Kerouac, S., Sandhu, B. K., Ducharme, F., & Saulnier, P. (1997). Psychosocial determinants of burnout in geriatric nursing. *International Journal of Nursing Studies, 32,* 443–456.

Durazo-Arvizu, R. A., McGee, D. L., Cooper, R. S., Liao, Y., & Luke, A. (1998). Mortality and optimal body mass index in a sample of the US population. *American Journal of Epidemiology, 147,* 739–749.

Durlak, J. A. (1997). *Successful prevention programs for children and adolescents.* New York: Plenum Press.

Dwyer, J. H. (1995). Genes, blood pressure, and African heritage. *Lancet, 346,* 392.

Eaker, E. D., Pinsky, J., & Castelli, W. P. (1992). Myocardial infarction and coronary death among women: Psychosocial predictors from a 20-year follow-up of women in the Framingham Study. *American Journal of Epidemiology, 135,* 854–864.

Eakin, J. M. (1997). Work-related determinants of health behavior. In D. S. Gochman (Ed.), *Handbook of health behavior research I: Personal and social determinants* (pp. 337–357). New York: Plenum Press.

Eckardt, M. J., Harford, T. C., Kaelber, C. T., Parker, E. S., Rosenthal, L. S., Ryback, R. S., Salmoiraghi, G. C., Vanderveen, E., & Warren, K. R. (1981). Health hazards associated with alcohol consumption. *Journal of the American Medical Association, 246,* 648–666.

Eckert, E. D. (1983). Behavior modification in anorexia nervosa: A comparison of two reinforcement schedules. In P. L. Darby, P. E. Garfinkel, D. M. Garner, & D. V. Coscina (Eds.), *Anorexia nervosa: Recent developments in research.* New York: Liss.

Eckholm, E. (1977). *The picture of health: Environmental sources of disease.* New York: Norton.

Eckholm, E., & Tierney, J. (1990, September 16). AIDS in Africa: A killer rages on. *The New York Times,* pp. A1, A10.

Edwards, G. (1977). The alcohol dependence syndrome: Usefulness of an idea. In G. Edwards & M. Grant (Eds.), *Alcoholism: New knowledge and new responses.* London: Croom Helm.

Edwards, G., & Gross, M. M. (1976). Alcohol dependence: Provisional description of a clinical syndrome. *British Medical Journal,* 1058–1061.

Edwards, G., Gross, M. M., Keller, M., Moser, J., & Room, R. (1977). *Alcohol-related disabilities* (WHO Offset Pub. No. 32). Geneva, Switzerland: World Health Organization.

Eisenberg, D. M., Kessler, R. C., Foster, C., Norlock, F. E., Calkins, D. R., & Delbanco, T. L. (1993). Unconventional medicine in the United States: Prevalence, costs, and patterns of use. *New England Journal of Medicine, 328,* 246–252.

El-Faizy, M., & Reinsch, S. (1994). Home safety intervention for the prevention of falls. *Physical and Occupational Therapy in Geriatrics, 12,* 33–49.

Elkins, P. D., & Roberts, M. C. (1983). Psychological preparation for pediatric hospitalization. *Clinical Psychology Review, 3,* 275–295.

Ellenhorst-Ryan, J. M. (1997). The nature of cancer. In C. Varricchio, M. Pierce, C. Walker, & T. B. Ades (Eds.), *A cancer source book for nurses* (7th ed.) (pp. 27–34). Atlanta: The American Cancer Society.

Ellestad, M. H. (1996). *Stress testing* (4th ed.). Philadelphia: Davis.

Ellickson, P., Saner, H., & McGuigan, K. A. (1997). Profiles of violent youth: Substance use and other concurrent problems. *American Journal of Public Health, 87,* 985–991.

Elliott, T. E., & Elliott, B. A. (1992). Physician attitudes and beliefs about use of morphine for cancer pain. *Journal of Pain and Symptom Management, 7,* 141–148.

Ellis, A. (1962). *Reason and emotion in psychotherapy.* New York: Stuart.

Emery, C. F., Hauck, E. R., Blumethal, J. A. (1992). Exercise adherence or maintenance among older adults: 1-year follow-up study. *Psychology and Aging, 7,* 466–470.

Emmons, K. M., Wechsler, H., Dowdall, G., & Abraham, M. (1998). Predictors of smoking among U.S. college students. *American Journal of Public Health, 88,* 104–107.

Emrick, C. D., & Hansen, J. (1983). Assertions regarding effectiveness of treatment for alcoholism: Fact or fantasy? *American Psychologist, 38,* 1078–1088.

Engel, G. L. (1977). The need for a new medical model: A challenge for biomedicine. *Science, 196,* 129–136.

Ennett, S. T., Tobler, N. S., Ringwalt, C. L., & Flewelling, R. L. (1994). How effective is drug abuse resistance education? A meta-analysis of Project DARE outcome evaluations. *American Journal of Public Health, 84,* 1394–1401.

Enqvist, B. & Fischer, K. (1997). Preoperative hypnotic techniques reduce consumption of analgesics after surgical removal of third mandibular molars: A brief communication. *International Journal of Clinical and Experimental Hypnosis, 45,* 102–108.

Epstein, L. H., Valoski, A., Wing, R. R., & McCurley, J. (1994). Ten-year outcomes of behavioral family-based treatment for childhood obesity. *Health Psychology, 13,* 371–388.

Ernster, V. L., Grady, D., Müke, R., Black, D., Selby, J., & Kerlikowske, K. (1995). Facial wrinkling in men and women by smoking status. *American Journal of Public Health, 85,* 78–82.

Esplen, M. J., Toner, B., Hunter, J., Glendon, G., Butler, K., & Field, B. (1998). A group therapy approach to facilitate integration of risk information for women at risk for breast cancer. *Canadian Journal of Psychiatry, 43,* 375–380.

Esterling, B. A., Kiecolt-Glaser, J. K., Bodnar, J. C., & Glaser, R. (1994). Chronic stress, social support, and persistent alterations in the natural killer cell response to cytokines in older adults. *Health Psychology, 13,* 291–298.

Evans, D. A., Funkenstein, H., Albert, M. S., Scherr, P. A., Cook, N. R., Chown, M. J., Hebert, L. E., Hennekens, C. H., & Taylor, J. O. (1989). Prevalence of Alzheimer's disease in a community population of older persons: Higher than previously reported. *Journal of the American Medical Association, 262,* 2551–2556.

Evans, F. J. (1985). Expectancy, therapeutic instructions, and the placebo response. In L. White, B. Tursky, & G. E. Schwartz (Eds.), *Placebo: Theory, research, and mechanisms* (pp. 215–228). New York: Guilford Press.

Evans, G. W., Hygge, S., & Bullinger, M. (1995). Chronic noise and psychological stress. *Psychological Science, 6,* 333–338.

Evans, L. (1987). Fatality risk reduction from safety belt use. *Journal of Trauma, 27,* 746–749.

Evans, R. I. (1976). Smoking in children: Developing a social psychological strategy of deterrence. *Preventive Medicine, 5,* 122–127.

Evans, R. I., Rozelle, R. M., Maxwell, S. E., Raines, B. E., Dill, C. A., Guthrie, T. J., Henderson, A. H., & Hill, D. C. (1981). Social modeling films to deter smoking in adolescents: Results of a three year field investigation. *Journal of Applied Psychology, 66,* 399–414.

Evans, R. I., Smith, C. K., & Raines, B. E. (1984). Deterring cigarette smoking in adolescents: A psychosocial-behavioral analysis of an intervention strategy. In A. Baum, S. E. Taylor, & J. E. Singer (Eds.), *Handbook of psychology and health: Vol. 4. Social psychological aspects of health* (pp. 301–318). Hillsdale, NJ: Erlbaum.

Everhart, J., & Wright, D. (1995). Diabetes mellitus as a risk factor for pancreatic cancer: A meta analysis. *Journal of the American Medical Association, 273,* 1605–1609.

Everson, S. A., Kauhanen, J., Kaplan, G. A., Goldberg, D. E., Julkunen, J., Tuomilehto J., & Salonen, J. T. (1997). Hostility and increased risk of mortality and acute myocardial infarction: The mediating role of behavioral risk factors. *American Journal of Epidemiology, 146,* 142–152.

Fairburn, C. G., Hay, P. J., & Welch, S. L. (1993). Binge eating and bulimia nervosa: Distribution and determinants. In C. G. Fairburn & G. T. Wilson (Eds.), *Binge eating: Nature, assessment, and treatment* (pp. 123–143). New York: Guilford Press.

Falk, A., Hanson, B. S., Issacsson, S., & Ostergren, P. (1992). Job strain and mortality in elderly men: Social network, support, and influence as buffers. *American Journal of Public Health, 82,* 1136–1139.

Farley, C., Haddad, S., & Brown, B. (1996). The effects of a 4-year program promoting bicycle helmet use among children in Quebec. *American Journal of Public Health, 86,* 46–51.

Farrer, L. A., Cupples, A., Haines, J. L., Hyman, B., Kukull, W. A., Mayeaux, R., Myers, R. H., Pericak-Vance, M. A., Risch, N., & van Duijn, C. M. (1998). Effects of age, sex, and ethnicity on association between apolipoprotein E genotype and Alzheimer disease: A meta-analysis. *Journal of the American Medical Association, 278,* 1349–1356.

Fawzy, F. I., Fawzy, N. W., Hyun, C. S., Elashoff, R., Guthrie, D., Fahley, J. L., & Morton, D. L. (1993). Malignant melanoma: Effects of an early structures psychiatric intervention, coping, and affective state on recurrence and survival 6 years later. *Archives of General Psychiatry, 50,* 681–689.

Feist, J. & Feist G. J. (1998). *Theories of personality* (4th ed.). Boston: McGraw-Hill.

Feldman, J. (1966). *The dissemination of health information.* Chicago: Aldine.

Felson, D. T., Zhang, Y., Hannan, M. T., Kannel, W. B., & Kiel, D. P. (1995). Alcohol intake and bone mineral density in elderly men and women: The Framingham Study. *American Journal of Epidemiology, 142,* 485–492.

Ferguson, S. A., & Lund, A. K. (1995). Driver fatalities in 1985–1994 air bag cars. Arlington, VA: *Insurance Institute for Highway Safety.*

Fernandez, E., & Sheffield, J. (1996). Relative contributions of life events versus daily hassles to the frequency and intensity of headaches. *Headache, 36,* 595–602.

Ferraro, D. P. (1980). Acute effects of marijuana on human memory and cognition. In R. C. Peterson (Ed.), *Marijuana research findings.* National Institute on Drug Abuse. Washington, DC: U.S. Government Printing Office.

Fichten, C. S., Creti, L., Amsel, R., Brender, W., Weinstein, N., & Libman, E. (1995). Poor sleepers who do not complain of insomnia: Myths and realities about psychological and lifestyle characteristics of older good and poor sleepers. *Journal of Behavioral Medicine, 18,* 189–223.

Field, T. M. (1998). Massage therapy effects. *American Psychologist, 53,* 1270–1281.

Fielding, J. E. (1985). Smoking: Health effects and control. *New England Journal of Medicine, 313,* 491–498.

Fife, B. L. (1994). The conceptualization of meaning in illness. *Social Science in Medicine, 38,* 309–316.

Fife, B. L., Irick, N., & Painter, J. D. (1993). A comparative study of the attitudes of physicians and nurses toward the management of cancer pain. *Journal of Pain Symptom Management, 8,* 132–139.

Fingerhut, L. A. (1993). *Firearm mortality among children, youth, and young adults 1–34 years of age, trends and current status: United States, 1985–1990.* Advance Data from Vital and Health Statistics, No., 231. Washington, DC: U.S. Government Printing Office.

Finsen, V., Persen, L., Lovlien, M., Veslegaard, E., Simensen, M., Gasvann, A., & Benum, P. (1988). Transcutaneous electrical nerve stimulation after major amputation. *British Journal of Bone and Joint Surgery, 70*(B), 109–112.

Fiore, M. C., Bailey, W. C., Cohen, S. J., Dorfman, S. F., Goldstein, M. G., Gritz, E. R., Heyman, R. B., Holbrook, J., Jaén, C. R., Kottke, T. E., Lando, H. A., Mecklenburg, R., Mullen, P. D., Nett, L. M., Robinson, L., Stitzer, M. L., Tommasello, A. C., Villejo, L., & Wewers, M. E. (1996). *Smoking Cessation: Clinical Practice Guideline No. 18.* AHCPR Publication No. 69–0692. Rockville, MD: U.S. Department of Health and Human Services. Public Health Service, Agency for Health Care Police and Research.

Fishbein, M. & Ajzen, I. (1975). *Belief, attitude, intention, and behavior: An introduction to theory and research.* Reading, MA: Addison-Wesley.

Fisher, E. B., Jr., Arfken, C. L., Heins, J. M., Houston, C. A., Jeffe, D. B., & Sykes, R. K. (1997). Acceptance of diabetes regimens in adults. In D. S. Gochman (Ed.), *Handbook of health behavior research II: Provider determinants* (pp. 189–212). New York: Plenum Press.

Fisher, M. J. (1995, April 3). Health coverage lacking among minority-Americans. *National Underwriter Property & Casualty-Risk & Benefits Management, 14,* 3.

Fitzgerald, T. E., Tennen, H., Afflect, G., & Pransky, G. S. (1993). The relative importance of dispositional optimism and control appraisals in quality of life after coronary artery bypass surgery. *Journal of Behavioral Medicine, 16,* 25–43.

Fixx, J. F. (1977). *The complete book of running.* New York: Random House.

Fixx, J. F. (1980). *Jim Fixx's second book of running.* New York: Random House.

Flanders, W. D., & Rothman, K. J. (1982). Interaction of alcohol and tobacco in laryngeal cancer. *American Journal of Epidemiology, 115,* 371–379.

Flay, B. R., Koepke, D., Thomson, S. J., Santi, S., Best, A., & Brown, S. (1989). Six-year follow-up of the first Waterloo school smoking prevention trial. *American Journal of Public Health, 79,* 1371–1376.

Flegal, K. M., Troiano, R. P., Pamuk, E. R., Kuczmarski, R. J., & Campbell, S. M. (1995). The influence of smoking cessation on the prevalence of overweight in the United States. *New England Journal of Medicine, 333,* 1165–1170.

Fleishman, J. A., & Fogel, B. (1994). Coping and depressive symptoms among people with AIDS. *Health Psychology, 13,* 156–169.

Flett, G. L., Hewitt, P. L., Blankstein, K. R., & Mosher, S. W. (1995). Perfectionism, life events, and depressive symptoms: A test of a diathesis-stress model. *Current Psychology: Developmental Learning, Personality-Social, 14,* 112–137.

Fleury, J. (1992). The application of motivational theory to cardiovascular risk reduction. *Image: Journal of Nursing Scholarship, 24,* 229–239.

Flor, H., & Birbaumer, N. (1993). Comparison of the efficacy of electromyographic biofeedback, cognitive-behavioral therapy, and conservative medical interventions in the treatment of chronic musculoskeletal pain. *Journal of Consulting and Clinical Psychology, 61,* 653–658.

Folkman, S. (1993). Psychosocial effects of HIV infection. In L. Goldberger & S. Breznitz (Eds.), *Handbook of stress: Theoretical and clinical aspects* (2nd ed., pp. 658–681). New York: Free Press.

Folsom, A. R., Kaye, S. A., Sellers, T. A., Hong, C. P., Cerhan, J. D., Potter, J. D., & Prineas, R. J. (1993). Body fat distribution and 5-year risk of death in older women. *Journal of the American Medical Association, 269,* 483–487.

Fontana, A. F., Kerns, R. D., Rosenberg, R. L., & Colonese, K. L. (1989). Support, stress, and recovery from coronary heart disease: A longitudinal causal model. *Health Psychology, 8,* 175–193.

Fontham, E. T. H., Correa, P., Reynolds, P., Wu-Williams, A., Buffler, P. A., Greenberg, R. S., Chen, V. W., Alterman, T., Boyd, P., Austin, D. F., & Liff, J. (1994). Environmental tobacco smoke and lung cancer in nonsmoking women: A multicenter study. *Journal of the American Medical Association, 271,* 1952–1959.

Forbes, G. B. (1992). Exercise and lean weight: The influence of body weight. *Nutrition Reviews, 50,* 147–161.

Forde, D. R. (1993). Perceived crime, fear of crime, and walking alone at night. *Psychological Reports, 73,* 403–407.

Fordyce, W. E. (1974). Pain viewed as learned behavior. In J. J. Bonica (Ed.), *Advances in neurology* (Vol. 4). New York: Raven Press.

Fordyce, W. E. (1976). *Behavioral methods for chronic pain and illness.* St. Louis: Mosby.

Fordyce, W. E. (1990a). Contingency management. In J. J. Bonica (Ed.), *The management of pain* (2nd ed., pp. 1702–1710). Malvern, PA: Lea & Febiger.

Fordyce, W. E. (1990b). Learned pain: Pain as behavior. In J. J. Bonica (Ed.), *The management of pain* (2nd ed., pp. 291–299). Malvern, PA: Lea & Febiger.

Fordyce, W. E., Brockway, J. A., Bergman, J. A., & Spengler, D. (1986). Acute back pain: A control-group comparison of behavioral vs. traditional management methods. *Journal of Behavioral Medicine, 9,* 127–140.

Fordyce, W. E., Shelton, J. L., & Dundore, D. E. (1982). The modification of avoidance learning pain behavior. *Journal of Behavioral Medicine, 5,* 405–414.

Fortmann, S. P., & Killen, J. D. (1994). Who shall quit? Comparisons of volunteer and population-based recruitment in two minimal-contact smoking cessation studies. *American Journal of Epidemiology, 140,* 39–51.

Francis, M. E., & Pennebaker, J. W. (1992). Putting stress into words: The impact of writing on physiological, absentee, and self-reported emotional well-being measures. *American Journal of Health Promotion, 6,* 280–287.

Frank, E., Winkleby, M. A., Altman, D. G., Rockhill, B., & Fortmann, S. P. (1991). Predictors of physicians' smoking cessation advice. *Journal of the American Medical Association, 266,* 3139–3144.

Frank, R. G., Bouman, D. E., Cain, K., & Watts, C. (1992). A preliminary study of a traumatic injury program. *Psychology and Health, 8,* 129–140.

Franz, I. D. (1913). On psychology and medical education. *Science, 38,* 555–566.

Frasure-Smith, N., Lespérance, F., & Talajic, M. (1995). The impact of negative emotions on prognosis following myocardial infarction: Is it more than depression? *Health Psychology, 14,* 388–398.

Freedman, D. S., Williamson, D. F., Croft, J. B., Ballew, C., & Byers, T. (1995). Relationship of body fat distribution to ischemic heart disease: The National Health and Nutrition Examination Survey I (NHANES I): Epidemiologic Follow-up Study. *American Journal of Epidemiology, 142,* 53–63.

Freeman, R. C., Rodriguez, G. M., & French, J. F. (1994). A comparison of male and female intravenous drug users' risk behaviors for HIV infection. *American Journal of Drug and Alcohol Abuse, 20,* 129–157.

French, S. A., Perry, C. L., Leon, G. R., & Fulkerson, J. A. (1994). Weight concerns, dieting behavior and smoking initiation among adolescents: A prospective study. *American Journal of Public Health, 84,* 1818–1820.

French, S. A., Story, M., Downes, B., Resnick, M. D., & Blum, R. W. (1995). Frequent dieting among adolescents: Psychosocial and health behavior correlates. *American Journal of Public Health, 85,* 695–701.

Freund, K. M., D'Agostino, R. B., Belanger, A. J., Kannel, W. B., & Stokes, J., III. (1992). Predictors of smoking cessation: The Framingham Study. *American Journal of Epidemiology, 135,* 957–964.

Frezza, M., di Padova, C., Pozzato, G., Terpin, M., Baraona, E., & Lieber, C. S. (1990). High blood alcohol levels in women: The role of decreased gastric alcohol dehydrogenase activity and first-pass metabolism. *New England Journal of Medicine, 322,* 95–99.

Fried, L. P., Kronmal, R. A., Newman, A. B., Bild, D. E., Mittelmark, M. B., Polak, J. F., Robbins, J. A., & Gardin, J. M. (1998). Risk factors for 5-year mortality in older adults: The Cardiovascular Health Study. *Journal of the American Medical Association, 279,* 585–592.

Friedländer, L. (1968). *Roman life and manners under the early empire.* New York: Barnes & Noble.

Friedman, Edward S., Clark, D. B., & Gershon, S. (1992). Stress, anxiety, and depression: Review of biological, diagnostic, and nosologic issues. *Journal of Anxiety Disorders, 6,* 337–363.

Friedman, L. A., & Kimball, A. W. (1986). Coronary heart disease mortality and alcohol consumption in Framingham. *American Journal of Epidemiology, 124,* 481–489.

Friedman, M., & Rosenman, R. H. (1974). *Type A behavior and your heart.* New York: Knopf.

Fries, J. F. (1998). Reducing the need and demand for medical services. *Psychosomatic Medicine, 60,* 140–142.

Froland, S. S., Jenum, P., Lendboe, C. F., Wefring, K. W., Linnestad, P. J., & Bohmer, T. (1988). HIV-1 infection in a Norwegian family before 1970. *Lancet, i,* 1344–1345.

Frost, K., Frank, E., & Maibach, E. (1997). Relative risk in the news media: A quantification of misrepresentation. *American Journal of Public Health, 87,* 842–845.

Fuchs, C. S., Stampfer, M. J., Colditz, G. A., Giovannucci, E. L., Manson, J. E., Kawachi, I., Hunter, D. J., Hankinson, S. E., Hennekens, C. H., Rosner, B., Speizer, F. E., & Willett, W. C. (1995). Alcohol consumption and mortality among women. *New England Journal of Medicine, 332*, 1245–1250.

Fuller, R. K., Branchey, L., Brightwell, D. R., Derman, R. M., Emrick, C. D., Iber, F. L., James, K. E., Lacoursiere, R. B., Lee, K. K., Lowenstam, I., Maany, I., Neiderhiser, D., Nocks, J. J., & Shaw, S. (1986). Disulfiram treatment of alcoholism: A Veterans Administration cooperative study. *Journal of the American Medical Association, 256*, 1449–1455.

Fuller, T. D., Edwards, J. N., Vorakitphokatorn, S., & Sermsri, S. (1996). Chronic stress and psychological well-being: Evidence from Thailand on household crowding. *Social Science and Medicine, 42*, 265–280.

Funk, S. C. (1992). Hardiness: A review of theory and research. *Health Psychology, 11*, 335–345.

Furnham, A., & Kramers, M. (1989). Eating-problem patients conceptions of normality. *Journal of Genetic Psychology, 150*, 147–153.

Futterman, A. D., Kemeny, M. E., Shapiro, D., & Fahey, J. L. (1994). Immunological and physiological changes associated with induced positive and negative mood. *Psychosomatic Medicine, 56*, 499–511.

Gallagher, E. J., Viscoli, C. M., & Horwitz, R. I. (1993). The relationship of treatment adherence to the risk of death after myocardial infarction in women. *Journal of the American Medical Association, 270*, 742–743.

Galton, F. (1879). Psychometric experiments. *Brain, 2*, 149–162.

Galton, F. (1883). *Inquiries into human faculty and its development*. London: Macmillan.

Gammon, M. D., John, E. M., & Britton, J. A. (1998). Recreational and occupational physical activities and risk of breast cancer. *Journal of the National Cancer Institute, 90*, 100–117.

Gao, F., Bailes, E., Robertson, D. L., Chen, Y., Rodenburg, C. M., Michael, S. F., Cummins, L. B., Arthur, L. O., Peeters, M., Shaw, G. M., Sharp, P. M., & Hahn, B. H. (1999). Origin of HIV-1 in the chimpanzee Pan tryoglodytes troglodytes. *Nature, 397*, 436–441.

Garbarino, J., & Kostelny, K. (1997). What children can tell us about living in a war zone. In J. D. Osofsky (Ed.), *Children in a violent society* (pp. 32–41). New York: Guilford Press.

Garfinkel, P. E., & Garner, D. M. (1982). *Anorexia nervosa: A multidimensional perspective*. New York: Brunner/Mazel.

Garfinkel, P. E., & Garner, D. M. (1984). Bulimia in anorexia nervosa. In R. C. Hawkins, II, W. J. Fremouw, & P. F. Clement (Eds.), *The binge-purge syndrome: Diagnosis, treatment and research*. New York: Springer.

Garfinkel, P. E., Moldofsky, H., & Garner, D. M. (1977). The outcome of anorexia nervosa: Significance of clinical features, body image, and behavior modification. In R. A. Vigersky (Ed.), *Anorexia nervosa* (pp. 315–329). New York: Raven Press.

Garland, A. F., & Zigler, E. F. (1994). Psychological correlates of help-seeking attitudes among children and adolescents. *American Journal of Orthopsychiatry, 64*, 586–593.

Garner, D. M., & Garfinkel, P. E. (1980). Social-cultural factors in the development of anorexia nervosa. *Psychological Medicine, 10*, 647–656.

Garner, D. M., Garfinkel, P. E., & Bemis, K. M. (1982). A multidimensional psychotherapy for anorexia nervosa. *International Journal of Eating Disorders, 1*, 3–46.

Garner, D. M., Garfinkel, P. E., Schwartz, D., & Thompson, M. (1980). Cultural expectations of thinness in women. *Psychological Reports, 47*, 483–491.

Garrison, W. T., & McQuiston, S. (1989). *Chronic illness during childhood and adolescence: Psychological aspects*. Newbury Park, CA: Sage.

Gastorf, J. W., & Galanos, A. N. (1983). Patient compliance and physicians' attitude. *Family Practice Research Journal, 2*, 190–198.

Gatchel, R. J. (1993). Psychophysiological disorders: Past and present perspectives. In R. J. Gatchel & E. B. Blanchard (Eds.), *Psychophysiological disorders: Research and clinical applications* (pp. 1–21). Washington, DC: American Psychological Association.

Gatchel, R. J. (1996). Psychological disorders and chronic pain: Cause-and-effect relationships. In R. J. Gatchel & D. C. Turk (Eds.), *Psychological approaches to pain management: A practitioner's handbook*. New York: Guilford Press.

Gaziano, J. M., Buring, J. E., Breslow, J. L., Goldhaber, S. Z., Rosner, B., VanDenburgh, M., Willett, W., & Hennekens, C. H. (1993). Moderate alcohol intake, increased levels of high-density lipoprotein and its subfractions, and decreased risk of myocardial infarction. *New England Journal of Medicine, 329*, 1829–1834.

Genuis, M. L. (1995). The use of hypnosis in helping cancer patients control anxiety, pain, and emesis: A review of recent empirical studies. *American Journal of Clinical Hypnosis, 37*, 316–326.

Gibbons, A. (1991). Does war on cancer equal war on poverty? *Science, 253*, 260.

Gibbons, F. X., Eggleston, T. J., & Benthin, A. C. (1997). Cognitive reactions to smoking relapse: The reciprocal relation between dissonance and self-esteem. *Journal of Personality and Social Psychology, 72*, 184–195.

Gilbar, O. (1989). Who refuses chemotherapy: A profile. *Psychological Reports, 64*, 1291–1297.

Gilbert, D. G. (1995). *Smoking: Individual differences, psychopathology, and emotion*. Washington DC: Taylor & Francis.

Gillum, R. F., Mussolino, M. E., & Ingram, D. D. (1996). Physical activity and stroke incidence in women and men: The NHANES Epidemiologic Follow-Up Study. *American Journal of Epidemiology, 143*, 660–869.

Gillum, R. F., Mussolino, M. E., & Madans, J. H. (1998). Coronary heart disease risk factors and attributable risks in African-American women and men: NHANES I Epidemiologic Follow-Up Study. *American Journal of Public Health, 88*, 913–917.

Giovannucci, E., (1999). Tomatoes, tomato-based products, lycopene, and cancer: Review of the epidemiologic literature. *Journal of the National Cancer Institute, 91,* 317–331.

Giovino, G. A., Schooley, M. W., Zhu, B., Chrismon, J. H., Tomar, S. L., Peddicord, J. P., Merritt, R. K., Houston, C. G., & Eriksen, M. P. (1994). Surveillance for selected tobacco use behaviors—United States, 1900–1994. *Morbidity and Mortality Weekly Report, 43,* No. SS-3.

Glanz, K., Patterson, R. E., Kristal, A. R., DiClemente, C. C., Heimendinger, J., Linnan, L., & McLerran, D. F. (1994). Stages of change in adopting healthy diets: Fat, fiber, and correlates of nutrient intake. *Health Education Quarterly, 21,* 499–519.

Glascoff, M. A., Knight, S. M., & Jenkins, L. K. (1994). Designated driver programs: College students' experiences and opinions. *Journal of American College Health, 43,* 65–70.

Glasner, P. D., & Kaslow, R. A. (1990). The epidemiology of human immunodeficiency virus infection. *Journal of Consulting and Clinical Psychology, 58,* 13–21.

Glass, D. C., & Singer, J. E. (1972). *Urban stress: Experiments on noise and social stressors.* New York: Academic Press.

Glasser, R. J. (1976). *The body is the hero.* New York: Random House.

Glasser, W. (1976). *Positive addiction.* New York: Harper & Row.

Goedert, M., Strittmatter, W. J., & Roses, A. D. (1994). Risky apolipoprotein in brain. *Nature, 372,* 45.

Goffman, E. (1961). *Asylums.* Garden City, NY: Doubleday.

Gold, D. R., Wang, X., Wypij, D., Speizer, F. E., Ware, J. H., & Dockery, D. W. (1996). Effects of cigarette smoking on lung function in adolescent boys and girls. *New England Journal of Medicine, 335,* 931–937.

Goldberg, L., Elliot, D., Clarke, G. N., MacKinnon, D. P. Moe, E., Zoref, L., Green, C., Wolf, S. L., Greffrath, E., Miller, D. J., & Lapin, A. (1996). Effects of a multidimensional anabolic steroid prevention intervention: The Adolescents Training and Learning to Avoid Steroids (ATLAS) program. *Journal of the American Medical Association, 276,* 1555–1562.

Goldman, L. S., & Kimball, C. P. (1985). Cardiac surgery: Enhancing postoperative outcomes. In A. M. Razin (Ed.), *Helping cardiac patients: Biobehavioral and psychotherapeutic approaches* (pp. 113–155). San Francisco: Jossey-Bass.

Goldman, S. L., Whitney-Saltiel, D., Granger, J., & Rodin, J. (1991). Children's representations of "everyday" aspects of health and illness. *Journal of Pediatric Psychology, 16,* 747–766.

Goldner, E. M., & Birmingham, C. L. (1994). Anorexia nervosa: methods of treatment. In L. Alexander-Mott & D. B. Lumsden (Eds.), *Understanding eating disorders: Anorexia nervosa, bulimia nervosa, and obesity* (pp. 135–157). Washington, DC: Taylor & Francis.

Goldstein, A. (1976). Opioid peptides (endorphins) in pituitary and brain. *Science, 193,* 1081–1086.

Goldston, D. B., Kovacs, M., Obrosky, D. S. & Iyengar, S. (1995). A longitudinal study of life events and metabolic control among youths with insulin-dependent diabetes mellitus. *Health Psychology, 14,* 409–414.

Gomberg, E. S. L. (1989). Suicide risk among women with alcohol problems. *American Journal of Public Health, 79,* 1363–1365.

Gonder-Frederick, L. A., Cox, D. J., Bobbitt, S. A., & Pennebaker, J. W. (1986). Blood glucose symptom beliefs of diabetic patients: Accuracy and implications. *Health Psychology, 5,* 327–341.

Goodall, T. A., & Halford, W. K. (1991). Self-management of diabetes mellitus: A critical review. *Health Psychology, 10,* 1–8.

Goodwin, D. G. (1976). *Is alcoholism hereditary?* New York: Oxford University Press.

Goodwin, D. W., Schulsinger, F., Hermansen, L., Guze, S. B., & Winoker, G. (1973). Alcohol problems in adoptees raised apart from alcoholic biological parents. *Archives of General Psychiatry, 28,* 238–243.

Goodwin, J. S., Hunt, W. C., Key, C. R., & Samet, J. M. (1987). The effect of marital status on stage, treatment, and survival of cancer patients. *Journal of the American Medical Association, 258,* 3125–3130.

Gordon, T., Castelli, W. P., Hjortland, M. C., Kannel, W. B., & Dawber, T. R. (1977). High density lipoprotein as a protective factor against coronary heart disease. The Framingham study. *American Journal of Medicine, 62,* 707–714.

Gordon, T. & Kannel, W. B. (1984). Drinking and mortality: The Framingham Study. *American Journal of Epidemiology, 120,* 97–107.

Gore, J. M., & Fallon, J. T. (1994). Case records of the Massachusetts General Hospital: A 25-year-old man with the recent onset of diabetes mellitus and congestive heart failure. *New England Journal of Medicine, 331,* 460–466.

Gorman, C. (1991, September 16). Why do Blacks die young?. *Time, 138,* 50–52.

Gottlieb, B. H. (1996). Theories and practices of mobilizing support in stressful circumstances. In C. L. Cooper (Ed.), *Handbook of stress, medicine, and health* (pp. 339–356). Boca Raton, FL: CRC Press.

Gottman, J. M. (1991). Predicting the longitudinal course of marriages. *Journal of Marital and Family Therapy, 17,* 3–7.

Gould, K. L., Ornish, D., Scherwitz, L., Brown, S., Edens, R. P., Hess, M. J., Mullani, N., Bolomey, L., Dobbs, F., Armstrong, W. T., Merritt, T., Ports, T., Sparler, S., Billings, J. (1995). Changes in myocardial perfusion abnormalities by positron emission tomography after long-term, intense risk factor modification. *Journal of the American Medical Association, 274,* 894–901.

Grady, D., & Ernster, V. (1992). Does cigarette smoking make you ugly and old? *American Journal of Epidemiology, 135,* 839–842.

Graig, E. (1993). Stress as a consequence of the urban physical environment. In L. Goldberger & S. Breznitz (Eds.), *Handbook of stress: Theoretical and clinical aspects* (2nd ed., pp. 316–332). New York: Free Press.

Graham, R. B. (1990). *Physiological psychology*. Belmont, CA: Wadsworth.

Greenberg, M. R., & Schneider, D. (1994). Violence in American cities: Young Black males is the answer, but what was the question? *Social Science and Medicine, 39,* 179–187.

Greenberger, E., & O'Neil, R. (1993). Spouse, parent, worker: Role commitments and role-related experiences in the construction of adults' well-being. *Developmental Psychology, 29,* 181–197.

Greendale, G. A., Barrett-Connor, E., Edelstein, S., Ingles, S., & Halle, R. (1995). Lifetime leisure exercise and osteoporosis: The Rancho Bernardo Study. *American Journal of Epidemiology, 141,* 951–959.

Greenley, J. R., & Davidson, R. E. (1988). Organizational influences on patient health behavior. In D. S. Gochman (Ed.), *Health behavior: Emerging research perspectives* (pp. 215–229). New York: Plenum Press.

Greenwood, J., Love, E. R., & Pratt, O. E. (1983). The effects of alcohol or of thiamine deficiency upon reproduction in the female rat and fetal development. *Alcohol and Alcoholism, 18,* 45–51.

Greer, S., & Morris, T. (1978). The study of psychological factors in breast cancer: Problems of method. *Social Science and Medicine, 12,* 129–134.

Greist, J. H. (1984). Exercise in the treatment of depression. *Coping with mental stress: The potential and limits of exercise intervention*. Washington, DC: National Institute of Mental Health.

Greist, J. H., Eischens, R. R., Klein, M. H., & Linn, D. (1981). Addendum to "Running through your mind." In M. H. Sacks & M. L. Sachs (Eds.), *Psychology of running*. Champaign, IL: Human Kinetics Publishers.

Greist, J. H., & Greist, T. H. (1979). *Antidepressant treatment: The essentials*. Baltimore: Williams & Wilkins.

Greist, J. H., Klein, M. H., Eischens, R. R., Faris, J., Gurman, A. S., & Morgan, W. P. (1978). Running through your mind. *Journal of Psychosomatic Research, 22,* 259–294.

Greist, J. H., Klein, M. H., Eischens, R. R., Faris, J., Gurman, A. S., & Morgan, W. P. (1979). Running as treatment of depression. *Comprehensive Psychiatry, 20,* 41–54.

Grinspoon, L., & Bakalar, J. B. (1995). Marihuana as medicine: A plea for reconsideration. *Journal of the American Medical Association, 273,* 1875–1876.

Gross, N. J. (1994). Lung health study: Disappointment and triumph. *Journal of the American Medical Association, 272,* 1539.

Grossman, D. C., Krieger, J. W., Sugarman, J. R., & Forquera, R. A. (1994). Health status of urban American Indians and Alaska Natives: A population-based study. *Journal of the American Medical Association, 271,* 845–850.

Grover, S. A., Gray-Donald, K., Joseph, L., Abrahamowicz, M., & Coupal, L. (1994). Life expectancy following dietary modification or smoking cessation. *Archives of Internal Medicine, 154,* 1697–1704.

Grunau, R. V. E., & Craig, K. D. (1988). Pain. In W. Linden (Ed.), *Biological barriers in behavioral medicine* (pp. 257–279). New York: Plenum Press.

Gugler, R., Rohner, H-G., Kratochvil, P., Branditätter, G., & Schmitz, H. (1982). Effects of smoking on duodenal ulcer healing with cimetidine and ormetidine. *Gut, 23,* 866–871.

Gull, W. W. (1874). Anorexia nervosa (apepsia hysterica, anorexia hysterica). *Transactions of the Clinical Society of London, 7,* 22–28. (Reprinted in R. M. Kaufman & M. Heiman [Eds.], *Evolution of psychosomatic concepts: Anorexia nervosa, A paradigm*. New York: International University Press, 1964.)

Gullette, E. C. D., Blumenthal, J. A., Babyak, M., Jiang, W., Waugh, R. A., Frid, D. J., O'Connor, C. M., Morris, J. J., & Krantz, D. S., (1997). Effects of mental stress on myocardial ischemia during daily life. *Journal of the American Medical Association, 277,* 1521–1526.

Gureje, O., Von Korff, M., Simon, G. E., & Gater, R. (1996). Persistent pain and well-being: A World Health Organization study in primary care. *Journal of the American Medical Association, 280,* 147–151.

Gwinup, G., Chelvam, R., & Steinberg, T. (1971). Thickness of subcutaneous fat and activity of underlying muscles. *Annals of Internal Medicine, 74,* 408–411.

Haddon, W. H., Jr. (1970). On the escape of tigers: An ecologic note. *Technology Reviews, 72,* 3–7.

Haddon, W. H., Jr. (1972). A logical framework for categorizing highway safety phenomena and activity. *Journal of Trauma, 12,* 193–207.

Haddon, W. H., Jr. (1980, September-October). The basic strategies for reducing damage from hazards of all kinds. *Hazard Prevention, 6,* 16–22.

Haglund, B., & Cnattingius, S. (1990). Cigarette smoking as a risk factor for sudden infant death syndrome: A population-based study. *American Journal of Public Health, 80,* 29–32.

Hains, A. A., & Ellmann, S. W. (1994). Stress inoculation training as a preventive intervention for high school youths. *Journal of Cognitive Psychotherapy, 8,* 219–232.

Hakim, A. A., Petrovitch, H., Burchfiel, C. M., Ross, G. W., Rodriguez, B. L., White, L. R., Yano, K., Curb, J. D., & Abbott, R., D. (1998). Effects of walking on mortality among nonsmoking retired men. *New England Journal of Medicine, 338,* 94–99.

Hale-Carlsson, G., Hutton, B., Fuhrman, J., Morse, D., McNutt, L., & Clifford, A. (1996). Physical violence and injuries in intimate relationships—New York, Behavioral Risk Factor Surveillance System, 1994. *Morbidity and Mortality Weekly Report, 45,* 765–767.

Hales, D. (1997). *An invitation to health* (7th ed.). Pacific Grove, CA: Brooks/Cole.

Hall, G. R. (1994). Caring for people with Alzheimer's disease using the conceptual model of Progressively lowered Stress Threshold in the clinical setting. *Nursing Clinics of North America, 27,* 129–141.

Hall, H. I., May, D. S., Lew, R. A., Koh, H. K., & Nadel, M. (1997). Sun protection behaviors in the U.S. White population. *Preventive Medicine, 26,* 401–407.

Hall, J. A., Irish, J. T., Roter, D. L., Ehrlich, C. M., & Miller, L. H. (1994). Gender in medical encounters: An analysis of physician and patient communication in a primary care setting. *Health Psychology, 13,* 384–392.

Hall, N. R., & Goldstein, A. L. (1981). Neurotransmitters and the immune system. In R. Ader (Ed.), *Psychoneuroimmunology* (pp. 521–543). New York: Academic Press.

Halmi, K. A., Falk, J. R., & Schwartz, E. (1981). Binge-eating and vomiting: A survey of a college population. *Psychological Medicine, 11,* 697–706.

Hansen, W. B., Graham, J. W., Sobel, J. L., Shelton, D. R., Flay, B. R., & Johnson, C. A. (1987). The consistency of peer and parent influences on tobacco, alcohol, and marijuana use among young adolescents. *Journal of Behavioral Medicine, 10,* 559–579.

Hansen, W. B., Raynor, A. E., & Wolkenstein, B. H. (1991). Perceived personal immunity to the consequences of drinking alcohol: The relationship between behavior and perception. *Journal of Behavioral Medicine, 14,* 205–224.

Hanvik, L. J. (1951). MMPI profiles in patients with low back pain. *Journal of Consulting and Clinical Psychology, 15,* 350–353.

Hardy, J. D., & Smith, T. W. (1988). Cynical hostility and vulnerability to disease: Social support, life stress, and physiological response to conflict. *Health Psychology, 7,* 447–459.

Harrell, E. H., Kelly, K., & Stutts, W. A. (1996). Situational determinants of correlations between serum cortisol and self reported stress measures. *Psychology: A Journal of Human Behavior, 33,* 22–25.

Harris, M. A., & Lustman, P. J. (1998). The psychologist in diabetes care. *Clinical Diabetes, 16*(2), 91–93.

Harris, M. B. (1981). Runners' perceptions of the benefits of running. *Perceptual and Motor Skills, 52,* 153–154.

Harris, R. E., & Wynder, E. L. (1988). Breast cancer and alcohol consumption: A study in weak associations. *Journal of the American Medical Association, 259,* 2867–2871.

Harris, S. S., Caspersen, C. J., DeFriese, G. H., & Estes, H. (1989). Physical activity counseling for healthy adults as a primary preventive intervention in the clinical setting: Report for the US Preventive Services Task Force. *Journal of the American Medical Association, 261,* 3590–3598.

Harris, T. B., Ballard-Barbasch, R., Madans, J., Makuc, D. M., & Feldman, J. J. (1993). Overweight, weight loss and risk of coronary heart disease in older women: The NHANES I Epidemiologic Follow-up Study. *American Journal of Epidemiology, 137,* 1318–1327.

Hartz, A. J., Rupley, D. C., & Rimm, A. A. (1984). The association of girth measurements with disease in 32,856 women. *American Journal of Epidemiology, 119,* 71–80.

Hatch, J. P. (1993). Headache. In R. J. Gatchel & E. B. Blanchard (Eds.), *Psychophysiological disorders: Research and clinical applications* (pp. 111–149). Washington, DC: American Psychological Association.

Hausenblas, H. A., Carron, A. V., & Mack, D. E. (1997). Application of the theories of reasoned action and planned behavior to exercise behavior: A meta-analysis. *Journal of Sport and Exercise Psychology, 19,* 36–51.

Hawkins, W. E. (1992). Problem behaviors and health-enhancing practices of adolescents: A multivariate analysis. *Health Values: The Journal of Health Behavior, Education and Promotion, 16,* 46–54.

Hayashida, M., Alterman, A. I., McLellan, A. T., O'Brien, C. P., Purtill, J. J., Volpicelli, J. R., Raphaelson, A. H., & Hall, C. P. (1989). Comparative effectiveness and costs of inpatient and outpatient detoxification of patients with mild-to-moderate alcohol withdrawal syndrome. *New England Journal of Medicine, 320,* 358–365.

Haynes, R. B. (1976a). A critical review of the "determinants" of patient compliance with therapeutic regimens. In D. L. Sackett & R. B. Haynes (Eds.), *Compliance with therapeutic regimens* (pp. 26–39). Baltimore: Johns Hopkins University Press.

Haynes, R. B. (1976b). Strategies for improving compliance: A methodological analysis and review. In D. L. Sackett & R. B. Haynes (Eds.), *Compliance with therapeutic regimens* (pp. 69–82). Baltimore: Johns Hopkins University Press.

Haynes, R. B. (1979a). Determinants of compliance: The disease and the mechanics of treatment. In R. B. Haynes, D. W. Taylor, & D. L. Sackett (Eds.), *Compliance in health care* (pp. 49–62). Baltimore: Johns Hopkins University Press.

Haynes, R. B. (1979b). Introduction. In R. B. Haynes, D. W. Taylor, & D. L. Sackett (Eds.), *Compliance in health care* (pp. 1–7). Baltimore: Johns Hopkins University Press.

Haynes, R. B., McKibbon, K. A., & Kanani, R. (1996). Systematic review of randomized trials of interventions to assist patients to follow prescriptions for medications. *Lancet, 348,* 383–386.

Haynes, R. B., Wang, E., & da Mota Gomes, M. (1987). A critical review of interventions to improve compliance with prescribed medications. *Patient Education and Counseling, 10,* 155–166.

Haynes, S. G., Feinleib, M., & Kannel, W. B. (1980). The relationship of psychosocial factors to coronary heart disease in the Framingham study: III. Eight-year incidence of coronary heart disease. *American Journal of Epidemiology, 111,* 37–58.

Hays, R. D., Kravitz, R. L., Mazel, R. M., Sherbourne, C. D., DiMatteo, M. R., Rogers, W. H., & Greenfield, S. (1994). The impact of patient adherence on health outcomes for patients with chronic disease in the Medical Outcomes Study. *Journal of Behavioral Medicine, 17,* 347–360.

Haythornthwaite, J. S. (1992–93). Behavioral stress, sodium intake, and blood pressure. *Homeostasis in Health and Disease, 34,* 302–312.

Hearn, W. L., Flynn, D. D., Hime, G. W., Rose, S., Cofino, J. C., Mantero-Atienza, E., Wetli, C. V., & Mash, D. C. (1991). Cocaethylene: A unique cocaine metabolite displays high affinity for the dopamine transporter. *Journal of Neurochemistry, 56,* 698–701.

Heather, N., & Robertson, I. (1990). *Problem drinking* (2nd ed.). Oxford, England: Oxford University Press.

Hebert, L. E., Scherr, P. A., Beckett, L. A., Albert, M. S., Pilgrim, D. M., Chown, M. J., Feenkenstein, H., & Evans, D. A. (1995). Age-specific incidence of Alzheimer's disease in a community population. *Journal of the American Medical Association, 273,* 1354–1359.

Hebert, L. E., Scherr, P. A., Beckett, L. A., Albert, M. S., Rosner, B., Taylor, J. O. & Evans, D. A. (1993). Relation of smoking and low-to-moderate alcohol consumption to change in cognitive function: A longitudinal study in a defined community of older persons. *American Journal of Epidemiology, 137,* 881–891.

Hebert, P. R., Gaziano, J. M., Chan, K. S., & Hennekens, C. H. (1997). Cholesterol lowering with statin drugs, risk of stroke, and total mortality: An overview of randomized trials. *Journal of the American Medical Association, 278,* 313–321.

Hegel, M. T., Ayllon, T., Thiel, G., & Oulton, B. (1992). Improving adherence to fluid restrictions in male hemodialysis patients: A comparison of cognitive and behavioral approaches. *Health Psychology, 11,* 324–330.

Helby, E. M., Gafarian, C. T., & McCann, S. C. (1989). Situational and behavioral correlates of compliance to a diabetic regimen. *Journal of Compliance in Health Care, 4,* 101–116.

Helgeson, V. S., Cohen, S., & Fritz H. L. (1998). Social ties and cancer. In J. C. Holland (Ed.), *Psychooncology* (pp. 99–109). New York: Oxford University Press.

Helgeson, V. S. (1993). The onset of chronic illness: Its effect on the patient-spouse relationship. *Journal of Social and Clinical Psychology, 12,* 406–428.

Hellmich, N. (1995, May 25). Wake-up call for the sleep deprived. *USA Today,* pp. D1, D2.

Helmrich, S. P., Ragland, D. R., Leung, R. W., & Paffenbarger, R. S., Jr. (1991). Physical activity and reduced occurrence of non-insulin-dependent diabetes mellitus. *New England Journal of Medicine, 325,* 147–152.

Helzer, J. E., Robins, L. N., & McEvoy, L. (1987). Post-traumatic stress disorder in the general population: Findings of the Epidemiologic Catchment Area survey. *New England Journal of Medicine, 317,* 1630–1634.

Hennekens, C. H., Buring, J. E., Manson, J. E., Stampfer, M. J., Rosner, B., Cook, N. F., Belanger, C., LaMatte, F., Gaziano, J. M., Ridker, P. M., Willett, W., & Peto, R. (1996). Lack of long-term supplementations with beta carotene on the incidence of malignant neoplasms and cardiovascular disease. *New England Journal of Medicine, 394,* 1145–1149.

Hepler, R. S., & Frank, I. M. (1971). Marijuana smoking and intraocular pressure. *Journal of the American Medical Association, 217,* 1392.

Herbert, T. B., & Cohen, S. (1993a). Depression and immunity: A meta-analytic review. *Psychological Bulletin, 113,* 472–486.

Herbert, T. B., & Cohen, S. (1993b). Stress and immunity in humans: A meta-analytic review. *Psychosomatic Medicine, 55,* 364–379.

Herbert, T. B., & Cohen, S. (1994). Stress and illness. In V. S. Ramachandran (Ed.), *Encyclopedia of human behavior, Vol. 4* (pp. 325–332). San Diego, CA: Academic Press.

Hermann, C., Kim M., & Blanchard, E. B. (1995). Behavioral and prophylactic pharmacological intervention studies of pediatric migraine: A exploratory meta-analysis. *Pain, 60,* 139–255.

Herning, R. I., Jones, R. T., Bachman, J., & Mines, A. H. (1981). Puff volume increases when low-nicotine cigarettes are smoked. *British Medical Journal, 283,* 187–189.

Herring, L. (1997, May/June). CDC arms with behavioral science in war on disease and injury. *American Psychological Society Observer, 10*(1), 5–6.

Herschbach, P., Duran, G., Waadt, S., Zettler, A., Amm, C., Marten-Mittag, B., & Strian, F. (1997). Psychometric properties of the Questionnaire on Stress in Patients with Diabetes—Revised (QSD—R). *Health Psychology, 16,* 171–174.

Heston, L. L., & White, J. A. (1991). *The vanishing mind: A practical guide to Alzheimer's disease and other dementias* (2nd ed.). New York: Freeman.

Heszen-Klemens, I. (1987). Patients' noncompliance and how doctors manage this. *Social Science and Medicine, 24,* 409–416.

Hetherington, M. M., & Rolls, B. J. (1996). Sensory-specific satiety: Theoretical frameworks and central characteristics. In E. D. Capaldi (Ed.), *Why we eat what we eat: The psychology of eating* (pp. 267–290). Washington, DC: American Psychological Association.

Heusinkveld, K. B. (1997). Cancer prevention and risk assessment. In C. Varricchio, M. Pierce, C. Walker, & T. B. Ades (Eds.), *A cancer source book for nurses* (7th ed.) (pp. 35–42). Atlanta: The American Cancer Society.

Hewitt, P. L., Flett, G. L., & Mosher, S. W. (1992). The Perceived Stress Scale: Factor structure and relation to depression symptoms in a psychiatric sample. *Journal of Psychopathology and Behavioral Assessment, 14,* 247–257.

Higgins, M. W., Kjelsberg, M., & Metzner, H. (1967). Characteristics of smokers and nonsmokers in Tecumseh, Michigan. I: The distribution of smoking habits in persons and families and their relationship to social characteristics. *American Journal of Epidemiology, 86,* 45–59.

Higgins, R. L., & Marlatt, G. A. (1973). Effects of anxiety arousal on the consumption of alcohol by alcoholics and social drinkers. *Journal of Consulting and Clinical Psychology, 41,* 426–433.

Higgins, R. L., & Marlatt, G. A. (1975). Fear of interpersonal evaluation as a determinant of alcohol consumption in male social drinkers. *Journal of Abnormal Psychology, 84,* 644–651.

Hilgard, E. R. (1978). Hypnosis and pain. In R. A. Sternbach (Ed.), *The psychology of pain.* New York: Raven Press.

Hilgard, E. R., & Hilgard, J. R. (1994). *Hypnosis in the relief of pain* (Rev. ed.). Los Altos, CA: Kaufmann.

Hill, A. J., Boudreau, F., Amyot, E., Dery, D., & Godin, G. (1997). Predicting the stages of smoking acquisition according to the theory of planned behavior. *Journal of Adolescent Health, 21,* 107–115.

Hill, C. S., Jr. (1995). When will adequate pain treatment be the norm? *Journal of the American Medical Association, 274,* 1881–1882.

Hill, J. O., Drougas, H. J., & Peters, J. C. (1994). Physical activity, fitness, and moderate obesity. In C. Bouchard, R. J. Shephard, & T. Stephens (Eds.), *Physical activity, fitness, and health: International proceedings and consensus statement* (pp. 684–695). Champaign, IL: Human Kinetics.

Hobfoll, S. E., & Vaux, A. (1993). Social support: Resources and context. In L. Goldberger & S. Breznitz (Eds.), *Handbook of stress: Theoretical and clinical aspects* (2nd ed., pp. 685–705). New York: Free Press.

Hochbaum, G. (1958). *Public participation in medical screening programs* (DHEW Publication No. 572, Public Health Service). Washington, DC: U. S. Government Printing Office.

Hochschild, A. (with Machung, A.). (1989). *The second shift: Working parents and the revolution at home.* New York: Viking.

Hoek, H. W. (1993). Review of the epidemiological studies of eating disorders. *International Review of Psychiatry, 5,* 61–74.

Hoffmann, P. (1997). The endorphin hypothesis. In W. P. Morgan (Ed.), *Physical activity and mental health* (pp. 163–177). Washington, DC: Taylor & Francis.

Hofmann, D. A., & Stetzer, A. (1996). A cross-level investigation of factors influencing unsafe behaviors and accidents. *Personnel Psychology, 49,* 307–339.

Holahan, C. J., Moos, R. H., Holahan, C. K., & Brennan, P. L. (1995). Social support, coping, and depressive symptoms in a late-middle-aged sample of patients reporting cardiac illness. *Health Psychology, 14,* 152–163.

Holderness, C. C., Brooks-Gunn, J., & Warren, M. P. (1994). Co-morbidity of eating disorders and substance abuse: Review of the literature. *International Journal of Eating Disorders, 16,* 1–34.

Holland, J. C., & Lewis, S. (1993). Emotions and cancer: What do we really know? In D. Goleman & J. Gurin (Eds.), *Mind/body medicine: How to use your mind for better health* (pp. 85–109). Yonkers, NY: Consumer Reports Books.

Hollis, J. F., Connett, J. E., Stevens, V. J., & Greenlick, M. R. (1990). Stressful life events, Type A behavior, and the prediction of cardiovascular and total mortality over six years. *Journal of Behavioral Medicine, 13,* 263–280.

Holme, I. (1990). An analysis of randomized trials evaluating the effect of cholesterol reduction on total mortality and coronary heart disease incidence. *Circulation, 82,* 1916–1924.

Holmes, D. T., Tariot, P. N., & Cox, C. (1998). Preliminary evidence of psychological distress among reservists in the Persian Gulf War. *Journal of Nervous and Mental Disease, 186,* 166–173.

Holmes, M. D., Hunter, D. J., Colditz, G. A., Stampfer, M. J., Hankinson, S. E., Speizer, F. E., Rosner, B., & Willett, W. C. (1999). Association of dietary intake of fat and fatty acids with risk of breast cancer. *Journal of the American Medical Association, 281,* 914–920.

Holmes, T. H., & Masuda, M. (1974). Life change and illness susceptibility. In B. S. Dohrenwend & B. P. Dohrenwend (Eds.), *Stressful life events: Their nature and effects* (pp. 45–72). New York: Wiley.

Holmes, T. H., & Rahe, R. H. (1967). The Social Readjustment Rating Scale. *Journal of Psychosomatic Research, 11,* 213–218.

Holmes, W. C., Bix, B., Meritz, M., Turner, J., & Hutelmyer, C. (1997). Human immunodeficiency virus (HIV) infection and quality of life: the potential impact of Axis I psychiatric disorders in a sample of 95 HIV seropositive men. *Psychosomatic Medicine, 59,* 187–192.

Holroyd, K. A., & Penzien, D. B. (1990). Pharmacological versus non-pharmacological prophylaxis of recurrent migraine headache: A meta-analytic review of clinical trials. *Pain, 42,* 1–13.

Holt, N. L., Daling, J. R., McKnight, B., Moore, D. E., Stergachis, A., & Weiss, N. S. (1994). Cigarette smoking and functional ovarian cysts. *American Journal of Epidemiology, 139,* 781–786.

Holt, R. R. (1993). Occupational stress. In L. Goldberger & S. Breznitz (Eds.), *Handbook of stress: Theoretical and clinical aspects* (2nd ed., pp. 333–367). New York: Free Press.

Honkanen, R. (1993). Alcohol in home and leisure injuries. International Symposium on Alcohol-related Accidents and Injuries (1991, Yverdon-les-Bains, Switzerland). *Addiction, 88,* 939–944.

Hopper, J. L., & Seeman E. (1994). The bone density of female twins discordant for tobacco use. *New England Journal of Medicine, 330,* 387–392.

Horan, J. J. (1973). "In vivo" emotive imagery: A technique for reducing childbirth anxiety and discomfort. *Psychological Reports, 32,* 1328.

Horan, J. J., & Dellinger, J. K. (1974). "In vivo" emotive imagery: A preliminary test. *Perceptual and Motor Skills, 39,* 359–362.

Horan, J. J., Layng, F. C., & Pursell, C. H. (1976). Preliminary study of effects of "in vivo" emotive imagery on dental discomfort. *Perceptual and Motor Skills, 42,* 105–106.

Hornbrook, M. C., Stevens, V. J., Wingfield, D. J., Hollis, J. F., Greenlick, M. R., & Ory, M. G. (1994). Preventing falls among community-dwelling older persons: Results from a randomized trial. *Gerontologist, 34,* 16–23.

Horwitz, R. I., Viscoli, C. M., Berkman, L., Donaldson, R. M., Horwitz, S. M., Murray, C. J., Ransohoff, D. F., & Sindelar, J. (1990). Treatment adherence and risk of death after myocardial infraction. *Lancet, 336,* 542–545.

Houston, B. K. (1986). Psychological variables and cardiovascular and neuroendocrine reactivity. In K. A. Matthews, S. M. Weiss, T. Detre, T. M. Dembroski, B. Falkner, S. B. Manuck, & R. B. Williams, Jr. (Eds.), *Handbook of stress, reactivity, and cardiovascular disease* (pp. 207–209). New York: Wiley-Interscience.

Howard, G., Wagenknecht, L. E., Burk, G. L., Diez-Roux, A., Evans, G. W., McGovern, P., Nieto, J., & Tell, G. S. (1998). Cigarette smoking and progression of atherosclerosis: The Atherosclerosis Risk in Communities (ARIC) Study. *Journal of the American Medical Society, 279,* 119–124.

Hsu, J. S. J., & Williams, S. D. (1991). Injury prevention awareness in an urban Native American population. *American Journal of Public Health, 81,* 1466–1468.

Hsu, L. K. G. (1990). *Eating disorders.* New York: Guilford Press.

Huang, Z., Hankinson, S. E., Colditz, G. A., Stampfer, M. J., Hunter, D. J., Manson, J. E., Hennekens, C. H., Rosner, B., Speizer, F. E., & Willett, W. C. (1997). Dual effects of weight and weight gain on breast cancer risk. *Journal of the American Medical Association, 278,* 1407–1411.

Hughes, J. (1975). Isolation of an endogenous compound from the brain with pharmacological properties similar to morphine. *Brain Research, 88,* 295–308.

Hughes, J. R., Gulliver, S. B., Fenwick, J. W., Valliere, W. A., Cruser, K., Pepper, S., Shea, P., Solomon, L. J., & Flynn, B. S. (1992). Smoking cessation among self-quitters. *Health Psychology, 11,* 331–334.

Hughes, J. R., Gust, S. W., Keenan, R. M., Fenwick, J. W., & Healey, M. L. (1989). Nicotine vs placebo gum in general medical practice. *Journal of the American Medical Association, 261,* 1300–1305.

Hull, J. G. (1981). A self-awareness model of the causes and effects of alcohol consumption. *Journal of Abnormal Psychology, 90,* 586–600.

Hull, J. G. (1987). Self-awareness model. In H. T. Blane & K. E. Leonard (Eds.), *Psychological theories of drinking and alcoholism* (pp. 272–304). New York: Guilford Press.

Hull, J. G., & Bond, C. F. (1986). Social and behavioral consequences of alcohol consumption and expectancy: A meta-analysis. *Psychological Bulletin, 99,* 347–360.

Hull, J. G., Van Treuren, R. R., & Virnelli, S. (1987). Hardiness and health: A critique and alternative approach. *Journal of Personality and Social Psychology, 53,* 518–530.

Hulley, S., Grady, D., Bush, T., Furberg, C., Herrington, D., Riggs, B., & Vittinghoff, E. (1998). Randomized trial of estrogen plus progestin for secondary prevention of coronary heart disease in postmenopausal women. *Journal of the American Medical Association, 280,* 605–613.

Human Capital Initiative Report. (1996, April). Doing the right thing: A research plan for healthy living. *American Psychological Society Observer,* Special Issue, Report 4.

Humphries, S. A., Johnson, M. H., & Long, N. R. (1996). An investigation of the gate control theory of pain using the experimental pain stimulus of potassium iontophoresis. *Perception and Psychophysics, 58,* 693–703.

Hunink, M. G., Goldman, L., Tosteson, N. A., Mittlemen, M. A., Goldman, P. A., Williams, L. W., Tsevat, J., & Weinstein, M. C. (1997). The recent decline in mortality from coronary heart disease, 1980–1990: The effect of secular trends in risk factors and treatment. *Journal of the American Medical Association, 277,* 535–542.

Hunt, L. M., Jordan, B., Irwin, S., & Browner, C. H. (1989). Compliance and the patient's perspective: Controlling symptoms in everyday life. *Culture, Medicine, and Psychiatry, 13,* 315–334.

Hunt, W. A., Barnett, L. W., & Branch, L. G. (1971). Relapse rates in addiction programs. *Journal of Clinical Psychology, 27,* 455–456.

Hunter, C., Jr. (1982). Freestanding alcohol treatment centers—A new approach to an old problem. *Psychiatric Annals, 12,* 396–408.

Hunter, D. J., Manson, J. E., Colditz, G. A., Stampfer, M. J., Rosner, B., Hennekens, C. H., Speizer, F. E., & Willett, W. C. (1993). A prospective study of the intake of vitamins C, E, and A and the risk of breast cancer. *New England Journal of Medicine, 329,* 234–240.

Hunter, M., & Philips, C. (1981). The experience of headache: An assessment of the qualities of tension headache pain. *Pain, 10,* 209–219.

Husten, C.G., Warren, C. W., Crossett, L., & Sharp, D. (1998). Trends in tobacco use among high school students in the United States, 1991–1995. *Journal of School Health, 68,* 137–140.

Hyland, A., Cummings, K. M., Shopland, D. R., & Lynn, W. R. (1998). Prevalence of cigar use in 22 North American communities: 1989 and 1993. *American Journal of Public Health, 88,* 1086–1089.

Hyman, R. B., Baker, S., Ephraim, R., Moadel, A., & Philip, J. (1994). Health Belief Model variables as predictors of screening mammography utilization. *Journal of Behavior Medicine, 17,* 391–406.

Ickovics, J. R., Druley, J. A., Grigorenko, E. L., Morrill, A. C., Beren, S. E., & Rodin, J. (1998). Long-term effects of HIV counseling and testing for women: Behavioral and psychological consequences are limited at 18 months posttest. *Health Psychology, 17,* 395–402.

Ikard, F. F., Green, D., & Horn, D. A. (1969). A scale to differentiate between types of smoking as related to the management of affect. *International Journal of Addictions, 4,* 649–659.

Ikegami, N. (1992). The economics of health care in Japan. *Science, 258,* 614–618.

Ilacqua, G. E. (1994). Migraine headaches: Coping efficacy of guided imagery training. *Headache, 34,* 99–102.

International Association for the Study of Pain (IASP), Subcommittee on Taxonomy. (1979). Pain terms: A list with definitions and notes on usage. *Pain, 6,* 249–252.

International Society of Sport Psychology. (1992). Physical activity and psychological benefits: A position statement from the International Society of Sport Psychology. *Journal of Applied Sport Psychology, 4,* 94–98.

Irwin, M., Mascovich, M., Gillin, C., Willoughby, R., Pike, J., & Smith, T. L. (1994). Partial sleep deprivation reduces natural killer cell activity in humans. *Psychosomatic Medicine, 56,* 493–498.

Ismail, A. I., Burt, B. A., & Eklund, S. A. (1983). Epidemiologic patterns of smoking and peridontal disease in the United States. *Journal of the American Dental Association, 106,* 617–621.

Iso, H., Jacobs, D. R., Jr., Wentworth, P., Neaton, J. D., & Cohen, J. D. (1989). Serum cholesterol levels and six-year mortality from stroke in 350,977 men screened for the Multiple Risk Factor Intervention Trial. *New England Journal of Medicine, 320,* 904–910.

Jablon, S., Hrubec, Z., & Boise, J. D. (1991). Cancer in populations living near nuclear facilities. *Journal of the American Medical Association, 265,* 1403–1408.

Jackson, R., Scragg, R., & Beaglehole, R. (1992). Does recent alcohol consumption reduce the risk of acute myocardial infarction and coronary death in regular drinkers? *American Journal of Epidemiology, 136,* 819–824.

Jacobs, A. L., Kurtz, R. M., & Strube, M. J. (1995). Hypnotic analgesia, expectancy effects, and choice of a design: A reexamination. *International Journal of Clinical and Experimental Hypnosis, 43,* 55–68.

Jacobs, D., Blackburn, H., Higgins, M., Reed, D., Iso, H., McMillian, G., Neaton, J., Nelson, J., Potter, J., Rifkind, B., Jossouw, J., Shekelle, R., & Yusuf, S. (1992). Report of the conference on low blood cholesterol: Mortality associations. *Circulation, 86,* 1046–1060.

Jacobs, D. R., Jr., Muldoon, M. F., & Rästam, L. (1995). Invited Commentary: Low blood cholesterol, non-illness mortality, and other nonatherosclerotic disease mortality: A search for causes and confounders. *American Journal of Epidemiology, 141,* 518–122.

Jacobsen, P. B. & Hann, D. M. (1998). Cognitive-behavioral interventions. In J. C. Holland (Ed.), *Psycho-oncology* (pp. 717–729). New York: Oxford University Press.

Jacobson, E. (1934). *You must relax.* New York: McGraw-Hill.

Jacobson, E. (1938). *Progressive relaxation: A physiological and clinical investigation of muscle states and their significance in psychology and medical practice* (2nd ed.). Chicago: University of Chicago Press.

Jagal, S. B., Kreiger, N., & Darlington, G. (1993). Past and recent physical activity and risk of hip fracture. *American Journal of Epidemiology, 138,* 107–118.

Jamison, K. R., & Akiskal, H. (1983). Medication compliance in patients with bipolar disorder. *Psychiatric Clinics of North America, 6,* 175–192.

Janis, I. L. (1958). *Psychological stress.* New York: Wiley.

Janis, I. L. (1984). Improving adherence to medical recommendations: Prescriptive hypotheses derived from recent research in social psychology. In A. Baum, S. E. Taylor, & J. E. Singer (Eds.), *Handbook of psychology and health: Vol. 4. Social psychological aspects of health* (pp. 113–148). Hillsdale, NJ: Erlbaum.

Janis, I. L., & Rodin, J. (1979). Attribution, control, and decision making: Social psychology and health care. In G. C. Stone, F. Cohen, & N. E. Adler (Eds.), *Health psychology—A handbook* (pp. 487–521). San Francisco: Jossey-Bass.

Japsen, B. (1994). Indians seek supplemental fundings. *Modern Healthcare, 24,* 78.

Jarvik, M. (1977). Biological factors underlying the smoking habit. In M. Jarvik, J. Cullen, E. Gritz, T. Vogt, & L. West (Eds.), *Research on smoking and behavior* (NIDA Publication No. ADM 78-581). Rockville, MD: National Institute on Drug Abuse.

Jay, S. M., Elliott, C. H., Woody, P. D., & Siegel, S. (1991). An investigation of cognitive-behavior therapy combined with oral Valium for children undergoing painful medical procedures. *Health Psychology, 10,* 317–322.

Jeffery, R. W., & French, S. A. (1996). Socioeconomic status and weight control practices among 20- to 45-year-old women. *American Journal of Public Health, 86,* 1005–1010.

Jeffery, R. W. & French, S. A. (1998). Epidemic obesity in the United States: Are fast foods and television viewing contributing? *American Journal of Public Health, 88,* 277–280.

Jellinek, E. M. (1960). *The disease concept of alcoholism.* New Haven, CT: College and University Press.

Jemmott, J. B., III, & Locke, S. E. (1984). Psychosocial factors, immunologic mediation, and human susceptibility to infectious diseases: How much do we know? *Psychological Bulletin, 95,* 78–108.

Jenkins, C. D. (1998). Cardiovascular disease. In E. A. Blechman & K. D. Brownell (Eds.), *Behavioral medicine and women: A comprehensive handbook* (pp. 604–614). New York: Guilford.

Jenkins, E. J., & Bell, C. C. (1997). Exposure and response to community violence among children and adolescents. In J. D. Osofsky (Ed.), *Children in a violent society* (pp. 9–31). New York: Guilford Press.

Jennings, G. L. R., Reid, C. M., Christy, I., Jennings, J., Anderson, W. P., Dart, A. (1998). Animals and cardiovascular health. In C. C. Wilson & D. C. Turner (Eds.), *Companion animals in human health* (pp. 161–171). Thousand Oaks, CA: Sage.

Jih, C-S., Sirgo, V. I., & Thomure, J. C., (1995). Alcohol consumption, locus of control, and self-esteem of high school and college students. *Psychological Reports, 76,* 851–857.

Johansen, C., & Olsen, J. H. (1998). Risk of cancer among Danish utility Workers—A nationwide cohort study. *American Journal of Epidemiology, 147,* 548–555.

John, E. M., Savitz, D. A., & Sandler, D. P. (1991). Prenatal exposure to parents' smoking and childhood cancer. *American Journal of Epidemiology, 133,* 123–132.

Johnson, J. V., & Hall, E. M. (1988). Job strain, work place social support, and cardiovascular disease: A cross-sectional study of a random sample of the Swedish working population. *American Journal of Public Health, 78,* 1336–1342.

Johnson, M., & Vögele, C. (1993). Benefits of psychological preparation for surgery: A meta-analysis. *Annals of Behavioral Medicine, 15,* 245–256.

Johnson, M. P. (1995). Patriarchal terrorism and common couple violence: Two forms of violence against women. *Journal of Marriage and the Family, 57,* 283–294.

Johnson, R. A., & Gerstein, D. R. (1998). Initiation of use of alcohol, cigarettes, marijuana, cocaine, and other substances in US birth cohorts since 1919. *American Journal of Public Health, 88,* 27–33.

Johnson, S. B., (1993). Chronic diseases of childhood: Assessing compliance with complex medical regimens. In N. A. Krasnegor, L. Epstein, Johnson, S. B., & Yaffe, S. J. (Eds.), *Developmental aspects of health compliance behavior* (pp.167–184). Hillsdale, NJ: Erlbaum.

Johnson, S. B., Freund, A., Silverstein, J., Hansen, C. A., & Malone, J. (1990). Adherence-health status relationships in childhood diabetes. *Health Psychology, 9,* 606–631.

Johnson, S. B., Tomer, A., Cunningham, W. R., & Henretta, J. C. (1990). Adherence in childhood diabetes: Results of a confirmatory factor analysis. *Health Psychology, 9,* 493–501.

Johnston, L. D., O'Malley, P. M., & Bachman, J. G. (1997). *National survey results on drug use from the Monitoring the Future study, 1975–1995, Vol. II: College students and young adults.* NIH Publication No. 98-4140. Rockville, MD: National Institute on Drug Abuse.

Johnston, L. D., O'Malley, P. M., & Bachman, J. G. (1998). *National survey results of drug use from the Monitoring the Future, 1975–1997, Vol. I: Secondary School Students.* National Institute on Drug Abuse No. 98-4345. Rockville, MD: National Institute on Drug Abuse.

Joiner, T. E., Jr., Heatherton, T. F., Rudd, M. D., & Schmidt, N. E. (1997). Perfectionism, perceived weight status, and bulimic symptoms: Two studies testing a diathesis-stress model. *Journal of Abnormal Psychology, 106,* 145–153.

Jones, J. A., Eckhardt, L. E., Mayer, J. A., Bartholomew, S., Malcarne, V. L., Hovell, M. F., & Elder, J. P. (1993). The effects of an instructional audiotape on breast self-examination proficiency. *Journal of Behavioral Medicine, 16,* 225–235.

Jorenby, D. E., Leischow, S. J., Nides, M. A., Rennard, S. I., Johnston, J. A., Hughes, A. R., Smith, S. S., Muramoto, M. L., Daughton, D. M., Doan, K., Fiore, M. C., & Baker, T. B. (1999). A controlled trial of sustained-release bupropion, a nicotine patch, or both for smoking cessation. *New England Journal of Medicine, 340,* 685–691.

Jousilahti, P., Vartiainen, E., Toumilehto, J., Pekkanen, J., & Puska, P. (1995). Effect of risk factors and changes in risk factors on coronary mortality in three cohorts of middle-aged people in Eastern Finland. *American Journal of Epidemiology, 141,* 50–60.

Kabat, G. C., Stellman, S. D., & Wynder, E. L. (1995). Relation between exposure to environmental tobacco smoke and lung cancer in lifetime nonsmokers. *American Journal of Epidemiology, 142,* 141–148.

Kabat-Zinn, J. (1993). Mindfulness meditation: Health benefits of an ancient Buddhist practice. In D. Goleman & J. Gurin (Eds.), *Mind/body medicine: How to use your mind for better health* (pp. 259–275). Yonkers, NY: Consumer Reports Books.

Kabat-Zinn, J., & Chapman-Waldrop, A. (1988). Compliance with an outpatient stress reduction program: Rates and predictors of program completion. *Journal of Behavioral Medicine, 11,* 333–352.

Kabat-Zinn, J., Lipworth, L., & Burney, R. (1985). The clinical use of mindfulness meditation for the self-regulation of chronic pain. *Journal of Behavioral Medicine, 8,* 163–190.

Kabat-Zinn, J., Massion, A. O., Kristeller, J., Peterson, L. G., Fletcher, K. E., Pbert, L., Lenderking, W. R., & Santorelli, S. F. (1992). Effectiveness of a meditation-based stress reduction program in the treatment of anxiety disorders. *American Journal of Psychiatry, 149,* 936–943.

Kahn, H. A. (1963). The relationship of reported coronary heart disease mortality to physical activity of work. *American Journal of Public Health, 53,* 1058–1067.

Kahn, H. S., Tatham, L. M., Rodriquez, C., Calle, E. E., Thun, M. J., & Heath, C. W., Jr. (1997). Stable behaviors associated with adults' 10-year change in body mass index and likelihood of gain at the waist. *American Journal of Public Health, 87,* 747–754.

Kalafat, J. (1997). Prevention of youth suicide. In R. P. Weissberg, T. P. Gullotta, R. L. Hampton, B. A. Ryan, & G. R. Adams (Eds.), *Enhancing children's wellness* (pp. 175–213). Thousand Oaks, CA: Sage.

Kalafat, J., & Elias, M. (1994). An evaluation of a school-based suicide awareness intervention. *Suicide and Life Threatening Behavior, 24,* 224–233.

Kalat, J. W. (1998). *Biological psychology* (6th ed.). Pacific Grove, CA: Brooks/Cole.

Kamarck, T. W., Jennings, R., Pogue-Geile, M., & Manuck, S. B. (1994). A multidimensional measurement model for cardiovascular reactivity: Stability and cross-validation in two adult samples. *Health Psychology, 13,* 471–478.

Kaminski, P. L., & McNamara, K. (1996). A treatment for college women at risk for bulimia: A controlled evaluation. *Journal of Counseling & Development, 74,* 288–294.

Kamiya, J. (1969). Operant control of the EEG alpha rhythm and some of its reported effects on consciousness. In C. Tart (Ed.), *Altered states of consciousness.* New York: Wiley.

Kann, L., Kinchen, S. A., Williams, B. I., Ross, J. G., Lowry, R., Hill, C. V., Grunbaum, J. A., Blumson, P. S., Collins, J. L., & Kolbe, L. J. (1998). Youth Risk Behavior Surveillance—United States, 1997. *Morbidity and Mortality Weekly Report, 47,* No. SS-3.

Kann, L., Warren, C. W., Harris, W. A., Collins, J. L., Douglas, K. A., Collins, M. E., Williams, B. I., Ross, J. G., & Kolbe, L. J. (1995). Youth Risk Behavior Surveillance—United States, 1993. *Morbidity and Mortality Weekly Report, 44,* No. SS-1.

Kanner, A. D., Coyne, J. C., Schaefer, C., & Lazarus, R. S. (1981). Comparison of two modes of stress measurement: Daily hassles and uplifts versus major life events. *Journal of Behavioral Medicine, 4,* 1–39.

Kaplan, G. A., Strawbridge, W. J., Cohen, R. D., & Hungerford, L. R. (1996). Natural history of leisure-time physical activity and its correlates: Association with mortality from all causes and cardiovascular disease over 28 years. *American Journal of Epidemiology, 144,* 793–797.

Kaplan, H. I. (1985). Psychological factors affecting physical conditions (psychosomatic disorders). In H. I. Kaplan & B. J. Saddock (Eds.), *Comprehensive textbook of psychiatry IV* (pp. 1106–1113). Baltimore: Williams & Wilkins.

Kaplan, J. R., Fontenot, M. B., Manuck, S. B., & Muldoon, M. F. (1996). Influence of dietary lipids on agonistic and affirmative behavior in macaca fascicularis. *American Journal of Primatology, 38,* 333–347.

Kaplan, J. R., Shively, C. A., Fontenot, M. B., Morgan, T. M., Howell, S. M., Manuck, S. B., Muldoon, M. F., & Mann, J. J. (1994). Demonstration of an association among dietary cholesterol, central serotonergic activity, and social behavior in monkeys. *Psychosomatic Medicine, 56,* 479–484.

Kaplan, R. M. (1984). The connection between clinical health promotion and health status. *American Psychologist, 39,* 755–765.

Kaplan, R. M. (1994). Measures of health outcome in social support research. In S. A. Shumaker & S. M. Czajkowski (Eds.), *Social support and cardiovascular disease* (pp. 65–94). New York: Plenum Press.

Kaplan, R. M., & Bush, J. W. (1982). Health-related quality of life measurement for evaluation research and policy analysis. *Health Psychology, 1,* 61–80.

Karasek, R. A., Theorell, T., Schwartz, J. E., Schnall, P. L., Pieper, C. F., & Michela, J. L. (1988). Job characteristics in relation to the prevalence of myocardial infarction in the U. S. Health Examination Survey (HES) and the Health and Nutrition Examination Survey (HANES). *American Journal of Public Health, 78,* 910–918.

Kasl, S. V. (1996). Theory of stress and health. In C. L. Cooper (Ed.), *Handbook of stress, medicine, and health* (pp. 13–26). Boca Raton, FL: CRC Press.

Kasl, S. V., & Cobb, S. (1966a). Health behavior, illness behavior, and sick role behavior I. Health and illness behavior. *Archives of Environmental Health, 12,* 246–266.

Kasl, S. V., & Cobb, S. (1966b). Health behavior, illness behavior, and sick role behavior II. Sick role behavior. *Archives of Environmental Health, 12,* 531–541.

Katan, M. B., Grundy, S. M., & Willett, W. C. (1997). Beyond low fat diets. *New England Journal of Medicine, 337,* 563–567.

Katerndahl, D. A., & Lawler, W. R. (1999). Variability in meta-analytic results concerning the value of cholesterol reduction in coronary heart disease: A meta-meta-analysis. *American Journal of Epidemiology, 149,* 429–441.

Katz, R. C., Ashmore, J., Barboa, E., Trueblood, K., McLaughlin, V., & Mathews, L. (1998). Knowledge of disease and dietary compliance in patients with end-stage renal disease. *Psychological Reports, 82,* 331–336.

Kavanagh, T., & Shepard, R. J. (1973). The immediate antecedents of myocardial infarction in active men. *Canadian Medical Association Journal, 109,* 19–22.

Kawachi, I., Colditz, G. A., Stampfer, M. J., Willett, W. C., Manson, J. E., Rosner, B., Speizer, F. E., & Hennekens, C. H. (1993). Smoking cessation and decreased risk of stroke in women. *Journal of the American Medical Association, 269,* 232–236.

Kawachi, I., Colditz, G. A., Ascherio, A., Rimm, E. B., Giovannucci, E., Stampfer, M. J., & Willett, W. C. (1994). Prospective study of phobic anxiety and risk of coronary heart disease in men. *Circulation, 89,* 1992–1997.

Kawachi, I., Sparrow, D., Vokonas, P. S., & Weiss, S. T. (1994). Symptoms of anxiety and risk of coronary heart disease: The Normative Aging Study. *Circulation, 90,* 2225–2229.

Kawachi, I., Troist, R. J., Robnitzky, A. G., Coakley, E. H., & Colditz, G. A. (1996). Can physical activity minimize weight gain in women after smoking cessation? *American Journal of Public Health, 86,* 999–1004.

Kazak, A. E., Meeske, K., Penati, B., Barakat, L. P., Christakis, D., Meadows, A. T., Casey, R., & Stuber, M. L. (1997). Posttraumatic stress, family functioning, and social support in survivors of childhood leukemia and their mothers and fathers. *Journal of Consulting and Clinical Psychology, 65,* 120–129.

Keefe, F. J. (1982). Behavioral assessment and treatment of chronic pain: Current status and future directions. *Journal of Consulting and Clinical Psychology, 50,* 896–911.

Keefe, F. J., & Block, A. R. (1982). Development of an observation method for assessing pain behavior in chronic low back pain patients. *Behavior Therapy, 13,* 363–375.

Keefe, F. J., Brown, G. K., Wallston, K. A., & Caldwell, D. S. (1989). Coping with rheumatoid arthritis pain: Catastrophizing as a maladaptive strategy. *Pain, 37,* 51–56.

Keefe, F. J., & Van Horn, Y. (1993). Cognitive-behavioral treatment of rheumatoid arthritis pain: Maintaining treatment gains. Special Issue: The challenges of pain in arthritis. *Arthritis Care and Research, 6,* 213–222.

Keil, C. P. (1998). Loneliness, stress, and human-animal attachment among older adults. In C. C. Wilson & D. C. Turner (Eds.), *Companion animals in human health* (pp. 123–134). Thousand Oaks, CA: Sage.

Keller, S. E., Shiflett, S. C., Schleifer, S. J., & Bartlett, J. A. (1994). Stress, immunity, and health. In R. Glaser & J. K. Kiecolt-Glaser (Eds.), *Handbook of human stress and immunity* (pp. 217–244). San Diego, CA: Academic Press.

Kelly, J. A., St. Lawrence, J. S., Brasfield, T. L., Lemke, A., Amideé, T., Roffman, R. E., Hood, H. V., Smith, J. E., Kilgore, H., & McNeill, C., Jr. (1990). Psychological factors that predict AIDS high-risk versus AIDS precautionary behavior. *Journal of Consulting and Clinical Psychology, 58,* 117–120.

Kelly, J. A., & Kalichman, S. C. (1998). Reinforcement value of unsafe sex as a predictor of condom use and continued HIV/AIDS risk behavior among gay and bisexual men. *Health Psychology, 17,* 328–335.

Kelly, J. A., Otto-Salaj, L. L., Sikkema, K. J., Pinkerton, S. D., & Bloom, F. R. (1998). Implications of HIV treatment advances for behavioral research on AIDS: Protease inhibitors and new challenges in HIV secondary prevention. *Health Psychology, 17,* 310–319.

Kelly, M. A., McKinty, H. R., & Carr, R. (1988). Utilization of hypnosis to promote compliance with routine dental flossing. *American Journal of Clinical Hypnosis, 31,* 57–60.

Keltikangas-Järvinen, L., & Räikkönen, K. (1990a). Developmental trends in Type A behavior as predictors for the development of somatic coronary heart disease risk factors. *Psychotherapy and Psychosomatics, 51,* 210–215.

Keltikangas-Järvinen, L., & Räikkönen, K. (1990b). Type A factors as predictors of somatic risk factors of coronary heart disease in young Finns: A six-year follow-up study. *Journal of Psychomatic Research, 34,* 89–97.

Kempe, R. S. (1997). A developmental approach to the treatment of abused children. In M. E. Helfer, R. S. Kempe, & R. D. Krugman (Eds.), *The battered child* (5th ed.; pp. 543–565). Chicago: University of Chicago Press.

Kendall, P. C., & Watson, D. (1981). Psychological preparation for stressful medical procedures. In C. K. Prokop & L. A. Bradley (Eds.), *Medical psychology: Contributions to behavioral medicine* (pp. 197–221). New York: Academic Press.

Kenford, S. L., Fiore, M. C., Jorenby, D. E., Smith, S. S., Wetter, D., & Baker, T. B. (1994). Predicting smoking cessation: Who will quit with and without the nicotine patch. *Journal of the American Medical Association, 271,* 589–604.

Kent, D. (1997). Healthcare's redefinition drives research on relation between health and wealth. *American Psychology Society Observer, 10*(3), 12–13, 38.

Kerns, R. D., Turk, D. C., & Rudy, T. E. (1985). The West Haven-Yale Multidimensional Pain Inventory. *Pain, 23,* 345–356.

Kerr, G., & Goss, J. (1996). The effects of a stress management program on injuries and stress levels. *Journal of Applied Sport Psychology, 8,* 109–117.

Kessler, R. C. (1997). The effects of stressful life events on depression. *Annual Review of Psychology, 48,* 191–124.

Keys, A. (1980). *Seven countries: A multivariate analysis of death and coronary heart disease.* Cambridge, MA: Harvard University Press.

Keys, A., Brozek, J., Henschel, A., Mickelsen, O., & Taylor, H. L. (1950). *The biology of human starvation.* 2 vols. Minneapolis: University of Minnesota Press.

Khiefets, L. I., London, S. J., & Peters, J. M. (1997). Leukemia risk and occupational electric field exposure in Los Angles County, California. *American Journal of Epidemiology, 146,* 82–90.

Kiecolt-Glaser, J. K., Dura, J. R., Speicher, C. E., Trask, J., & Glaser, R. (1991). Spousal caregivers of dementia victims: Longitudinal changes in immunity and health. *Psychosomatic Medicine, 53,* 345–362.

Kiecolt-Glaser, J. K., Dyer, C. S., & Shuttleworth, E. C. (1988). Upsetting social interactions and distress among Alzheimer's disease family caregivers: A replication and extension. *American Journal of Community Psychology, 16,* 825–837.

Kiecolt-Glaser, J. K., Fisher, L., Ogrocki, P., Stout, J. C., Speicher, C. E., & Glaser, R. (1987). Marital quality, marital disruption, and immune function. *Psychosomatic Medicine, 49,* 13–35.

Kiecolt-Glaser, J. K., & Glaser, R. (1989). Psychoneuroimmunology: Past, present, and future. *Health Psychology, 8,* 677–682.

Kiecolt-Glaser, J. K., & Glaser, R. (1993). Mind and immunity. In D. Goleman & J. Gurin (Eds.), *Mind/body medicine: How to use your mind for better health* (pp. 39–61). Yonkers, NY: Consumer Reports Books.

Kiecolt-Glaser, J. K., Glaser, R., Cacioppo, J. T., MacCallum, R. C., Snydersmith, M., Cheongtag, K., & Malarkey, W. B. (1996). Marital conflict in older adults: Endocrine and immunological correlates. *Psychosomatic Medicine, 59,* 339–349.

Kiecolt-Glaser, J. K., Glaser, R., Dyer, C., Shuttleworth, E. C., Ogrocki, P., & Speicher, C. E. (1987). Chronic stress and immune function in family caregivers of Alzheimer's disease victims. *Psychosomatic Medicine, 49,* 523–535.

Kiecolt-Glaser, J. K., Malarkey, W. B., Cacioppo, J. T. & Glaser, R. (1994). Stressful personal relationships: Immune and endocrine function. In R. Glaser & J. K. Kiecolt-Glaser (Eds.), *Handbook of human stress and immunity* (pp. 321–339). San Diego, CA: Academic Press.

Kiecolt-Glaser, J. K., Marucha, P. T., Malarkey, W. B., Mercado, A. M., & Glaser, R. (1995). Slowing of wound healing by psychological stress. *Lancet, 346,* 1194–1196.

Kiecolt-Glaser, J. K., Newton, T., Cacioppo, J. T., MacCallum, R. C., Glaser, R., & Malarkey, W. B. (1997). Marital conflict and endocrine function: Are men really more physiologically affected than women? *Journal of Consulting and Clinical Psychology, 64,* 324–332.

Kiely, D. K., Wolf, P. A., Cupples, L. A., Beiser, A. S., & Kannel, W. B. (1994). Physical activity and stroke risk: The Framingham Study. *American Journal of Epidemiology, 140,* 608–620.

Kiernan, M., Rodin, J., Brownell, K. D., Wilmore, J. H., & Crandall, C. (1992). Relation of level of exercise, age, and weight-cycling history to weight and eating concerns in male and female runners. *Health Psychology, 11,* 418–421.

Kimball, C. P. (1981). *The biopsychosocial approach to the patient.* Baltimore: Williams & Wilkins.

King, A. C., Oman, R. F., Brassington, G. S., Bliwise, D. L., & Haskell, W. L. (1997). Moderate-intensity exercise and self-rated quality of sleep in older adults: A randomized controlled trial. *Journal of the American Medical Association, 277,* 32–37.

Kinney, R. D., Gatchel, R. J., Polatin, P. B., Fogarty, W. T., & Mayer, T. G. (1993). Prevalence of psychopathology in acute and chronic low back pain patients. *Journal of Occupational Rehabilitation, 3,* 95–103.

Kirschenbaum, K. S. (1997). Prevention of sedentary lifestyles: Rationale and methods. In W. P. Morgan (Ed.), *Physical activity and mental health* (pp. 33–48). Washington, DC: Taylor & Francis.

Kitamura, A., Hiroyasu, I., Sankai, T., Naito, Y., Sato, S., Klyama, M., Okamura, T., Nakagawa, Y., Lida, T., Shimamoto, T., & Komachi, Y. (1998) Alcohol intake and premature coronary heart disease in urban Japanese men. *American Journal of Epidemiology, 147,* 59–65.

Kiyak, H. A., Vitalinao, P. P., & Crinean, J. (1988). Patients' expectations as predictors of orthognathic surgery outcomes. *Health Psychology, 7,* 251–268.

Kizer, W. M. (1987). *The healthy workplace: A blueprint for corporate action.* New York: Wiley.

Klag, M. J., Ford, D. E., Mead, L. A., He, J., Whelton, Liang, K., & Levine, D. M. (1993). Serum cholesterol in young men and subsequent cardiovascular disease. *New England Journal of Medicine, 328,* 313–318.

Klatsky, A. L., & Armstrong, M. A. (1992). Alcohol, smoking, coffee, and cirrhosis. *American Journal of Epidemiology, 136,* 1248–1257.

Klatsky, A. L., Friedman, G. D., & Siegelaub, A. B. (1981). Alcohol and mortality: A ten-year Kaiser-Permanente experience. *Annals of Internal Medicine, 95,* 139–145.

Klein, D. N., & Rubovits, D. R. (1987). The reliability of subjects' reports of stressful life events inventories: A longitudinal study. *Journal of Behavioral Medicine, 10,* 501–512.

Klein, R., Klein, B. E. K. & Moss, S. E. (1998). Relation of smoking to the incidence of age-related maculopathy: The Beaver Dam Eye Study. *American Journal of Epidemiology, 147,* 103–110.

Klohn, L. S., & Rogers, R. W. (1991). Dimensions of the severity of a health threat: The persuasive effects of visibility, time of onset, and rate of onset on young women's intentions to prevent osteoporosis. *Health Psychology, 10,* 323–329.

Klonoff, E. A., & Landrine, H. (1993). Cognitive representations of bodily parts and products: Implications for health behavior. *Journal of Behavioral Medicine, 16,* 497–508.

Klonoff, E. A., & Landrine, H. (1994). Culture and gender diversity in commonsense beliefs about the causes of six illnesses. *Journal of Behavioral Medicine, 17,* 407–418.

Kluger, R. (1996). *Ashes to ashes; America's hundred-year cigarette war, the public health and the unabashed triumph of Philip Morris.* New York: Knopf.

Knekt, P., Järvinen, R., Seppänen, R., Hellövaara, M., Teppo, L., Pukkala, E. & Aromaa, A. (1997). Dietary flavonoids and the risk of lung cancer and other malignant neoplasms. *American Journal of Epidemiology, 146,* 223–230.

Knopp, R. H., Walden, C. E., Retzlaff, B. M., McCann, B. S., Dowdy, A. A., Albers, J. J., Gey, G. O., & Cooper, M. N. (1997). Long-term cholesterol-lowering effects of 4 fat-restricted diets in hypercholesterolemic and combined hyperlipidemic men. *Journal of the American Medical Association, 278,* 1509–1515.

Kobasa, S. C. (1979). Stressful life events, personality, and health: An inquiry into hardiness. *Journal of Personality and Social Psychology, 37,* 1–11.

Kobasa, S. C. O., & Maddi, S. R. (1977). Existential personality theory. In R. Corsini (Ed.), *Current personality theories* (pp. 242–276). Itasca, IL: Peacock.

Kobasa, S. C., Maddi, S. R., & Courington, S. (1981). Personality and constitution as mediators in the stress-illness relationship. *Journal of Health and Social Behavior, 22,* 368–378.

Kobasa, S. C., Maddi, S. R., & Kahn, S. (1982). Hardiness and health: A prospective study. *Journal of Personality and Social Psychology, 42,* 168–177.

Kog, E., & Vandereycken, W. (1985). Family characteristics of anorexia nervosa and bulimia: A review of the research literature. *Clinical Psychology Review, 5,* 159–180.

Koh, H. K., Bak, S. M., Geller, A. C., Mangione, T. W., Hingson, R. W., Levenson, S. M., Miller, D. R., Lew, R. A., & Howland, J. (1997). Sunbathing habits and sunscreen use among White adults: Results of a national survey. *American Journal of Public Health, 87,* 1214–1217

Koniak-Griffin, D. (1994). Aerobic exercise, psychological well-being, and physical discomforts during adolescent pregnancy. *Research in Nursing and Health, 17,* 253–268.

Koplan, J. P., Powell, K. E., Sikes, R. K., Shirley, R. W., & Campbell, C. C. (1982). An epidemiologic study of the benefits and risks of running. *Journal of the American Medical Association, 248,* 3118–3121.

Koski-Jannes, A. (1994). Drinking-related locus of control as a predictor of drinking after treatment. *Addictive Behaviors, 19,* 491–495.

Kovacs, M., Iyengar, S., Goldston, D., Obrosky, D. S., Stewart, J., & Marsh, J. (1990). Psychological functioning among mothers of children with insulin-dependent diabetes mellitus: A longitudinal study. *Journal of Consulting and Clinical Psychology, 58,* 189–195.

Kozlowski, L. T., Wilkinson, A., Skinner, W., Kent, C., Franklin, T., & Pope, M. (1989). Comparing tobacco cigarette dependence with other drug dependencies. *Journal of the American Medical Association, 261,* 898–901.

Kral, J. G. (1992). Overview of surgical techniques for treating obesity. *American Journal of Clinical Nutrition, 55,* 552S–555S.

Kramer, A. M. (1995). Health care for elderly persons—myths and realities. *New England Journal of Medicine, 332,* 1027–1029.

Kramsch, D. M., Aspen, A. J., Abramowitz, B. M., Kreimendahl, T., & Hood, W. B., Jr. (1981). Reduction of coronary atherosclerosis by moderate conditioning exercise in monkeys on an atherogenic diet. *New England Journal of Medicine, 305,* 1483–1489.

Krause, N. (1991). Stress and isolation from close ties in later life. *Journals of Gerontology, 46,* S183–S184.

Kremer, E. F., Atkinson, J. H., Jr., & Ignelzi, R. J. (1981). Measurement of pain: Patient preference does not confound pain measurement. *Pain, 10,* 241–248.

Krieger, N., & Sidney, S. (1996). Racial discrimination and blood pressure: The CARDIA study of young Black and White adults. *American Journal of Public Health, 86,* 1370–1378.

Krieger, N., Sidney, S., & Coakley, E. (1998). Racial discrimination and skin color in the CARDIA study: Implications for public health research. *American Journal of Public Health, 88,* 1308–1313.

Krokosky, N. J., & Reardon, R. C. (1989). The accuracy of nurses' and doctors' perception of patient pain. In S. G. Funk, E. M. Tornquist, M. T. Champagne, L. A. Copp, & R. A. Wiese (Eds.), *Key aspects of comfort: Management of pain, fatigue, and nausea* (pp. 127–140). New York: Springer.

Kronmal, R. A., Cain, K. C., Ye, Z., & Omenn, G. (1993). Total serum cholesterol levels and mortality risk as a function of age: A report based on the Framingham data. *Archives of Internal Medicine, 153,* 1065–1073.

Kujala, U. M., Kaprio, J., Sarna, S., & Koskenvuo, M. (1998). Relationship of leisure-time physical activity and mortality: The Finnish Twin Cohort. *Journal of the American Medical Association, 279,* 440–444.

Kulik, J. A., & Carlino, P. (1987). The effect of verbal commitment and treatment choice on medication compliance in a pediatric setting. *Journal of Behavioral Medicine, 10,* 367–376.

Kulik, J. A., & Mahler, H. I. M. (1993). Emotional support as a moderator of adjustment and compliance after coronary artery bypass surgery: A longitudinal study. *Journal of Behavioral Medicine, 16,* 48–63.

Kurz, D. (1997). Physical assaults by male partners: A major social problem. In M. R. Walsh (Ed.), *Men, women, and gender: Ongoing debates* (pp. 222–231). New Haven, CT: Yale University Press.

Kushi, L., Fee, R. M., Folsom, A. R., Mink, P. J., Anderson, K. E., & Sellers, T. A. (1997). Physical activity and mortality in postmenopausal women. *Journal of the American Medical Association, 227,* 1287–1292.

Lachs, M. S., Williams, C., O'Brien, S., Hurst, L., & Horwitz, R. (1997). Risk factors for reported elder abuse and neglect: A nine-year observational cohort study. *The Gerontologist, 37,* 469–474.

Laforge, R. G., Greene, G. W., & Prochaska, J. O. (1994). Psychosocial factors influencing low fruit and vegetable consumption. *Journal of Behavioral Medicine, 17,* 361–374.

Lakka, T. A., & Salonen, J. T. (1992). Physical activity and serum lipids: A cross-sectional population study in Eastern Finnish men. *American Journal of Epidemiology, 136,* 806–816.

Lakka, T. A., Venäläinen, J. M., Rauramaa, R., Salonen, R., Tuomilehto, J., & Salonen, J. T. (1994). Relations of leisure-time physical activity and cardiorespiratory fitness to the risk of acute myocardial infarction in men. *New England Journal of Medicine, 330,* 1549–1554.

Lam, T. H., He, Y., Li, L. S., Li, L. S., He, S. F., & Liang, B. Q. (1997). Mortality attributable to cigarette smoking in China. *Journal of the American Medical Association, 278,* 1505–1508.

Lambert, S. A. (1996). The effects of hypnosis/guided imagery on the postoperative course of children. *Journal of Developmental and Behavioral Pediatrics, 17,* 307–310.

Landrine, H., & Klonoff, E. A. (1994). Cultural diversity in causal attributions for illness: The role of the supernatural. *Journal of Behavioral Medicine, 17,* 181–193.

Langer, E. J., & Rodin, J. (1976). The effects of choice and enhanced personal responsibility for the aged: A field experiment in an institutional setting. *Journal of Personality and Social Psychology, 34,* 191–198.

Langford, H. G., Blaufox, D., Oberman, A., Hawkins, M., Curb, J. D., Cutter, G. R., Wassertheil-Smoller, S., Pressel, S., Babcock, C., Abernethy, J. D., Hotchkiss, J., & Tyler, M. (1985). Dietary therapy slows the return of hypertension after stopping prolonged medication. *Journal of the American Medical Association, 253,* 657–664.

Lantz, P. M., House, J. S., Lepkowsi, J. M., Williams, D. R., Mero, R. P., & Chen, J. (1998). Socioeconomic factors, health behaviors, and mortality: Results from a nationally representative prospective study of US adults. *Journal of the American Medical Association, 279,* 1703–1708.

Laporte, R., Brenes, G., & Dearwarter, S. (1983). HDL-cholesterol across a spectrum of physical activity from quadriplegia to marathon running. *Lancet, I,* 1212–1213.

LaRosa, J. H. (1990). Executive women and health: Perceptions and practices. *American Journal of Public Health, 80,* 1450–1454.

Larroque, B., Kaminski, M., Dehaene, P., Subtil, D., Delfosse, M-J., & Querleu, D. (1995). Moderate prenatal alcohol exposure and psychomotor development at preschool age. *American Journal of Public Health, 85,* 1654–1661.

Lash, T. L., & Aschengrau, A. (1999). Active and passive cigarette smoking and the occurrence of breast cancer. *American Journal of Epidemiology, 149,* 5–12.

Lau, R. R. (1997). Cognitive representations of health and illness. In D. S. Gochman (Ed.), *Handbook of health behavior research I: Personal and social determinants* (pp. 51–69). New York: Plenum Press.

Lau, R. R., & Hartman, K. A. (1983). Common sense representations of common illnesses. *Health Psychology, 2,* 167–185.

Launer, L. J., Feskens, E. J. M., Kalmjin, S., & Kromhout, D. (1996). Smoking, drinking, and thinking: The Zuphen Elderly Study. *American Journal of Epidemiology, 143,* 219–227.

Lavey, R. S., & Taylor, C. B. (1985). The nature of relaxation therapy. In S. R. Burchfield (Ed.), *Stress: Psychological and physiological interactions.* Washington, DC: Hemisphere.

Law, A., Logan, H., & Baron, R. S. (1994). Desire for control, felt control, and stress intervention training during dental treatment. *Journal of Personality and Social Psychology, 67,* 926–936.

Lazarus, R. S. (1984a). Puzzles in the study of daily hassles. *Journal of Behavioral Medicine, 7,* 375–389.

Lazarus, R. S. (1984b). The trivialization of distress. In B. L. Hammonds & C. J. Scheirer (Eds.), *Psychology and health: The Master Lecture Series* (pp. 125–144). Washington, DC: American Psychological Association.

Lazarus, R. S. (1993). From psychological stress to the emotions: A history of changing outlooks. *Annual Review of Psychology, 44,* 1–21.

Lazarus, R. S., & DeLongis, A. (1983). Psychological stress and coping in aging. *American Psychologist, 38,* 245–254.

Lazarus, R. S., DeLongis, A., Folkman, S., & Gruen, R. (1985). Stress and adaptational outcomes. *American Psychologist, 40,* 770–779.

Lazarus, R. S., & Folkman, S. (1984). *Stress, appraisal, and coping.* New York: Springer.

Lee, I-M., Hsieh, C-c., & Paffenbarger, R. S., Jr. (1995). Exercise intensity and longevity in men. *Journal of the American Medical Association, 273,* 1179–1184.

Lee, I-M., & Paffenbarger, R. S., Jr. (1992). Change in body weight and longevity. *Journal of the American Medical Association, 268,* 2045–2049.

Lee, I-M., Paffenbarger, R. S., Jr., & Hsieh, C-c. (1992). Physical activity and risk of prostatic cancer among college alumni. *American Journal of Epidemiology, 135,* 169–179.

Lee, J. A. H. (1997). Declining effect of latitude on melanoma mortality rates in the United States: A preliminary study. *American Journal of Epidemiology, 146,* 413–417.

Leevy, C. M., Gellene, R., & Ning, M. (1964). Primary liver cancer in cirrhosis of the alcoholic. *Annals of the New York Academy of Science, 114,* 1026–1020.

Lehman, A. K., & Rodin, J. (1989). Styles of self-nurturance and disordered eating. *Journal of Consulting and Clinical Psychology, 57,* 117–122.

Lehrer, P. M., Carr, R., Sargunaraj, D., & Woolfolk, R. L. (1994). Stress management techniques: Are they all equivalent, or do they have specific effects? *Biofeedback and Self-Regulation, 19,* 353–401.

Leibel, R. L., Rosenbaum, M., & Hirsch, J. (1995). Changes in energy expenditure resulting from altered body weight. *New England Journal of Medicine, 332,* 621–629.

Le Marchand, L., Kolonel, L. N., & Yoshizawa, C. N. (1991). Lifetime occupational physical activity and prostate cancer risk. *American Journal of Epidemiology, 133,* 103–111.

Leproult, R., Copinschi, G., Buxton, O., & Van Cauter, E. (1997). Sleep loss results in an elevation of cortisol levels the next evening. *Sleep, 20,* 865–870.

Lerner, W. D., & Fallon, H. J. (1985). The alcohol withdrawal syndrome. *New England Journal of Medicine, 313,* 951–952.

LeRoy, P. L., & Filasky, R. (1990). Thermography. In J. J. Bonica (Ed.), *The management of pain* (2nd ed., pp. 610–621). Malvern, PA: Lea & Febiger.

Lescohier, L., & Gallagher, S. S. (1996). Unintentional injury. In R. J. DiClemente, W. B. Hansen, & L. E. Ponton (Eds.), *Handbook of adolescent health risk behavior* (pp. 225–258). New York: Plenum Press.

Lester, D. (1994). Are there unique features of suicide in adults of different ages and developmental stages? *Omega Journal of Death and Dying, 29,* 337–348.

Leutwyler, K. (1995, April). The price of prevention. *Scientific American, 272,* 124–129.

Levenson, R. L., & Mellins, C. A. (1992). Pediatric HIV disease: What psychologists need to know. *Professional Psychology Research and Practice, 23,* 410–415.

Levenson, R. W., Sher, K. J., Grossman, L. M., Newman, J., & Newlin, D. B. (1980). Alcohol and stress response dampening: Pharmacological effects, expectancy, and tension reduction. *Journal of Abnormal Psychology, 89,* 528–538.

Leventhal, H. (1970). Findings and theory in the study of fear communications. *Advances in Experimental Social Psychology, 5,* 119–186.

Leventhal, H., & Avis, N. (1976). Pleasure, addiction, and habit: Factors in verbal report or factors in smoking behavior? *Journal of Abnormal Psychology, 85,* 478–488.

Leventhal, H., & Cleary, P. D. (1980). The smoking problem: A review of the research and theory in behavioral risk modification. *Psychological Bulletin, 88,* 370–405.

Leventhal, H., & Diefenbach, M. (1991). The active side of illness cognition. In J. A. Skelton & R. T. Croyle (Eds.), *Mental representation in health and illness* (pp. 247–272). New York: Springer-Verlag.

Leventhal, H., Nerenz, D. R., & Steele, D. J. (1984). Illness representations and coping with health threats. In A. Baum, S. E. Taylor, & J. E. Singer (Eds.), *Handbook of psychology and health Vol. 4 Social psychological aspect of health* (pp. 219–252). Hillsdale, NJ: Erlbaum.

Levi, L. (1974). Psychosocial stress and disease: A conceptual model. In E. K. E. Gunderson & R. H. Rahe (Eds.), *Life stress and illness* (pp. 8–33). Springfield, IL: Thomas.

Levy, R. K. (1997). The transtheoretical model of change: An application to bulimia nervosa. *Psychotherapy, 34,* 278–285

Levy, S. M. (1985). *Behavior and cancer: Life-style and psychosocial factors in the initiation and progression of cancer.* San Francisco: Jossey-Bass.

Ley, P. (1997). Compliance among patients. In A. Baum, S. Newman, J. Weinman, R. West, & C. McManus (Eds.), *Cambridge handbook of psychology, health and medicine* (pp. 281–284). Cambridge, United Kingdom: Cambridge University Press.

Li, G., & Baker, S. P. (1994). Alcohol in fatally injured bicyclists. 37th Annual Meeting of the Association for Advancement of Automotive Medicine (1993, San Antonio, Texas). *Accident Analysis and Prevention, 26,* 543–548.

Liao, Y., Cooper, R. S., Cao, G., Durazo-Arivizu, R., Kaufman, J. S., Luke, A., & McGee, D. L. (1998). Mortality patterns among adult Hispanics: Findings from the NHIS, 1986 to 1990. *American Journal of Public Health, 88,* 227–232.

Lichtenstein, E. L., Hollis, J. F., Severson, H. H., Stevens, V. J., Vogt, T. M., Glasgow, R. E., & Andrews, J. A. (1996). Tobacco cessation interventions in health care settings: Rationale, model, outcomes. *Addictive Behaviors, 21,* 709–720.

Liddell, A. (1990). Personality characteristics versus medical and dental experiences of dentally anxious children. *Journal of Behavioral Medicine, 13,* 183–194.

Lierman, L. M., Kasprzyk, D., Benoliel, J. Q. (1991). Understanding adherence to breast self-examination in older women. *Western Journal of Nursing Research, 13,* 46–66.

Light, K. C., Kopke, J. P., Obrist, P. A., & Willis, P. W. (1983). Psychological stress induces sodium fluid retention in men at high risk for hypertension. *Science, 220,* 429–431.

Light, K. C., Turner, J. R., Hinderliter, A. L., & Sherwood, A. (1993a). Race and gender comparisons: I. Hemodynamic responses to a series of stressors. *Health Psychology, 12,* 354–365.

Light, K. C., Turner, J. R., Hinderliter, A. L., & Sherwood, A. (1993b). Race and gender comparisons: II. Predictions of work blood pressure from laboratory baseline and cardiovascular reactivity measures. *Health Psychology, 12,* 366–375.

Lilienfeld, A. M., & Lilienfeld, D. E. (1980). *Foundations of epidemiology* (2nd ed.). New York: Oxford University Press.

Linden, W. (1988). Biopsychological barriers to the behavioral treatment of hypertension. In W. Linden (Ed.), *Biological barriers in behavioral medicine* (pp. 163–191). New York: Plenum Press.

Linden, W., Stossel, C., & Maurice, J. (1996). Psychosocial interventions for patients with coronary artery disease: A meta-analysis. *Archives of Internal Medicine, 156,* 745–752.

Lindsted, K. D., & Singh, P. N. (1997). Body mass and 26-year risk of mortality among women who never smoked: Findings from the Adventist Mortality study. *American Journal of Epidemiology, 146,* 1–11.

Linn, R. (1976). *The last chance diet.* New York: Bantam.

Linn, S., Carroll, M., Johnson, C., Fulwood, R., Kalsbeek, W., & Briefel, R. (1993). High-density lipoprotein cholesterol and alcohol consumption in US White and Black adults: Data from NHANES II. *American Journal of Public Health, 83,* 811–816.

Linton, S. J., & Bradley, L. A. (1996). Strategies for the prevention of chronic pain. In R. J. Gatchel, & D. C. Turk (Eds.), *Psychological approaches to pain management: A practitioner's handbook* (pp. 438–457). New York: Guilford Press.

Lipton, R. I. (1994). The effects of moderate alcohol use on the relationship between stress and depression. *American Journal of Public Health, 84,* 1913–1917.

Liska, A. E., & Baccaglini, W. (1990). Feeling safe by comparison: Crime in the newspapers. *Social Problems, 37,* 360–374.

Lissner, L., Odell, P. M., D'Agostino, R. B., Stokes, J., III, Kreger, B. E., Belanger, A. J., & Brownell, K. D. (1991). Variability of body weight and health outcomes in the Framingham population. *New England Journal of Medicine, 324,* 1839–1844.

Liu, S., Siegel, P. Z., Brewer, R. D., Mokdad, A. H., Sleet, D. A., & Serdula, M. (1997). Prevalence of alcohol-impaired driving: Results from a national self-reported survey of health behaviors. *Journal of the American Medical Association, 277,* 122–125.

Loeser, J. D. (1989). Chronic pain. In F. C. Seitz, J. E. Carr, & M. Covey (Eds), *Issues in behavioral medicine* (pp. 16–20). Bozeman, MT: Clinical Management Consultants.

Loeser, J. D. (1990). Pain after amputation: Phantom limb and stump pain. In J. J. Bonica (Ed.), *The management of pain* (2nd ed., pp. 244–256). Malvern, PA: Lea & Febiger.

Loomis, D., & Richardson, D. (1998). Race and the risk of fatal injury at work. *American Journal of Public Health, 88,* 40–44.

Loomis, D. P., Richardson, D. B., Wolf, S. H., Runyan, C. W., & Butts, J. D. (1997). Fatal occupational injuries in a southern state. *American Journal of Epidemiology, 145,* 1089–1099.

Lorber, J. (1975). Good patients and problem patients: Conformity and deviance in a general hospital. *Journal of Health and Social Behavior, 16,* 213–225.

Lovallo, William R. (1997). *Stress & health: Biological and psychological interactions.* Thousand Oaks, CA: Sage.

Lovastatin Study Group III. (1988). A multicenter comparison of lovastatin and cholestyramine therapy for severe hypercholesterolemia. *Journal of the American Medical Association, 260,* 359–366.

Lowry, R., Holtzman, D., Truman, B. I., Kann, L., Collins, J. L., & Kolbe, L. J. (1994). Substance use and HIV-related sexual behaviors among US high school students: Are they related? *American Journal of Public Health, 84,* 1116–1120.

Loxley, W. M., & Hawks, D. V. (1994). AIDS and injecting drug use: Very risky behaviour in a Perth sample of injecting drug users. *Drug and Alcohol Review, 13,* 21–30.

Lubin, J. H., Blot, W. J., Berrino, F., Flamant, R., Gillis, C. R., Kunzer, M., Schmahl, D., & Visco, G. (1984). Patterns of lung cancer according to type of cigarette smokers. *International Journal of Cancer, 33,* 569–576.

Lubin, J. H., Richter, B. S., & Blot, W. J. (1984). Lung cancer risk with cigar and pipe use. *Journal of the National Cancer Institute, 73,* 377–381.

Lucas, A. R., Beard, C. M., O'Fallon, W. M., & Kurland, L. T. (1991). 50-year trends in the incidence of anorexia nervosa in Rochester, Minn.: A population-based study. *American Journal of Psychiatry, 7,* 917–922.

Lucchesi, B. R., Schuster, C. R., & Emley, G. S. (1967). The role of nicotine as a determinant of cigarette smoking frequency in man with observations of certain cardiovascular effects associated with the tobacco alkaloid. *Clinical Pharmacology and Therapeutics, 8,* 791.

Luecken, L. J., Suarez, E. C., Kuhn, C. M., Barefoot, J. C., Blumenthal, J. A., Siegler, I. C., & Williams, R. B. (1997). Stress in employed women: Impact of marital status and children at home on neurohormone output and home strain. *Psychosomatic Medicine, 59,* 352–359.

Lundberg, U. (1998). Work and stress in women. In K. Orth-Gomér, M. Chesney, & N. K. Wenger (Eds.), *Women, stress, and heart disease* (pp. 41–56). Mahwah, NJ: Erlbaum.

Lutgendorf, S. K., Antoni, M. H., Ironson, G., Starr, K., Costello, N., Zuckerman, M., Klimas, N., Fletcher, M. A., & Schneiderman, N. (1998). Changes in cognitive coping skills and social support during cognitive behavioral stress management intervention and distress outcomes in symptomatic human immunodeficiency virus (HIV)-seropositive gay men. *Psychosomatic Medicine, 60,* 204–214.

Lutz, R. W., Silbret, M., & Olshan, W. (1983). Treatment outcome and compliance with therapeutic regimens: Long-term follow-up of a multidisciplinary pain program. *Pain, 17,* 301–308.

Lyles, J. N., Burish, T. G., Krozely, M. G., & Oldham, R. K. (1982). Efficacy of relaxation training and guided imagery in reducing the aversiveness of cancer chemotherapy. *Journal of Consulting and Clinical Psychology, 50,* 509–524.

Lynch, D. J., Birk, T. J., Weaver, M. T., Gohara, A. F., Leighton, R. F., Repka, F. J., & Walsh, M. E. (1992). Adherence to exercise interventions in the treatment of hypercholesterolemia. *Journal of Behavior Medicine, 15,* 365–377.

Macarthur, C., Saunders, N., & Feldman, W. (1995). *Helicobacter pylori,* gastroduodenal disease, and recurrent abdominal pain in children. *Journal of the American Medical Association, 273,* 729–734.

MacDorman, M. F., Cnattingius, S., Hoffman, H. J., Kramer, M. S., & Haglund, B. (1997). Sudden infant death syndrome and smoking in the United States and Sweden. *American Journal of Epidemiology, 146,* 249–257.

MacDougal, J. M., Dembroski, T. M., Dimsdale, J. E., & Hackett, T. P. (1985). Components of Type A, hostility, and anger-in: Further relationships to angiographic findings. *Health Psychology, 4,* 137–142.

Macharia, W. M., Leon, G., Rowe, B. H., Stephenson, B. J., & Haynes, R. B. (1992). An overview of interventions to improve compliance with appointment keeping for medical services. *Journal of the American Medical Association, 267,* 1813–1817.

MacLean, D., & Reichlin, S. (1981). Neuroendocrinology and the immune process. In R. Ader (Ed.), *Psychoneuroimmunology* (pp. 475–520). New York: Academic Press.

Maclure, M. (1993). Demonstration of deductive meta-analysis: Ethanol intake and risk of myocardial infarction. *Epidemiology Review, 15,* 328–351.

Maes, M., Hendricks, D., Van Gastel, A., Demedts, P., Wauters, A., Neels, H., Janca, A., & Scharpe, S. (1997). Effects of psychological stress on serum immunoglobulin, complement and acute phase protein concentrations in normal volunteers. *Psychoneuroendocrinology, 22,* 397–410.

Magdol, L., Moffitt, T. E., Caspi, A., Newman, D. L., Fagan, J., & Silva, P. A. (1997). Gender differences in partner violence in a birth cohort of 21-year-olds bridging the gap between clinical and epidemiological approaches. *Journal of Consulting and Clinical Psychology, 65,* 68–78.

Maher, R. A., & Rickwood, D. (1997). The theory of planned behavior, domain specific self-efficacy and adolescent smoking. *Journal of Child and Adolescent Substance Abuse, 6,* 57–76.

Maier, S. F., Watkins, L. R., & Fleshner, M. (1994). Psychoneuroimmunology: The interface between behavior, brain, and immunity. *American Psychologist, 49,* 1004–1017.

Mairs, D. A. E. (1995). Hypnosis and pain in childbirth. *Contemporary Hypnosis, 12,* 111–118.

Malley, P. B., Kush, F., & Bogo, R. J. (1994). School-based adolescent suicide prevention and intervention programs: A survey. *School Counselor, 42,* 130–136.

Malmivaara, A., Hakkinen, U., Aro, T., Heinrichs, M., Koskenniemi, L., Klosma, E., Lappi, S., Paloheimo, R., Servo, C., Vaaranen, V., & Hernberg, S. (1995). The treatment of acute low back pain—bed rest, exercise, or ordinary activity. *New England Journal of Medicine, 332,* 351–355.

Mancuso, R. A., & Pennebaker, J. W. (1994). *Resolving vs. dredging up past traumas: The effects of writing.* Paper presented at the convention of the American Psychological Association, Los Angeles, CA.

Manczak, D. W. (1997, December). Hospitalization: Helping a child cope. *Clinical Reference Systems,* p. 1477.

Manne, S. L., Bakeman, R., Jacobsen, P. B., Gorfinkle, K., Bernstein, D., & Redd, W. H. (1992). Adult-child interaction during invasive medical procedures. *Health Psychology, 11,* 241–249.

Mannino, D. M., Klevens, R. M., & Flanders, W. D. (1994). Cigarette smoking: An independent risk factor for impotence? *American Journal of Epidemiology, 140,* 1003–1008.

Manson, J. E., Nathan, D. M., Krolewski, A. S., Stampfer, M. J., Willett, W. C., & Hennekens, C. H. (1992). A prospective study of exercise and incidence of diabetes among US male physicians. *Journal of the American Medical Association, 268,* 63–67.

Manson, J. E., Willett, W. C., Stampfer, M. J., Colditz, G. A., Hunter, D. J., Hankinson, S. E., Hennekens, C. H., & Speizer, F. E. (1995). Body weight and mortality among women. *New England Journal of Medicine, 333,* 677–685.

Markovitz, J. H., Matthews, K. A., Kannel, W. B., Cobb, J. L., & D'Agostino, R. B. (1993). Psychological predictors of hypertension in the Framingham study: Is there tension in hypertension? *Journal of the American Medical Association, 270,* 2439–2443.

Marlatt, G. A. (1987). Alcohol, the magic elixir: Stress, expectancy, and the transformation of emotional states. In E. Gottheil, K. A. Druly, S. Pashko, & S. P. Weinstein (Eds.), *Stress and addiction* (pp. 302–322). New York: Brunner/Mazel.

Marlatt, G. A., Demming, B., & Reid, J. (1973). Loss of control drinking in alcoholics: An experimental analogue. *Journal of Abnormal Psychology, 81,* 233–241.

Marlatt, G. A., & Gordon, J. R. (1980). Determinants of relapse: Implication for the maintenance of behavior change. In P. O. Davidson & S. M. Davidson (Eds.), *Behavioral medicine: Changing health lifestyles* (pp. 410–452). New York: Brunner/Mazel.

Marlatt, G. A., & Rohsenow, D. J. (1980). Cognitive processes in alcohol use: Expectancy and the balanced placebo design. In N. Mello (Ed.), *Advances in substance abuse: Behavioral and biological research.* Greenwich, CT: JAI Press.

Marlowe, N. (1998). Stressful events, appraisal, coping and recurrent headache. *Journal of Clinical Psychology, 54,* 247–256.

Maron, D. J., & Fortmann, S. P. (1987). Nicotine yield and measures of cigarette smoke exposure in a large population: Are lower-yield cigarettes safer? *American Journal of Public Health, 77,* 546–549.

Marques-Vidal, P., Ducimetiere, P., Evans, A., Campou, J-P., & Arveiler, D. (1996). Alcohol consumption and myocardial infarction: A case-control study in France and Northern Iceland. *American Journal of Epidemiology, 143,* 1089–1093.

Marshall, B. J. (1995). Helicobacter pylori: The etiologic agent for peptic ulcers. *Journal of the American Medical Association, 274,* 1064–1066.

Martikainen, P., & Valkomen, T. (1996). Mortality after the death of a spouse: Rates and causes of death in a large Finnish cohort. *American Journal of Public Health, 86,* 1087–1093.

Martin, J. E., & Dubbert, P. M. (1985). Adherence to exercise. In R. L. Terjung (Ed.), *Exercise and sport sciences reviews* (Vol. 13). New York: Macmillan.

Martin, P. R., Adinoff, B., Weingarter, H., Mukherjee, A. B., & Eckardt, M. J. (1986). Alcoholic organic brain disease: Nosology and pathophysiologic mechanisms. *Progress in Neuropsychopharmacolgy and Biological Psychiatry, 10,* 147–164.

Martin, T. R., & Bracken, M. B. (1986). Association of low birth weight with passive smoke exposure in pregnancy. *American Journal of Epidemiology, 124,* 633–642.

Martinsen, E. W., & Morgan, W. P. (1997). Antidepressant effects of physical activity. In W. P. Morgan (Ed.), *Physical activity and mental health* (pp. 93–106). Washington, DC: Taylor & Francis.

Marucha, P. T., Kiecolt-Glaser, J. K., & Favagehi, M. (1998). Mucosal wound healing is impaired by examination stress. *Psychosomatic Medicine, 60,* 362–365.

Maslach, C. (1997). Burnout in health professionals. In A. Baum, S. Newman, J. Weinman, R. West, & C. McManus (Eds.), *Cambridge handbook of psychology, health and medicine* (pp. 275–278). Cambridge, United Kingdom: Cambridge University Press.

Mason, J. W. (1971). A reevaluation of the concept of "non-specificity" in stress theory. *Journal of Psychiatric Research, 8,* 323–333.

Mason, J. W. (1975). A historical view of the stress field. Pt. 2. *Journal of Human Stress, 1,* 22–36.

Masur, F. T., III. (1981). Adherence to health care regimens. In C. K. Prokop & L. A. Bradley (Eds.), *Medical psychology: Contributions to behavioral medicine.* New York: Academic Press.

Matanoski, G., Kanchanaraksa, S., Lantry, D., & Chang, Y. (1995). Characteristics of nonsmoking women in NHANES I and NHANES I Epidemiologic Follow-up Study with exposure to spouses who smoke. *American Journal of Epidemiology, 142,* 149–157.

Matarazzo, J. D. (1980). Behavioral health and behavioral medicine: Frontiers for a new health psychology. *American Psychologist, 35,* 807–817.

Matarazzo, J. D. (1982). Behavioral health's challenge to academic, scientific, and professional psychology. *American Psychologist, 37,* 1–14.

Matarazzo, J. D. (1984). Behavioral health: A 1990 challenge for the health sciences professions. In J. D. Matarazzo, S. M. Weiss, J. A. Herd, N. E. Miller, & S. M. Weiss (Eds.), *Behavioral health: A handbook of health enhancement and disease prevention* (pp. 3–40). New York: Wiley.

Matarazzo, J. D. (1987a). Postdoctoral education and training of service providers in health psychology. In G. C. Stone, S. M. Weiss, J. D. Matarazzo, N. E. Miller, J. Rodin, C. D. Belar, M. J. Follick, & J. E. Singer (Eds.), *Health psychology: A discipline and a profession* (pp. 371–388). Chicago: University of Chicago Press.

Matarazzo, J. D. (1987b). Relationships of health psychology to other segments of psychology. In G. C. Stone, S. M. Weiss, J. D. Matarazzo, N. E. Miller, J. Rodin, C. D. Belar, M. J. Follick, & J. E. Singer (Eds.), *Health psychology: A discipline and a profession* (pp. 41–59). Chicago: University of Chicago Press.

Matarazzo, J. D. (1994). Health and behavior: The coming together of science and practice in psychology and medicine after a century of benign neglect. *Journal of Clinical Psychology in Medical Settings, 1,* 7–39.

Maton, K. I. (1988). Social support, organizational characteristics, psychological well-being, and group appraisal in three self-help group populations. *American Journal of Community Psychology, 16*, 53–77.

Matthews, K. A. (1989). Interactive effects of behavior and reproductive hormones on sex differences in risk for coronary heart disease. *Health Psychology, 8*, 373–387.

Matthews, K. A., Shumaker, S. A., Bowen, D. J., Langer, R. D., Hunt, J. R., Kaplan, R. M., Klesges, R. C., & Ritenbaugh, C. (1997). Women's health initiative: Why now? What is it? What's new? *American Psychologist, 52*, 101–116.

Mayeux, R., & Schupf, N. (1995). Apolipoprotein E and Alzheimer's disease; The implications of progress in molecular medicine. *American Journal of Public Health, 85*, 1280–1284.

Mayfield, D. (1976). Alcoholism, alcohol intoxication, and assaultive behavior. *Diseases of the Nervous System, 37*, 228–291.

McAuley, E. (1993). Self-efficacy and the maintenance of exercise participation in older adults. *Journal of Behavioral Medicine, 16*, 103–113.

McAuley, E. (1994). Physical activity and psychosocial outcomes. In C. Bouchard, R. J. Shephard, & T. Stephens (Eds.), *Physical activity, fitness, and health: International proceedings and consensus statement* (pp. 551–568). Champaign, IL: Human Kinetics.

McBride, C. M., Curry, S. J., Grothaus, L. C., Nelson, J. C., Lando, H., & Pirie, P. L. (1998). Partner smoking status and pregnant smoker's perceptions of support for the likelihood of smoking cessation. *Health Psychology, 17*, 63–69.

McCaffery, M. (1979). *Nursing management of the patient with pain* (2nd ed.). Philadelphia: Lippincott.

McCaul, K. D., Monson, N., & Maki, R. H. (1992). Does distraction reduce pain-produced distress among college students? *Health Psychology, 11*, 210–217.

McCaul, K. D., Sandgren, A. K., O'Neill, H. K., & Hinsz, V. B. (1993). The value of the theory of planned behavior, perceived control, and self-efficacy for predicting health-protective behaviors. *Basic and Applied Social Psychology, 14*, 231–252.

McClintic, J. R. (1978). *Physiology of the human body* (2nd ed.). New York: Wiley.

McCracken, L. M. (1997). "Attention" to pain in persons with chronic pain: A behavioral approach. *Behavior Therapy, 28*, 271–284.

McCutchan, J. A. (1990). Virology, immunology, and clinical course of HIV infection. *Journal of Consulting and Clinical Psychology, 58*, 5–12.

McGinnis, J. M., & Foege, W. H. (1993). Actual causes of death in the United States. *Journal of the American Medical Association, 270*, 2207–2212.

McGrady, A. (1994). Effects of group relaxation training and thermal biofeedback on blood pressure and related physiological and psychological variables in essential hypertension. *Biofeedback and Self Relaxation, 19*, 51–66.

McHugh, S., & Vallis, M. (1986). Illness behavior: Operationalization of the biopsychosocial model. In S. McHugh & J. M. Vallis (Eds.), *Illness behavior: A multidisciplinary model* (pp. 1–31). New York: Plenum Press.

McKinnon, W., Weisse, C. S., Reynolds, C. P., Bowles, C. A., & Baum, A. (1989). Chronic stress, leucocyte subpopulations, and humoral response to latent viruses. *Health Psychology, 8*, 389–402.

McLean., S., Skirboll, L. R., & Pert, C. B. (1985). Comparison of substance P and enkephalin distribution in rat brain: An overview using radioimmunocytochemistry. *Neuroscience, 14*, 837–852.

McLellan, A. T., Arndt, I. O., Metzger, D. S., Woody, G. E., & O'Brien, C. P. (1993). The effects of psychosocial services in substance abuse treatment. *Journal of the American Medical Association, 269*, 1953–1959.

McMurran, M. (1994). *The psychology of addiction*. London: Taylor & Francis.

McMurray, R. G., Sheps, D. S., & Guinan, D. M. (1984). Effects of naloxone on maximal stress testing in females. *Journal of Applied Physiology, 56*, 436–440.

Mechanic, D. (1978). *Medical sociology* (2nd ed.). New York: Free Press.

Medical Essay (1993, June). Cholesterol. In Supplement to *Mayo Clinic Health Letter*, pp. 1–8. Also reprinted in R. Yarian (Ed.), *Health: Annual editions 95/96* (pp. 177–180). Guilford, CT: Dushkin.

Meichenbaum, D., & Cameron, R. (1983). Stress inoculation training: Toward a general paradigm for training coping skills. In D. Meichenbaum & M. E. Jaremko (Ed.), *Stress reduction and prevention* (pp. 115–154). New York: Plenum Press.

Meichenbaum, D., & Turk, D. C. (1976). The cognitive-behavioral management of anxiety, anger and pain. In P. O. Davidson (Ed.), *The behavioral management of anxiety, depression, and pain*. New York: Brunner/Mazel.

Melamed, B. G. (1984). Health intervention: Collaboration for health and science. In B. L. Hammonds & C. J. Scheirer (Eds.), *Psychology and health: The Master Lecture Series Vol. 3* (pp. 49–119). Washington, DC: American Psychological Association.

Melzack, R. (1973). *The puzzle of pain*. New York: Basic Books.

Melzack, R. (1975a). How acupuncture can block pain. In M. Weisenberg (Ed.), *Pain: Clinical and experimental perspectives* (pp. 251–257). St. Louis: Mosby.

Melzack, R. (1975b). The McGill Pain Questionnaire: Major properties and scoring methods. *Pain, 1*, 277–299.

Melzack, R. (1987). The short-form McGill Pain Questionnaire. *Pain, 30*, 191–197.

Melzack, R. (1992, April). Phantom limbs. *Scientific American, 266*, 120–126.

Melzack, R. (1993). Pain: Past, present and future. *Canadian Journal of Experimental Psychology, 47*, 615–629.

Melzack, R., & Wall, P. D. (1965). Pain mechanisms: A new theory. *Science, 150*, 971–979.

Melzack, R., & Wall, P. D. (1982). *The challenge of pain.* New York: Basic Books.

Melzack, R., & Wall, P. D. (1988). *The challenge of pain* (rev. ed.). London: Penguin.

Mendes de Leon, C. F. (1992). Anger and impatience/irritability in patients of low socioeconomic status with acute coronary heart disease. *Journal of Behavioral Medicine, 15,* 273–284.

Mermelstein, R., Cohen, S., Lichtenstein, E., Baer, J. S., & Kamarck, T. (1986). Social support and smoking cessation and maintenance. *Journal of Consulting and Clinical Psychology, 54,* 447–453.

Metropolitan Life Insurance Company. (1959). New weight standards for men and women. *Statistical Bulletin, 40,* 1.

Meyer, A. K., & Northup, W. B. (1997). What is violence prevention, anyway? *Educational Leadership, 54,* 31–33.

Meyer, D., Leventhal, H., & Gutman, M. (1985). Common-sense models of illness: The example of hypertension. *Health Psychology, 4,* 115–135.

Meyer, T. J., & Mark, M. M. (1995). Effects of psychosocial interventions with adult cancer patients: A meta-analysis of randomized experiments. *Health Psychology, 14,* 101–108.

Meyerowitz, B. E., Richardson, J., Hudson, S., & Leedham, B. (1998). Ethnicity and cancer outcomes: Behavioral and psychosocial considerations. *Psychological Bulletin, 123,* 47–70.

Michela, J. L. (1987). Interpersonal and individual impacts of a husband's heart attack. In A. Baum & J. E. Singer (Eds.), *Handbook of psychology and health: Vol. 5. Stress* (pp. 255–301). Hillsdale, NJ: Erlbaum.

Michie, S., Marteau, T. M., & Kidd, J. (1992). Predicting antenatal class attendance: Attitudes of self and others. *Psychology and Health, 7,* 225–234.

Mikail, S. F., DuBreuil, S. C., & D'Eon, J. L. (1993). A comparative analysis of measures used in the assessment of chronic pain patients. *Psychological Assessment, 5,* 117–120.

Millar, M. G., & Millar, K. (1995). Negative affective consequences of thinking about disease detection behaviors. *Health Psychology, 14,* 141–146.

Millar, W. J. (1983). Sex differentials in mortality by income level in urban Canada. *Canadian Journal of Public Health, 74,* 329–334.

Miller, A. L. (1993, March). *The U. S. smoking-material fire problem through 1990: The role of lighted tobacco products in fire.* Paper presented at the meeting of the National Fire Protection Association, Quincy, MA.

Miller, B. A., Kolonel, L. N., Bernstein, L., Young, J. L., Swanson, G. M., West. D., Key C. R., Liff, J. M., Glover, C. S., & Alexander, G. A. (Eds.). (1996). *Racial/ethnic patterns of cancer in the United States 1988–1992.* (National Institutes of Health Publication No. 96–4104). Bethesda, MD: U. S. Department of Health and Human Services, Public Health Service, and National Institutes of Health. National Cancer Institute.

Miller, J. D., & Cisin, I. H. (1983). *Highlights from the National Survey on Drug Abuse: 1982.* (DHHS Publication No. ADM 83–1277). Washington, DC: U.S. Government Printing Office.

Miller, J. J., Fletcher, K., & Kabat-Zinn, J. (1995). Three year follow-up and clinical implications of a mindfulness meditation-based stress reduction intervention in the treatment of anxiety disorders. *General Hospital Psychiatry, 17,* 192–200.

Miller, M. F., Barabasz, A. F., & Barabasz, M. (1991). Effects of active alert and relaxation hypnotic inductions on cold pressor pain. *Journal of Abnormal Psychology, 100,* 223–226.

Miller, N. E. (1969). Learning of visceral and glandular responses. *Science, 163,* 434–445.

Miller, S. B., Friese, M., Dolgoy, L., Sita, A., Lavoie, K., & Campbell, T. (1998). Hostility, sodium consumption, and cardiovascular response to interpersonal stress. *Psychosomatic Medicine, 60,* 71–77.

Miller, T. W. (1996). Current measures in the assessment of stressful life events. In T. W. Miller (Ed.), *Theory and assessment of stressful life events* (pp. 209–233). Madison, CT: International Universities Press.

Miller, W. R., & Hester, R. K. (1980). Treating the problem drinker: Modern approaches. In W. R. Miller (Ed.), *The addictive behaviors* (pp. 11–141). Oxford, England: Pergamon Press.

Mills, L. G. (1998). Mandatory arrest and prosecution policies for domestic violence: A critical literature review and the case for more research to test victim empowerment approaches. *Criminal Justice and Behavior, 25,* 306–318.

Millstein, S. G., & Irwin, C. E. (1987). Concepts of health and illness: Different constructs or variations on a theme? *Health Psychology, 6,* 515–524.

Mitchell, J. E., & de Zwaan, M. (1993). Pharmacological treatments of binge eating. In C. G. Fairburn & G. T. Wilson (Eds.), *Binge eating: Nature, assessment, and treatment* (pp. 250–269). New York: Guilford Press.

Mittelmark, M. B., Murray, D. M., Luepker, R. V., Pechacek, T. F., Pirie, P. L., & Pallonen, U. E. (1987). Predicting experimentation with cigarettes: The Childhood Antecedents of Smoking Study (CASS). *American Journal of Public Health, 77,* 206–208.

Mittleman, H. A., Maclure, M., Tofler, G. H., Sherwood, J. B., Goldberg, R. J., & Muller, J. E. (1993). Triggering of acute myocardial infarction by heavy physical exertion: Protection against triggering by regular exertion. *New England Journal of Medicine, 329,* 1677–1683.

Mobily, P. R., Herr, K. A., Clark, M. K., & Wallace, R. B. (1994). An epidemiologic analysis of pain in the elderly: The Iowa 65+ Rural Health Study. *Journal of Aging and Health, 6,* 139–154.

Modesti, D. G., & Tryon, W. W. (1994, August). *Emotional strain on adult children of a parent with Alzheimer's disease.* Paper presented at the American Psychological Association convention, Los Angeles, CA.

Moffatt, S., Phillimore, P., Bhopal, J., & Foy, C. (1995). "If this is what it is doing to our washing, what is it doing to our lungs?" Industrial pollution and public understanding in North East England. *Social Science and Medicine, 41,* 883–891.

Monane, M., Bohn, R. L., Gurwitz, J. H., Glynn, R. J., Levin, R., & Avorn, J. (1996). Compliance with anti-hypertensive therapy among elderly Medicaid enrollees: The rates of age, gender, and race. *American Journal of Public Health, 86,* 1805–1808.

Monroe, S. M. (1982). The assessment of life events: Event-symptom associations and the cause of disorder. *Journal of Abnormal Psychology, 91,* 14–24.

Monroe, S. M., & Simons, A. D. (1991). Diathesis-stress theories in the context of life stress research: Implications for the depressive disorders. *Psychological Bulletin, 110,* 406–425.

Monson, R. R., & Lyon, J. L. (1975). Proportional mortality among alcoholics. *Cancer, 36,* 1077–1079.

Montano, D. E., Thompson, B., Taylor, V. M., & Mahloch, J. (1997). Understanding mammography intention and utilization among women in an inner city public hospital clinic. *Preventive Medicine, 26,* 817–824.

Moos, R. H. (1984). The crisis of illness: Chronic conditions. In R. H. Moos (Ed.), *Coping with physical illness 2: New perspectives* (pp. 139–143). New York: Plenum Press.

Moos, R. H., & Schaefer, J. A. (1984). The crisis of physical illness: An overview and conceptual analysis. In R. H. Moos (Ed.), *Coping with physical illness 2: New perspectives* (pp. 3–25). New York: Plenum Press.

Morabia, A., Bernstein, M., Héritier, S., & Khatchatrian, N. (1996). Relation of breast cancer with passive and active exposure to tobacco smoke. *American Journal of Epidemiology, 143,* 918–928.

Morey, S. S. (1998). NIH issues consensus statement on acupuncture. *American Family Physician, 57,* 2545–2546.

Morgan, D. (1996). *Sleep secrets for shift workers & people with off-beat schedules.* Duluth, MN: Whole Person Associates.

Morgan, R. E., Palinkas, L. A., Barrett-Connor, E. L., & Wingard, D. L. (1993). Plasma cholesterol and depressive symptoms in older men. *Lancet, 341,* 75–79.

Morgan, W. P. (1973). Influence of acute physical activity on state anxiety. In *Proceedings of the College Physical Education Association,* Pittsburgh, PA.

Morgan, W. P. (1979, February). Negative addiction in runners. *The Physician and Sportsmedicine,* pp. 56–63, 67–70.

Morgan, W. P. (1981). Psychological benefits of physical activity. In F. J. Nagle & H. J. Montoye (Eds.), *Exercise in health and disease.* Springfield, IL: Thomas.

Morgan, W. P. (1997a). Methodological considerations. In W. P. Morgan (Ed.), *Physical activity and mental health* (pp. 3–32). Washington, DC: Taylor & Francis.

Morgan, W. P. (1997b). Preface. In W. P. Morgan (Ed.), *Physical activity and mental health* (pp. xiii–xv). Washington, DC: Taylor & Francis.

Morris, D. B. (1994, Autumn). Pain's dominion: What we make of pain. *Wilson Quarterly,* pp. 8–33.

Morris, D. L., Kritchevsky, S. B., & Davis, C. E. (1994). Serum carotenoids and coronary heart disease: The Lipid Research Clinics Coronary Primary Prevention Trial and Follow-up Study. *Journal of the American Medical Association, 272,* 1439–1441.

Morris, J. N., Heady, J. A., Raffle, P. A. B., Roberts, C. G., & Parks, J. W. (1953). Coronary heart-disease and physical activity of work. *Lancet, ii,* 1053–1057, 1111–1120.

Mosbach, P., & Leventhal, H. (1988). Peer group identification and smoking: Implications for intervention. *Journal of Abnormal Psychology, 97,* 238–245.

Moser, R., McCance, K. L., & Smith, K. R. (1991). Results of a national survey of physicians' knowledge and application of prevention capabilities. *American Journal of Preventive Medicine, 7,* 384–390.

Moss, M., Bucher, B., Moore, F. A., Moore, E. E., & Parsons, P. E. (1996). The role of chronic alcohol abuse in the development of Acute Respiratory Distress Syndrome. *Journal of the American Medical Association, 275,* 50–54.

Moy, C. S., Songer, T. J., LaPorte, R. E., Dorman, J. S., Kriska, A. M., Orchard, T. J., Becker, D. J., & Drash, A. L. (1993). Insulin-dependent diabetes mellitus, physical activity, and death. *American Journal of Epidemiology, 137,* 74–81.

Moyer, M. A. (1989). Use of patient-controlled analgesia for burn pain. In S. C. Funk, E. M. Tornquist, M. T. Champagne, L. A. Copp, & R. A. Wiese (Eds.), *Key aspects of comfort: Management of pain, fatigue, and nausea* (pp. 135–140). New York: Springer.

Mufti, R. M., Balon, R., & Arfken, C. L. (1998). Low cholesterol and violence. *Psychiatric Services, 49,* 221–224.

Muldoon, M. F., Manuck, S. B., & Matthews, K. M. (1992). Lowering cholesterol concentrations and mortality: A quantitative review of primary prevention trials. *British Medical Journal, 301,* 309–314.

Mulsant, B. H., Pollock, B. G., Nebes, R. D., Hoch, C. C., & Reynolds, C. F., III. (1997). Depression in Alzheimer's dementia. In L. L. Heston (Ed.), *Progress in Alzheimer's disease and similar conditions* (pp. 161–175). Washington, DC: American Psychiatric Press.

Multiple Risk Factor Intervention Trial Research Group. (1977). Statistical design considerations in the NHLI Multiple Risk Factor Intervention Trial. *Journal of Chronic Diseases, 30,* 261–275.

Multiple Risk Factor Intervention Trial Research Group. (1982). Risk factor changes and mortality. *Journal of the American Medical Association, 248,* 1465–1477.

Multiple Risk Factor Intervention Trial Research Group. (1990). Mortality rates after 10.5 years for participants in the Multiple Risk Factor Intervention Trial. *Journal of the American Medical Association, 263,* 1795–1801.

Murphy, D. A., Mann, T., O'Keefe, Z., & Rotherram-Borus, M. J. (1998). Number of pregnancies, outcome expectancies, and social norms among HIV-

Peay, M. Y., & Peay, E. R. (1998). The evaluation of medical symptoms by patients and doctors. *Journal of Behavioral Medicine, 21,* 57–81.

Peele, S. (1993). The conflict between public health goals and the temperance mentality. *American Journal of Public Health, 83,* 805–810.

Pell, S., & Fayerweather, W. E. (1985). Trends in the incidence of myocardial infarction and in associated mortality and morbidity in a large employed population, 1957–1983. *New England Journal of Medicine, 312,* 1005–1011.

Pelleymounter, M. A., Cullen, M. J., Baker, M. B., Hecht, R., Winters, D., Boone, T., & Collins, F. (1995). Effects of *obese* gene production body weight regulation in *ob/ob* mice. *Science, 269,* 540–543.

Pemberton, A. R., Vernon, S. W., & Lee, E. S. (1996). Prevalence and correlates of bulimia nervosa and bulimic behaviors in a racially diverse sample of undergraduate students in two universities in southeast Texas. *American Journal of Epidemiology, 144,* 450–455.

Penkower, L., Dew, M. A., Kingsley, L., Becker, J. T., Satz, P., Schaerf, F. W., & Sheridan, K. (1991). Behavioral, health and psychosocial factors and risk for HIV infection among sexually active homosexual men: The Multicenter AIDS Cohort Study. *American Journal of Public Health, 81,* 194–196.

Pennebaker, J. W. (1982). *The psychology of physical symptoms.* New York: Springer-Verlag.

Pennebaker, J. W. (1993). Putting stress into words: Health, linguistic, and therapeutic implications. *Behavior Research and Therapy, 31,* 539–548.

Pennebaker, J. W. (1997a). *Opening up: The healing power of expressing emotions* (rev. ed.). New York, Guilford Press.

Pennebaker, J. W. (1997b). Writing about emotional experiences as a therapeutic process. *Psychological Science, 8,* 162–168.

Pennebaker, J. W., Barger, S. D., & Tiebout, J. (1989). Disclosure of traumas and health among Holocaust survivors. *Psychosomatic Medicine, 51,* 577–589.

Pennebaker, J. W., Colder, M., & Sharp, L. K. (1990). Accelerating the coping process. *Journal of Personality and Social Psychology, 58,* 528–537.

Pennebaker, J. W., Kiecolt-Glaser, J. K., & Glaser, R. (1988). Disclosure of trauma and immune function: Health implications for psychotherapy. *Journal of Consulting and Clinical Psychology, 56,* 239–245.

Perera, F. P. (1997). Environment and cancer: Who are susceptible? *Science, 278,* 1068–1073.

Perkins, K. A., Dubbert, P. M., Martin, J. E., Faulstich, M. E., & Harris, J. K. (1986). Cardiovascular reactivity to psychological stress in aerobically trained versus untrained mild hypertensives and normotensives. *Health Psychology, 5,* 407–421.

Perkins, K. A., Epstein, L. H., Marks, B. L., Stiller, R. L., & Jacob, R. G. (1989). The effect of nicotine on energy expenditure during light physical activity. *New England Journal of Medicine, 320,* 898–903.

Perl, E. R., & Kruger, L., (1996). Nociception and pain: Evolution of concepts and observations. In L. Kruger (Ed.), *Pain and touch* (pp. 180–211). San Diego, CA: Academic Press.

Perri, M. G., McAllister, D. A., Gange, J. J., Jordan, R. C. McAdoo, W. G., & Nezu, A. M. (1988). Effects of four maintenance programs on the long-term management of obesity. *Journal of Consulting and Clinical Psychology, 56,* 529–534.

Persky, V. W., Kempthrone-Rawson, J., & Shekelle, R. B. (1987). Personality and risk of cancer: 20-year followup of the Western Electric Study. *Psychosomatic Medicine, 49,* 435–439.

Persons, J. B., & Rao, P. A. (1985). Longitudinal study of cognitions, life events, and depression in psychiatric inpatients. *Journal of Abnormal Psychology, 94,* 51–63.

Pert, C. B., & Snyder, S. H. (1973). Opiate receptor: Demonstration in nervous tissue. *Science, 179,* 1011–1014.

Peterson, C., Seligman, M. E. P., Yurko, K. H., Martin, L. R., & Friedman, H. S. (1998). Catastrophizing and untimely death. *Psychological Science, 9,* 127–130.

Peterson, L., & Gable, S. (1997). Holistic injury prevention. In J. R. Lutzker (Ed.), *Handbook of child abuse research and treatment* (pp. 291–316).

Peterson, L., Gillies, R., Cook, S. C., Schick, B., & Little, T. (1994). Developmental patterns of expected consequences for simulated bicycle injury events. *Health Psychology, 13,* 218–223.

Peterson, L., & Schick, B. (1993). Empirically derived injury prevention rules. Special section: Behavioral pediatrics. *Journal of Applied Behavior Analysis, 26,* 451–460.

Peto, R., Doll, R., Buckley, J. D., & Spron, M. B. (1981). Can dietary beta-carotene materially reduce human cancer rates? *Nature, 290,* 201–208.

Pettingale, K. W., Morris, T., Greer, S., & Haybittle, J. L. (1985). Mental attitudes to cancer: An additional prognostic factor. *Lancet, i,* 750.

Pfohl, B., Barrash, J., True, B., & Alexander, B. (1989). Failure of two Axis II measures to predict medication noncompliance among hypertensive outpatients. *Journal of Personality Disorders, 3,* 45–52.

Pierce, E. F., & Pate, D. W. (1994). Mood alterations in older adults following acute exercise. *Perceptual and Motor Skills, 79,* 191–194.

Pierce, J. P., Choi ,W. S., Gilpin, E. A., Farkas, A. J., & Berry, C. C. (1998). Tobacco industry promotion of cigarettes and adolescent smoking. *Journal of the American Medical Association, 279,* 511–515.

Pietschmann, R. J. (1984, November). Probing death on the run. *Runner's World,* pp. 38–44, 90–94.

Pike, J. L., Smith, T. L., Hauger, R. L., Nicassio, P. M., & Irwin, M. R. (1994, August). *Immunologic effects of acute stress: Chronic life stress as a moderator.* Presented at the American Psychological Association convention, Los Angeles, CA.

Pinel, J. P. J. (1997). *Biopsychology* (3rd ed.). Boston: Allyn and Bacon.

infected young women. *Health Psychology, 17,* 470–475.

Murphy, J. K., Stoney, C. M., Alpert, B. S., & Walker, S. S. (1995). Gender and ethnicity in children's cardiovascular reactivity: 7 years of study. *Health Psychology, 14,* 48–55.

Murphy, L. R. (1996). Stress management in work settings: A critical review of the health effects. *American Journal of Health Promotion, 11,* 112–135.

Murray, D. M., Davis-Hearn, M., Goldman, A. I., Pirie, P., & Luepker, R. V. (1988). Four- and five-year follow-up results from four seventh-grade smoking prevention strategies. *Journal of Behavioral Medicine, 11,* 395–405.

Murray, D. M., Richards, P. S., Luepker, R. V., & Johnson, C. A. (1987). The prevention of cigarette smoking in children: Two- and three-year follow-up comparisons of four prevention strategies. *Journal of Behavioral Medicine, 10,* 595–611.

Murray, M. E., Guerra, N. G., & Williams, K. R. (1997). Violence prevention for the 21st century. In R. P. Weissberg, T. P. Gullotta, R. L. Hampton, B. A. Ryan, & G. R. Adams (Eds.), *Enhancing children's wellness* (pp. 105–128). Thousand Oaks, CA: Sage.

Mustard, T. R., & Harris, A. V. E. (1989). Problems in understanding prescription labels. *Perceptual and Motor Skills, 69,* 291–299.

Myers, L., Coughlin, S. S., Webber, L. S., Srinivasan, S. R., Berenson, G. S. (1995). Prediction of adult cardiovascular multifactorial risk status from childhood risk factor levels: The Bogalusa Heart Study. *American Journal of Epidemiology, 142,* 918–924.

Nakao, M., Nomura, S., Shimosawa, T., Yoshiuchi, K., Kumano, H., Kuboki, T., Suematsu, H., & Fujita, T. (1997). Clinical effects of blood pressure biofeedback treatment on hypertension by auto-shaping. *Psychosomatic Medicine, 59,* 331–338.

National Center for Health Statistics. (1994). *Health, United States.* Hyattsville, MD: U. S. Government Printing Office.

National Center for Injury Prevention and Control (1998). 10 leading causes of deaths by age group—1995. http://www.cdc.gov/ncipc/images

National Education Association. (1998). What can we do about school violence? *NEA Today, 17,* 19.

National Highway Traffic Safety Administration. (1993–1996). *Fatality analysis reporting system, 1992–1995.* Washington, DC: U.S. Department of Transportation.

National Highway Traffic Safety Administration. (1998). Presidential initiative for increasing seat belt use nationwide. http://www.nhtsa.dot.gov/people/injury

National Institute on Alcohol Abuse and Alcoholism (NIAAA). (1988). Alcohol and aging. *Alcohol Alert, 2,* 1–4.

National Safe Kids Campaign. (1997). The National Safe Kids Campaign motor vehicle occupant injury fact sheet. http://www.safekids.org/fact97/

Navarro, V. (1990). Race or class versus race and class: Mortality differentials in the United States. *Lancet, 336,* 1238–1240.

Neighbors, H. W. (1997). Husbands, wives, family, and friends: Sources of stress, sources of support. In R. J. Taylor, J. S. Jackson, & L. M. Chatters (Eds.), *Family life in Black America* (pp. 277–292). Thousand Oaks, CA: Sage.

Neimark, J., Conway, C., & Doskoch, P. (1994, September/October). Back from the drink. *Psychology Today, 27,* 46–49.

Nelson, H. D., Nevitt, M. C., Scott, J. C., Stone, K. L., & Cummings, S. R. (1994). Smoking, alcohol, and neuromuscular and physical functioning of older women. *Journal of the American Medical Association, 272,* 1825–1831.

Nelson, M. E., Fiatarone, M. A., Marganti, C. M., Trice, I., Greenberg, R. A., & Evans, W. J. (1994). Effects of high-intensity strength training on multiple risk factors for osteoporotic fractures. *Journal of the American Medical Association, 272,* 1909–1914.

Nemeroff, C. J. (1995). Magical thinking about illness virulence: Conceptions of germs from "safe" versus "dangerous" others. *Health Psychology, 14,* 147–151.

Nestle, M. (1997). Alcohol guidelines for chronic disease prevention: From Prohibition to moderation. *Nutrition Today, 32*(2), 86–92.

Neugebauer, R. (1984). The reliability of life-event reports. In B. S. Dohrenwend & B. P. Dohrenwend (Eds.), *Stressful life events & their contexts* (pp. 85–107). New Brunswick, NJ: Rutgers University Press.

Neuman, P. A., & Halvorson, P. A. (1983). *Anorexia nervosa and bulimia.* New York: Van Nostrand Reinhold.

Neumarker, K. J. (1997). Mortality and sudden death in anorexia nervosa. *International Journal of Eating Disorders, 21,* 202–212.

Newacheck, P. W., & Taylor, W. R. (1992). Childhood chronic illness: Prevalence, severity, and impact. *American Journal of Public Health, 82,* 364–371.

Newberne, P. M., & Suphakarn, V. (1983). Nutrition and cancer: A review, with emphasis on the role of vitamins C and E and selenium. *Nutrition and Cancer, 5,* 107–119.

Ng, B., Dimsdale, J. E., Shragg, G. P., & Deutsch, R. (1996). Ethnic differences in analgesic consumption for postoperative pain. *Psychosomatic Medicine, 58,* 125–129.

Nicholas, M. K., Wilson, P. H., & Goyen, J. (1991). Operant-behavioral and cognitive-behavioral treatment for chronic low back pain. *Behavior Research and Therapy, 29,* 235–238.

Nicholson, N. L., & Blanchard, E. B. (1993). A controlled evaluation of behavioral treatment of chronic headache in the elderly. *Behavior Therapy, 24,* 395–408.

Nides, M., Rand, C., Dolce, J., Murray, R., O'Hara, P., Voelker, H., & Connett, J. (1994). Weight gain as a function of smoking cessation and 2-mg nicotine gum use among middle-aged smokers with mild lung impairment in the first 2 years of the Lung Health Study. *Health Psychology, 13,* 354–361.

Nigl, A. J. (1984). *Biofeedback and behavioral strategies in pain treatment.* New York: Medical and Scientific Books.

NIH Technology Assessment Conference Panel. (1993). Methods for voluntary weight loss and control. *Annals of Internal Medicine, 119,* 764–770.

Nikiforov, S. V., & Mamaev, V. B. (1998). The development of sex differences in cardiovascular disease mortality: A historical perspective. *American Journal of Public Health, 88,* 1345–1353.

Nisbett, R. E. (1972). Hunger, obesity, and the ventromedial hypothalamus. *Psychological Review, 79,* 433–453.

Nivision, M. E., & Endresen, I. M. (1993). An analysis of relationships among environmental noise, annoyance and sensitivity to noise, and the consequences for health and sleep. *Journal of Behavior Medicine, 16,* 257–276.

Nolen-Hoeksema, S. (1994, August). *Rumination in response to depression.* Presented at the American Psychological Association convention, Los Angeles, CA.

Norman, P., & Conner, M. (1993). The role of social cognition models in predicting attendance at health checks. *Psychology and Health, 8,* 447–462.

Norris, F.H. (1997). Frequency and structure of precautionary behavior in the domains of hazard preparedness, crime prevention, vehicular safety, and health maintenance. *Health Psychology, 16,* 566–575.

Norvell, N., & Belles, D. (1993). Psychological and physical benefits of circuit weight training in law enforcement personnel. *Journal of Consulting and Clinical Psychology, 61,* 520–527.

Novelli, P. (1997). Knowledge about causes of peptic ulcer disease—United States, March–April 1997. *Morbidity and Mortality Weekly Reports, 46,* 985–987.

O'Brien, M. K. (1997). Compliance among health professionals. In A. Baum, S. Newman, J. Weinman, R. West, & C. McManus (Eds.), *Cambridge handbook of psychology, health and medicine* (pp. 278–281). Cambridge, United Kingdom: Cambridge University Press.

O'Brien, R. W., & Bush, P. J. (1997). Health behavior in children. In D. S. Gochman (Ed.), *Handbook of health behavior research III: Demography, development, and diversity* (pp. 49–71). New York: Plenum Press.

O'Callaghan, F. V., Chant, D. C., Callan, V. J. & Baglioni, A. (1997). Models of alcohol use by young adults: A examination of various attitude-behavior theories. *Journal of Studies on Alcohol, 58,* 502–507.

Occupational Safety and Health Administration. (1996). *Guidelines for preventing workplace violence for health care and social service workers.* Washington, DC: OSHA Publications Office.

Occupational Safety and Health Administration. (1998). OSHA facts: Common sense at work. http://www.osha-slc.gov/OshDoc/OSHFacts

O'Connor, P. J. (1997). Overtraining and staleness. In W. P. Morgan (Ed.), *Physical activity and mental health* (pp. 145–160). Washington, DC: Taylor & Francis.

O'Donnell, C. R. (1995). Firearm deaths among children and youth. *American Psychologist, 50,* 771–776.

Ohannessian, C. M., Stabenau, J. R., & Hesselbrock, V. M. (1995). Childhood and adulthood temperament and problem behaviors and adulthood substance use. *Addictive Behaviors, 20,* 77–86.

Oldridge, N. B., Guyatt, G. H., Fischer, M. E., & Rimm, A. A. (1988). Cardiac rehabilitation after myocardial infarction. *Journal of the American Medical Association, 260,* 945–950.

O'Leary, A. (1990). Stress, emotion, and human immune function. *Psychological Bulletin, 108,* 363–382.

Olkkonen, S., & Honkanen, R. (1990). The role of alcohol in nonfatal bicycle injuries. *Accident Analysis and Prevention, 22,* 89–96.

Olness, K. (1993). Hypnosis: The power of attention. In D. Goleman & J. Gurin (Eds.), *Mind/body medicine: How to use your mind for better health* (pp. 277–290). Yonkers, NY: Consumer Reports Books.

Olsen, R., & Sutton, J. (1998). More hassle, more alone: Adolescents with diabetes and the role of formal and informal support. *Child Care, Health and Development, 24,* 31–39.

Olshansky, S. J., Carnes, B. A., & Cassel, C. K. (1993, April). The aging of the human species. *Scientific American, 268,* 46–52.

Omenn, G. G., Goodman, G. E., Thornquist, M. D., Balmes, J., Cullen, M. R., Glass, A., Keogh, J. P., Meyskens, F. L., Valanis, B., Williams, J. H., Jr., Barnhart, S., & Hammar, S. (1996). Effects of a combination of beta carotene and vitamin A on lung cancer and cardiovascular disease, *New England Journal of Medicine, 334,* 1150–1155.

Orme, C. M., & Binik, Y. M. (1989). Consistency of adherence across regimen demands. *Health Psychology, 8,* 27–43.

Orne, M. T. (1980). Hypnotic control of pain: Toward a clarification of the different psychological processes involved. In J. J. Bonica (Ed.), *Pain* (pp. 155–172). New York: Raven Press.

Ornish, D. (1993). *Eat more, weigh less.* New York: Harper Collins.

Ornish, D. (1995, May). *Reversing heart disease.* Presented by St. Patrick's Hospital, Lake Charles, LA.

Ornish, D., Brown, S. E., Scherwitz, L. W., Billings, J. H., Armstrong, W. T., Ports, T., McLanahan, S. M., Kirkeeide, R. L., Brand, R. J., & Gould, K. L. (1990). Can lifestyle changes reverse coronary heart disease? The Lifestyle Heart Trial. *Lancet, 336,* 129–133.

Ornish, D., Scherwitz, L. W., Billings, J. H., Gould, L., Merritt, T. A., Sparler, S., Armstrong, W. T., Ports, T. A., Kirkeeide, R. L., Hogeboom, C., & Brand, R. J. (1998). Intensive lifestyle changes for reversal of coronary heart disease. *Journal of the American Medical Association, 280,* 2001–2007.

Orth-Gomér, K. (1998). Psychosocial risk factor profile in women with coronary heart disease. In K. Orth-Gomér, M. Chesney, & N. K. Wenger (Eds.), *Women, stress, and heart disease* (pp. 25–38). Mahwah, NJ: Erlbaum.

Osofsky, J. D. (1997). Prevention and policy: Directions for the future. In J. D. Osofsky (Ed.), *Children in a violent society* (pp. 323–328). New York: Guilford Press.

Ott, P. J., & Levy, S. M. (1994). Cancer in women. In V. J. Adesso, D. M. Reddy, & R. Fleming (Eds.), *Psychological perspectives on women's health* (pp. 83–98). Washington, DC: Taylor & Francis.

Ouellette, S. C. (1993). Inquiries into hardiness. In L. Goldberger & S. Breznitz (Eds.), *Handbook of stress: Theoretical and clinical aspects* (2nd ed., pp. 77–100). New York: Free Press

Oxman, T. E., Berkman, L. F., Kasl, S., Freeman, D. H., Jr., & Barrett, J. (1992). Social support and depressive symptoms in the elderly. *American Journal of Epidemiology, 135,* 356–368.

Padian, N. S., Shiboski, S. C., Glass, S. O., & Vittinghoff, E. (1997). Heterosexual transmission of human immunodeficiency virus (HIV) in Northern California: Results from a ten-year study. *American Journal of Epidemiology, 146,* 350–357.

Paffenbarger, R. S., Jr., Gima, A. S., Laughlin, M. E., & Black, R. A. (1971). Characteristics of longshoremen related to fatal coronary heart disease and stroke. *American Journal of Public Health, 61,* 1362–1370.

Paffenbarger, R. S., Jr., Hyde, R. T., & Wing, A. L. (1987). Physical activity and incidence of cancer in diverse populations: A preliminary report. *American Journal of Clinical Nutrition, 45,* 312–315.

Paffenbarger, R. S., Jr., Hyde, R. T., Wing, A. L., & Hsieh, C-c. (1986). Physical activity, all-cause mortality, and longevity of college alumni. *New England Journal of Medicine, 314,* 605–613.

Paffenbarger, R. S., Jr., Hyde, R. T., Wing, A. L., Lee, I-M., Jung, D., & Klampert, J. B. (1993). The association of changes in physical activity level and other lifestyle characteristics with mortality among men. *New England Journal of Medicine, 328,* 538.

Paffenbarger, R. S., Jr., Laughlin, M. E., Gima, A. S., & Black, R. A. (1970). Work activity of longshoremen as related to death from coronary heart disease and stroke. *New England Journal of Medicine, 282,* 1109–1114.

Paffenbarger, R. S., Jr., Wing, A. L., & Hyde, R. T. (1978). Physical activity as an index of heart attack risk in college alumni. *American Journal of Epidemiology, 108,* 161–175.

Palmblad, J., Petrini, B., Wasserman, J., & Åkerstedt, T. (1979). Lymphocyte and granulocyte reactions during sleep deprivation. *Psychosomatic Medicine, 41,* 273–278.

Palmer, S. E., Canzona, L., & Wai, L. (1984). Helping families respond effectively to chronic illness: Home dialysis as a case example. In R. H. Moos (Ed.), *Coping with physical illness 2: New perspectives* (pp. 283–294). New York: Plenum Press.

Pamuk, E. R., Williamson, D. F., Serdula, M. K., Madans, J., & Byers, T. E. (1993). Weight loss and subsequent death in a cohort of U.S. adults. *Annals of Internal Medicine, 119,* 744–748.

Pappas, G. (1994). Elucidating the relationships between race, socioeconomic status, and health. *American Journal of Public Health, 84,* 892–893.

Paran, E., Amir, M., & Yaniv, N. (1996). Evaluating the response of mild hypertensives to biofeedback-assisted relaxation using a mental stress test. *Journal of Behavior Therapy and Experimental Psychiatry, 27,* 157–167.

Park, C. L. (1998). Stress-related growth and thriving through coping: The roles of personality and cognitive processes. *Journal of Social Issues, 54*(2), 267–277.

Parker, D. R., McPhillips, J. V., Derby, C. A., Gans, K. M., Lasater, T. M., & Carleton, R. A. (1996). High-density-lipoprotein cholesterol and types of alcoholic beverages consumed among men and women. *American Journal of Public Health, 86,* 1022–1027.

Parsons, T. (1951). *The social system.* New York: Free Press.

Parsons, T. (1978). *Action theory and the human condition.* New York: Free Press.

Pate, R. R., Heath, G. W., Dowda, M., & Trost, S. G. (1996). Associations between physical activity and other health behaviors in a representative sample of US adolescents. *American Journal of Public Health, 86,* 1477–1581.

Pate, R. R., Pratt, M., Blair, S. N., Haskell, W. L., Macera, C. A., Bouchard, C., Buchner, D., Ettinger, W., Heath, G. W., King, A. C., Kriska, A., Leon, A. S., Marcus, B. H., Morris, J., Paffenbarger, R. S., Jr., Patrick, K., Pollock, M. L., Rippe, J. M., Sallis, J., & Wilmore, J. H. (1995). Physical activity and public health: A recommendation from the Centers for Disease Control and Prevention and the American College of Sports Medicine. *Journal of the American Medical Association, 273,* 402–407.

Patterson, D. R., & Ptacek, J. T. (1997) Baseline pain as a moderator of hypnotic analgesia for burn injury treatment. *Journal of Consulting and Clinical Psychology, 65,* 60–67.

Pattishall, E. G. (1989). The development of behavioral medicine: Historical models. *Annals of Behavioral Medicine, 11,* 43–48.

Paul, C. L., Sanson-Fisher, R. W., Redman, S., & Carter, S. (1994). Preventing accidental injury to young children in the home using volunteers. *Health Promotion International, 9,* 241–249.

Pauling, L. (1980). Vitamin C therapy of advanced cancer. *New England Journal of Medicine, 302,* 694–698.

Paulus, P. B., McCain, G., & Cox, V. C. (1978). Death rates, psychiatric commitments, blood pressure, and perceived crowding as a function of institutional crowding. *Environmental Psychology and Nonverbal Behavior, 3,* 107–116.

Pbert, L., Doerfler, L. A., & DeCosimo, D. (1992). An evaluation of the Perceived Stress Scale in two clinical populations. *Journal of Psychopathology and Behavioral Assessment, 14,* 363–375.

Pearce, J. M. S. (1994). Headache. *Journal of Neurology, Neurosurgery and Psychiatry, 57,* 134–143.

Pearlin, L. I., Turner, H., & Semple, S. (1989). Coping and the mediation of caregiver stress. In E. Light B. D. Lebowitz (Eds.), *Alzheimer's disease treatmen and family stress: Directions for research* (pp. 198–2 (DHHS Publication No. ADM 89-1569). Washin ton, DC: U.S. Government Printing Office.

Pinto, R. P., & Hollandsworth, J. G., Jr. (1989). Using videotape modeling to prepare children psychologically for surgery: Influence of parents and costs versus benefits of providing preparation services. *Health Psychology, 8*, 79–95.

Piotrowski, C. (1998). Assessment of pain: A survey of practicing clinicians. *Perceptual and Motor Skills, 86*, 181–182.

Pipho, C. (1998). Living with zero tolerance. *Phi Delta Kappan, 79*, 725–726.

Pirie, P. L., Murray, D. M., & Luepker, R. V. (1991). Gender differences in cigarette smoking and quitting in a cohort of young adults. *American Journal of Public Health, 81*, 324–327.

Plaud, J. J., Mosely, T. H., & Moberg, M. (1998). Alzheimer's disease and behavioral gerontology. In J. J. Plaud & G.H. Eifert (Eds.), *From behavior theory to behavior therapy* (pp. 223–245). Boston: Allyn and Bacon.

Plaut, S. M., & Friedman, S. B. (1981). Psychosocial factors in infectious disease. In R. Ader (Ed.), *Psychoneuroimmunology* (pp. 3–30). New York: Academic Press.

Polatin, P. B. (1996). Integration of pharmacotherapy with psychological treatment of chronic pain. In R. J. Gatchel & D. C. Turk (Eds.), *Psychological approaches to pain management: A practitioner's handbook* (pp. 305–328). New York: Guilford Press.

Polich, J. M., Armor, D. J., & Braiker, H. B. (1980). *The course of alcoholism: Four years after treatment.* Santa Monica, CA: Rand.

Polivy, J. (1996). Psychological consequences of food restriction. *Journal of the American Dietetic Association, 96*, 589–594.

Polivy, J., & Herman, C. P. (1983). *Breaking the diet habit: The natural weight alternative.* New York: Basic Books.

Polivy, J., & Herman, C. P. (1995). Dieting and its relation to eating disorders. In K. D. Brownell & C. G. Fairburn. *Eating disorders and obesity: A comprehensive handbook* (pp. 83–92). New York: Guilford Press.

Poll: Over 40 percent of homes with kids have guns. (1998, November 14). *Lake Charles American Press,* p. D10).

Pollock, M. L., Wilmore, J. H., & Fox, S. M., III. (1978). *Health and fitness through physical activity.* New York: Wiley.

Pols, M. A., Peeters, P. H. M., Twisk, J. W. R., Kemper, H. C. G. & Grobbee, D. E. (1997). Physical activity and cardiovascular disease risk profile in women. *American Journal of Epidemiology, 146*, 322–328.

Pomerleau, O. F. (1980). Why people smoke: Current psycho-biological models. In P. O. Davidson & S. M. Davidson (Eds.), *Behavioral medicine: Changing health lifestyles* (pp. 94–115). New York: Brunner/Mazel.

Pomerleau, O. F. (1982). A discourse on behavioral medicine: Current status and future trends. *Journal of Consulting and Clinical Psychology, 50*, 1030–1039.

Pomerleau, O. F., Fertig, J. B., Seyler, E. L., & Jaffe, J. (1983). Neuroendocrine reactivity to nicotine in smokers. *Psychopharmacology, 81*, 61–67.

Pope, H. G., Jr., & Hudson, J. I. (1984). *New hope for binge eaters: Advances in the understanding and treatment of bulimia.* New York: Harper & Row.

Pope, H. G., Jr., Hudson, J. I., & Yurgelun-Todd, D. (1984). Anorexia nervosa and bulimia among 300 suburban women shoppers. *American Journal of Psychiatry, 141*, 292–293.

Popham, R. E. (1978). The social history of the tavern. In Y. Israel, F. B. Glaser, H. Kalant, R. E. Popham, W. Schmidt, & R. G. Smart (Eds.), *Research advances in alcohol and drug problems* (Vol. 2, pp. 225–302). New York: Plenum Press.

Popham, R. E., Schmidt, W., & Israelstam, S. (1984). Heavy alcohol consumption and physical health problems: A review of the epidemiologic evidence. In R. G. Smart, H. D. Cappell, F. B. Glaser, Y. Israel, H. Kalant, R. E. Popham, W. Schmidt, & E. M. Sellers (Eds.), *Research advances in alcohol and drug problems* (Vol. 8). New York: Plenum Press.

Porter, J., & Jick, H. (1980). Addiction rate in patients treated with narcotics. *New England Journal of Medicine, 302*, 123.

Pratt, M. (1999). Benefits of lifestyle activity vs structured exercise. *Journal of the American Medical Association, 281*, 375–376.

Prochaska, J. O. (1994). Strong and weak principles for progressing from precontemplation to action on the basis of twelve problem behaviors. *Health Psychology, 13*, 47–51.

Prochaska, J. O., DiClemente, C. C., & Norcross, J. C. (1992). In search of how people change: Applications to addictive behaviors. *American Psychologist, 47*, 1102–1114.

Prochaska, J. O., Redding, C. A., Harlow, L. L., Rossi, J. S., & Velicer, W. F. (1994). The transtheoretical model of change and HIV prevention: A review. *Health Education Quarterly, 21*, 471–486.

Prochaska, J. O., Velicer, W. F., Rossi, J. S., Goldstein, M. G., Marcus, B. H., Rakowski, W., Flore, C., Harlow, L. L., Redding, C. A., Rosenbloom, D., & Rossi, S. R. (1994). Stages of change and decisional balance for 12 problem behaviors. *Health Psychology, 13*, 39–46.

Prohaska, T. R., Keller, U. L., Leventhal. E. A., & Leventhal, H. (1987). Impact of symptoms and aging attribution on emotions and coping. *Health Psychology, 6*, 495–514.

Ptacek, J. T., Smith, R. E., & Zanas, J. (1992). Gender, appraisal, and coping: A longitudinal analysis. *Journal of Personality, 60*, 747–770.

Pugliese, K., & Shook, S. L. (1998). Gender, ethnicity, and network characteristics: Variation in social support resources. *Sex Roles, 38*, 215–238.

Pukish, M. M., & Tucker, J. A. (1994, August). *Natural recovery from alcoholism: Contexts surrounding abstinent and moderation outcomes.* Paper presented at the 102nd convention of the American Psychological Association, Los Angeles, CA.

Puska, P., & Mustaniemi, H. (1975). Incidence and presentation of myocardial infarction in North Karelia, Finland. *Acta Medicus Scandinavia, 197*, 211–216.

Pyle, R. L., Mitchell, J. E., & Eckert, E. D. (1981). Bulimia: A report of 34 cases. *Journal of Clinical Psychiatry, 42,* 60–64.

Pyle, R. L., Mitchell, J. E., Eckert, E. D., Halvorson, P. A., Neuman, P. A., & Goff, G. M. (1983). The incidence of bulimia in freshman college students. *International Journal of Eating Disorders, 2,* 75–85.

Rabins, P. V. (1989). Behavior problems in the demented. In E. Light & B. D. Lebowitz (Eds.), *Alzheimer's disease treatment and family stress: Directions for research* (pp. 322–339). (USDHHS Publication No. ADM 89-1569). Washington, DC: U.S. Government Printing Office.

Rabins, P. V. (1996). Developing treatment guidelines for Alzheimer's disease and other dementias. *Journal of Clinical Psychiatry, 57,* 37–38.

Rabkin, J. G. (1993). Stress and psychiatric disorders. In L. Goldberger & S. Breznitz (Eds.), *Handbook of stress: Theoretical and clinical aspects* (2nd ed., pp. 477–495). New York: Free Press.

Rabkin, J. G., & Struening, E. L. (1976). Life events, stress, and illness. *Science, 194,* 1013–1020.

Ragland, D. R., & Brand, R. J. (1988). Type A behavior and mortality from coronary heart disease. *New England Journal of Medicine, 318,* 65–69.

Raglin, J. S. (1997). Anxiolytic effects of physical activity. In W. P. Morgan (Ed.), *Physical activity and mental health* (pp.107–126). Washington, DC: Taylor & Francis.

Rahe, R. H. (1984). Developments in life change measurement: Subjective life change unit scaling. In B. S. Dohrenwend & B. R. Dohrenwend (Eds.), *Stressful life events and their contexts.* New Brunswick, NJ: Rutgers University Press.

Rahe, R. H., Romo, M., Bennett, L., & Siltanen, P. (1974). Recent life changes, myocardial infarction, and abrupt coronary death. *Archives of Internal Medicine, 133,* 221–228.

Raitakari, O. T., Porkka, V. K., Taimela, S., Telama, R., Räsänen, L. & Vükai, J. S. A. (1994). Effects of persistent physical activity and inactivity on coronary risk factors in children and young adults: The Cardiovascular Risk in Young Finns study. *American Journal of Epidemiology, 140,* 195–205.

Ramsay, D. S., Seeley, R. J., Bolles, R. C., & Woods, S. C. (1996). Ingestive homeostasis: The primacy of learning. In E. D. Capaldi (Ed.), *Why we eat what we eat: The psychology of eating* (pp. 11–27). Washington, DC: American Psychological Association.

Ranchor, A. V., Sanderman, R., Bouma, J., Buunk, B. P., & van den Heuvel, W. J. A. (1997). An exploration of the relation between hostility and disease. *Journal of Behavioral Medicine, 20,* 223–240.

Rand, C. S. W., & Stunkard, A. J. (1983). Obesity and psychoanalysis: Treatment and four-year follow-up. *American Journal of Psychiatry, 140,* 1140–1144.

Rankin, R. (1969). Air pollution control and public apathy. *Journal of the Air Pollution Control Association, 19,* 565–569.

Raphael, K. G., Cloitre, M., & Dohrenwend, B. P. (1991). Problems of recall and misclassification with checklist methods of measuring stressful life events. *Health Psychology, 10,* 62–74.

Rasmussen, B. K. (1993). Migraine and tension-type headache in a general population: Precipitating factors, female hormones, sleep pattern and relation to lifestyle. *Pain, 53,* 65–72.

Ratliff-Crain, J., Temoshok, L., Kiecolt-Glaser, J. K., & Tamarkin, L. (1989). Issues in psychoneuroimmunology. *Health Psychology, 8,* 747–752.

Ratner, H., Gross, L., Casas, J., & Castells, S. (1990). A hypnotherapeutic approach to improvement of compliance in adolescent diabetics. *American Journal of Clinical Hypnosis, 32,* 154–159.

Reed, D. M., LaCroix, A. Z., Karasek, R. A., Miller, D., & MacLean, C. A. (1989). Occupational strain and the incidence of coronary heart disease. *American Journal of Epidemiology, 129,* 495–502.

Reed, D. M., MacLean, C. J., & Hayash, T. (1987). Predictors of atherosclerosis in the Honolulu Heart Program: Biologic, dietary, and lifestyle characteristics. *American Journal of Epidemiology, 126,* 214–225.

Rehm, J. T., Bondy, S. J., Sempos, C. T., & Vuong, C. V. (1997). Alcohol consumption and coronary heart disease morbidity and mortality. *American Journal of Epidemiology, 146,* 495–501.

Rejeski, W. J., Brubaker, P. H., Herb, R. A., Kaplan, J. R., & Koritnik, D. (1988). Anabolic steroids and aggressive behavior in Cynomolgus monkeys. *Journal of Behavioral Medicine, 11,* 95–105.

Rejeski, W. J., Thompson, A., Brubaker, P. H., & Miller, H. S. (1992). Acute exercise: Buffering psychosocial stress responses in women. *Health Psychology, 11,* 355–362.

Remafedi, G., French, S., Story, M., Resnick, M. D., & Blum, R. (1998). The relationship between suicide risk and sexual orientation: Results of a population-based study. *American Journal of Public Health, 88,* 57–60.

Rembolt, C. (1998). Making violence unacceptable. *Educational Leadership, 56,* 32–38.

Repetti, R. L. (1993a). The effects of workload and the social environment at work on health. In L. Goldberger & S. Breznitz (Eds.), *Handbook of stress: Theoretical and clinical aspects* (2nd ed. pp. 368–385). New York: Free Press.

Repetti, R. L. (1993b). Short-term effects of occupational stressors on daily mood and health complaints. *Health Psychology, 12,* 125–131.

Reppucci, J. D., Revenson, T. A., Aber, M., & Reppucci, N. D. (1991). Unrealistic optimism among adolescent smokers and nonsmokers. *Journal of Primary Prevention, 11,* 227–236.

Resnick, H. S., Kilpatrick, D. G., Best, C. L., & Kramer, T. L. (1992). Vulnerability-stress factors in development of posttraumatic stress disorder. *Journal of Nervous and Mental Disease, 180,* 424–430.

Resnick, M. D., Bearman, P. S., Blum, R. W., Bauman, K. E., Harris, K. M., Jones, J., Tabor, J., Beuhring, T., Sieving, R. E., Shew, M., Ireland, M., Bearinger,

L. H., & Udry, J. R. (1997). Protecting adolescents from harm: Findings from the National Longitudinal Study on Adolescent Health. *Journal of the American Medical Association, 278,* 823–832.

Revicki, D. A., & May, H. J. (1985). Occupational stress, social support, and depression. *Health Psychology, 4,* 61–77.

Rexrode, K. M., Carey, V. J., Hennekens, C. H., Walters, E. E., Colditz, G. A., Stampher, M. J., Willett, W. C., & Manson, J. E. (1998). Abdominal adiposity and coronary heart disease in women. *Journal of the American Medical Association, 280,* 1843–1948.

Rexrode, K. M., Hennekens, C. H., Willett, W. C., Colditz, G. A. Stampfer, M. J., Rich-Edwards, J. W., Speizer, F. E., & Manson, J. E. (1997). A prospective study of body mass index, weight change, and risk of stroke in women. *Journal of the American Medical Association, 277,* 1539–1545.

Reynolds, P., & Kaplan, G. A. (1990). Social connections and risk for cancer: Prospective evidence from the Alameda County Study. *Behavioral Medicine, 16,* 101–110.

Ricciuti, C. G. (1997). Cardiac catheterization. In S. VanRiper & J. VanRiper (Eds.), *Cardiac diagnostic tests: A guide for nurses* (pp. 265–296). Philadelphia: Saunders.

Ridker, P. M., Vaughan, D. E., Stampfer, M. J., Glynn, R. J., & Hennekens, C. H. (1994). Association of moderate alcohol consumption and plasma concentration of endogenous tissue-type plasminogen activator. *Journal of the American Medical Association, 272,* 929–933.

Riger, S. (1985). Crime as an environmental stressor. *Journal of Community Psychology, 13,* 270–280.

Rimm, E. B., Stampfer, M. J., Ascherio, A., Giovannucci, E., Colditz, G. A., & Willett, W. C. (1993). Vitamin E consumption and risk of coronary heart disease in men. *New England Journal of Medicine, 328,* 1450–1456.

Rimm, E. B., Stampfer, M. J., Giovannucci, E., Ascherio, A., Spiegelman, D., Colditz, G. A., & Willett, W. C. (1995). Body size and fat distribution as predictors of coronary heart disease among middle-age and older U.S. men. *American Journal of Epidemiology, 141,* 1117–1127.

Ritchie, K., & Kildea, D. (1995). Is senile dementia "age-related" or "ageing-related"?—Evidence from meta-analysis of dementia prevalence in the oldest old. *Lancet, 346,* 931–934.

Rivara, F., Mueller, B. A., Somes, G., Mendoza, C. T., Rushforth, N. B., & Kellermann, A. L. (1997). Alcohol and illicit drug abuse and the risk of violent death in the home. *Journal of the American Medical Association, 278,* 569–575.

Roberts, S. S. (1998). Working toward a world without Type I diabetes. *Diabetes Forecast, 51*(7), 85–87.

Robertson, L. S. (1983). *Injuries: Causes, control strategies, and public policy.* Lexington, MA: Heath.

Robine, J-M., & Ritchie, K. (1991). Healthy life expectancy: Evaluation of global indicator of change in population health. *British Medical Journal, 302,* 457–460.

Robins, L. N. (1995). Editorial: The natural history of substance use as a guide to setting drug policy. *American Journal of Public Health, 85,* 12–13.

Rodin, J. (1992). *Body traps.* New York: William Morrow.

Rodin, J., & Langer, E. J. (1977). Long-term effects of a control-relevant intervention with the institutionalized aged. *Journal of Personality and Social Psychology, 35,* 897–902.

Rodin, J., & Salovey, P. (1989). Health psychology. *Annual Review of Psychology, 40,* 533–579.

Rodin, J., & Stone, G. C. (1987). Historical highlights in the emergence of the field. In G. C. Stone, S. M. Weiss, J. D. Matarazzo, N. E. Miller, J. Rodin, C. D. Belar, M. J. Follick, & J. E. Singer (Eds.), *Health psychology: A discipline and a profession* (pp. 15–26). Chicago: University of Chicago Press.

Rogers, R. G. (1992). Living and dying in the U.S.A.: Sociodemographic determinants of death among Blacks and Whites. *Demography, 29,* 287–303.

Rohsenow, D. J. (1982). Social anxiety, daily moods, and alcohol use over time among heavy social drinking men. *Addictive Behaviors, 7,* 311–315.

Room, R., & Day, N. (1974). Alcohol and mortality. In M. Keller (Ed.), *Second special report to the U.S. Congress: Alcohol and health.* Washington, DC: U.S. Government Printing Office.

Room, R., & Greenfield, T. (1993). Alcoholics Anonymous, other 12-step movements and psychotherapy in the US population, 1990. *Addiction, 88,* 555–562.

Rorer, B., Tucker, C. M., & Blake, H. (1988). Long-term nurse-patient interactions: Factors in patient compliance or noncompliance to the dietary regimen. *Health Psychology, 7,* 35–46.

Rosch, P. J. (1996). Stress and sleep: Some startling and sobering statistics. *Stress Medicine, 12,* 207–210.

Rosellini, L. (1997, November 10). How far should you go to stay fit? The battle between tough and tame. *U.S. News & World Report, 123,* 95–96.

Rosenberg, E. L., Ekman, P., & Blumenthal, J. A. (1998). Facial expression and the affective component of cynical hostility in male coronary heart disease patients. *Health Psychology, 17,* 376–380.

Rosenberg, H. (1993). Prediction of controlled drinking by alcoholics and problem drinkers. *Psychological Bulletin, 113,* 129–139.

Rosenberg, P. S., & Biggar, R. J. (1998). Trends in HIV incidence among young adults in the United States. *Journal of the American Medical Association, 279,* 1894–1899.

Rosenfeld, I. (1998, August 16). Acupuncture goes mainstream (Almost). *Parade,* 10–11.

Rosenfield, S. (1992). The costs of sharing: Wives' employment and husbands' mental health. *Journal of Health and Social Behavior, 33,* 213–225.

Rosengren, A., Tibblin, G., & Wilhelmsen, L. (1991). Self-perceived psychological stress and incidence of coronary artery disease in middle-aged men. *American Journal of Cardiology, 68,* 1171–1175.

Rosenman, R. H., Brand, R. J., Jenkins, C. D., Friedman, M., Straus, R., & Wurm, M. (1975). Coronary heart disease in the Western Collaborative Group Study: Final follow-up of 8½ years. *Journal of the American Medical Association, 233,* 872–877.

Rosenstock, I. M. (1990). The health belief model: Explaining health behavior through expectancies. In K. Glanz, F. M. Lewis, & B. K. Rimer (Eds.), *Health behavior and health education: Theory, research, and practice* (pp. 39–62). San Francisco: Jossey-Bass.

Ross, C. E. (1993). Fear of victimization and health. *Journal of Quantitative Criminology, 9,* 159–175.

Ross, M. J., & Berger, R. S. (1996). Effects of stress inoculation training on athletes' postsurgical pain and rehabilitation after orthopedic injury. *Journal of Consulting and Clinical Psychology, 64,* 406–410.

Rost, K., Carter, W., & Innui, T. (1989). Introduction of information during the initial medical visit: Consequences for patient follow-through with physician recommendations for medication. *Social Science and Medicine, 28,* 315–321.

Roter, D. L. (1988). Reciprocity in the medical encounter. In D. S. Gochman (Ed.), *Health behavior: Emerging research perspectives* (pp. 293–303). New York: Plenum Press.

Roth, D. L., & Holmes, D. S. (1985). Influence of physical fitness in deterring the impact of stressful events on physical and psychologic health. *Psychosomatic Medicine, 47,* 164–173.

Roth, H. P. (1987). Measurement of compliance. *Patient Education and Counseling, 10,* 107–116.

Roth, S., Newman, E., Pelcovitz, D., van der Kolk, B., & Mandel, F. S., (1997). Complex PTSD in victims exposed to sexual and physical abuse: Results from the DSM-IV field trial for posttraumatic stress disorder. *Journal of Traumatic Stress, 101,* 539–555.

Rotter, J. B. (1966). Generalized expectancies for internal versus external control of reinforcement. *Psychological Monographs, 80* (Whole No. 609).

Rotter, J. B. (1982). *The development and applications of social learning theory: Selected papers.* New York: Praeger.

Rotton, J., Yoshikawa, J., & Kaplan, F. (1979). *Perceived control, malodorous air pollution and behavioral aftereffects.* Paper presented at the annual meeting of the Southeastern Psychological Association, New Orleans.

Rouse B. A. (Ed.). (1998). *Substance abuse and mental health statistics source book.* Rockville, MD: Department of Health and Human Services: Substance Abuse and Mental Health Services Administration.

Routh, D. K., & Sanfilippo, M. D. (1991). Helping children cope with painful medical procedures. In J. P. Bush & S. W. Harkins (Eds.), *Children in pain: Clinical and research issues from a developmental perspective* (pp. 397–424). New York: Springer-Verlag.

Rowe, M. M. (1997). Hardiness, stress, temperament, coping, and burnout in health professionals. *American Journal of Health Behavior, 21,* 163–171.

Rozin, P. (1996). Sociocultural influences on human food selection. In E. D. Capaldi (Ed.), *Why we eat what we eat: The psychology of eating* (pp. 233–263). Washington, DC: American Psychological Association.

Ruback, R. B., & Pandey, J. (1996). Gender differences in perceptions of household crowding: Stress, affiliation, and role obligations in rural India. *Journal of Applied Social Psychology, 26,* 417–436.

Ruback, R. B., Pandey, J., & Begum, H. A. (1997). Urban stressors in South Asia: Impact on male and female pedestrians in Delhi and Dhaka. *Journal of Cross-Cultural Psychology, 28,* 23–43.

Rudy, T. E., Turk, D. C., Zaki, H. S., & Curtin, H. D. (1989). An empirical taxometric alternative to traditional classification of temporomandibular disorders. *Pain, 36,* 311–320.

Rueter, M. A., & Harris, D. V. (1980, August). *The effects of running on individuals who are clinically depressed.* Paper presented at the annual meeting of the American Psychological Association, Montreal.

Ruiz, P., & Ruiz, P. P. (1983). Treatment compliance among Hispanics. *Journal of Operational Psychiatry, 14,* 112–114.

Runyon, C. W., & Runyon, D. K. (1991). How can physicians get kids to wear bicycle helmets? A prototypic challenge in injury prevention. *American Journal of Public Health, 81,* 972–973.

Russell, N. K., & Roter, D. L. (1993). Health promotion counseling of chronic-disease patients during primary care visits. *American Journal of Public Health, 83,* 979–982.

Ruuskanen, J. M., & Parkatti, T. (1994). Physical activity and related factors among nursing home residents. *Journal of the American Geriatrics Society, 42,* 987–991.

Ruzicka, L. T. (1995). Suicide mortality in developed countries. In A. D. Lopez, G. Caselli, & T. Valkonen (Eds.), *Adult mortality in developed countries: From description to explanation* (pp. 83–110). Oxford, UK: Clarendon Press.

Ryan, W. (1971). *Blaming the victim.* New York: Pantheon.

Sacco, R. L., Elkind, M., Boden-Albala, B., I-Feng, L., Kargman, D. E., Hauser, W. A., Shea, S., & Paik, M. C. (1999). The protective effect of moderate alcohol consumption on ischemic stroke. *Journal of the American Medical Association, 281,* 53–60.

Sachs, M. L. (1982). Compliance and addiction to exercise. In R. C. Cantu (Ed.), *The exercising adult* (pp. 19–27). Lexington, MA: Collamore Press.

Sackett, D. L., & Snow, J. C. (1979). The magnitude of compliance and noncompliance. In R. B. Haynes, D. W. Taylor, & D. L. Sackett (Eds.), *Compliance in health care* (pp. 11–22). Baltimore: Johns Hopkins University Press.

Sacks, J. J., Holingreen, P., Smith, S. M., & Sosin, D. M. (1991). Bicycle-associated head injuries and deaths in the United States from 1984 through 1988. *Journal of the American Medical Association, 266,* 3016–3018.

Sacks, J. J., & Nelson, D. E. (1994). Smoking and injuries: An overview. *Preventive Medicine, 23,* 515–520.

Saldana, L., Peterson, L. (1997). Preventing injury in children: The need for parental involvement. In T. S. Watson & F. M. Gresham (Eds.), pp. 221–238. *Handbook of child behavior therapy.* New York: Plenum Press.

Sallan, S. E., Zinberg, N. E., & Frei, E., III. (1975). Antiemetic effect of delta-9-tetrahydrocannabinol in patients receiving cancer chemotherapy. *New England Journal of Medicine, 293,* 795–797.

Salonen, J. T., Alfthan, G., Huttunen, J. K., & Puska, P. (1984). Association between serum selenium and the risk of cancer. *American Journal of Epidemiology, 120,* 342–349.

Sanders, M. R., Shepherd, R. W., Cleghorn, G., & Woolford, H. (1994). The treatment of recurrent abdominal pain in children: A controlled comparison of cognitive-behavioral family intervention and standard pediatric care. *Journal of Consulting and Clinical Psychology, 62,* 306–314.

Sandler, D. P., Comstock, G. W., Helsing, K. J., & Shore, D. L. (1989). Deaths from all causes in non-smokers who lived with smokers. *American Journal of Public Health, 79,* 163–167.

Sarason, B. R., & Sarason, I. G. (1994). Assessment of social support. In S. A. Shumaker & S. M. Czajkowski (Eds.), *Social support and cardiovascular disease* (pp. 41–63). New York: Plenum Press.

Saunders, T., Driskell, J. E., Johnston, J. H., & Sales, E. (1996). The effects of stress inoculation training on anxiety and performance. *Journal of Occupational Health Psychology, 1,* 170–186.

Schachter, S. (1980). Urinary pH and the psychology of nicotine addiction. In P. O. Davidson & S. M. Davidson (Eds.), *Behavioral medicine: Changing health lifestyles* (pp. 70–93). New York: Brunner/Mazel.

Schachter, S. (1982). Recidivism and self-cure of smoking and obesity. *American Psychologist, 37,* 436–444.

Scharff, L., & Marcus, D. A. (1994). Interdisciplinary outpatient group treatment of intractable headache. *Headache, 34,* 73–78.

Scheier, M. F., Matthews, K. A., Owens, J. F., Magovern, G. J., Sr., Lefebvre, R. C., Abbott, R. A., & Carver, C. S. (1989). Dispositional optimism and recovery from coronary artery bypass surgery: The beneficial effects on physical and psychological well-being. *Journal of Personality and Social Psychology, 57,* 1024–1040.

Scherwitz, L., Perkins, L., Chesney, M., & Hughes, G. (1991). Cook-Medley Hostility Scale and subsets: Relationship to demographic and psychosocial characteristics in young adults in the CARDIA study. *Psychomatic Medicine, 53,* 36–49.

Schleifer, S. J., Keller, S. E., Camerino, M., Thorton, J. C., & Stein, M. (1983). Suppression of lymphocyte stimulation following bereavement. *Journal of the American Medical Association, 250,* 374–377.

Schmaling, K. B. (1998). Asthma. In E. A. Blechman & K. D. Brownell (Eds.), *Behavioral medicine and women: A comprehensive handbook* (pp. 566–569). New York: Guilford.

Schmelkin, L. P., Wachtel, A. B., Schneiderman, B. E., & Hecht, D. (1988). The dimensional structure of medical students' perception of diseases. *Journal of Behavioral Medicine, 11,* 171–183.

Schmied, L. A., & Lawler, K. A., (1986). Hardiness, Type A behavior, and the stress-illness relation in working women. *Journal of Personality and Social Psychology, 51,* 1218–1223.

Schnall, P. L., Pieper, C., Schwartz, J. E., Karasek, R. A., Schlussel, Y., Devereaux, R. B., Ganau, A., Alderman, M., Warren, K., & Pickering, T. G. (1990). The relationship between "jobstrain" workplace diastolic blood pressure, and left ventricular mass index. *Journal of the American Medical Association, 263,* 1929–1935.

Schoenbaum, M. (1997). Do smokers understand the mortality effects of smoking? Evidence from the Health Retirement Survey. *American Journal of Public Health, 87,* 755–759.

Schoenberg, J. B., Wilcox, H. B., Mason, T. J., Bill, J., & Stemhagen, A. (1989). Variation in smoking-related lung cancer risk among New Jersey women. *American Journal of Epidemiology, 130,* 688–695.

Schofield, W. (1969). The role of psychology in the delivery of health services. *American Psychologist, 24,* 568–584.

Schulz, T. F., Boshoff, C. H., & Weiss, R. A. (1996). HIV infection and neoplasia. *Lancet, 348,* 587–591.

Schwartz, B. S., Stewart, W. F., Simon, D., & Lipton, R. B. (1998). Epidemiology of tension-type headache. *Journal of the American Medical Association, 279,* 381–383.

Schwartz, G. E., & Weiss, S. M. (1978). Behavioral medicine revisited: An amended definition. *Journal of Behavioral Medicine, 1,* 249–251.

Schwarz, D. E. (1993). Adolescent trauma: Epidemiologic approach. *Adolescent Medicine: State of the Art Reviews, 4,* 11–22.

Schwarz, D. F., Grisso, J. A., Miles, C., Holmes, J. H., & Sutton, R. L. (1993). An injury prevention program in an urban African-American community. *American Journal of Public Health, 83,* 675–680.

Schwarzer, R., & Leppin, A. (1989). Social support and health: A meta-analysis. *Psychology and Health, 3,* 1–15.

Schwarzer, R., & Leppin, A. (1992). Possible impact of social ties and support on morbidity and mortality. In H. O. E. Veiel & U. Baumann (Eds.), *The meaning and measurement of social support* (pp. 65–83). New York: Hemisphere.

Sclafani, A., & Springer, D. (1976). Dietary obesity in adult rats: Similarities to hypothalamic and human obesity. *Physiology and Behavior, 17,* 461–471.

Seddon, J., Willett, W. C., Speizer, F. E., & Hankinson, S. E. (1997). A prospective study of cigarette smoking and age-related macular degeneration in women. *Journal of the American Medical Association, 276,* 1141–1146.

Sedlacek, K., & Taub, E. (1996). Biofeedback treatment of Raynaud's disease. *Professional Psychology: Research and Practice, 27,* 549–553.

Segall, A. (1997). Sick role concepts and health behavior. In D. S. Gochman (Ed.), *Handbook of health behavior research I: Personal and social determinants* (pp. 289–301). New York: Plenum Press.

Seligman, M. E. P. (1975). *Helplessness*. San Francisco: Freeman.

Sellwood, W., & Tarrier, N. (1994). Demographic factors associated with extreme non-compliance in schizophrenia. *Social Psychiatry and Psychiatric Epidemiology, 29,* 172–177.

Selye, H. (1956). *The stress of life*. New York: McGraw-Hill.

Selye, H. (1976). *Stress in health and disease*. Reading, MA: Butterworths.

Selye, H. (1982). History and present status of the stress concept. In L. Goldberger & S. Breznitz (Eds.), *Handbook of stress: Theoretical and clinical aspects* (pp. 7–17). New York: Free Press.

Serdula, M. K., Collins, M. E., Williamson, D. F., Anda, R. F., Pamuk, E., & Byers, T. E. (1993). Weight control practices of U.S. adolescents and adults. *Annals of Internal Medicine, 119,* 667–671.

Shaffer, J. W., Graves, P. L., Swank, R. T., & Pearson, T. A. (1987). Clustering of personality traits in youth and the subsequent development of cancer among physicians. *Journal of Behavioral Medicine, 10,* 441–447.

Sharma, S., & Kumaraiah, V., & Mishra, H. (1996). Behavioral intervention in test anxiety. *NIMHANS Journal, 14,* 57–60.

Shaw, C. R. (1981). What is cancer and how much is caused by occupational exposure? In C. R. Shaw (Ed.), *Prevention of occupational cancer*. Boca Raton, FL: CRC Press.

Sheidler, V. R. (1987). New methods in analgesic delivery. In D. B. McGuire & C. H. Yarbro (Eds.), *Cancer pain management* (pp. 203–222). Philadelphia: Saunders.

Shekelle, R. B., Raynar, W. J., Ostfield, A. M., Garron, D. C., Bieliauskas, L. A., Liu, S. C., Maliza, C., & Paul, O. (1981). Psychological depression and 17-year risk of death from cancer. *Psychosomatic Medicine, 43,* 117–125.

Shekelle, R. B., Rossof, A. H., & Stamler, J. (1991). Dietary cholesterol and incidence of lung cancer: The Western Electric study. *American Journal of Epidemiology, 134,* 480–484.

Sher, K. J. (1987). Stress response dampening. In H. T. Blane & K. E. Leonard (Eds.), *Psychological theories of drinking and alcoholism* (pp. 227–271). New York: Guilford Press.

Sher, K. J., & Levenson, R. W. (1982). Risk for alcoholism and individual differences in the stress-response-dampening effect of alcohol. *Journal of Abnormal Psychology, 91,* 350–367.

Sherbourne, C. D., Hays, R. D., Ordway, L., DiMatteo, M. R., & Kravitz, R. L. (1992). Antecedents of adherence to medical recommendations: Results from the Medical Outcomes Study. *Journal of Behavioral Medicine, 15,* 447–468.

Sherman, J. E., & Liebeskind, J. C. (1980). An endorphinergic centrifugal substrate of pain modulation: Recent findings, current concepts, and complexities. In J. J. Bonica (Ed.), *Pain*. New York: Raven Press.

Sherman, R. A. (1997). History of treatment attempts. In R. A. Sherman (Ed.), *Phantom pain* (pp. 143–147). New York: Plenum Press.

Sherman, R. A., Katz, J., Marbach, J. J., & Heermann-Do, K. (1997). Locations, characteristics, and descriptions. In R. A. Sherman (Ed.), *Phantom pain* (pp. 1–32). New York: Plenum Press.

Sherwood, R. J. (1983). Compliance behavior of hemodialysis patients and the role of the family. *Family Systems Medicine, 1,* 60–72.

Shipley, R. H., Butt, J. H., Horwitz, B., & Farbry, J. E. (1978). Preparation for a stressful medical procedure: Effects of amount of stimulus preexposure and coping style. *Journal of Consulting and Clinical Psychology, 46,* 499–507.

Shore, E. R., Gregory, T., & Tatlock, L. (1991). College students' reactions to a designated driver program: An exploratory study. *Journal of Alcohol and Drug Education, 37,* 1–6.

Shroyer, J. A. (1990). Getting tough on anabolic steroids: Can we win the battle? *The Physician and Sportsmedicine, 18*(2), 106–118.

Sidney, S. Beck, J. E., Tekawa, I. S., Quesenberry, C. P., & Friedman, G. D. (1997). Marijuana use and mortality. *American Journal of Public Health, 87,* 585–590.

Sidney, S., Friedman, G. D., & Siegelaub, A. B. (1987). Thinness and mortality. *American Journal of Public Health, 77,* 317–322.

Siegel, D., & Lopez, J. (1997). Trends in antihypertensive drug use in the United States: Do the JNC V recommendations affect prescribing? *Journal of the American Medical Association, 278,* 1745–1748.

Siegel, J. M. (1990). Stressful life events and use of physician services among the elderly: The moderating role of pet ownership. *Journal of Personality and Social Psychology, 58,* 1081–1086.

Siegel, M. (1993). Involuntary smoking in the restaurant workplace: A review of employee exposure and health effects. *Journal of the American Medical Association, 270,* 490–493.

Siegler, I. C., Peterson, B. L., Barefoot, J. C., & Williams, R. B. (1992). Hostility during late adolescence predicts coronary risk factors at mid-life. *American Journal of Epidemiology, 136,* 146–154.

Siegman, A. W. (1994). From Type A to hostility to anger: Reflections on the history of coronary-prone behavior. In A. W. Siegman & T. W. Smith (Eds.), *Anger, hostility, and the heart* (pp. 1–21). Hillsdale, NJ: Erlbaum.

Siegman, A. W., Anderson, R., Herbst, J., Boyle, S., & Wilkinson, J. (1992). Dimensions of anger-hostility and cardiovascular reactivity in provoked and angered men. *Journal of Behavioral Medicine, 15,* 257–272.

Siegman, A. W., Dembroski, T. M., & Ringel, N. (1987). Components of hostility and the severity of coronary artery disease. *Psychosomatic Medicine, 49,* 127–135.

Siegman, A. W., & Snow, S. C. (1997). The outward expression of anger, the inward experience of anger and CVR: The role of vocal expression. *Journal of Behavioral Medicine, 20,* 29–45.

Simone, C. B. (1983). *Cancer and nutrition.* New York: McGraw-Hill.

Sims, E. A. H. (1974). Studies in human hyperphagia. In G. Bray & J. Bethune (Eds.), *Treatment and management of obesity.* New York: Harper & Row.

Sims, E. A. H. (1976). Experimental obesity, dietary-induced thermogenesis, and their clinical implications. *Clinics in Endocrinology and Metabolism, 5,* 377–395.

Sims, E. A. H., Danforth, E., Jr., Horton, E. S., Bray, G. A., Glennon, J. A., & Salans, L. B. (1973). Endocrine and metabolic effects of experimental obesity in man. *Recent Progress in Hormonal Research, 29,* 457–496.

Sims, E. A. H., & Horton, E. S. (1968). Endocrine and metabolic adaptation to obesity and starvation. *American Journal of Clinical Nutrition, 21,* 1455–1470.

Sinyor, D., Golden, M., Steinert, Y., & Seraganian, P. (1986). Experimental manipulation of aerobic fitness and the response to psychosocial stress: Heart rate and self-report measures. *Psychosomatic Medicine, 48,* 324–337.

Siscovick, D. S., Fried, L., Mittelmark, M., Rutan, G., Bild, D., & O'Leary, D. H. (1997). Exercise intensity and subclinical cardiovascular disease in the elderly: The Cardiovascular Health Study. *American Journal of Epidemiology, 145,* 977–988.

Sjöström, L. V. (1992a). Morbidity of severely obese subjects. *American Journal of Clinical Nutrition, 55,* 508S–515S.

Sjöström, L. V. (1992b). Mortality of severely obese subjects. *American Journal of Clinical Nutrition, 55,* 516S–523S.

Skelton, J. A. (1991). Laypersons' judgments of patient credibility and the study of illness representations. In J. A. Skelton & R. T. Croyle (Eds.), *Mental representation in health and illness* (pp. 108–131). New York: Springer-Verlag.

Skinner, B. F. (1953). *Science and human behavior.* New York: Macmillan.

Skinner, B. F. (1987). *Upon further reflection.* Englewood Cliffs, NJ: Prentice-Hall.

Slater, J., & Depue, R. A. (1981). The contribution of environmental events and social support to serious suicide attempts in primary depressive disorder. *Journal of Abnormal Psychology, 90,* 275–285.

Slattery, M. L., Boucher, K. M., Caan, B. J., Potter, J. D., & Ma, K-N. (1998). Eating patterns and risk of colon cancer. *American Journal of Epidemiology, 148,* 4–16.

Slattery, M. L., & Kerber, R. A. (1993). A comprehensive evaluation of family history and breast cancer risk. *Journal of the American Medical Association, 270,* 1563–1568.

Slattery, M. L., Schumacher, M. C., Smith, K. R., West, D. W., & Abd-Elghany, N. (1990). Physical activity, diet, and risk of colon cancer in Utah. *American Journal of Epidemiology, 128,* 989–999.

Slay, H. A., Hayaki, J., Napolitano, M. A., & Brownell, K. D. (1998). Motivations for running and eating attitudes in obligatory versus nonobligatory runners. *International Journal of Eating Disorders, 23,* 267–275.

Smith, J. T., Barabasz, A., & Barabasz, M. (1996). Comparison of hypnosis and distraction in severely ill children undergoing painful medical procedures. *Journal of Counseling Psychology, 43,* 187–195.

Smith, M., Colligan, M., Horning, R. W., & Hurrel, J. (1978). *Occupational comparison of stress-related disease incidence.* Cincinnati: National Institute for Occupational Safety and Health.

Smith, R. (1997). The future of healthcare systems: Information technology and consumerism will transform health care worldwide. *British Medical Journal, 314,* 495–496.

Smith, T. W. (1994). Concepts and methods in the study of anger, hostility, and health. In A. W. Siegman & T. W. Smith (Eds.), *Anger, hostility, and the heart* (pp. 23–42). Hillsdale, NJ: Erlbaum.

Smith, T. W., & Brown, P. C. (1991). Cynical hostility, attempts to exert social control, and cardiovascular reactivity in married couples. *Journal of Behavioral Medicine, 14,* 581–592.

Smith-Warner, S. A., Spiegelman, D., Shaw-Shyuan, Y., van den Brandt, P. A., Folsom, A. R., Goldbohm, R. A., Graham, S., Holmberg, L., Howe, G. R., Marshall, J. R., Miller, A. B., Potter, J. D., Speizer, F. E., Willett, W. C., Wolk, A., & Hunter, D. J. (1998). Alcohol and breast cancer in women: A pooled analysis of cohort studies. *Journal of the American Medical Association, 279,* 535–540.

Smoking Cessation Clinical Practice Guideline Panel and Staff (1996). The Agency for Health Care Policy and Research: *Smoking Cessation Clinical Practice Guideline. Journal of the American Medical Association, 275,* 1270–1280.

Snyder, S. H. (1977, March). Opiate receptors and internal opiates. *Scientific American, 236,* 44–56.

Sobel, D. S. (1995). Rethinking medicine: Improving health outcomes with cost-effective psychosocial interventions. *Psychosomatic Medicine, 57,* 234–244.

Sobell, L. C., Cunningham, J. A., & Sobell, M. B. (1996). Recovery from alcohol problems with and without treatment: Prevalence in two population surveys. *American Journal of Public Health, 86,* 966–972.

Solomon, C. M. (1998). Picture this: A safer workplace. Polaroid addresses family violence to combat workplace violence. *Workforce, 77*(2), 82–86.

Solomon, G. F. (1987). Psychoneuroimmunology: Interactions between central nervous system and immune system. *Journal of Neuroscience Research, 18,* 1–9.

Solomon, G. F., & Moos, R. L. (1964). Emotions, immunity, and disease: A speculative theoretical integration. *Archives of General Psychiatry, 11,* 657–674.

Sonstroem, R. J. (1984). Exercise and self-esteem. *Exercise and Sport Sciences Reviews, 12,* 123–155.

Sonstroem, R. J. (1997). Physical activity and self esteem. In W. P. Morgan (Ed.), *Physical activity and mental health* (pp. 127–143). Washington, DC: Taylor & Francis.

Sontag, S., Graham, D. Y., Belsito, A., Weiss, J., Farley, A., Grunt, R., Cohen, N., Kinnear, D., Davis, W., Archabault, A., Achord, J., Thayer, W., Gillies, R., Sidorov, J., Sadesin, S. M., Dyck, W., Fleshler, B., Cleator, I., Wenger, J., & Opekun, A., Jr. (1984). Cimetidine, cigarette smoking, and recurrence of duodenal ulcer. *New England Journal of Medicine, 311,* 689–693.

Sorenson, S. B., Upchurch, D. M., & Shen, H. (1996). Violence and injury in marital arguments: Risk patterns and gender differences. *American Journal of Public Health, 86,* 35–40.

Sotile, W. M. (1996). *Psychosocial interventions for cardiopulmonary patients.* Champaign, IL: Human Kinetics.

Soukup, J. E. (1996). *Alzheimer's disease: A guide to diagnosis, treatment, and management.* Westport, CT: Praeger.

Sours, J. A. (1980). *Starving to death in a sea of objects: The anorexia nervosa syndrome.* New York: Aronson.

Spiegel, D. (1993). Social support: How friends, family, and groups can help. In D. Goleman & J. Gurin (Eds.), *Mind/body medicine: How to use your mind for better health* (pp. 331–349). Yonkers, NY: Consumer Reports Books.

Spiegel, D., Bloom, J. R., & Yalom, I. D. (1981). Group support for patients with metastatic cancer. *Archives of General Psychiatry, 38,* 527–533.

Spiegel, D., & Kato, P. (1996). Psychosocial influences on cancer incidence and progression. *Harvard Review of Psychiatry, 4,* 10–26.

Spiegel, D., Kraemer, H. C., Bloom, J. R., & Gottheil, E. (1989). Effect of psychosocial treatment on survival of patients with metastatic breast cancer. *Lancet, ii,* 888–891.

Stall, R. (1986). Respondent-identified reasons for change and stability in alcohol consumption as a concomitant of the aging process. In C. R. Janes, R. Stall, & S. M. Gifford (Eds.), *Anthropology and epidemiology: Interdisciplinary approaches to the study of health and disease* (pp. 275–302). Boston: Reidel.

Stall, R., McKusick, L., Wiley, J., Coates, T. J., & Ostrow, D. G. (1986). Alcohol and drug use during sexual activity and compliance with safe sex guidelines for AIDS: The AIDS Behavioral Research Project. *Health Education Quarterly, 13,* 359–371.

Stamler, J., Wentworth, D., & Neaton, J. D. (1986). Is relationship between serum cholesterol and risk of premature death from coronary heart disease continuous and graded? Findings in 356, 222 primary screenees of the Multiple Risk Factor Intervention Trial (MRFIT). *Journal of the American Medical Association, 256,* 2823–2828.

Stampfer, M. J., Hennekens, C. H., Manson, J. E., Colditz, G. A., Rosner, D., & Willett, W. C. (1993). Vitamin E consumption and the risk of coronary heart disease in women. *New England Journal of Medicine, 328,* 1444–1449.

Stanton, A. L. (1987). Determinants of adherence to medical regimens by hypertensive patients. *Journal of Behavioral Medicine, 10,* 377–394.

Stanton, W. R., Mahalski, P. A., McGee, R., & Silva, P. A. (1993). Reasons for smoking or not smoking in early adolescence. *Addictive Behaviors, 18,* 321–329.

Stason, W., Neff, R., Miettinen, O., & Jick, H. (1976). Alcohol consumption and nonfatal myocardial infarction. *American Journal of Epidemiology, 104,* 603–608.

Steele, C. M., & Josephs, R. A. (1990). Alcohol myopia: Its prized and dangerous effects. *American Psychologist, 45,* 921–933.

Steele, C. M., Southwick, L., & Pagano, R. (1986). Drinking your troubles away: The role of activity in mediating alcohol's reduction of psychological stress. *Journal of Abnormal Psychology, 95,* 173–180.

Steenland, K. (1992). Passive smoking and the risk of heart disease. *Journal of the American Medical Association, 267,* 94–99.

Stein, M., Schleifer, S. J., & Keller, S. E. (1981). Hypothalamic influences on immune response. In R. Ader (Ed.), *Psychoneuroimmunology* (pp. 429–447). New York: Academic Press.

Stein, P. N., & Motta, R. W. (1992). Effects of aerobic and nonaerobic exercise on depression and self-concept. *Perceptual and Motor Skills, 74,* 79–89.

Steinhausen, H. C., Winkler, C., & Meier, M. (1997). Eating disorders in adolescence in a Swiss epidemiological study. *International Journal of Eating Disorders, 22,* 247–151.

Steinmetz, H. M., & Hobson, S. J. G. (1994). Prevention of falls among the community-dwelling elderly: An overview. *Physical and Occupational Therapy in Geriatrics, 12,* 13–29.

Steinmetz, K. A., Kushi, L. H., Bostick, R. M., Folsom, A. R., & Potter, J. D. (1994). Vegetables, fruit, and colon cancer in the Iowa Women's Health Study. *American Journal of Epidemiology, 139,* 1–15.

Sternbach, R. A. (1978). Clinical aspects of pain. In R. A. Sternbach (Ed.), *The psychology of pain.* New York: Raven Press.

Stevens, J., Cai, J., Pamuk, E. R., Williamson, D. F., Thun, M., & Wood, J. L. (1998). The effect of age on the association between body-mass index and mortality. *New England Journal of Medicine, 338,* 1–7.

Stevenson, T., & Lennie, J. (1992). Empowering school students in developing strategies to increase bicycle helmet wearing. *Health Education Research, 7,* 555–566.

Stewart, A., Greenfield, S., Hays, R. D., Wells, K., Rogers, W. H., Berry, S. D., McGlynn, E. A., & Ware, J. E., Jr. (1989). Functional status and well-being of patients with chronic conditions. *Journal of the American Medical Association, 262,* 907–913.

Stewart, W. F., Lipton, R. B., Celentano, D. D., & Reed, M. L. (1992). Prevalence of migraine headache in the United States. *Journal of the American Medical Association, 267,* 64–69.

Stiffman, A. R., Earls, F., Dore, P., Cunningham, R., & Farber, S. (1996). Adolescent violence. In R. J. Di Clemente, W. B. Hansen, & L. E. Ponton (Eds.),

Handbook of adolescent health risk behavior (pp. 289–312). New York: Plenum Press.

Stoddard, J. J., & Miller, T. (1995). Impact of parental smoking on the prevalence of wheezing respiratory illness in children. *American Journal of Epidemiology, 141*, 96–102.

Stofan, J. R., DiPietro, L., Davis, D., Kohl, H. W., III, & Blair, S. N. (1998). Physical activity patterns associated with cardiorespiratory fitness and reduced mortality: The Aerobics Center Longitudinal Study. *American Journal of Public Health, 88*, 1807–1813.

Stokols, D. (1972). On the distinction between density and crowding: Some implications for future research. *Psychological Review, 79*, 275–277.

Stone, A. A., Bovbjerg, D. H., Neale, J. M., Napoli, A., Valdimarsdottir, H., Cox, D., Hayden, F. G., & Gwaltney, J. M., Jr. (1992). Development of the common cold symptoms following experimental rhinovirus is related to prior stressful life events. *Behavior Medicine, 18*, 115–120.

Stone, A. A., Reed, B. R., & Neale, J. M. (1987). Changes in daily event frequency precedes episodes of physical symptoms. *Journal of Human Stress, 13*, 70–74.

Stone, G. C. (1982). *Health Psychology:* A new journal for a new field. *Health Psychology, 1*, 1–6.

Stone, G. C. (1984). A final word [editorial]. *Health Psychology, 3*, 585–589.

Stone, G. C. (1987). The scope of health psychology. In G. C. Stone, S. M. Weiss, J. D. Matarazzo, N. E. Miller, J. Rodin, C. D. Belar, M. J. Follick, & J. E. Singer (Eds.), *Health psychology: A discipline and a profession* (pp. 27–40). Chicago: University of Chicago Press.

Stone, R., Cafferata, G. L., & Sangl, J. (1987). Caregivers of the frail elderly: A national profile. *Gerontologist, 27*, 616–626.

Stout, N. A., Jenkins, E. L., & Pizatella, T. J. (1996). Occupational injury mortality rates in the United States: Changes from 1980 to 1989. *American Journal of Public Health, 86*, 73–77.

Strain, E. C., Mumford, G. K., Silverman, K., & Griffiths, R. R. (1994). Caffeine dependence syndrome: Evidence from case histories and experimental evaluation. *Journal of the American Medical Association, 272*, 1043–1047.

Straus, M. A., Gelles, R. J., & Steinmetz, S. K. (1980). *Behind closed doors: Violence in the American family.* Garden City, NY: Anchor.

Strecher, V. J., Champion, V. L., & Rosenstock, I. M. (1997). The health belief model and health behavior. In D. S. Gochman (Ed.), *Handbook of health behavior research I: Personal and social determinants* (pp. 71–91). New York: Plenum Press.

Strecher, V. J., & Rosenstock, I. M. (1997). The health belief model. In A. Baum, S. Newman, J. Weinman, R. West, & C. McManus (Eds.), *Cambridge handbook of psychology, health and medicine* (pp. 113–117). Cambridge, United Kingdom: Cambridge University Press.

Streissguth, A. P., Barr, H. M., Kogan, J., & Bookstein, F. L. (1996). *Understanding the occurrence of secondary disabilities in clients with fetal alcohol syndrome (FAS) and fetal alcohol effects (FAE).* Seattle, WA: University of Washington Publication Services.

Streltzer, J. (1997). Pain. In W-S. Tseng & J. Streltzer (Eds.), *Culture and psychopathology: A guide to clinical assessment* (pp. 87–100). New York: Brunner/Mazel.

Strong, C. A. (1895). The psychology of pain. *Psychological Review, 2*, 329–347.

Stuart, R. B. (1967). Behavioral control of overeating. *Behavior Research and Therapy, 5*, 357–365.

Stunkard, A. J. (1989). Perspectives on human obesity. In A. J. Stunkard & A. Baum (Eds.), *Perspectives on behavioral medicine: Eating, sleeping, and sex* (pp. 9–30). Hillsdale, NJ: Erlbaum.

Stunkard, A. J., Harris, J. R., Pedersen, N. L., & McClean, G. E. (1990). The body-mass index of twins who have been reared apart. *New England Journal of Medicine, 322*, 1483–1487.

Stunkard, A. J., Sørensen, T. I. A., Hanis, C., Teasdale, T. W., Chakraborty, R., Schull, W. J., & Schulsinger, F. (1986). An adoption study of human obesity. *New England Journal of Medicine, 314*, 193, 198.

Suarez, E. C., Kuhn, C. M., Schanberg, S. M., Williams, R. B., Jr., & Zimmermann, E. A. (1998). Neuroendocrine, cardiovascular, and emotional responses of hostile men: The role of interpersonal challenge. *Psychosomatic Medicine, 60*, 78–88.

Suchman, E. A. (1965). Social patterns of illness and medical care. *Journal of Health and Human Behavior, 6*, 2–16.

Sundstrom, E. (1978). Crowding as a sequential process: Review of research on the effects of population density on humans. In A. Baum & Y. M. Epstein (Eds.), *Human response to crowding* (pp. 31–116). Hillsdale, NJ: Erlbaum.

Susser, M. (1991). What is a cause and how do we know one? A grammar for pragmatic epidemiology. *American Journal of Epidemiology, 133*, 635–648.

Sweet, J. J., Rozensky, R. H., & Tovian, S. M. (1991). Clinical psychology in medical settings: Past and present. In J. J. Sweet, R. H. Rozensky, & S. M. Tovian (Eds.), *Handbook of clinical psychology in medical settings.* New York: Plenum Press.

Syrjala, K. L., & Chapman, C. R. (1984). Measurement of clinical pain: A review and integration of research findings. In C. Benedetti, C. R. Chapman, & G. Moricca (Eds.), *Advances in pain research and therapy: Vol. 7. Recent advances in the management of pain.* New York: Raven Press.

Sytkowski, P. A., D'Agostino, R. B., Belanger, A., & Kannel, W. B. (1996). Sex and time trends in cardiovascular disease incidence and mortality: The Framingham Heart Study, 1950–1989. *American Journal of Epidemiology, 143*, 338–350.

Szmukler, G. I., Eisler, I., Russell, G. F. M., & Dare, C. (1985). Anorexia nervosa, parental "expressed emotion" and dropping out of treatment. *British Journal of Psychiatry, 147*, 265–271.

Talbott, E., Helmkamp, J., Matthews, K., Kuller, L., Cottington, E., & Redmond, G. (1985). Occupational noise exposure, noise-induced hearing loss, and the epidemiology of high blood pressure. *American Journal of Epidemiology, 121,* 501–514.

Tang, J-L., Morris, J. K., Wald, N. J., Hole, D., Shipley, M., & Tunstall-Pedoe, H. (1995). Mortality in relation to tar yield of cigarettes: A prospective study of four cohorts. *British Medical Journal, 311,* 1530–1533.

Tanji, J. L. (1997). Sports medicine. *Journal of the American Medical Association, 277,* 1901–1902.

Tanner, E. K. W., & Feldman, R. H. L. (1997). Strategies for enhancing appointment keeping in low-income chronically ill clients. *Nursing Research, 46,* 342–344.

Tavris, C. (1992). *The mismeasure of women.* New York: Simon and Schuster.

Taylor, S. E. (1979). Hospital patient behavior: Reactance, helplessness, or control? *Journal of Social Issues, 35*(1), 156–184.

Taylor, S. E. (1982). The impact of health organizations on recipients of services. In A. W. Johnson, O. Grusky, & B. H. Raven (Eds.), *Contemporary health services: Social science perspectives* (pp. 103–137). Boston: Auburn House.

Taylor, S. E., & Aspinwall, L. G. (1993). Coping with chronic illness. In L. Goldberger & S. Breznitz (Eds.), *Handbook of stress: Theoretical and clinical aspects* (2nd ed., pp. 511–531). New York: Free Press.

Taylor, S. E., Repetti, R. L., & Seeman, T. (1997). Health psychology: What is an unhealthy environment and how does it get under the skin? *Annual Review of Psychology, 48,* 411–447.

Taylor, S. P., Gammon, C. B., & Capasso, D. R. (1976). Aggression as a function of alcohol and threat. *Journal of Personality and Social Psychology, 34,* 938–941.

Taylor, S. P., & Leonard, K. E. (1983). Alcohol and human physical aggression. In R. G. Geen & E. I. Donnerstein (Eds.), *Aggression: Theoretical and empirical reviews* (Vol. 2, pp. 77–101). New York: Academic Press.

Tedesco, L. A., Keffer, M. A., Davis, E. L., & Christersson, L. A. (1993). Self-efficacy and reasoned action: Predicting oral health status and behaviour at one, three, and six month intervals. *Psychology and Health, 8,* 105–121.

Tedesco, L. A., Keffer, M. A., & Fleck-Kandath, C. (1991). Self-efficacy, reasoned action, and oral health behavior reports: A social cognitive approach to compliance. *Journal of Behavioral Medicine, 14,* 341–355.

Telch, C. F., & Telch, M. J. (1985). Psychological approaches for enhancing coping among cancer patients: A review. *Clinical Psychology Review, 5,* 325–344.

ten Bensel, R. W., Rheinberger, M. M., & Radbill, S. X. (1997). Children in a world of violence: The roots of child maltreatment. In M. E. Helfer, R. S. Kempe, & R. D. Krugman (Eds.), *The battered child* (5th ed. pp. 3–28). Chicago: University of Chicago Press.

ter-Kuile, M. M., Spinhoven, P., Linssen, A., Corry, G., Zitman, F. G., & Rooijmans, H. G. M. (1994). Autogenic training and cognitive self-hypnosis for the treatment of recurrent headaches in three different subject groups. *Pain, 58,* 331–340.

Thayer, R. E., Newman, J. R., & McClain, T. M. (1994). Self-regulation of mood: Strategies for changing a bad mood, raising energy, and reducing tension. *Journal of Personality and Social Psychology, 67,* 910–925.

Thomas, W., White, C. M., Mah, J., Geisser, M. S., Church, T. R., & Mandel, J. S. (1995). Longitudinal compliance with annual screening for fecal occult blood. *American Journal of Epidemiology, 142,* 176–182.

Thompson, B. W. (1994). *A hunger so wide and so deep: American women speak out on eating problems.* Minneapolis: University of Minnesota Press.

Thompson, D. C., Nunn, M. E., Thompson, R. S., & Rivara, F. P. (1996). Effectiveness of bicycle safety helmets in preventing serious facial injury. *Journal of the American Medical Association, 276,* 1994–1995.

Thompson, D. C., Rivara, F. P., Thompson, R. S. (1996). Effectiveness of bicycle safety helmets in preventing head injuries: A case-control study. *Journal of the American Medical Association, 276,* 1968–1973.

Thompson, D. R., & Meddis, R. (1990a). A prospective evaluation of in-hospital counseling for first time myocardial infarction in men. *Journal of Psychosomatic Research, 34,* 237–248.

Thompson, D. R., & Meddis, R. (1990b). Wives' responses to counseling early after myocardial infarction. *Journal of Psychosomatic Research, 34,* 249–258.

Thompson, E. L. (1978). Smoking education programs 1960–1976. *American Journal of Public Health, 68,* 250–257.

Thompson, L., & Walker, A. J. (1989). Gender in families: Women and men in marriage, work, and parenthood. *Journal of Marriage and the Family, 51,* 845–871.

Thompson, P. D. (1982). Cardiovascular hazards of physical activity. *Exercise and Sports Sciences Reviews, 10,* 208–235.

Thompson, P. D., Funk, E. J., Carleton, R. A., & Sturner, W. Q. (1982). The incidence of death during jogging in Rhode Island joggers from 1975 through 1980. *Journal of the American Medical Association, 247,* 2535–2538.

Thompson, R. A., & Sherman, R. T. (1993). *Helping athletes with eating disorders.* Champaign, IL: Human Kinetics Publishers.

Thun, M. J., Day-Lally, C. A., Calle, E. E., Flanders, W. D., & Heath, C. W., Jr. (1995). Excess mortality among cigarette smokers: Changes in a 20-year interval. *American Journal of Public Health, 85,* 1223–1230.

Thune, I., Brenn, T., Lund, E., & Gaard, M. (1997). Physical activity and the risk of breast cancer. *New England Journal of Medicine, 336,* 1269–1275.

Tinker, J. E., & Tucker, J. A. (1994, August). *Environmental contexts surrounding natural recovery from obesity.* Paper presented at the American Psychological Association Convention, Los Angeles, CA.

Tobler, N. S. (1986). Meta-analysis of 143 adolescent drug prevention programs: Quantitative outcome results of program participants compared to a control or comparison group. *Journal of Drug Issues, 16,* 537–567.

Tomar, S. L., & Giovino, G. A. (1998). Incidence and predictors of smokeless tobacco use among U.S. youth. *American Journal of Public Health, 88,* 20–26.

Tomkins, S. S. (1966). Psychological model for smoking behavior. *American Journal of Public Health, 56* (Suppl. 12), 17–20.

Tomkins, S. S. (1968). A modified model of smoking behavior. In E. F. Borgatta & R. R. Evans (Eds.), *Smoking, health and behavior* (pp. 165–188). Chicago: Aldine.

Toniolo, P., Riboli, E., Protta, F., Charrel, M., & Coppa, A. P. (1989). Calorie-providing nutrients and risk of breast cancer. *Journal of the National Cancer Institute, 81,* 278–286.

Toobert, D. J., & Glasgow, R. E. (1991). Problem solving and diabetes self-care. *Journal of Behavioral Medicine, 14,* 71–86.

Traven, N. D., Kuller, L. H., Ives, D. G., Rutan, G. H., & Perper, J. (1995). Coronary heart disease mortality and sudden death: Trends and patterns in 35- to 44-year-old white males, 1970–1990. *American Journal of Epidemiology, 142,* 45–52.

Travis, J. (1995, August 19). One Alzheimer's gene leads to another. *Science News, 148,* 118.

Treiber, F. A., Davis, H., Musante, L., Raunikar, R. A., Strong, W. G., McCaffrey, F., Meeks, M. C., & Vandernoord, R. (1993). Ethnicity, gender, family history of myocardial infarction, and menodynamic responses to laboratory stressors in children. *Health Psychology, 12,* 6–15.

Tremblay, A., Plourde, G., Després, J-P., & Bouchard, C. (1989). Impact of dietary fat content and fat oxidation on energy intake in humans. *American Journal of Clinical Nutrition, 49,* 799–805.

Treviño, F. M., Moyer, E., Valdez, B., & Stroup-Benham, C. A. (1991). Health insurance coverage and utilization of health services by Mexican Americans, mainland Puerto Ricans, and Cuban Americans. *Journal of the American Medical Association, 265,* 233–237.

Trevisan, M., Krogh, V., Freudanheim, J., Blake, A., Muti, P., Panico, S., Farinaro, E., Mancini, M., Menotti, A., Ricci, G., & Research Group ATS-RF 2 of the Italian National Research Council. (1990). Consumption of olive oil, butter, and vegetable oils and coronary heart disease risk factors. *Journal of the American Medical Association, 263,* 688–692.

Tsoh, J. Y., McClure, J. B., Skaar, K. L., Wetter, D. W., Cinciripini, P. M., Prokhorov, A. V., Friedman, K., & Gritz, E. (1997). Smoking cessation 2: Components of effective intervention, *Behavioral Medicine, 23,* 15–27.

Tucker, L. A. (1989). Use of smokeless tobacco, cigarette smoking, and hypercholesterolemia. *American Journal of Public Health, 79,* 1048–1050.

Turk, D. C. (1978). Cognitive behavioral techniques in the management of pain. In J. P. Foreyt & D. P. Rathjen (Eds.), *Cognitive behavior therapy.* New York: Plenum Press.

Turk, D. C. (1996). Biopsychosocial perspective on chronic pain. In R. J. Gatchel & D. C. Turk (Eds.), *Psychological approaches to pain management: A practitioner's handbook* (pp. 3–32). New York: Guilford Press.

Turk, D. C. (1997). Pain: A multidimensional perspective. In A. Baum, S. Newman, J. Weinman, R. West, & C. McManus (Eds.), *Cambridge handbook of psychology, health and medicine* (pp. 146–150). Cambridge, United Kingdom: Cambridge University Press.

Turk, D. C., Meichenbaum, D., & Genest, M. (1983). *Pain and behavioral medicine: A cognitive behavioral perspective.* New York: Guilford Press.

Turk, D. C., & Nash, J. M. (1993). Chronic pain: New ways to cope. In D. Goleman & J. Gurin (Eds.), *Mind/body medicine: How to use your mind for better health* (pp. 111–130). Yonkers, NY: Consumer Reports Books.

Turk, D. C., & Rudy, T. E. (1988). Toward an empirically derived taxonomy of chronic pain patients: Integration of psychological assessment data. *Journal of Consulting and Counseling Psychology, 56,* 233–238.

Turk, D. C., & Rudy, T. E. (1992). Classification logic and strategies in chronic pain. In D. C. Turk & R. Melzack (Eds.), *Handbook of pain assessment* (pp. 409–428). New York: Guilford Press.

Turk, D. C., Sist, T. C., Okifuji, A., Miner, M. F., Florio, G., Harrison, P., Massey, J., Lema, M. L., & Zevon, M. A. (1998). Adaptation to metastatic cancer pain, regional/local cancer pain and non-cancer pain: Role of psychological and behavioral factors. *Pain, 74,* 247–256.

Turner, J. A., & Chapman, C. R. (1982a). Psychological interventions for chronic pain: A critical review. I: Relaxation training and biofeedback. *Pain, 12,* 1–21.

Turner, J. A., & Chapman, C. R. (1982b). Psychological interventions for chronic pain: A critical review. II: Operant conditioning, hypnosis, and cognitive-behavior therapy. *Pain, 12,* 23–46.

Turner, J. A., & Clancy, S. (1988). Comparison of operant behavioral and cognitive-behavioral group treatment for chronic low back pain. *Journal of Consulting and Clinical Psychology, 56,* 261–266.

Turner, J. A., Deyo, R. A., Loeser, J. D., Von Korff, M., & Fordyce, W. E. (1994). The importance of placebo effects in pain treatment and research. *Journal of the American Medical Association, 271,* 1609–1614.

Turner, J. A., & Jensen, M. P. (1993). Efficacy of cognitive therapy for chronic low back pain. *Pain, 52,* 169–177.

Twisk, J. W. R., Kemper, H. C. G., van Mechelen, W., & Post, G. B. (1997). Tracking of risk factors for coronary heart disease over a 14-year period: A comparison between lifestyle and biologic risk factors with data from the Amsterdam Growth and Health Study. *American Journal of Epidemiology, 145,* 688–696.

Uchino, B. N., & Garvey, T. S. (1997). The availability of social support reduces cardiovascular reactivity to acute psychological stress. *Journal of Behavioral Medicine, 20,* 15–27.

USA Today Magazine. (1997, October). Clues that you may need a new doctor. *USA Today Magazine, 126* (2629), 1–2.

U.S. Bureau of the Census (USBC). (1973). *Statistical abstracts of the United States, 1973* (94th ed.). Washington, DC: U.S. Government Printing Office.

U.S. Bureau of the Census (USBC). (1975). *Historical statistics of the United States: Colonial times to 1970, Part 1.* Washington, DC: U.S. Government Printing Office.

U.S. Bureau of the Census (USBC). (1979) *Statistical abstracts of the United States, 1974* (100th ed.). Washington, DC: U. S. Government Printing Office.

U.S. Bureau of the Census (USBC). (1997). *Statistical abstracts of the United States: 1997* (117th ed.). Washington, DC: U.S. Government Printing Office.

U.S. Bureau of the Census (USBC). (1998). *Statistical abstracts of the United States: 1998* (118th ed.). Washington, DC: U.S. Government Printing Office.

U.S. Department of Health and Human Services (USDHHS). (1984). *The health consequences of smoking: Chronic obstructive lung disease. A report of the Surgeon General* (DHHS Publication No. PHS-50205). Washington DC: U.S. Government Printing Office.

U.S. Department of Health and Human Services (USDHHS). (1989). *Reducing the health consequences of smoking: 25 years of progress. A report of the Surgeon General* (DHHS Publication No. CDC 89-8411). Rockville, MD: U.S. Government Printing Office.

U.S. Department of Health and Human Services (USDHHS). (1990). *The health benefits of smoking cessation: A report of the Surgeon General* (DHHS Publication No. CDC 90-8416). Washington, DC: U.S. Government Printing Office.

U.S. Department of Health and Human Services (USDHHS). (1991). *Healthy people 2000: National health promotion and disease prevention objectives.* (PHS Publication No. 91-50212). Washington, DC: Author.

U.S. Department of Health and Human Services (USDHHS). (1993). *National Institutes of Health fact book.* Washington, DC: U.S. Government Printing Office.

U.S. Department of Health and Human Services (USDHHS). (1995). *Healthy people 2000 review, 1994* (DHHS Publication No. 95-1256-1). Washington, DC: U.S. Government Printing Office.

U. S. Department of Health and Human Services (USDHHS). (1996). *Physical activity and health: A report of the Surgeon General.* Atlanta, GA: Centers for Disease Control and Prevention.

U.S. Department of Health and Human Services (USDHHS). (1997). *Ninth special report to the U.S. Congress on alcohol and health* by NIAAA. Washington, DC: U.S. Government Printing Office.

U.S. Department of Health and Human Services (USDHHS). (1998a). *Health, United States, 1998* (DHHS publication No. PHS 98-1232). Washington, DC: U.S. Government Printing Office.

U.S. Department of Health and Human Services (USDHHS). (1998b). *Healthy people 2010 objectives; Draft for public comment.* Washington, DC: U.S. Government Printing Office.

U.S. Department of Health and Human Services (USDHHS). (1998c). *Preliminary results from the 1997 National Household Survey on Drug Abuse* (DHHS publication No. SMA 98-3251). Washington, DC: U.S. Government Printing Office.

U.S. Department of Health and Human Services (USDHHS). (1998d). *Tobacco use among U.S. racial/ethnic minority groups: A report of the Surgeon General.* Atlanta: Centers for Disease Control and Prevention.

U.S. Public Health Service (USPHS). (1964). *Smoking and health: Public Health Service report of the Advisory Committee to the Surgeon General of the Public Health Service* (PHS Publication No. 1103). Washington, DC: U.S. Government Printing Office.

Vaeth, P. A. C., & Satariano, W. A. (1998). Alcohol consumption and breast cancer stage at diagnosis. *Alcoholism: Clinical and Experimental Research, 22,* 928–934.

Vaillant, G. E. (1983). *The natural history of alcoholism: Causes, patterns, and paths to recovery.* Cambridge, MA: Harvard University Press.

van Assema, P., Pieterse, M., Kok, G., Eriksen, M., & de Vries, H. (1993). The determinants of four cancer-related risk behaviours. *Health Education Research, 8,* 461–472.

Van der Does, A. J., & Van Dyck, R. (1989). Does hypnosis contribute to the care of burn patients? Review of evidence. *General Hospital Psychiatry, 11,* 119–124.

van Lenthe, F. J., van Mechelen, W., Kemper, H. C. G., & Twisk, J. W. R. (1998). Association of a central pattern of body fat with blood pressure and lipoproteins from adolescence into adulthood. *American Journal of Epidemiology, 147,* 686–693.

Vartianen, E., Paavola, M., McAlister, A., & Puska, P. (1998). Fifteen-year follow-up of smoking prevention effects in the North Karelia Youth Project. *American Journal of Public Health, 88,* 81–85.

Vena, J. E., Graham, S., Zielezny, M., Swanson, M. K., Barnes, R. E., & Nolan, J. (1985). Lifetime occupational exercise and colon cancer. *American Journal of Public Health, 75,* 357–365.

Ventura, S. J., Anderson, R. N., Martin, J. A. & Smith, B. L. (1998). Births and deaths: Preliminary data for 1997. *National Vital Statistics Report, 47*(4), 1–42.

Verbrugge, L. M. (1983). Multiple roles and physical health of women and men. *Journal of Health and Social Behavior, 24,* 16–30.

Verbrugge, L. M. (1989). The twain meet: Empirical explanation of sex differences in health and mortality. *Journal of Health and Social Behavior, 30,* 282–304.

Verschuren, W. M. M., & Kromhout, D. (1995). Total cholesterol concentration and mortality at a relatively young age: Do men and women differ? *British Medical Journal, 311,* 779–783.

Vincent, P. (1971). Factors influencing patient noncompliance: A theoretical approach. *Nursing Research, 20,* 509–516.

Vita, A. J., Terry, R. B., Hubert, H. B., & Fries, J. F. (1998). Aging, health risks, and cumulative disability. *New England Journal of Medicine, 338,* 1035–1041.

Vitaliano, P. P., Maiuro, R. D., Russo, J., Mitchell, E. S., Carr, J. E., & Van Citters, R. L. (1988). A biopsychosocial model of medical student distress. *Journal of Behavioral Medicine, 11,* 311–331.

Voegele, C., Jarvis, A., & Cheeseman, K. (1997). Anger suppression, reactivity, and hypertension risk: Gender makes a difference. *Annals of Behavioral Medicine, 19,* 61–69.

Voelker, R. (1998). A "family heirloom" turns 50. *Journal of the American Medical Association, 279,* 1241–1245.

Von Korff, M., Barlow, W., Cherkin, D., & Deyo, R. A. (1994). Effects of practice style in managing back pain. *Annals of Internal Medicine, 121,* 187–195.

Wagenaar, A. C., Maybee, R. G., & Sullivan, K. P. (1988). Mandatory seat belt laws in eight states. A time-series evaluation. *Journal of Safety Research, 19,* 51–70.

Waldron, I. (1997). Changing gender roles and gender differences in health behavior. In D. S. Gochman (Ed.), *Handbook of health behavior research I: Personal and social determinants* (pp. 303–328). New York: Plenum Press.

Walker, S. P., Rimm, E. B., Ascherio, A., Kawachi, I., Stampfer, M. J., & Willett, W. C. (1996). Body size and fat distribution as predictors of stroke among US men. *American Journal of Epidemiology, 144,* 1143–1150.

Wall, P. D. (1980). The role of the substantia gelatinosa as a gate control. In J. J. Bonica (Ed.), *Pain.* New York: Raven Press.

Wall, P. D., & Jones, M. (1991). *Defeating pain: The war against a silent epidemic.* New York: Plenum Press.

Walsh, J. M. E., & Grady, D. (1995). Treatment of hyperlipidemia in women. *Journal of the American Medical Association, 274,* 1152–1158.

Walsh, T. D., & Leber, B. (1983). Measurement of chronic pain: Visual Analog Scales and McGill Pain Questionnaire compared. In J. J. Bonica, U. Lindblom, & A. Iggo (Eds.), *Advances in pain research and therapy* (Vol. 5). New York: Raven Press.

Walter, L., & Brannon, L. (1991). A cluster analysis of the Multidimensional Pain Inventory. *Headache, 31,* 476–479.

Wannamethee, G., & Shaper, A. G. (1992). Physical activity and stroke in British middle-aged men. *British Medical Journal, 304,* 597–601.

Wannamethee, G., Shaper, A. G. & Macfarlane, P. W. (1993). Heart rate, physical activity, and mortality from cancer and other noncardiovascular diseases. *American Journal of Epidemiology, 137,* 735–748.

Ward, A., & Morgan, W. (1984). Adherence patterns of healthy men and women enrolled in an adult exercise program. *Journal of Cardiac Rehabilitation, 4,* 143–152.

Ward, E. M. (1997, December). Dealing with diabetes: Diet and exercise hold key to control. *Environmental Nutrition, 20,* 1–2.

Waters, A. J., Jarvis, M. J., & Sutton, S. R. (1998, July 9). Nicotine withdrawal and accident rates. *Nature, 394,* 137.

Watson, M. & Greer, S. (1998). Personality and coping. In J. C. Holland (Ed.), *Psycho-oncology* (pp. 91–98). New York: Oxford University Press.

Webster, D. W., Gainer, P. S., & Champion, H. P. (1993). Weapon carrying among inner-city junior high school students: Defensive behavior vs aggressive delinquency. *American Journal of Public Health, 83,* 1604–1608.

Weinstein, N. D. (1980). Unrealistic optimism about future life events. *Journal of Personality and Social Psychology, 39,* 806–820.

Weinstein, N. D. (1983). Reducing unrealistic optimism about illness susceptibility. *Health Psychology, 2,* 11–20.

Weinstein, N. D. (1984). Why it won't happen to me: Perceptions of risk factors and susceptibility. *Health Psychology, 3,* 431–457.

Weinstein, N. D. (1988). The precaution adoption process. *Health Psychology, 7,* 355–386.

Weinstein, N. D., Rothman, A. J., & Sutton, S. R. (1998). Stage theories of health behavior: Conceptual and methodological issues. *Health Psychology, 17,* 290–299.

Weisner, C., Greenfield, T., & Room, R. (1995). Trends in the treatment of alcohol problems in the US general population, 1979 through 1990. *American Journal of Public Health, 85,* 55–60.

Weisner, C., & Schmidt, L. (1992). Gender disparities in treatment for alcohol problems. *Journal of the American Medical Association, 228,* 1872–1876.

Weitz, R. (1996). *The sociology of health, illness, and health care: A critical approach.* Belmont, CA: Wadsworth.

Welch, S. L., Doll, H. A., & Fairburn, C. G. (1997). Life events and the onset of bulimia nervosa: A controlled study. *Psychological Medicine, 27,* 515–522.

Wellisch, D. K. (1981). Intervention with the cancer patient. In C. K. Prokop & L. A. Bradley (Eds.), *Medical psychology: Contributions to behavioral medicine* (pp. 230–240). New York: Academic Press.

Werner, R. M., & Pearson, T. A., (1998). What's so passive about passive smoking? Secondhand smoke as a cause of atherosclerotic disease. *Journal of the American Medical Association, 179,* 157–158.

Wertlieb, D. L., Jacobson, A., & Hauser, S. (1990). The child with diabetes: A developmental stress and coping perspective. In *Psychological aspects of serious illness: Chronic conditions, fatal diseases, and clinical care* (pp. 61–101). Washington, DC: American Psychological Association.

Wesch, D., Lutzker, J. R., Frisch, L., & Dillon, M. M. (1987). Evaluating the impact of a service fee on patient compliance. *Journal of Behavioral Medicine, 10*, 91–101.

Wetter, D. W., Fiore, M. C., Gritz, E. R., Lando, H. A., Stitzer, M. L., Hasselblad, V., & Baker, T. B. (1998). The Agency for Health Care Policy and Research *Smoking Cessation Clinical Practice Guideline:* Findings and implications for psychologists. *American Psychologist, 53*, 657–669.

Whalen, C. K., Henker, B., O'Neil, R., Hollingshead, J., Holman, A., & Moore, B. (1994). Optimism in children's judgments of health and environmental risks. *Health Psychology, 13*, 319–323.

White, D. R., & White, N. M. (1988). Causes and effects of obesity: Implications for behavioral treatment. In W. Linden (Ed.), *Biological barriers in behavioral medicine* (pp. 35–62). New York: Plenum Press.

White, E., Jacobs, E. J., & Daling, J. R. (1996). Physical activity in relation to colon cancer in middle-aged men and women. *American Journal of Epidemiology, 144*, 42–50.

Whitemore, A. S., Perlin, S. A., & DiCiccio, Y. (1995). Chronic obstructive pulmonary disease in lifetime nonsmokers: Results from NHANES. *American Journal of Public Health, 85*, 702–706.

Wiens, A. N., & Menustik, C. E. (1983). Treatment outcome and patient characteristics in an aversion therapy program for alcoholism. *American Psychologist, 38*, 1089–1096.

Wiley, J. A., & Camacho, T. C. (1980). Life-style and future health: Evidence from the Alameda County Study. *Preventive Medicine, 9*, 1–21.

Willett, W. C., Hunter, D. J., Stampfer, M. J., Colditz, G., Manson, J. E., Spiegelman, D., Rosner, B., Hennekens, C. H., & Speizer, F. E., (1992). Dietary fat and fiber in relation to risk of breast cancer. *Journal of the American Medical Association, 268*, 2037–2044.

Willett, W. C., Manson, J. E., Stampfer, M. J., Colditz, G. A., Rosner, B., Speizer, F. E., & Hennekens, C. H. (1995). Weight, weight change, and coronary heart disease in women: Risk within the "normal" weight range. *Journal of the American Medical Association, 273*, 461–465.

Williams, A. F., & Lund, A. K. (1992). Injury control: What psychologists can contribute. *American Psychologist, 47*, 1036–1039.

Williams, B. K., & Knight, S. M. (1994). *Healthy for life: Wellness and the art of living.* Pacific Grove, CA: Brooks/Cole.

Williams, D. A. (1996). Acute pain management. In R. J. Gatchel & D. C. Turk (Eds.), *Psychological approaches to pain management: A practitioner's handbook* (pp. 55–77). New York: Guilford Press.

Williams, G. C., Grow, U. M., Freedman, Z. R., Ryan, R. M., & Deci, E. L. (1996). Motivational predictors of weight loss and weight-loss maintenance. *Journal of Personality and Social Psychology, 70*, 115–126.

Williams, Paul, & Dickinson, J. (1993). Fear of crime: Read all about it? The relationship between newspaper crime reporting and fear of crime. *British Journal of Criminology, 33*, 33–56.

Williams, Paul T. (1996). High-density lipoprotein cholesterol and other risk factors for coronary heart disease in female runners. *New England Journal of Medicine, 334*, 1298–1303.

Williams, Paula G., Wiebe, D. J., & Smith, T. W. (1992). Coping processes as mediators of the relationship between hardiness and health. *Journal of Behavior Medicine, 15*, 237–255.

Williams, R. B., Jr. (1989). *The trusting heart: Great news about Type A behavior.* New York: Times Books.

Williams, R. B., Jr. (1993). Hostility and the heart. In D. Goleman & J. Gurin (Eds.), *Mind/body medicine: How to use your mind for better health* (pp. 65–83). Yonkers, NY: Consumer Reports Books.

Williams, R. B., Barefoot, J. C., Califf, R. M., Haney, T. L., Saunders, W. B., Pryor, D. B., Hlatky, M. A., Siegler, I. C., & Mark, D. B. (1992). Prognostic importance of social and economic resources among medically treated patients with angiographically documented coronary artery disease. *Journal of the American Medical Association, 267*, 520–524.

Williams, R. B., Jr., Haney, T. L., Lee, K. L., Kong, Y., Blumenthal, J. A., & Whalen, R. E. (1980). Type A behavior hostility and coronary atherosclerosis. *Psychosomatic Medicine, 42*, 539–549.

Williams, T., & Clarke, V. A. (1997). Optimistic bias in beliefs about smoking. *Australian Journal of Psychology, 49*, 106–112.

Williamson, D. F. (1993). Descriptive epidemiology of bodyweight and weight change in U.S. adults. *Annals of Internal Medicine, 119*, 646–649.

Williamson, D. F., Madans, J., Anda, R. F., Kleiman, J. C., Giovino, G. A., & Byers, T. (1991). Smoking cessation and severity of weight gain in a national cohort. *New England Journal of Medicine, 324*, 739–745.

Williamson, D. F., & Pamuk, E. R. (1993). The association between weight loss and increased longevity: A review of the evidence. *Annals of Internal Medicine, 119*, 731–736.

Williamson, D. F., Pamuk, E., Thun, M., Flanders, D., Byers, T., & Heath, C. (1995). Prospective study of intentional weight loss and mortality in never-smoking overweight UD white women aged 40–64 years. *American Journal of Epidemiology, 141*, 1128–1141.

Willich, S. N., Lewis, M., Lowell, H., Arntz, H., Schubert, F., & Schröder, R. (1993). Physical exertion as a trigger of acute myocardial infarction. *New England Journal of Medicine, 329*, 1684–1690.

Wills, T. A. (1998). Social support. In E. A. Blechman & K. D. Brownell (Eds.), *Behavioral medicine and women: A comprehensive handbook* (pp. 118–128). New York: Guilford Press.

Wills, T. A., Pierce, J. P., & Evans, R. I. (1996). Large-scale environmental risk factors for substance use. *American Behavioral Scientist, 39*, 800–822.

Wilson, G. T. (1987). Cognitive studies in alcoholism. *Journal of Consulting and Clinical Psychology, 55*, 325–331.

Wilson, G. T. (1989). The treatment of bulimia nervosa: A cognitive-social learning analysis. In A. J. Stunkard & A. Baum (Eds.), *Perspectives in behavioral medicine: Eating, sleeping, and sex* (pp. 73–98). Hillsdale, NJ: Erlbaum.

Wilson, P. W. F., Christiansen, J. C., Anderson, K. M., & Kannel, W. B. (1989). Impact of national guidelines for cholesterol risk factor screening. *Journal of the American Medical Association, 262,* 41–44.

Winett, R. A. (1995). A framework for health promotion and disease prevention programs. *American Psychologist, 50,* 341–350.

Wing, R. R. (1992). Behavioral treatment of severe obesity. *American Journal of Clinical Nutrition, 55,* 545S–551S.

Wingard, D. L., Berkman, L. F., & Brand, R. J. (1982). A multivariate analysis of health-related practices: A nine-year mortality follow-up of the Alameda County study. *American Journal of Epidemiology, 116,* 765–775.

Winkelstein, W. (1995). A new perspective on John Snow's communicable disease theory. *American Journal of Epidemiology, 142,* (Suppl.), S3–S9.

Winkleby, M. A., Flora, J. A., & Kraemer, H. C. (1994). A community-based heart disease intervention: Predictors of change. *American Journal of Public Health, 84,* 767–772.

Winkleby, M. A., Kraemer, H. C., Ahn, D. K., & Varady, A. N. (1998). Ethnic and socioeconomic differences in cardiovascular disease risk factors: Findings for women from the Third National Health and Nutrition Examination Survey, 1988–1994. *Journal of the American Medical Association, 280,* 356–362.

Winkleby, M. A., Robinson, T. N., Sundquist, J., & Kraemer, H. C. (1999). Ethnic variation in cardiovascular disease risk factors among children and young adults: Findings from the third National Health and Nutrition Examination survey, 1988–1994. *Journal of the American Medical Association, 281,* 1006–1013.

Winter, R. (1994, September-October). Which pain relievers work best? *Consumers Digest, 33,* 76–79.

Wiseman, C. V., Gray, J. J., Mosimann, J. E., & Ahrens, A. H. (1992). Cultural expectations of thinness in women: An update. *International Journal of Eating Disorders, 11,* 85–89.

Wisocki, P. A. (1998). Arthritis and osteoporosis. In E. A. Blechman & K. D. Brownell (Eds.), *Behavioral medicine & women: A comprehensive handbook* (pp. 562–565). New York: Guilford Press.

Witkin, G., Tharp, M., Schrof, J. M., Toch, T., & Scattarella, C. (1998, June 1). Again: School shooting in Springfield, Oregon. *U.S. News & World Report, 124,* 16–19.

Wolf, S. L., Nacht, M., & Kelly, J. L. (1982). EMG feedback training during dynamic movement for low back pain patients. *Behavior Therapy, 13,* 395–406.

Wonderlich, S. A., Brewerton, T. D., Jocic, Z., Dansky, B. S., & Abbott, D. W. (1997). Relationships of childhood sexual abuse and eating disorders. *Journal of the American Academy of Child and Adolescent Psychiatry, 36,* 1107–1113.

Wonderlich, S. A., Wilsnack, R. W., Wilsnack, S. C., & Harris, T. R. (1996). Childhood sexual abuse and bulimic behavior in a nationally representative sample. *American Journal of Public Health, 86,* 1082–1086.

Wolfgang, M. E. (1957). Victim precipitated criminal homicide. *Journal of Criminal Law and Criminology, 48,* 1–11.

Wong, M., & Kaloupek, D. G. (1986). Coping with dental treatment: The potential impact of situational demands. *Journal of Behavioral Medicine, 9,* 579–597.

Wood, P. D., Stefanick, M. L., Dreon, D. M., Frey-Hewitt, B., Garay, S. C., Williams, P. T., Superko, H. R., Fortmann, S. P., Albers, J. J., Vranizan, K. M., Ellsworth, N. M., Terry, R. B., & Haskell, W. L. (1988). Changes in plasma lipids and lipoproteins in overweight men during weight loss through dieting compared with exercise. *New England Journal of Medicine, 319,* 1173–1179.

World Health Organization. (1998). *The world health report 1998: Life in the twenty-first century: A vision for all.* Geneva, Switzerland.

Wright, L. K. (1997). Health behavior of caregivers. In D. S. Gochman (Ed.), *Handbook of health behavior research III: Demography, development, and diversity* (pp. 267–284). New York: Plenum Press.

Wu, J. M. (1990). Summary and concluding remarks. In J. M. Wu (Ed.), *Environmental tobacco smoke: Proceedings of the international symposium at McGill University 1989* (pp. 367–375). Lexington, MA: Heath.

Wyden, P. (1965). *The overweight society.* New York: Morrow.

Wynder, E. L. (1997). Tobacco as a cause of lung cancer: Some reflections. *American Journal of Epimemiology, 146,* 687–694.

Wylie-Rosett, J. (1998). Diabetes: Medical aspects. In E. A. Blechman & K. D. Brownell (Eds.), *Behavioral medicine and women: A comprehensive handbook* (pp. 623–627). New York: Guilford.

Wysocki, T. (1989). Impact of blood glucose monitoring on diabetic control: Obstacles and interventions. *Journal of Behavioral Medicine, 12,* 183–205.

Wysocki, T., Green, L., & Huxtable, K. (1989). Blood glucose monitoring by diabetic adolescents: Compliance and metabolic control. *Health Psychology, 8,* 267–284.

Wysocki, T., Harris, M. A., Greco, P., Harvey, L. M., McDonell, D., Danda, C. L. E., Bubb, J., & White, N. H. (1997). Social validity of support group and behavior therapy interventions for families of adolescents with insulin-dependent diabetes mellitus. *Journal of Pediatric Psychology, 22,* 635–649.

Yaari, S., & Goldbourt, U. (1998). Voluntary and involuntary weight loss: Associations with long term mortality in 9,228 middle-aged and elderly men. *American Journal of Epidemiology, 148,* 546–555.

Yager, J., Grant, I., Sweetwood, H. L., & Gerst, M. (1981). Life event reports by psychiatric patients, nonpatients, and their partners. *Archives of General Psychiatry, 38,* 343–347.

Yano, K., Rhoads, G. G., Kagan, A., & Tillotson, J. (1978). Dietary intake and risk of coronary heart disease in Japanese men living in Hawaii. *American Journal of Clinical Nutrition, 31,* 1270–1279.

Yarnold, P. R., Michelson, E. A., Thompson, D. A., & Adams, S. L. (1998). Predicting patient satisfaction: A study of two emergency departments. *Journal of Behavioral Medicine, 21,* 545–563.

Yates, A., Leehey, K., & Shisslak, C. M. (1983). Running —an analogue of anorexia? *New England Journal of Medicine, 308,* 251–255.

Yong, L-C., Brown, C. C., Schatzkin, A., Dresser, C. M., Siesinski, M. J., Cox, C. S., & Taylor, P. R. (1997). Intake of vitamins E, C, and A and risk of lung cancer: The NHANES I Epidemiologic Followup Study. *American Journal of Epidemiology, 146,* 231–243.

Young, D. R., Haskel, W. L., Jalulis, D. E., & Fortmann, S. P. (1993). Associations between changes in physical activity and risk factors for coronary heart disease in a community-based sample of men and women: The Stanford Five-City Project, *American Journal of Epidemiology, 138,* 205–216.

Young, L. D. (1993). Rheumatoid arthritis. In R. J. Gatchel & E. B. Blanchard (Eds.), *Psychophysiological disorders: Research and clinical applications* (pp. 269–298). Washington, DC: American Psychological Association.

Zador, P. L., & Ciccone, M. A. (1993). Automobile driver fatalities in frontal impacts: Air bags compared with manual belts. *American Journal of Public Health, 83,* 661–666.

Zautra, A. J. (1998). Arthritis: Behavioral and psychosocial aspects. In E. A. Blechman & K. D. Brownell (Eds.), *Behavioral medicine and women: A comprehensive handbook* (pp. 554–558). New York: Guilford.

Zeanah, C. H., & Scheeringa, M. S. (1997). The experience and effects of violence in infancy. In J. D. Osofsky (Ed.), *Children in a violent society* (pp. 97–123). New York: Guilford Press.

Zhang, J., Feldblum, P. J., & Fortney, J. A. (1992). Moderate physical activity and bone density among perimenopausal women. *American Journal of Public Health, 82,* 736–738.

Zimbardo, P. G. (1969). The human choice: Individuation, reason, and order versus deindividuation, impulse, and chaos. In W. J. Arnold & D. Levine (Eds.), *Nebraska symposium on motivation.* Lincoln: University of Nebraska Press.

Zimmerman, M. (1983). Methodological issues in the assessment of life events: A review of issues and research. *Clinical Psychology Review, 3,* 339–370.

Zimmerman, R. S., & Olson, K. (1994). AIDS-related risk behavior and behavior change in a sexually active heterosexual sample: A test of three models of prevention. *AIDS Education and Prevention, 6,* 189–204.

Zinberg, N. E. (1984). *Drug, set, and setting: The basis for controlled intoxicant use.* New Haven, CT: Yale University Press.

Zonderman, A. B., Costa, P. T., & McCrae, R. R. (1989). Depression as a risk for cancer morbidity and mortality in a nationally representative sample. *Journal of the American Medical Association, 262,* 1191–1195.

Zubin, J., & Spring, B. (1977). Vulnerability—a new view of schizophrenia. *Journal of Abnormal Psychology, 86,* 103–127.

Zuckerman, M., Ball, S., & Black, J. (1990). Influences of sensation seeking, gender, risk appraisal, and situational motivation on smoking. *Addictive Behaviors, 15,* 209–220.

Zyazema, N. Z. (1984). Toward better patient drug compliance and comprehension: A challenge to medical and pharmaceutical services in Zimbabwe. *Social Science and Medicine, 18,* 551–554.

NAME INDEX

SUBJECT INDEX

PHOTO CREDITS

Chapter 1, 9, Corbis; **13**, Corbis; **Chapter 2, 29**, Corbis; **37**, Jerry Berndt/Stock Boston; **Chapter 3, 60**, PhotoDisc; **66**, PhotoDisc; **69**, Stephen Derr/The Image Bank; **73**, Corbis; **75**, Corbis; **Chapter 4, 88**, Corbis; **91**, Corbis; **94**, Bob Daemmrich/The Image Works; **96**, Corbis; **103**, PhotoDisc; **Chapter 5, 125**, Corbis; **126**, Corbis; **128**, Michael Siluk/The Image Works; **129**, Corbis; **131**, Corbis; **Chapter 6, 153**, Corbis; **154**, Corbis; **157**, Corbis; **Chapter 7, 178**, Corbis; **180**, Corbis; **181**, Sepp Seitz/Woodfin Camp & Associates; **185**, FPG International; **191**, Corbis; **195**, PhotoDisc; **196**, Corbis; **Chapter 8, 209**, Corbis; **212**, Robert Kalman/The Image Works; **219**, Norman R. Rowan/The Image Works; **Chapter 9, 251**, Hazel Hankin/Stock Boston; **258**, Leinwand/Monkmeyer Press; **Chapter 10, 282**, Michael Melford/The Image Bank; **284**, Michael Siluk/The Image Works; **285**, Corbis; **Chapter 11, 297**, Corbis; **306**, Corbis; **309**, Frank Keillor/Jeroboam; **316**, Rhoda Sidney/Stock Boston; **325**, PhotoDisc; **Chapter 12, 333**, Michael Siluk/The Image Works; **336**, Corbis; **339**, R.S. Uzzell/Woodfin Camp & Associates; **344**, Corbis; **350**, Corbis; **353**, Corbis; **Chapter 13, 376**, Corbis; **381**, Penny Tweedy/Tony Stone Images; **393**, Corbis; **Chapter 14, 409**, Corbis; **411**, Courtesy of the U. of Washington School of Medicine, FAS Research Fund; **422**, Schneider/Monkmeyer Press; **431**, Corbis; **Chapter 15, 446**, Wallace Kirkland/Life Magazine; **454**, Topham/The Image Works; **459**, Corbis; **465**, Susan Rosenberg/Photo Researchers, Inc.; **Chapter 16, 481**, M. Bernsau/The Image Works; **496**, Corbis; **502**, Corbis; **Chapter 17, 509**, Corbis; **519**, Paula Lerner/Woodfin Camp & Associates.